OPERATIVE TECHNIC
IN
GENERAL SURGERY

OPERATIVE TECHNIC

IN

GENERAL SURGERY

Edited by

WARREN H. COLE, M.D., F.A.C.S.

PROFESSOR AND HEAD OF THE DEPARTMENT OF SURGERY, UNIVERSITY
OF ILLINOIS COLLEGE OF MEDICINE; DIRECTOR OF SURGICAL
SERVICE, ILLINOIS RESEARCH AND EDUCATIONAL
HOSPITALS, CHICAGO

Introduction by

FRANK H. LAHEY, M.D., F.A.C.S.

APPLETON-CENTURY-CROFTS, INC.

NEW YORK

TO MY WIFE, CLARA,

WITHOUT WHOSE PATIENCE AND UNDERSTANDING,
EDITORSHIP OF THIS WORK COULD NOT HAVE
BEEN ACCOMPLISHED

AUTHORS

W. E. ADAMS, M.D.
PROFESSOR OF SURGERY, UNIVERSITY OF CHICAGO MEDICAL SCHOOL;
ATTENDING SURGEON, ALBERT MERRITT BILLINGS HOSPITAL

Esophagus

HARVEY S. ALLEN, M.D.
ASSISTANT PROFESSOR, NORTHWESTERN UNIVERSITY MEDICAL SCHOOL;
ATTENDING SURGEON, PASSAVANT MEMORIAL HOSPITAL AND
COOK COUNTY HOSPITAL, CHICAGO

Surgery of the Hand and Its Tendons

B. MARDEN BLACK, M.D.
HEAD OF A SECTION, GENERAL SURGERY,
MAYO CLINIC, ROCHESTER, MINNESOTA

The Thyroid and Parathyroid Glands

JAMES BARRETT BROWN, M.D., F.A.C.S.
PROFESSOR OF CLINICAL SURGERY, WASHINGTON UNIVERSITY SCHOOL OF MEDICINE;
SURGEON TO BARNES AND BARNARD HOSPITALS

The Face, Mouth and Jaws

ALEXANDER BRUNSCHWIG, M.D., F.A.C.S.
PROFESSOR OF CLINICAL SURGERY, CORNELL UNIVERSITY MEDICAL COLLEGE;
ATTENDING SURGEON, MEMORIAL HOSPITAL FOR THE TREATMENT OF
CANCER AND ALLIED DISEASES, NEW YORK CITY

The Pancreas and Adrenal

WARREN H. COLE, M.D., F.A.C.S.
PROFESSOR AND HEAD OF THE DEPARTMENT OF SURGERY, UNIVERSITY
OF ILLINOIS COLLEGE OF MEDICINE; DIRECTOR OF SURGICAL
SERVICE, ILLINOIS RESEARCH AND EDUCATIONAL
HOSPITALS, CHICAGO

The Gallbladder and Bile Ducts
Splenectomy

FREDERICK A. COLLER, M.S., M.D., F.A.C.S.
PROFESSOR OF SURGERY AND CHAIRMAN OF THE DEPARTMENT,
UNIVERSITY OF MICHIGAN MEDICAL SCHOOL,
ANN ARBOR, MICHIGAN

Abdominal Incisions

vii

AUTHORS

CHARLES E. DAVIS, JR., M.D.
FORMERLY INSTRUCTOR IN SURGERY AND GYNECOLOGY, UNIVERSITY OF VIRGINIA
MEDICAL SCHOOL; FORMERLY CHIEF SURGEON, BECKLEY HOSPITAL, BECKLEY,
WEST VIRGINIA; ATTENDING SURGEON, NORFOLK GENERAL HOSPITAL,
DE PAUL AND LEIGH MEMORIAL HOSPITALS, NORFOLK, VIRGINIA

Abdominal Hernia

MICHAEL E. DeBAKEY, M.D.
PROFESSOR OF SURGERY AND CHAIRMAN OF DEPARTMENT OF SURGERY,
BAYLOR UNIVERSITY COLLEGE OF MEDICINE, HOUSTON, TEXAS

The Liver and Subphrenic Space

The Blood Vessels

CLARENCE DENNIS, M.D.
PROFESSOR OF SURGERY, UNIVERSITY OF MINNESOTA MEDICAL SCHOOL;
ASSOCIATE CHIEF OF SURGERY, UNIVERSITY HOSPITAL

Surgery of the Small Intestine

CLAUDE F. DIXON, M.D.
DIVISION OF SURGERY, MAYO CLINIC,
ROCHESTER, MINNESOTA

The Lower Part of the Sigmoid, the Rectum and Anus

LESTER R. DRAGSTEDT, M.D., Ph.D.
PROFESSOR OF SURGERY AND CHAIRMAN OF THE DEPARTMENT OF SURGERY,
THE UNIVERSITY OF CHICAGO; ATTENDING SURGEON,
THE ALBERT MERRITT BILLINGS HOSPITAL

Gastric Vagotomy in the Treatment of Peptic Ulcer

DANIEL C. ELKIN, M.D.
WHITEHEAD PROFESSOR OF SURGERY, EMORY UNIVERSITY;
SURGEON-IN-CHIEF, EMORY UNIVERSITY HOSPITAL

The Blood Vessels

ROBERT ELMAN, M.D., F.A.C.S.
PROFESSOR OF CLINICAL SURGERY, WASHINGTON UNIVERSITY SCHOOL OF MEDICINE;
ASSISTANT SURGEON, BARNES HOSPITAL; ASSOCIATE SURGEON, ST. LOUIS
CHILDREN'S HOSPITAL; DIRECTOR OF SURGICAL SERVICE,
H. G. PHILLIPS HOSPITAL, ST. LOUIS

Preoperative and Postoperative Care

R. K. GILCHRIST, M.D.
CLINICAL ASSOCIATE PROFESSOR OF SURGERY (RUSH), UNIVERSITY OF ILLINOIS
COLLEGE OF MEDICINE; ATTENDING SURGEON, COOK COUNTY HOSPITAL;
ASSOCIATE ATTENDING SURGEON, PRESBYTERIAN HOSPITAL

Lymphatic System

FRANK GLENN, M.D.
PROFESSOR OF SURGERY AND CHAIRMAN OF DEPARTMENT, CORNELL UNIVERSITY
MEDICAL COLLEGE; SURGEON-IN-CHIEF, THE NEW YORK HOSPITAL

The Skin and Subcutaneous Tissue

ROSCOE R. GRAHAM, M.D., F.R.C.S. (C.)
THE LATE ASSISTANT PROFESSOR OF SURGERY, UNIVERSITY OF TORONTO;
SENIOR SURGEON, THE TORONTO GENERAL HOSPITAL

The Colon and Appendix

JESSIE GRAY, M.D.
SURGEON-IN-CHIEF, WOMEN'S COLLEGE HOSPITAL, TORONTO

The Colon and Appendix

EDWARD L. HOWES, M.D.
ASSOCIATE CLINICAL PROFESSOR OF SURGERY, COLUMBIA UNIVERSITY;
ASSISTANT ATTENDING SURGEON, PRESBYTERIAN HOSPITAL

Wounds and Wound Healing

SUMNER L. KOCH, M.D.
PROFESSOR OF SURGERY, NORTHWESTERN UNIVERSITY MEDICAL SCHOOL;
ATTENDING SURGEON, PASSAVANT MEMORIAL HOSPITAL, CHICAGO

Surgery of the Hand and Its Tendons

EDWIN P. LEHMAN, M.D.
PROFESSOR OF SURGERY AND GYNECOLOGY, DEPARTMENT OF MEDICINE,
UNIVERSITY OF VIRGINIA; CHIEF SURGEON AND GYNECOLOGIST,
UNIVERSITY OF VIRGINIA HOSPITAL

Abdominal Hernia

STANLEY M. LEVENSON, M.D.
SURGICAL SCIENTIST (RADIOBIOLOGY), MEDICAL NUTRITION LABORATORY,
UNDER THE SURGEON GENERAL, DEPARTMENT OF THE ARMY; INSTRUCTOR
IN SURGERY, UNIVERSITY OF ILLINOIS COLLEGE OF MEDICINE

Burns

AUTHORS

A. LEE LICHTMAN, M.D., M.S. and Ph.D. in SURGERY
FORMERLY ASSISTANT SURGEON, MAYO CLINIC, ROCHESTER, MINNESOTA;
ADJUNCT PROFESSOR OF SURGERY, POLYCLINIC MEDICAL SCHOOL AND
HOSPITAL; ASSISTANT SURGEON, GOUVERNEUR HOSPITAL, NEW YORK

The Lower Part of the Sigmoid, the Rectum and Anus

CHARLES C. LUND, M.D., F.A.C.S.
ASSISTANT PROFESSOR OF SURGERY, HARVARD MEDICAL SCHOOL;
VISITING SURGEON, III SURGICAL SERVICE, BOSTON CITY
HOSPITAL; RESEARCH FELLOW, THORNDIKE MEMORIAL
LABORATORY

Burns

KENNETH F. MACLEAN, M.D.
FORMERLY INSTRUCTOR IN SURGERY, UNIVERSITY OF
MICHIGAN MEDICAL SCHOOL

Abdominal Incisions

FRANK McDOWELL, M.D.
ASSISTANT PROFESSOR OF CLINICAL SURGERY, WASHINGTON UNIVERSITY
SCHOOL OF MEDICINE; ASSISTANT SURGEON, BARNES AND
ST. LOUIS CHILDREN'S HOSPITALS; CONSULTING
SURGEON, FRISCO HOSPITAL

The Face, Mouth and Jaws

FRANCIS M. McKEEVER, M.D.
ASSOCIATE PROFESSOR OF SURGERY (ORTHOPEDIC), UNIVERSITY OF
SOUTHERN CALIFORNIA SCHOOL OF MEDICINE, LOS ANGELES;
SENIOR ORTHOPEDIC SURGEON, LOS ANGELES COUNTY
GENERAL HOSPITAL AND CHILDREN'S HOSPITAL,
LOS ANGELES

Amputations

HARRISON L. McLAUGHLIN, M.D., C.M., F.A.C.S.
PROFESSOR OF CLINICAL ORTHOPEDIC SURGERY, COLLEGE OF PHYSICIANS AND
SURGEONS, COLUMBIA UNIVERSITY; ATTENDING ORTHOPEDIC SURGEON,
PRESBYTERIAN HOSPITAL, NEW YORK; CONSULTING SURGEON,
NORTHERN WESTCHESTER HOSPITAL, MOUNT KISCO, N. Y.

The Muscles, Fasciae, Tendons and Bursae

ALTON OCHSNER, B.A., M.D., ScD., F.A.C.S.

WILLIAM HENDERSON PROFESSOR OF SURGERY AND CHAIRMAN OF THE DEPARTMENT
OF SURGERY, SCHOOL OF MEDICINE, TULANE UNIVERSITY; DIRECTOR
OF DIVISION OF GENERAL SURGERY, OCHSNER CLINIC; CHIEF
OF SURGICAL SERVICE, FOUNDATION HOSPITAL; SENIOR
VISITING SURGEON, CHARITY HOSPITAL AND TOURO
INFIRMARY; CONSULTING SURGEON, ILLINOIS
CENTRAL HOSPITAL

The Liver and Subphrenic Space

THOMAS G. ORR, M.D., F.A.C.S.

PROFESSOR OF SURGERY, UNIVERSITY OF KANSAS SCHOOL OF MEDICINE;
SURGEON-IN-CHIEF, UNIVERSITY OF KANSAS MEDICAL CENTER

The Breast

JOHN DEJ. PEMBERTON, M.D.

HEAD OF A SECTION IN SURGERY, MAYO CLINIC;
PROFESSOR OF SURGERY, MAYO FOUNDATION,
ROCHESTER, MINNESOTA

The Thyroid and Parathyroid Glands

JOHN D. STEWART, M.D.

PROFESSOR OF SURGERY AND CHAIRMAN OF THE DEPARTMENT,
UNIVERSITY OF BUFFALO MEDICAL SCHOOL

Hemorrhage and Shock

WALTMAN WALTERS, M.D.

HEAD OF A SECTION IN SURGERY, MAYO CLINIC; PROFESSOR OF
SURGERY, MAYO FOUNDATION, UNIVERSITY OF MINNESOTA;
SURGEON, ST. MARY'S HOSPITAL,
ROCHESTER, MINNESOTA

Surgery of Stomach and Duodenum

NATHAN A. WOMACK, M.D.

PROFESSOR OF SURGERY, STATE UNIVERSITY OF IOWA
COLLEGE OF MEDICINE, IOWA CITY

Portal Hypertension

Preface

Perhaps the greatest progress in the art of Surgery from the standpoint of introduction of new principles in operative technic was made in the latter part of the nineteenth century, and early part of the twentieth, due largely to the stimulus afforded by the advent of surgical asepsis. When it was discovered one or two decades ago that the last of the body cavities, namely the thorax, could be invaded successfully by the surgeons, it might have appeared to some, that additional progress in the field of technic would be slow in development. Such reasoning is obviously fallacious, and subsequent events have proved it so. For example, the improvements made in cardiovascular surgery in the treatment of arteriovenous fistula, coarctation of the aorta, patent ductus arteriosus, and lastly, pulmonary stenosis, are proof that introduction of new principles in technic will always be forthcoming.

One of the great contributions made during the past several years to the art of surgery, is the knowledge that refinement in technic of methods already existent may make sufficient difference in results to justify operations which otherwise might not be indicated except in unusual circumstances. The introduction of sulfonamides, penicillin and other antibiotic agents has been of great aid in improving results, but in reality, has had much less influence than assumed by most people, including physicians. These agents must not be allowed to displace sound surgical principles.

As important as operative technic is in surgical results, it is a well known fact that fundamental principles such as those involved in hemorrhage and shock, burns, treatment of open wounds, etc., are of vital importance and must be utilized. The necessity for a large amount of blood in long difficult operations (discovered only a short time ago) is an example of the importance of fundamental principles in surgery. Why it took the surgical profession so long to make this discovery is a mystery very difficult to explain. Because of the necessity of thorough knowledge of fundamental principles in surgical results these subjects are included in the text. Furthermore, such phases as anatomy, physiology, indications, precautions, etc., have also been presented in at least slight detail lest the young surgeon gain the idea that perfection in technic is so important as to displace other phases of surgical knowledge.

In addition to general surgery, many specialties including orthopedics, neurosurgery, plastic surgery, urology, thoracic surgery and gynecology have been presented; however, ophthalmology and otolaryngology have been omitted largely because these two specialties are less distinctly related to general surgery than those included.

The editor wishes to thank the various contributing authors for their splendid contributions and for their excellent cooperation. The most valuable suggestions made by numerous surgical friends are hereby acknowledged. The untiring effort of Miss Annabel Wheeler, Mrs. Helene Coleman and Dr. James Majarakis in the preparation of the text and index is likewise acknowledged. At all times the publishers have been most helpful and cooperative.

WARREN H. COLE

CONTENTS

_____

* Deceased

Introduction

In producing this book, *Operative Technic in General Surgery,* the authors, the editor and the publishers have ably met a real demand and that is the presentation of methods of performing surgical operations brought up to date by a variety of busy surgeons actively engaged in the performance of the operative procedures which they have described and in sufficient numbers from which to draw deductions and to advocate sound procedures.

We in surgery are interested in the investigative work upon which is established all sound surgical procedures. We are interested in the diagnosis upon which depends so much the selection of proper measures to meet the conditions which require treatment. We are interested in the decision for or against surgery. In spite of our interest in all of these points which constitute the foundation of a surgical problem, the ultimate controlling factors which will bring about surgical relief or failure to relieve are the selection of the operation and its proper technical performance.

In order to select the proper type of surgical procedure for any given case, one must obviously be familiar with all of the types of surgical operations applicable to that case in order to weigh one against the other and to make the proper choice of the type of operation for that patient.

Serious criticisms have at times been directed particularly against clinical surgeons because of their occasional overemphasis of technical procedures. There undoubtedly have been surgeons whose interest has been overbalanced on the side of technic, sometimes at the expense of more fundamental things. There undoubtedly have been surgeons who have become such adept technicians and so confident of their technical ability that they have been led into unwise decisions and unwise surgical procedures. Nevertheless, one must admit that the proper selection and the proper technical performance of the surgical operation are the final deciding factors in the attempt to cure any surgical lesion by an operation.

This book has the great advantage of having the various subjects presented by men who have had experience with the particular subject about which they write.

The field of surgery today is so wide and surgery itself is so complex that no one is capable of great technical expertness, really based upon a large experience, except in a relatively limited number and types of operative procedures. My own long and fairly large surgical experience has taught me with increasing contact with surgery that one must realize that it is impossible for a surgeon to attain great technical skill in any given operative procedure except by a special interest in the procedure and by performing it over and over again.

This contribution to operative technic in general surgery complies with all of these requirements. The names of these various authors appear frequently in the world literature on the subjects which they present in these volumes. They are still young enough to be flexible in their viewpoint and to be interested in newer and modern developments in surgery. They are, however, sufficiently mature to have had time and opportunity to acquire a volume of experience which makes them capable of presenting their subject with authority.

FRANK H. LAHEY

OPERATIVE TECHNIC

IN

GENERAL SURGERY

1

WOUND HEALING AND THE CARE OF WOUNDS

Edward L. Howes, M.D.

THE TISSUES REGENERATED

During wound healing only three tissues are regenerated; epithelium, fibrous tissue and blood vessels. These three tissues comprise the scar or cicatrix. An abundant new growth of blood vessels is essential for the regeneration of the other two tissues until after the scar is formed. Then only a maintenance blood supply is required and many of the new blood vessels are obliterated. As vessels are obliterated, the scar turns from red to white.

All of these tissues begin to regenerate after the exudative phase of healing. Regenerating epithelium recovers surfaces and the process is essentially the same for both skin and mucous membranes. Generated * fibrous tissue restores the continuity of the deeper tissues. Thus, wounded muscle, fat, liver, spleen, kidney, lung, and serosal surfaces are reunited and replaced by it.

The primary objective in the case of the healing wound is to establish conditions that will allow these tissues to properly regenerate; to restore continuity and function. Epithelium regenerates only from pre-existing epithelium; from that about the margins of the wound and from islands left in the wounded area. The process of epithelization consists of (1) hyperplasia and hypertrophy of pre-existing epithelium, (2) amoeboid motion of epithelial cells outward over the defect from the germinal layer of the old epithelium and (3) restratification and keratination of this single layer of cells to reform a new epithelial structure that incompletely resembles the original (Fig. 1).[1] Regenerated skin, for example, is without sebaceous glands or hair follicles. Restratification and keratinization, differentiation of the epithelial scar, occur promptly after the single layer of cells moves out from the germinal layer and the process is complete within a day or two after the area is covered with the single layer of cells. Thereafter, the only change that occurs in the epithelial scar is the regrowth of rudimentary nerve terminals into it, about six to twelve months later.[1a]

Fibroplasia, the process producing the fibrous tissue of the scar, begins with the multiplication of mononuclear cells and fibroblasts. These cells are brought to the site of injury during exudation and they also exist locally in embryonal nests (Fig. 2). The duration of multiplication is brief, one or two days, and the greater portion of the process, from the fourth day onward, is

---

* The term "generation" is used to emphasize that fibrous tissue appears in areas where it did not exist previously.

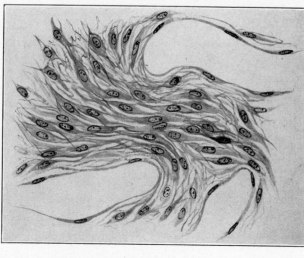

FIG. 2.

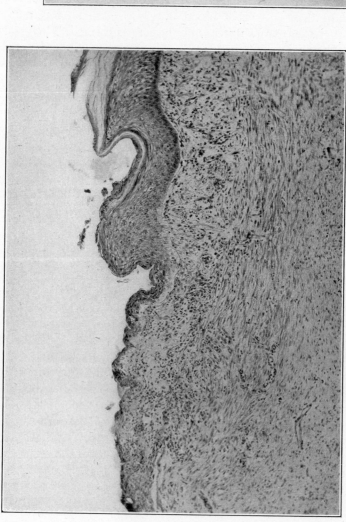

FIG. 1.

FIG. 1. Regeneration of skin. The defect is on the left. The single layer of cells advancing from the germinal layer can be seen in the middle of the photograph, extending for a considerable distance over the granulations, by following the germinal layer outward from the stratified thicker portion. Below, fibroblasts and reticulin are beginning to arrange themselves parallel to epithelium. (From Howes, *Surg., Gynec. & Obst.*, 76:738, 1943. By permission of Surgery, Gynecology and Obstetrics).

FIG. 2. Fibroblasts and intercellular fibers. Wound 10 days old. Vessels may be seen in the lower right hand, upper and lower left hand portions of illustration. (After Marchand.)

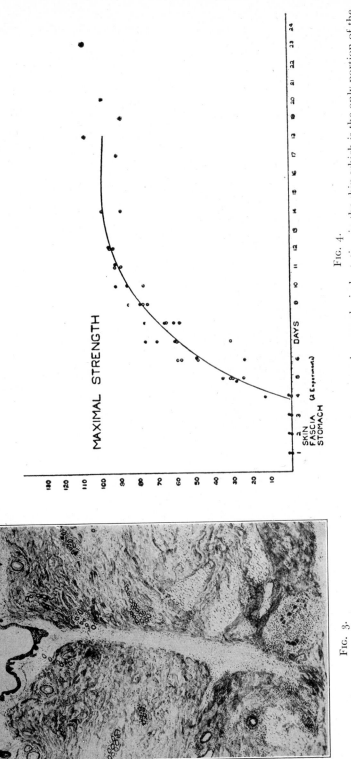

Fig. 3.

Fig. 3. Microscopic cross section of a healed sutured wound. Above may be seen the indentation in the skin which is the only portion of the scar visible externally. The white line down the middle is the new scar tissue. The normal tissues may be seen on either side.

Fig. 4. Tensile strength of a healing wound. After a period of 3 or 4 days when the wound, healing optimally, has only the strength given to it by the sutures, the wound begins to gather strength through fibroplasia. Actually, the wound loses some sutured strength on the second and third day because the tissues lose their capacity to hold sutures. (From Howes, *J.A.M.A.*, 92:42, 1929.)

concerned with the laying down of fibrils of reticulin.[2] A characteristic pattern of reticulin is produced in about 10 days. In the sutured wound, fibroplasia restores continuity (Fig. 3) and gives the wound strength (Fig. 4).[3] In the open wound, fibroplasia with its accompanying growth of blood vessels, produces "granulations."

After two weeks of healing the reticulin fibrils are arranged circularly about the blood vessels. They soon enlarge, however, into fibers that arrange themselves according to the stresses and strains affecting the area (Figs. 1 and 5). The change of the fibrils into fibers and their rearrangement in response to function comprise the pattern of differentiation of the generated fibrous tissue. Differentiation completes the strength of the wounded area, finally restoring its original strength.[4] In general, differentiation takes longer to complete in the fibrous than in the epithelial scar and the process exhibits great variability, depending on the nature of the tissues wounded and the direction of the wound. For example, in per primam healing of the skin, continuity is restored in two weeks but differentiation of generated connective tissue in the derma takes six months to be complete in order to restore the original strength of the skin. Wounds of ligaments, tendons, fascias and all tissues having great strength originally, also fall into the category of those requiring a long period of time for differentiation to restore original strength when the fibers were cut transversely (Fig. 6). On the other hand, in wounds of muscle and

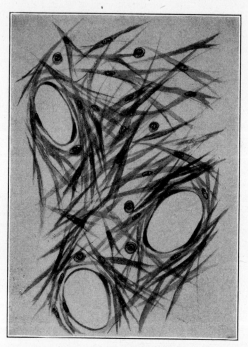

FIG. 5. Histologic features in the healing of a 20-day old wound. Note reticulin fibrils have increased in size, that there are fewer fibroblasts, and that vessels still remain large. (See figure 2.) (After Marchand.)

intestines, original strength is restored by the early deposition of reticulin because the strength of this reticulin is equivalent to that of undifferentiated connective tissue component in these structures. Original strength is always restored rapidly when the wound just separates the fibrous components of a tissue in contrast to cutting across the fibrous components. In other words, by planning the direction of the incision the surgeon can sometimes shorten the length of time when original strength is returned to the scar especially in those situations where considerable time is required. Moreover, differentiation is always hastened by graded function of the injured part. Physical and occupational therapy supply this function.

In the organs the fibrous scar has no function but only re-establishes continuity; function is carried on by hypertrophy of uninjured tissue of the same kind; *i.e.* by the remainder of the liver, the opposite kidney, etc.

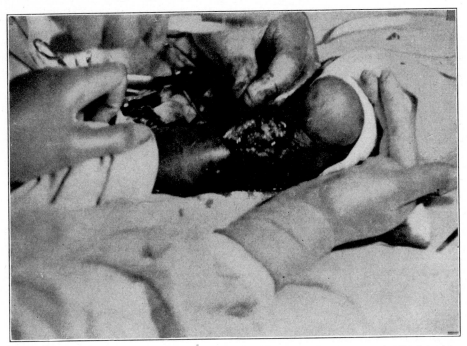

Fig. 6. Severed Achilles tendon. Cut transversely by a scythe. The longitudinal incision was made to pull down the tendon and to resuture it. Although continuity will be quickly restored by fibroplasia, a long period of differentiation will be required to support the weight of the body during walking.

THE CONTROL OF FIBROPLASIA

Every bit of deep tissue wounded or destroyed during the process of healing is replaced by generating fibrous tissue. Thus, infection and necrosis increase the amount of scarring.

This new fibrous tissue is laid down abundantly at first and binds planes of tissue together for a considerable distance in a soft tissue "callus." Because of initial abundance, fibroplasia is accused of interfering with function—an idea expressed in the term cicatrization. Actually, however, fibroplasia restores function and the job of the surgeon is to create the circumstances that allow the process to appear as early as possible and only in locations where it will contribute necessary strength to the tissues during healing. For example, in repair of the inguinal hernia, massive fibrosis could be instituted throughout the entire inguinal region by transplanting fascia or by injecting paraffin; yet, if the etiological defect in the transversalis fascia is not obliterated, the hernia recurs. Again, the surgeon could instigate fibrosis along the entire length of a cut tendon and bind the tendon to its sheath but the process is only needed between the severed ends.

Some of the fibrous tissue generated immediately after the injury is always partially reabsorbed during the period of differentiation. This absorption follows Wolff's law; namely, that regenerated and transplanted tissues continue to exist only in response to function. However, if an excessive amount of fibroplasia occurs initially as the result of the original injury or because an infection develops, then reabsorption will not be great enough to take away the large amount of fibrous scar that in turn interferes with function that might help to remove unnecessary scar tissue. Surgically, nothing can be done to change the amount of fibroplasia that follows accidental injury but it is possible by separating tissues composed of large collagen fibers to control the amount of fibroplasia responding to injury in wounds of election, and in all wounds, infection can be prevented (see chemotherapy).

RELATIONSHIP BETWEEN EPITHELIZATION AND FIBRO-PLASIA AND THE CONTROL OF EPITHELIZATION

Epithelization is a surface phenomena requiring a suitable granulating base. New epithelium extends across granulations like ice skims across a pond. If granulations are depressed below the surrounding skin edges or are elevated above them, the new epithelium will not extend outward unless the height of the granulations is corrected. If they are too high, the granulations must be cut down either with scissors (they are not sensitive) or by chemical cauterization. If they are too low, they must be encouraged to grow by reducing their bacterial flora, by mechanically removing sloughing bits of tissues, by preventing puddling of pus, and by the use of mild irritants. The last three can be accomplished by frequently changing moist dressings.

No drugs have been found to stimulate the rate of epithelization. However, an optimal rate of epithelization is obtained by keeping granulations of proper height in the correct physical state and at the same time, minimizing their bacterial flora. Granulations must not be allowed to dry or to macerate. By applying cholesterolized petrolatum containing a nontoxic antibacterial substance of low tissue toxicity, such as sulfamylon 5 per cent, granulations will not be injured, bacteriostasis will be obtained, and an optimal rate of epithelization will follow. Mont Reid [5] paraphrased the situation by saying; "Aid the growth of granulations by reducing the bacteria on their surfaces, but do not destroy the body by depriving it of the protection afforded by the granulations."

Even at its optimal rate, epithelization is a slow process—0.5 mm. per day (Fig. 7). Hence, the surgeon must learn to recognize the size of the granulating area that requires skin grafting. In general, any circular area with a diameter longer than 3 cm. requires grafting unless epithelial islands are still present within the area. Islands may be present in burns and varicose ulcer—deep epithelium remains uninjured about the hair follicles. Growth of these islands usually accounts for unusual stories of sudden regrowth of epithelium. If the defect is not circular, large areas may be recovered rather rapidly by the growth of epithelium from both sides of an angle. Another exception is the defect in the skin of the scrotum. The surrounding skin possesses sufficient elasticity to reduce an area of enormous size.

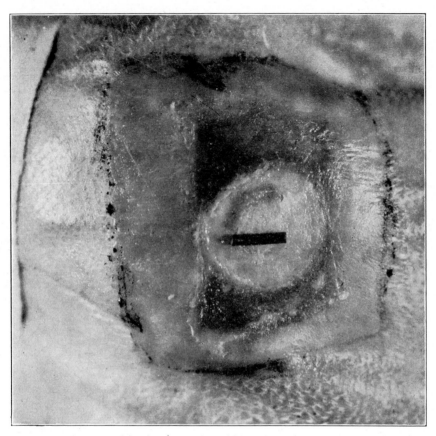

FIG. 7. A 13-day wound in the ear of the rabbit. The rod measures 0.5 centimeter. The outside black line denotes the original area of the wound. There has been no contraction. Inside this line is a rim of new epithelium (¾ to 1¼ cm.). The circle in the center was originally a square of epithelium (lying under the measuring rod) which has grown out into this shape. Between the circle and the rim are granulations appearing somewhat darker in color. The new growth of epithelium first appeared on the sixth day of healing. The rate of epithelization can be calculated from this photograph. The tip of the ear is toward the left. (From Howes, *Surg., Gynec. & Obst.,* 76:738, 1943. By permission of Surgery, Gynecology and Obstetrics).

Despite these exceptions, however, the principle is always to err on the side of early grafting; in fact, as soon as the granulations are bright red, not too moist and at the proper level. Moreover, if epithelial islands are present, early grafting does no harm. In some bone defects, even proper height can be neglected when granulations will not fill the cavity.

If early grafting of an area denuded of epithelium is not done, excessive contraction occurs. There is constant loss of blood serum; the patient's blood proteins become chronically depleted and amyloid disease results if the loss is long continued. Moreover, the blood vessels of the granulations soon start to obliterate and after a month, they become pale and then they no longer accept grafts. Besides, early skin grafting saves days and weeks of unnecessary hospitalization.

For these reasons, every general surgeon should know how to graft skin. Neither the procedure nor the necessary instruments should be segregated with the plastic surgeon. One of the pitiful sights to see in any hospital is the burned patient covered with old granulations, cachectic, dressed with salves reputed to stimulate epithelization, and developing contractures because: (1) the simple truth is not recognized that the area is too large to ever epithelize spontaneously; and (2) the surgeon is unskilled in doing the simple procedure of grafting skin. The criticism holds equally as well for large bed sores and leg ulcers that will not heal promptly.

THE EXUDATIVE PHASE

During the days immediately following wounding, the exudative phase of healing occurs. During it, hemorrhage is arrested, fibrin is deposited, bacterial invasion is resisted, dead tissue is liquefied and foreign bodies are sloughed. The injured area is corrected chemically to allow the propagation of cells. The initial care of all wounds is directed toward obtaining the shortest possible exudative phase of healing, thereby allowing tissues to regenerate as soon as possible.

Hemorrhage is arrested by the retraction of blood vessels and maintained by the deposition of fibrin in the cut ends of the severed vessels. Deposited fibrin also seals together tissue layers, acting as a glue between serosal surfaces. It provides a water-tight and air-tight seal; thus preventing leakage from wounds of hollow viscera immediately after suturing (Fig. 8). Fibrin anchors particulate matter, including bacteria, in one location in the wounded tissues.

Resistance to bacterial invasion and liquefaction of dead tissue is accomplished by the vascular and cellular reaction. After vasodilatation, exudate is poured into the injured area causing a transitory edema. Phagocytosis and antibacterial substances hinder the growth of, and destroy the bacteria, while enzymes liberated by the leukocytes liquefy dead tissue and thereby rid the area of food stuff for the growth of bacteria. Toxic by-products are carried away by the blood stream. The acidity of an area in which liquefaction of tissue proteins develops, gradually approaches neutrality, and new capillaries begin to sprout from old blood vessels in the surrounding healthy tissues. These capillaries start to grow about 48 hours after the injury but usually appear grossly on about the fourth day after the injury. Finally, with a correct chemical environment and nutrition furnished by the new capillaries, fibroplasia begins.

The exudative phase lasts about 4 days in healing per primam. During the exudative phase, the sutured wound has only the strength imparted by the sutures and deposited fibrin. In fact, the wound loses some of the immediate strength given by the sutures because the tissues partly lose their capacity to hold sutures through edema and liquefaction.

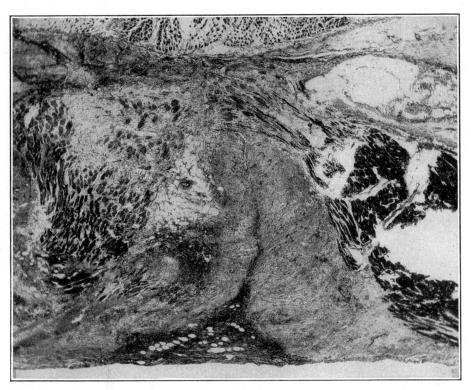

FIG. 8. Histologic features in the repair of peritoneum. In the center of the photograph can be seen the inverted approximated edges of the peritoneum. Stretching across the v-shaped cleft at the bottom of the photograph is deposited fibrin. Serosal surfaces should always be inverted when sutured, to place them in apposition so that fibrin can be deposited.

In the open wound, healing per primam, nothing seems to happen grossly during the exudative phase of healing except that a small amount of serum escapes. The phase terminates with the appearance of granulations and the wound begins to contract. Carrell and Du Nouy [6] called this period the latent period of healing—a stage of apparent inactivity when the mechanisms that bring about the redisintegration of the tissues are progressively set into motion.

The length of the exudative phase is dependent on the amount of dead tissue present in the wound, the efficiency of the blood supply and the degree and character of the bacterial contamination. An abundance of crushed tissue, a heavy or virulent bacterial contamination, and an inefficient blood supply prolong the exudative phase of healing. Infection lengthens this phase.

When frank suppuration occurs, the wound exhibits the classical signs of inflammation; *i.e.* redness, local heat and swelling. The surrounding tissues become indurated and tender, symptomatically the wound throbs. At first, spreading cellulitis develops about the wound but after 2 or 3 days,

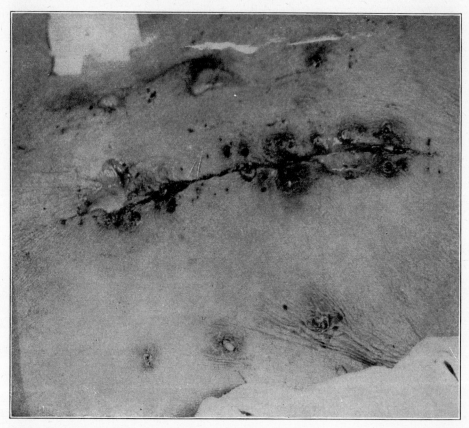

FIG. 9. Sutured right rectus wound, 9 days old, grossly infected. The sutures have been removed and the wound will shortly be laid wide open to provide drainage. At the left and right ends of the incision may be seen puddles of pus and the edges are already gaping spontaneously. Pus is also escaping from the retention suture holes situated above and below the incision. This wound was subsequently closed by secondary intention after adequate drainage was established. No postoperative herniation occurred because the infection was above the posterior rectus sheath.

the process begins to localize, pus escapes between the edges that begin to gape even though they are sutured (Fig. 9). Marked destruction of tissue substance occurs and blood vessels may become eroded to cause secondary hemorrhage. This liquefaction of tissue frees foreign bodies for extrusion. Tissues necrose in the following order: fat, nerve, muscle, and lastly the connective tissues and fascia. Bone remains. In fact, fascia, ligaments and

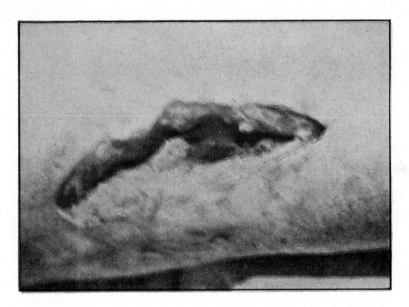

FIG. 10. Chronic suppuration in a wound with osteomyelitis in the bone beneath. The surrounding tissues are greatly scarred and indurated. The granulations are pale and hard. They do not bleed easily indicating that they have lost their rich blood supply. Contraction reduced the wound to this size, but will not reduce it any further.

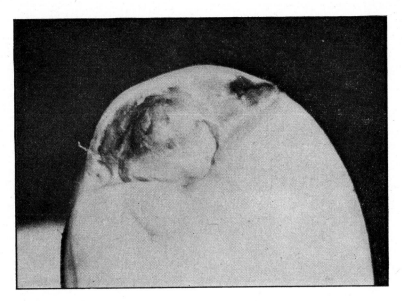

Fɪɢ. 11. Infected amputation stump. Wound filled with sloughing fascia that is stained green by the growth of pyocyaneus. End of the bone is protruding beyond the inflamed skin margins. All the soft tissues have retracted because of destruction of tissue by the infection. Slough had to be removed and the bone reamputated higher to allow closure of the wound.

tendons take so long to liquefy that they persist beyond the time when all other tissues have disappeared and then they are spoken of as "slough"—a misnomer meaning they have not sloughed. The persistency of slough, plus its capacity to support the growth of bacteria keeps up infection and conversely, infection subsides only when all slough has come away.

Granulations begin to appear in the infected wound shortly after localization has occurred and after a mechanism has been established for draining pus—a matter of 2 or 3 weeks sometimes. If drainage is adequate the infection quickly subsides, and the amount of discharge soon decreases. The pus becomes stickier and finally the discharge ceases.

The failure of bone to liquefy accounts for chronicity of osteomyelitis (Fig. 10). In some wounds, the infection, although chronic, may be severe enough to prevent granulations from growing into the area where slough exists while in other wounds, it may be so mild that granulations surround the slough and form a chronically draining sinus. In either case, the granulations do not correctly fill the wound until the slough comes away or is mechanically removed (Fig. 11).

Contraction likewise begins with the appearance of the granulations and hence, begins even when the wound is discharging pus. Purulency ceases only after all slough comes away. The resulting scar of the infected wound is always larger than it would be if the wound were not infected.

Between frank suppuration and optimal healing all degrees of untoward healing exists depending on the amount of dead tissue present, the inefficiency of the blood supply and the degree and nature of the bacterial contamination. The wound may become indurated, tender and slightly red and the entire process may subside without the wound discharging pus. This reaction can result, for example, from placing too much suture material in the subcutaneous fat.

In uncomplicated healing, the tissues surrounding the wound are soft and white all during the process and this "soft, white" healing is the type that must always be sought; it can be achieved by the surgeon, depending on how he cares for the wound. Infection and untoward healing are more easily prevented than cured.

CONTRACTION

Contraction occurs simultaneously with the regeneration of tissue. It is a powerful force for closing wounds resulting from the inward movement of the surrounding healthy tissues (Fig. 12). The process begins with the appearance of granulations; it starts at a maximal rate and gradually slows up as the size of the defect is reduced.[7] Because of contraction, the resulting scar is smaller than the original wound (Fig. 13). Because of contraction the amount of tissue that must be regenerated during healing is minimized. Sutures eliminate contraction. The process can close a large wound if it exists in freely movable tissues. On the other hand, contraction does not occur if the wounded tissues are fixed to underlying tissues or if they are stretched across bony structures. In such locations regeneration of tissue must account for the entire closure of the wound and the scar is then as great as the original wound. Anatomical areas, where contraction does not exist, are over the dorsum and palm of the hand, over the patella, the heel, and in the scalp.

A wound that can be approximated by sutures will be closed by contraction while a wound that cannot be closed by sutures will not be closed by contraction although greatly reduced in size and regenerated tissue must fill the remaining defect. The extent that contraction will close a wound depends on the elasticity of the surrounding tissues and the size of the defect to be closed. It is not unusual for contraction to advance the edge of a wound 4 cm. in freely movable tissues. To the contrary, old scar tissues do not contract nor do fascias, cartilage nor bone. The tissues wounded must be resilient like skin or muscle to exhibit contraction. Obviously, some defects are too large to close by contraction and as the process begins to terminate, progress becomes slower and finally stops. Clinically, this progress can be plotted.

5
4
3
AREA IN SQ CM
1 2 3 4 5 6 7 8 9 10 11 12 13 14 15 16
DAYS

FIG. 12.

I
LINE OF FORCE
II
III
IV
A
B
C
D
I Original incision.
II Gaping of wound.
III Early scar, contracted.
IV Late scar after retraction (in A and B, size equal to original incision.
A Parallel to direction of fibers.
B Oblique to direction of fibers.
C Horizontal to direction of fibers.
D All directions

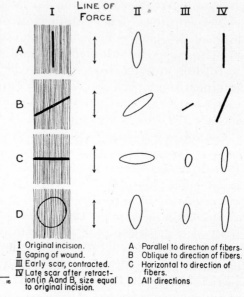

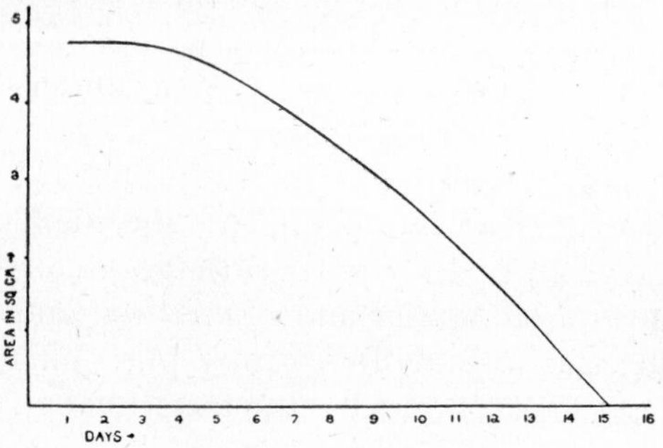

FIG. 13.

FIG. 12. Rate of healing in an open wound. For the first 4 days, there was no decrease in size of this open wound during the exudative phase of healing. After 4 days, the area decreases quickly in size due to (1) contraction and (2) regeneration of new tissue. Healing is occurring without infection. (From Howes, *Yale J. Biol. & Med.*, 285, 1930.)

FIG. 13. The original gaping of the wound is affected by the lines of force occurring in the surrounding tissues that are under tension. The early scar is always smaller than the original defect but the scar grows larger later. Scars in children grow with the child. (After Minervini.)

Many medications have been acclaimed as stimulants of wound healing because of the failure to control the propensity of contraction to close wounds.

Allowing contraction to occur in areas where tissues should be regenerated accounts for the phenomenon of contracture. For example, a contracture will fix the chin on the chest or the arm on the chest after a severe burn. Here contraction acts maximally, pulling all edges together whereas the necessary tissues should be grafted in order to establish two different planes of skin.

DEVELOPMENT OF WOUND INFECTION

The background for development of infection in the wound is usually more complicated than the simple entrance of bacteria between the cut edges. Actually, three factors are quantitatively involved; dead tissue, foreign bodies and bacteria. Bacteria are always required, of course, but unless they are really virulent, either dead tissue or foreign bodies or both are needed.

The possibility of infection increases with the extent of tissue damage and tissue death can result either from crushing the tissues directly or from interference with their blood supply. Thus, complete destruction of the blood supply of the wounded part for a period of time or sustained partial interference results in infection even when the bacterial contamination of the wound is minimal and avirulent. Various degrees of inadequacy of blood supply, anemia, shock, prolonged edema and thrombosis enhance the incidence of infection. On the other hand, an efficient blood supply is the best assurance against infection even though many bacteria are present in the wound.

Whether foreign bodies will help to initiate an infection in the presence of a moderate number of bacteria depends on their physical properties. If the foreign body helps initiate an infection, thereafter it becomes the nidus of this infection and the infection persists until the foreign body is extruded or liquefied. On the other hand, those foreign bodies that do not aid the onset of infection are eventually encapsulated in fibrous tissue. Foreign bodies that promote infection have the following characteristics: they have rough surfaces, porous interstices, are composed of organic material, are partially soluble and the soluble portion is chemically irritating to the tissues. To the contrary, those with the opposite physical properties; namely, insoluble smooth surfaces, nonporous, chemically and electrically inert, are less likely to act as an instigating factor in the development of infection in the presence of bacteria.

The size of the foreign body is also important but secondary to the physical properties mentioned. In the presence of minimal bacterial contamination tissues can sometimes encapsulate the foreign body with adverse physical properties if it is of small size, while with the same degree of bacterial contamination, a foreign body of large size with conducive physical properties can become encapsulated. A corollary is that the wound with the acceptable foreign body will heal without infection in the presence of a much larger bacterial contamination than the wound having foreign bodies with adverse physical properties. For these reasons, a detached piece of cancellous bone left in the traumatic wound will certainly produce an infection while a smooth steel jacketed bullet will become encapsulated. Again, a large smooth sheet of tantalum can be left in a wound while a small rough splinter of wood must be removed.

Viable wound edges free of dead tissue put up the best defense against the invasion of the bacteria. Bacteria grow in dead tissue in the wound just as they do in the test tube. Hence, good surgery ranks first in preventing infection and then an intelligent use of chemotherapy. The efficacy of surgical therapy rests on the completeness of removal of crushed tissue and the foreign bodies and the maintenance of an efficient blood supply.

The bacterial flora of the wound evolves and changes during the development of an infection in the wound. The original bacterial contamination of most wounds is a mixture of saprophytes, accounting for the 200 strains of bacteria that have been isolated from various wounds. Only a small percentage of wounds ever receive a single contaminant and then this is usually a virulent bacteria discharged from a pre-existing human infection.

The hay bacillus and other soil contaminants disappear from the mixed contamination of the wound within 24 hours usually leaving the staphylococci (the normal inhabitants of the skin) to dominate the flora. Hence, the commonest bacteria isolated from wounds is the staphylococcus.

The staphylococcus, though, may be displaced by the streptococcus and by gram-negative bacilli. Although the streptococci, the bacteria most feared, may enter the wound originally, there is good evidence that most streptococci enter the wound as secondary contaminants from the upper respiratory tract of the patient or from those who attend the wound. The streptococcus is feared because of its tendency to cause a spreading infection.

The gram-negative bacteria, pyocyaneus and proteus, come into the infected wound and dominate the flora about the seventh or tenth day after the infliction of the wound. These bacteria account for the green pus on dressings. They are of fecal origin and therefore, they enter the wound either from soiling or from the hands of those who attend the wound. Although these bacteria are seldom invasive and actually aid in proteolysis of slough, their importance has recently been reemphasized by their capacity to destroy penicillin. Thus, while they are not dangerous per se, they may aid more destructive bacteria to survive, and the pus they produce is abundant and difficult to eliminate.

In general, all the secondary bacterial contaminants are as important in the bacteriology of infection as the original bacterial contamination. While reduction in the amount of original bacterial contamination must be accomplished to prevent an immediate onset of infection, equally as important to preclude the possibility of its later appearance is to exclude the secondary contamination. This is particularly true when the recontamination occurs before granulations have appeared in the wound. A great deal of the success of the closed plaster method of treatment and the pressure treatment of burns originates from the fact that the original dressing is left in place for a length of time sufficient to allow granulations to grow. If recontamination takes place, then this rich protective vascular tissue becomes involved, and not necrosing tissue that readily supports the growth of bacteria. The flora of the granulations may change with the recontamination but reinfection is not initiated and the flora does not become mixed and better established as occurs when the recontamination takes place during the exudative phase of healing.

Anaerobic bacteria that cause serious infections such as tetanus and gas gangrene, survive in wounds when anaerobic conditions necessary for their growth exist. This may be in crushed tissue without blood supply but so often a pyogenic infection precedes the anaerobic infection and sets up the necessary conditions. Crushed or necrotic muscle is necessary for the development of gas gangrene. Therefore, if the initial surgical therapy turns the wounded area into one surrounded by viable cells, the possibility of starting an anaerobic infection is remote except in those rare instances where very virulent anaerobic bacteria are encountered. Specific antitoxin therapy lessens the danger of a fatal outcome. One of the great triumphs of World War II was the unplanned demonstration of the efficacy of immunization against tetanus. In the Philippines where both soldiers and natives were bombed alike, there were many deaths from tetanus reported by Glenn [8] in the unimmunized natives while not one death occurred among the immunized troops.

Failure of resolution of wound infection within two weeks indicates either an unusual bacterial infection; *i.e.* symbiosis, or the presence of a foreign body acting as the nidus of the infection or unextruded and unliquefied tissues; *i.e.* either fascia or bone.

GENERAL CONDITION OF THE PATIENT AND WOUND HEALING

Although most of the complications of healing arise locally from pathological conditions within the wound, the general condition of the patient has been increasingly recognized as contributing toward faulty healing.

Elimination of postoperative hemorrhage and hematoma in the wound has been accomplished by recognizing that the jaundiced patient has a prothrombin deficiency due to lack of absorption of vitamin K in the absence of bile. Giving bile salts and allowing absorption of vitamin K to occur from the food or hastening the process by giving extra vitamin K either orally or parenterally corrects the deficiency except when the liver is so badly damaged that prothrombin cannot be synthesized. Then fresh plasma must be given in the hope of supplying an adequate amount of prothrombin. At best, this supportive measure is a temporary expediency.

A deficient concentration of vitamin C in wounded tissues distorts fibroplasia. Fibroblasts appear but reticulin is poorly elaborated. The strands remain fine and short. The wounds gather strength at a slow rate and there is some tendency toward hemorrhage because new blood vessels are poorly supported. During healing, there is always mobilization of large quantities of vitamin C to the site of injury and if the area is large, the quantity moved is very large; much more than is found in the daily intake of food.

The amount of vitamin C in the blood does not disclose the true concentration of this vitamin in the tissues because an increased intake will temporarily elevate the blood level without appreciably changing the amount in the tissues. When there is doubt that tissue saturation does not exist, large amounts of vitamin C, *i.e.*, 2 or 3 hundred milligrams a day, should be given until nearly as much repeatedly reappears in the urine. Then the tissues are saturated. The vitamin is harmless and therefore can be taken in large amounts. Lund *et al.*,[9] have found that as much as 500 mg. a day are required to maintain tissue saturation in some severe burns. The route of administration is not important except that the parenteral route will be necessary if the patient is vomiting.

A deficient amount of serum protein [10] delays healing by two mechanisms: (1) an edema is produced in the wounded area and its circulation becomes inefficient; or (2) there may not be a sufficient or complete protein pattern for rebuilding new tissues. The first seems the more probable mechanism because starvation does not retard healing.[10a]

Adequate attention has not been given to the role of the combined deficiency of vitamin C and protein in delaying healing of wounds. Hartman has shown that a high percentage of patients with disrupted wounds exhibited this combination of deficiencies.

Dehydration [11] and anemia [12] retard the healing of wounds as well as an infection elsewhere in the body.[13] Uncontrolled diabetes predisposes a wound to infection through an unknown mechanism. There is no proof that syphilis distorts healing.

Wounds heal more rapidly in the young. The latent period is shorter and the rate of regeneration is more rapid. This tendency decreases with the slackening of growth. Once adult status is reached, however, there is no proof that wounds heal slower with advancing age.[14]

One fallacious form of therapy of wounds that is being repeatedly recommended is the local application of substances that affect growth through the general metabolism. Invariably, these substances, as for example the vitamins, are conjugated or split during intermediary metabolism to produce their influence on the growth of cells. In applying them locally, these mechanisms for their metabolism do not exist.

SUTURES

Use of Sutures. The function of sutures is to hold the edges of the wound together until healing occurs. Because they act as a splint they should provide a union of maximal strength; physically and chemically they should encourage healing to begin at the earliest possible moment after the repair of the wound. Moreover, they must be used correctly in order to encourage healing. The need to initiate the regeneration of tissue as soon as possible is repeatedly emphasized because the function of the suture is only taken over when this happens.[15] Serosal suturing prevents leakage (Fig. 16).

All sutures are foreign bodies in wounds and consequently, minimal amounts of them must be used. However, a balance must be obtained between using the least amount of suture material to obtain adequate hemostasis and consistent with giving the greatest amount of immediate sutured strength and promoting healing.[16]

Fortunately, maximal strength can be given to wounds immediately by means of the finest sutures. To do this, sutures should be used only in fascias and connective tissues where they hold, and not in muscle and fat where they serve only as foreign bodies. In addition, the bulk of the suture can be reduced by taking small bites of tissue and cutting sutures close to the knot. Large bite sutures leave long reaches exposed and there is a tendency to tie them tightly. Long ends of sutures beyond the knot are usually left either to give knot security or because the knot is not visible when the suture is cut. Thus, long ends are frequently left in the subcutaneous fat because the sutures are cut as far down as possible when the fat is not retracted and the knot is not seen.

Some surgeons are notorious for leaving long cut ends, up to ½ inch, beyond the knot. This is done on the theory that these long ends prevent the knots from becoming untied. Actually, as will be shown under the subject of "Knots," the form of the knot and the kind of suture material used are more important in determining knot security.

Requirements for Suturing. Not all wounds can be sutured primarily (see delayed primary closure). A wound should not be sutured unless it possesses the following properties. It must be free or nearly free of crushed tissues, the edges should have an efficient blood supply, and the numbers of foreign bodies included must be minimal and these must possess physical properties that favor encapsulation. Lastly, and most important, the number of bacteria present must be minimal. The incised wound, made under antiseptic conditions, possesses these properties.

Because tension reduces the blood supply to the edges of the wounds, tissues should not be sutured under tension. Instead, they should be "moved up" as far as possible.

To satisfy the requirements for suturing in traumatic wounds, crushed tissue is débrided to reduce its amount and they are irrigated to wash out bacteria on the surfaces of the tissues. Primary suturing of traumatic wounds should not be attempted later than ten hours after injury because the bacteria are already multiplying in the tissues. To meet the requirements for suturing in clean contaminated operative wounds (that is, those wounds that are made clean but become contaminated during the operation), the edges of wounds should be protected from contamination as much as possible by the use of pads before the infected site is broken into. This type of wound should also be irrigated free of bacteria after the peritoneum is closed and detached pieces of tissues should be débrided.

Objects of Suturing. Suturing not only reduces the size of the wound but also limits the amount of subsequent bacterial contamination. A wound completely sutured, for example, has the initial bacterial contamination "sealed in" and the tissues must deal with that amount of contamination.

Although some recontamination can take place during the first four days after suturing, thereafter it cannot occur as both DuMortier[17] and Berman et al.,[18] have shown.

Because of the importance of limiting the secondary bacterial contamination, suturing should always place the edges of the wounds in apposition wherever possible. However, if edges are to be moved up but left separated, buried small bite interrupted sutures should be used to fasten them to the underlying tissues at the points of maximum advancement (Fig. 14A), and

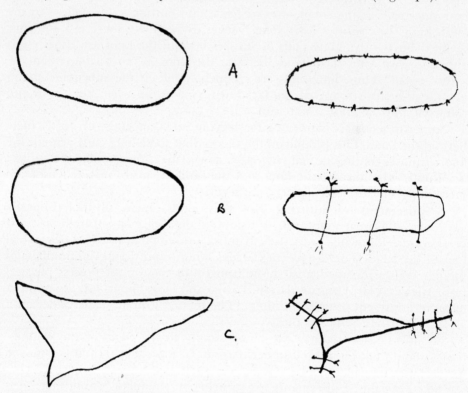

FIG. 14. A. Circular defect. The edges have been moved up to make a smaller defect by means of small bite, buried sutures around the edges. Unabsorbable suture material is best for this type of partial closure. The sutures to be removed after 8 or 10 days of healing. B. Partial closure of circular defect by means of sutures stretching across the wound. This is the type of closure that almost never works, as discussed in the text. C. Defect with angles. Method of partial closure on the right. Accurate approximation without tension obtained. Center left open.

not sutures bridging the defect—a technic unfortunately practiced too often, and vitiating every protective mechanism possessed by the tissues (Fig 14B). Bridging the defect with sutures places them exposed not only to bacteria, but without the proximity of cells capable of protecting and encapsulating them because these sutures are foreign bodies in the center of a wound healing by secondary intention. Such sutures only act as wicks to carry infection back into edges of the wound. The wound invariably becomes

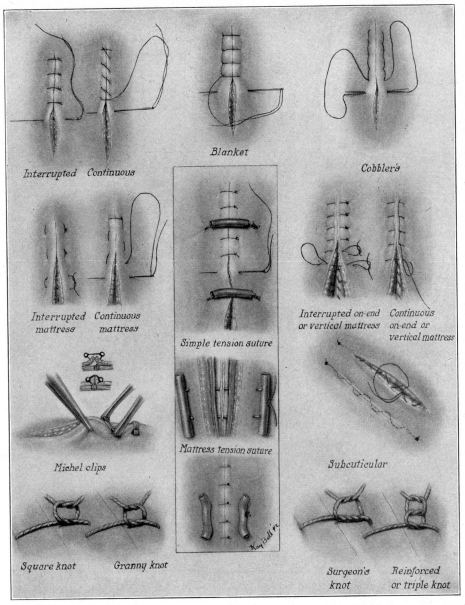

FIG. 15. Types of sutures and knots in common use. (From Orr, *Operations of General Surgery*. Courtesy of W. B. Saunders Co., Philadelphia, 1944.)

infected and the sutures have to be removed again, allowing the edges to gape wider than originally. To the contrary, when small bite interrupted sutures are used to advance the edges, they are completely buried and become encapsulated.

The size of a wound can also be reduced and the total amount of bacterial contamination can be limited by suturing the angles of the wound and leaving the center open (Fig. 14C). In the sutured angles, the edges are accurately approximated and therefore, all prerequisites for successful healing are satisfied.

The use of interrupted sutures completely eliminates the danger of a knot becoming untied. With a continuous suture, the integrity of the entire

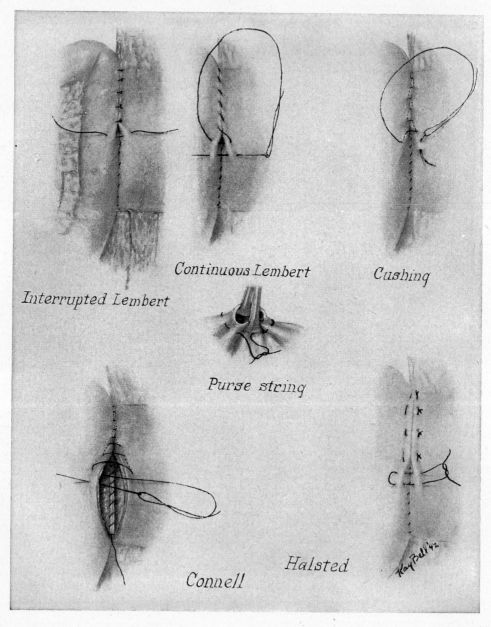

FIG. 16. Types of intestinal sutures in common use. (From Orr, *Operations of General Surgery*. Courtesy of W. B. Saunders Co., Philadelphia, 1944.)

suture line is in jeopardy if the knot on either end comes untied. On the other hand, if a knot becomes untied in an interrupted suture, the adjacent one on either side takes up its function.

Knots. The square knot has less tendency to untie than the granny knot. However, there is a tendency for all knots to slip in some suture materials. For example, monofilament nylon cannot hold the usual knots and in general, suture materials with slightly roughened surfaces hold knots better than the smooth variety. The roughened suture, on the other hand, pulls through the tissues with greater difficulty.

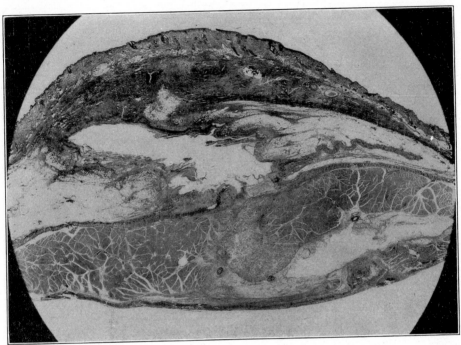

FIG. 17. Cross section of wound of the anterior abdominal wall. Blood clot fills the large open space in the subcutaneous fat above the muscle in the center of the photograph. The fascia in the anterior rectus sheath is still somewhat separated. Below, on the right, in the muscle is another cleared area where a hematoma existed.

Taylor [19] is one of the few individuals who has quantitatively studied the safety of knots. He found that three knots, all tied square, had the least tendency to untie and further, that the inclusion of a surgeon's knot definitely increased the possibility of slippage. When tension exists, a surgeon's knot (Fig. 15), is frequently used as the first throw while the second and third knots are being tied. He also discovered that knots are more secure in fine sutures than in the larger ones. Taylor believes that suture failures are due to insecure knots rather than to faulty suture material.

Suture Complications. In the sutured wound failure to obtain hemostasis results in a hematoma that may or may not clot (Fig. 17). If the blood clots and the area does not become infected the area is converted into a mass of fibrous tissue. If it does not clot the hematoma requires aspiration as soon as its presence is detected to collapse the dead space created and to prevent the formation of a cyst wall.

Transfixion of ligatures prevents hemorrhage from large vessels and neither large ligatures nor tight tying are required. In fact, both predispose to secondary hemorrhage.

Disruption and evisceration and postoperative herniation are the severest complications of suturing.[20]

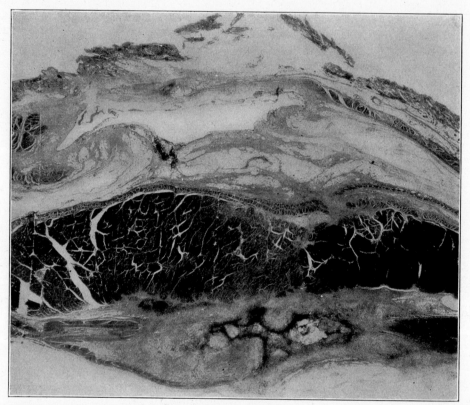

FIG. 18. Beneath the muscle can be seen small abscesses above the healed peritoneum. Failure of healing in this area starts a wedge of omentum that pushes outward with every increase in intra-abdominal tension.

Separation or disruption of skin may result from removing stitches before healing has occurred, but usually separation occurs when the edges are unintentionally inverted so that healing cannot occur. When the sutures are removed, separation must take place to allow healing to occur. A safe guard against too early removal of sutures is to remove alternate ones first and watch the degree of separation that occurs for the next 24 hours before removing all of them.

Separation of the anterior rectus fascia in wounds of the anterior abdominal wall is not a serious complication. Because of tone, sutured muscle, like tendon, always separates even when not contracting. Best maintenance of muscle is obtained by suturing its surrounding fascias or fibrous bands or septa within.

Separation or disruption of the posterior sheath of the rectus muscle in wounds of the anterior abdominal wall results either in postoperative hernia or evisceration. Postoperative herniation occurs when the sutures in the anterior rectus sheath hold. Evisceration is usually discovered when the skin sutures are removed although actually, revealing signs are present much sooner. The sudden appearance of an unexplained sero-sanguinous discharge from the wound, even when drained, about the fourth day of healing, is evidence and change in contour and tenderness are enough confirmation to justify treatment.

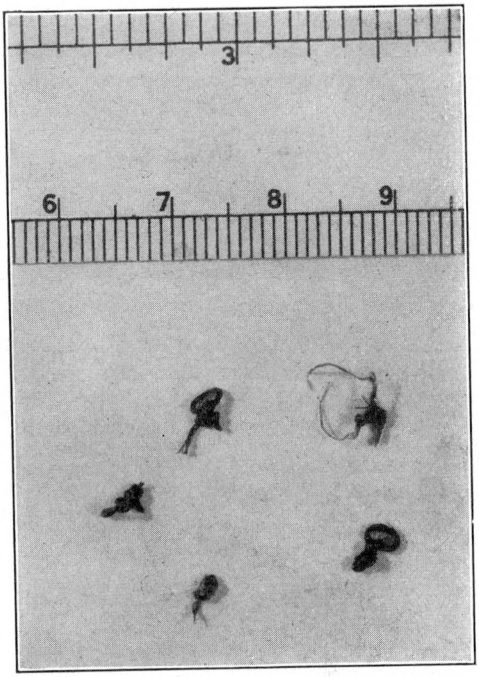

The usual postoperative evisceration of the wound is discovered at about the seventh or eighth day after operation when the wound should be healing. Generally, the patient has had a complicated convalescence. The disrupting force is an intermittent increase in intra-abdominal pressure caused by coughing, hiccoughing, distention or straining at stool. For these reasons, upper abdominal incisions are more susceptible because of the bellow action of the ribs.

FIG. 19. Stitches removed from patient with disrupted right rectus wound subsequent to repair of ruptured peptic ulcer 8 days before. Granulations covered sutures so that they were not visible. Three-fourths of them were pulled out of tissues and can be seen fully tied, and one-fourth broken. Cultures showed *Staph. aureus*.

The second factor is poor healing either because of low-grade infection (Fig. 18), lack of vitamin C, low-serum protein or improper hydration. Wounds in older patients with cancer are apt to heal poorly.
The third factor is that the wound possessed an insufficient immediate sutured strength. The tissues being thin the sutures easily cut through them, particularly when the patient is straining under a light anesthesia at the time of closure.

When the sutures break in a disruption, either because they cannot stand the strain or the knots untie or when the tissues are too thin, then the disruption occurs early, within the first 48 hours. In later disruptions, either the tissues gradually lose their capacity to hold the suture because of intermittent strain and gradual necrosis where the suture penetrates the tissue, combined with failure of the wound to gather its strength through healing (Fig. 19), or infection destroys the suture.

Patients with disrupted wounds are unfortunately quite sick and the mortality of a secondary repair is high, upwards to 20 per cent, depending on circumstances. Often times opening the skin and anterior fascia and tamponading back the viscera is a life saving procedure. Secondary repairs should be done earlier when the sanguinous discharge appears to prevent exhaustion. Correction of the factors that cause disruption is excellent prevention. Singleton [21] has shown that disruptions are less frequent in transverse than longitudinal incisions. Early ambulation of the patient has not increased the incidence of disruption.

DÉBRIDEMENT OF WOUND

Fredricka [22] demonstrated that an animal would not die of septicemia if the crushed tissues containing contaminating bacteria were cut away shortly after the injury was inflicted. This principle was carried into the treatment of traumatic wounds to prevent local infection of the wound as "débridement." An unnecessary amount of verbiage has been wasted on whether a traumatic wound should be excised or whether the lacerated tags of tissue devoid of blood supply should be trimmed away, indicating that the principles of débridement have not been understood. It matters not whether the wound is excised or loose tags are cut away as long as crushed tissue is removed and foreign bodies and healthy tissues are not needlessly sacrificed.

There has not been adequate instruction on the recognition of the tissue to be removed, nor has the relationship of débridement to time of suturing been properly taught.

In the first place, débridement of skin edges is always advised (Fig. 20); yet of all the tissues, skin has the least importance in preventing infection. Only the removal of irregularities that prevent satisfactory approximation is the object of skin débridement and many times it is advantageous, and just as good cosmetic result can be obtained by leaving the skin open. On the other hand, crushed muscle and fat are the two tissues that start infection in wounds and these are the tissues to remove. The amount of muscle to be débrided is easily recognized. Crushed muscle is dark red and it does not bleed, assuming of course, that the patient is not in shock. Removal of small amounts should be continued until the cut edge is of normal color and it bleeds readily. Crushed fat is difficult to recognize but certainly the débridement should be carried as far as the foreign bodies extend. Large amounts of fat can be cut away as long as "dead space" is not created; if a dead space is created in the subcutaneous fat, the skin edges should be left open to create a concave wound. Muscle cannot be removed excessively but it is surprising how much can be removed without creating a subsequent anatomical defect. Stimson [23] has warned against the too enthusiastic débridement of bone when it is fractured in small pieces. Only chips absolutely detached from periosteum should be removed, and always enough of the original architecture should be left to reestablish the continuity of the bone during healing. Tendons, nerves and blood vessels do not need débridement.

Lastly, it is important that débridement should cover the entire area of wounding and not remove excessive amounts of healthy tissue in available areas while leaving crushed tissues in areas reached with greater difficulty. Crushed tissue starts infection regardless of its location. For example, adequate débridement of muscle should be done on both sides of the bone in a compound fracture; the fracture site must be opened widely and the entire surrounding area débrided. All foreign bodies should be removed.

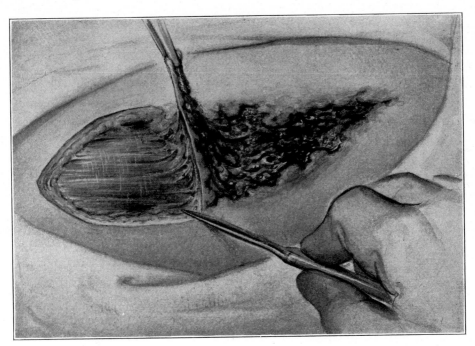

Fig. 20. Débridement of skin and subcutaneous tissue leaving uninjured muscle beneath.

There is no point in débriding wounds in limbs with destroyed blood supply. The limb should be débrided if the blood supply cannot be restored.

As has been stated, traumatic wounds should be sutured primarily only when débridement has been satisfactorily carried out. If any doubt exists as to the adequacy of débridement the wound should be left open for delayed primary closure. In general, there is less likelihood of obtaining a débridement satisfactory to permit suturing in the larger, more contused wounds than in the smaller ones cut by sharp weapons.

Débridement of traumatic wounds never should be omitted whenever the presence of crushed tissue is suspected and even when the wound is made with a sharp instrument and no dead tissue is seen. The depth of the wound must always be explored for foreign bodies. On the other hand, abuse of débridement must be discouraged. Wide excision of healthy tissue should always be avoided.

SECONDARY CLOSURE OF WOUNDS

During World War I, secondary closure of traumatic wounds gained some popularity. The procedure was carried out late, however, *i.e.*, when the wound was granulating and closure was no longer progressing. Skin was principally approximated to reduce the size of its defect and thereby eliminating grafting or at least, reducing the amount required.

Before delayed primary closure was introduced in World War II, another type of "secondary" closure was occasionally used on contaminated operative wounds to prevent infection. In this procedure, sutures were placed deep through the edges of the wound at the time of operation and it was packed open with gauze. Three or four days later, the gauze was removed and the sutures were tied. By this maneuver the wound is provided with open drainage during most of its exudative phase and the edges are brought together when young granulations are beginning to sprout. Recently, Coller and Valk [24] again have advocated the use of this type of secondary closure for wounds made for large bowel surgery.

These same physiological principles govern delayed primary closure popularized during World War II. Both methods provide open drainage during the exudative period of healing.

DELAYED PRIMARY CLOSURE OF TRAUMATIC WOUNDS

Previous experience had shown that if traumatic wounds were débrided and closed primarily, the procedure could be carried out successfully only when performed within 12 hours after injury. The length of this "safe period" was assumed to be determined by the activity of the bacteria, that were in general believed to be on the surface of the wound or ground into tissues during the first 7 or 8 hours, and thereafter multiplied and invaded the tissues. If the wound was débrided while the bacteria were invading the tissues, infection developed.

Encouraged by the possibility that the sulfonamides and penicillin might help delay the onset of infection, Olgivie in 1942 suggested that wounds could be débrided beyond this time limit but the procedure met with poor success. The closed plaster method of Trueta was also a failure when wounds were treated late and when all crushed tissues could not be débrided. Moreover, too much time was necessary to obtain healing with this procedure. Consequently, the old principle of secondary closure was employed again in World War II,[25a, 25b] but this time was correctly called delayed primary closure. Wounds were débrided in the initial treatment and they were packed open. Additional débridement was done, if necessary, at the time of the delayed closure. The procedure met with immediate success and the wounded could be quickly returned to duty. Stimson [23] and Churchill [26] reported 90 to 95 per cent of the wounds healed without infection. Sarjeant and Morton [27] reported 75 per cent healed in 14 days and 17 per cent healed in 21 days when the closure was done from the fifth to the ninth day after wounding. The total number of successes dropped to 80 per cent when closure was done from the tenth to twenty-first day.

At first, either the sulfonamides or penicillin were used, both locally and parenterally, but later, delayed primary closure was attempted without either drug and excellent percentage of primary healing was still obtained. In one group, 13,552 soft part wounds were so treated without loss of life or limb; no serious complications developed; and more than 90 per cent healed promptly (Churchill). Churchill attributes the success of the procedure largely to the surgery and he has repeatedly emphasized that chemotherapy with poor surgery will not accomplish the same results.

In doing the delayed closure, muscles were closed, then fascia. Skin was left open by some and closed by others. If the skin was closed, this had to be done very accurately. The tissues had to be closed without tension and without leaving dead space. The type of sutures employed was not important. The types of bacterial flora in the wound did not affect the outcome, but if any necrotic tissue was present, this was removed by additional débridement at the time of closure.

Churchill has warned that not all wounds of soft tissues can be closed; the percentage varying from 75 to 95 per cent depending on the nature of the wound. Those having deep recesses, those having received inadequate débridement originally, and of course, those with inadequate tissue cannot be closed. Sarjeant and Morton [27] add further contraindications. The surrounding tissues should be normal to palpation and the skin edges should not show any signs of inflammation. The appearance of the wound is the best guide for the proper time to do delayed closure. The edges should be red and relatively free of pus. If the wound is discharging much purulent exudate, the wound should be treated for 2 or 3 days with a chlorine solution until the exudate disappears. The patient's condition must allow the procedure to be done.

While emphasizing the importance of surgery Churchill advised the use of penicillin for cellulitis spreading from wounds and for certain wounds more prone than others to develop infection. For these he believed penicillin should be used throughout their treatment. Hence, complex wounds, compound fractures and those with nerve injuries should receive chemotherapy both before and after the delayed primary closure.

In many instances wounds treated by delayed primary closure were given first aid treatment locally by sulfonamides, the powder being dusted into the wound. The use of the sulfonamides early brings to mind that LeGroux [28] demonstrated that the length of time before bacteria began to multiply and to invade tissues is prolonged by the sulfonamides. On the other hand, the initial débridement would account for freeing many wounds of infection. Thus, in our military experience it cannot be said definitely whether chemotherapy helped decrease the number of infections obtained nor can it be said whether, in the future, fewer infections will be obtained when chemotherapy is correctly used. After all, in any consideration of delayed primary closure it must be remembered that, the sulfonamides are only bacteriostatic agents; they do not act quickly and only affect certain bacteria. Moreover, they were often used in concentrations that destroyed tissues. So too when penicillin alone was used, resistant strains of bacteria were encountered; again powder was placed in the wounds and careful statistical records were not kept of the results when penicillin was used immediately after the débridement (the time when penicillin would be most effective in preventing infection) or at the time of delayed closure.

Lastly, proof that chemotherapy may help prevent infection in delayed primary closure of wounds has been offered in the work of Hoerr.[29] He kept accurate statistics on the prophylactic use of oral sulfadiazine and penicillin in what he terms "secondary" closure of 197 soft tissue wounds in 138 patients. All were débrided shortly after infliction. Ninety-one wounds were closed, however, in less than 10 days and therefore, can be classified as "delayed primary closure." Of the total number of patients, 44 per cent had infected wounds and 28 per cent exhibited delayed healing when no chemotherapy was employed. These percentages are higher than in other reports where less rigid criteria for infection were followed. With oral sulfadiazine the incident of infection became 27 per cent, and of delayed healing 19 per cent. The same reduction was obtained with sulfadiazine plus penicillin. He found, as did Sarjeant and Morton,[27] that a greater percentage of infection occurred in real secondary closure; i.e. wounds older than 11 days that required excision of granulations and of scar tissue en bloc. Oral sulfadiazine reduced this rate to 13 per cent. In every other category also that tended to favor infection, the oral use of sulfadiazine reduced the incidence of infection. Adequate statistics are not available for the newer antibiotics.

The application of delayed primary closure of wounds finds its greatest usefulness in the treatment of compound fractures, notorious for becoming infected, (50 per cent). B. Stimson[23] in the British Army pioneered the use of this form of treatment during World War II. She emphasized that delayed closure can be employed only if the wound has been initially débrided, and that this débridement should not remove attached bone chips or bone fragments. The wound is best packed open with dry, fine-mesh gauze until the closure is carried out. Delayed primary closure cannot be used for compound fractures of the skull.

In civil surgery, the use of delayed primary closure will probably find its greatest application also in the treatment of compound fractures.

CHEMOTHERAPY OF WOUNDS

Chemotherapy can aid the healing of wounds by preventing infection from becoming established, by preventing spread of infection from the wound, and by hastening the resolution of the localized established infection.

Infection must be prevented in 3 types of wounds: (1) the clean operative wound; (2) the clean-contaminated operative wound; and (3) in the traumatic wound. The clean-contaminated operative wound is clean when made, but becomes contaminated by bacteria after opening into viscera or entering into a collection of pus. The traumatic wound differs from the clean-contaminated wound, not so much in the degree or character of bacterial contamination, but in the presence of larger amounts of crushed tissue and the possibility of a greater elapsed time before treatment is initiated. Because neither crushed tissue nor foreign bodies can be removed except by mechanical means, chemotherapy can only hope to prevent infection in traumatic wounds that contain a minimal amount of crushed tissue and no foreign bodies. By the same token, the clean-contaminated wound is ideal for testing the efficacy of chemotherapy to prevent infection in wounds.

With the introduction of the sulfonamides, spread of infection from wounds became preventable. Penicillin introduced later proved to be equally as effective for this purpose. Both agents acomplished this task best when given parenterally.

On the other hand, neither agent, as previously used, prevented the development of local infection in wounds. In an elaborate statistical study conducted for the Office of Scientific Research and Development under the guidance of Dr. Frank Meleney,[30] the sulfonamides employed systemically, locally, or combined, did not materially reduce the incidence or severity of local infection developing either in wounds or burns. The onset of the infection was not prolonged nor did the sulfonamides eliminate pathogenic bacteria from the wounds. Both traumatic wounds of soft parts and compound fractures were included in the group. The sulfonamides used were sulfathiazole and sulfadiazine.

Because penicillin unlike the sulfonamides acts in the presence of blood and after a short contact with the bacteria, penicillin should be more effective than the sulfonamides in preventing infection in wounds, particularly when the contamination is largely of gram-positive bacteria which are penicillin sensitive. It would not be expected that penicillin would be effective when the contamination is of mixed bacteria or when the gram-positive bacteria present are penicillin resistant. Moreover, gram-negative bacteria destroy penicillin by the elaboration of penicillinase. In experimental animals local infections in wounds have been held in abeyance by penicillin until the gram-negative bacteria appeared.

Penicillin, like the sulfonamides, failed to shorten the evolution of the established infection in the wound. Florey and Cairns [31] and a corps of bacteriologists treated battle casualties with localized infections with large amounts of penicillin. Initially, the number of gram-positive bacteria were reduced, but as soon as the gram-negative bacteria appeared this effect was lost.

Howes [32] has prevented infection in contaminated wounds by using streptomycin, 200 units per cc., and sulfamylon, 5 per cent. These concentrations kill bacteria but not cells and hence, it can be used as a subcutaneous antiseptic and can be injected about an infection. Moreover, the mixture is active against both gram-negative and gram-positive bacteria and yet does not interfere with wound healing. Clinically, the greatest success with this mixture has been in clean-contaminated wounds. Healing per primam has been obtained in all wounds that did not suffer repeated contamination. It has also been used in the peritoneal cavity when a fresh contamination occurs without causing harm. On the other hand, the evolution of the established infection is not hastened.[33]

Chemotherapy of the established wound infection requires adjunct therapy to remove slough and to provide chemical drainage. The most effective means found to date employs the use of an acid, and a demulcent. The acid explodes the leukocytes in the pus providing drainage; starts swelling and aids in the digestion of slough. Moreover, it attacks only dead tissue and is quickly neutralized by living tissue. Large loose pieces of slough, if readily available, should be cut away with the knife. The infected wound is washed for 10 minutes with the solution and then dressed subsequently with gauze soaked in the antibacterial mixture as mentioned above. General supportive treatment, especially heat, should be used. The amount of drainage is quickly reduced and the resolution of the infection is hastened.

Freshly prepared Dakin's solution also has the capacity to dissolve slough. This property is lost after 24 hours and the property is not possessed by other chlorine substitutes.

DRAINAGE OF WOUNDS

Only drainage of wounds of soft parts will be considered here. Drainage of peritoneum, joints and special anatomical locations will be discussed under the surgical technics employed for these areas. The clean contaminated wound and the traumatic wound are the two types that usually need drainage. The clean wound is generally sutured without drainage unless hemostasis has not been adequately obtained. Then two different types of drains are used depending on circumstances. A wick drain consisting of a sheath of rubber with or without a gauze center is used when it is thought that some slight oozing might continue. This drain can be removed in 24 or 48 hours depending on the character and the amount of drainage. At first, the drainage is sanguinous, then serosanguinous and gradually decreases in amount as the oozing stops. The drain should be removed when the drainage is a light pink and definitely decreasing in amount.

Packing is employed when the bleeding cannot be controlled by other means. Pressure is placed on the gauze, and fibrin clots in its meshes, completing the hemostasis. The packing is not removed early even if there is no further evidence of hemorrhage because bleeding will be reinitiated if the fibrin clot is disrupted. The superficial portion of the pack is first removed after 4 or 5 days and the innermost portion is not removed until the seventh or eighth day. At this time the gauze will usually have separated spontaneously by liquefaction of the fibrin clot, and no danger any longer exists on removing it. If, per chance, the innermost layer of gauze is adherent, a day or two longer should be waited before a vigorous attempt is made to remove it. Occasionally granulations will grow into the gauze and make it difficult to remove, but this complication is largely avoided if fine mesh or bandage gauze is used for the pack.

Fibrin foam and oxidized gauze control both types of hemorrhage, but should not be used if there is any danger of infection.

Ten years ago all traumatic wounds, if they were sutured, were invariably drained with a small wick of rubber. The object of this type of drainage was to "reverse lymph flow." Actually such drains probably recontaminated the wounded area as well. Now, either the traumatic wound is completely sutured without drainage if it has been débrided early or it is left open entirely for drainage by packing for 3 or 4 days and then closed completely without drainage, thus constituting the so-called delayed primary closure.

Drainage of the clean-contaminated wound can be briefly summarized as indicated below. The methods that have been employed are:

(1) Closure with wick drainage. Considered inadequate because of pocketing of pus. Various methods of placing drains have not been statistically evaluated.
(2) Packing open all layers above the sutured peritoneum—allowing these layers to close by secondary intention (Whipple).
(3) Delayed primary closure (Coller and others).
(4) Irrigation and débridement after closure of peritoneum. Primary closure of wound without drainage (Howes).
(5) Primary closure, but using a mixture of streptomycin and sulfamylon to irrigate the wound (Howes).

All five methods have been and are still being employed.

ANTISEPTICS AND WOUND HEALING

Antiseptics have only surface value for destroying bacteria; *i.e.* they are only able to kill bacteria on the surface of the skin or on the surfaces of inanimate objects. Antiseptics will not kill bacteria ground into tissues or bacteria situated deep in the hair follicles. Thus, even if the surface of the skin can be proven sterile after an antiseptic is applied, the first blood that runs from the wound after the skin is cut will invariably contain bacteria. These have escaped destruction because they were deep in the hair follicles.

Even for surface activity, antiseptics must also clean the surface of the skin and hence, the antibacterial substance is usually mixed with grease solvents such as acetone or alcohol in order to remove dirt and grease. Soap and water will likewise remove surface dirt and grease and wash away surface bacteria. Thus on the skin, soap and water can be substituted for antiseptic mixtures.[36] Newly isolated and not yet converted to the use of cleansing skin in surgery are many new powerful detergents that in small concentrations are much more efficient in removing grease and dirt than ordinary soap and water. Some of these also have antibacterial activity.

For example, Traub *et al.*[37] has found that with G 11 an extremely low resident bacterial population of the skin is obtained.

The ordinary antiseptics and especially alcohol and acetone mixtures definitely kill cells and interfere with wound healing. Shortly after Lister introduced the antiseptic era, their interference with wound healing became apparent and has never been denied, yet curiously most textbooks of surgery and first aid manuals still advise the use of antiseptics to prevent infection, especially in traumatic wounds, although these following facts are well known:

(1) That antiseptics will not kill bacteria in the presence of blood.

(2) That they will not kill bacteria ground into tissues and those on surfaces can be washed off by running water.

(3) That the solutions of iodine, bichloride mercury, lysol, the acriflavines, metholate etc., employed in wounds, not only kill additional cells in the fresh wound, but interfere with healing.

There is no objection to cleansing the surrounding skin with an antiseptic grease solvent mixture. Either running water or solutions of penicillin (up to 1000 units per cc.) or streptomycin (up to 200 units per cc.) or sulfamylon (up to 5 per cent) or a mixture of these should be the only antibacterials used to wash freshly damaged tissue. The solutions of penicillin must be made up fresh. Streptomycin does not have a complete bacterial spectrum so that the mixture with sulfamylon is better and seems to be more effective than sulfamylon alone.

CAN WOUND HEALING BE STIMULATED?

From what has been said about the phases of healing, it must be obvious that wound healing would be stimulated if the exudative phase of healing were shortened, if the rate of contraction were hastened, and if the rate of regeneration of new tissue were quickened.

Actually, the exudative phase of healing is more easily inhibited and prolonged than shortened; by infection, poor circulation, the poor general condition of the patient, etc., and one is generally satisfied if the therapy corrects the factors that impede progress. No method is known to hasten the rate of contraction, although it can be eliminated or the amount required minimized by the correct use of sutures and by grafting tissues.

This brings us to the question as to whether or not regeneration of tissues can be stimulated. When loss of tissue substance is great, even a greatly stimulated rate of healing would be inadequate, and grafting of tissue will be necessary.

These facts should be well known; yet hormones, plant substances and vitamins are constantly being pushed as stimulants for the entire process of wound healing. Their use is based on the fact that they hasten the division of cells when added to cultures of embryonal tissue, plants, or yeasts, growth phenomena having no relationship to wound healing. The optimistic clinical reports of stimulation of wound healing are always impressionistic.

Clinically, whenever the rate of regeneration of tissue after wounding has been accurately measured under the influence of these substances and contraction is adequately controlled, no stimulation of the rate of regeneration of tissue is ever found.[34] Favorite test objects for stimulation of wound healing are bed sores and varicose ulcers, actually representing inhibited rates of healing anyway. When the patient with varicose ulcer is put to bed, and the edema of the leg regresses and the area grows smaller, the small epithelial islands in the middle of the granulations sprout as the infection subsides and truly a remarkable bit of regeneration of tissue appears to occur. So, too, after the slough comes away at the base of the bed sore and the infection beneath is drained, granulations will spring up rapidly.

TRENDS IN THE THERAPY OF WOUNDS

Nonabsorbable sutures, such as silk and cotton are being employed by more surgeons and in increased numbers and types of wounds. To obtain the best results, however, with nonabsorbable material, a definite technic must be employed. The sutures must be interrupted, fine bites of tissue must be taken and fine sizes must be used. However, when catgut is used with this same technic, excellent healing is also obtained. The difference is technic.

There has been a consistent trend to employ smaller sizes of sutures. The stronger and larger sizes of catgut, No. 2 and No. 1, traditionally used by most surgeons to satisfy the mechanics of suturing, have been gradually supplanted by those with less thread strength such as, No. oo and No. ooo, which give as much strength to the tissue included in the suture. Small sutures cannot be tied too tightly, since they will break, thereby eliminating tissue necrosis. Elimination of tissue necrosis and reduction in the amount of foreign body suture material placed in the wound has resulted in more satisfactory healing as a sequence to the trend of employing sutures of smaller size. "Remember, you are suturing cells" is a good working rule.

Next, more transverse incisions in the abdomen have been employed—incisions that really hold the sutures more securely as described in Chapter 8. In fact, one wonders why longitudinal incisions ever became so popular and traditional. Undoubtedly, the reason was abhorrence of cutting muscle without the realization of how well it heals. Transverse incisions split or cut between the fascial bundles, especially in the important transversalis fascia and therefore, the sutures must pull at right angles to them or against these fibers. As a result, the wound of the anterior abdominal wall has greater initial strength and is better able to resist disrupting forces, particularly the suture line in the peritoneum and posterior sheath where disruptions and postoperative herniations start.

Confidence in obtaining greater initial strength of the wound and the realization that good healing could be obtained with regularity led to ready acceptance of early ambulation of the patient.

Powers[35] in 1944, concluded that by allowing a patient out of bed 24 or 48 hours after operation, the incidence of postoperative pulmonary and phlebitic complications was reduced. Constipation and gas pain were also less. There were misgivings, however, that wounds could not withstand this early activity without disruption or later, developing a hernia; these points had to be evaluated statistically. The score showed that the incidence of these postoperative complications did not increase, possibly because atrophy of surrounding muscles did not occur. Previously only "slick operators" practiced sending patients home 2 or 3 days after an appendectomy, whereas the more conservative surgeons required a full two weeks. European and South American surgeons always allowed their patients out of bed much earlier than the American surgeons. The principle of early ambulation was quickly adopted by the Armed Forces during the war because the soldier-patients were more readily reconditioned for duty if they were ambulated early. The suggestion for early ambulation came at the time also when there was a marked shortage of civilian hospital beds.

Contraindications to early ambulations are poor anatomical structures that tear easily while suturing and the development of infection in the wound. Patient with wounds of the extremity can be ambulated early but the involved limb must be kept elevated. "Too sick" is too inclusive a term to be used as a contraindication. Patients with partial anuria, those developing postoperative pneumonia, mild distention and postoperative fever have been benefited by early ambulation. The patients' attitude is improved, listlessness disappears, appetite improves and he becomes generally better. He usually objects to getting up the first day but thereafter, readily accepts the "new" method.

Hospitalization is going to be revolutionized by early ambulation when the system is developed properly. At present, in most instances, he is simply out of bed in the hospital and having someone serve him meals while he waits for the stitches to be taken out. After his locomotion is well established, he could be cared for at home if he were transported by ambulance and the arm of the hospital extended to his bedroom.

REFERENCES

1. HOWES, E. L.   Rate and Nature of Epithelization in Wounds with Loss of Substance, *Surg., Gynec. & Obst.*, 76:738-745, 1943.

1a. SPAIN, K. and LOEB, L.   A Quantitive Analysis of the Influence of the Size of Defect on Wound Healing, *J. Exper. Med.*, 23:107-122, [Jan. 1], 1916.

2. MARCHAND   *Der Process der Wundheilung*, F. Enke, Stuttgart, 1901.

3. HOWES, E. L., SOOY, J. and HARVEY, S. C.   The Healing of Wounds as Determined by their Tensile Strength, *J.A.M.A.*, 92:42-45, [Jan. 5], 1929.

4. HOWES, E. L., HARVEY, S. C. and HEWITT, C.   Rate of Fibroplasia and Differentiation in the Healing of Cutaneous Wounds, *Arch. Surg.*, 38:934-945, [May], 1939.

5. REID, M.   Some Considerations of the Problem of Wound Healing, *New England J. Med.*, 215:753-765, [Oct.], 1936.

6. CARREL, A. and DU NOUY, P. L.   Cicatrization of Wounds. The Latent Period, *J. Exper. Med.*, 34:339, [Oct.], 1921.

7. CARREL, A. and HARTMAN, A.   Cicatrization of Wounds. I. Relationship between Size of Wound and the Rate of Cicatrization, *J. Exper. Med.*, 24[No. 5]:429-450, 1916.

8. GLENN, F. Presented at the American Surgical Society, 1946. Paper to be printed.

9. LUND, C., GREEN, R., TAYLOR, L. and LEVENSON, S. Burns—A Collective Review, International Abstracts, *Surg., Gynec. & Obst.,* 82:443-478, [June], 1946.

10. THOMPSON, W. D., RAVDIN, I. S. and FRANK, I. Effect of Hypoproteinemia on Wound Disruption, *Arch. Surg.,* 36[No. 3]:500, 1938.

10a. THOMPSON, W. D., RAVDIN, I. S., RHOADS, J. E. and FRANK, I. L. Use of Lyophile Plasma in Correction of Hypoproteinemia and Prevention of Wound Disruption, *Arch. Surg.,* 36[No. 3]:509, 1938.

11. BIRD, C. E. and McKAY, E. M. The Healing of Wounds, *Surg., Gynec. & Obst.,* 54:872, 1932.

12. SANDBLOM, P. The Tensile Strength of Healing Wounds, *Acta chir. Scandinav.,* 90: [Supplement 89], Stockholm, 1944.

13. CARREL, A. Effet d'un Abces a Distance Sur la Cicatrisation d'une Plaie Aseptique, *Compt. rend. Soc. de biol.,* 90:333, 1924.

14. DU NOUY, P. L. Cicatrization of Wounds. III. The Relationship between Age of Patient, Area of Wound and Index of Cicatrization, *J. Exper. Med.,* 55:577, [April 1], 1932.

15. HOWES, E. L. A Renaissance of Suture Technique Needed, *Am. J. Surg.,* 47[No. 3]: 548-552, 1940.

16. HOWES, E. L. The Immediate Strength of the Sutured Wound, *Surgery,* 7[No. 1]: 24-31, 1940.

17. DuMORTIER, J. J. The Resistance of Healing Wounds to Infection, *Surg., Gynec. & Obst.,* 56:762, 1933.

18. BERMAN, J. K., HOUSER, A. and KURZ, W. Wound Immunity, *Surg., Gynec. & Obst.,* 77:205, 1943.

19. TAYLOR, F. N. Surgical Knots, *Ann. Surg.,* 107:458, 1938. See also *Surgery,* 5:498, 1939.

20. MELENEY, F. and HOWES, E. L. Disruption of Abdominal Wounds with Protrusion of Viscera, *Ann. Surg.,* 99:5-17, [Jan.], 1934.

21. SINGLETON, A. and BLOCKER, T. The Problem of Disruption of Abdominal Wounds and Postoperative Hernia, *J.A.M.A.,* 112[No. 2]:122-127, 1939.

22. FREDRICKA. Quoted after Walton Martin Surgical Infections, *Nelson's Surgery,* Vol. I, p. 367, Nelson and Son, New York.

23. STIMSON, B. Treatment of Compound Fractures in Italian Campaign, *Ann. Surg.,* 124:435, [Aug.], 1946.

24. COLLER, F. and WALK, W. C. The Delayed Closure of Contaminated Wounds, *Ann. Surg.,* 112:256-270, 1940.

25. EDWARDS, H. Revival of Early Wound Closure—Two Stage Operation, *Lancet,* 583, [May 12], 1945.

25a. STAMMERS, F. A. R. The Policy of Delay Suture, *Lancet,* 586, [May 12], 1945.

25b. CAPPER, W. M. Treatment of Battle Wounds—Two Stage Operation, *Idem.,* 587.

26. CHURCHILL, E. D. Surgical Management of Wounded in Mediterranean Theater at Time of Fall of Rome, *Ann. Surg.,* 120:268, [Sept.], 1944.

27. SARJEANT, T. R. and MORTON, W. A. Delayed Suture of Soft Tissue Wounds, *Lancet,* 332, [Sept. 2], 1944.

28. LEGROUX, M. R. Chimioprevention de L'infection bacteriere des Plaies de Guerre, *Memoires de L'acadamie de Chirurgie,* 66:415, 1940.

29. HOERR, STANLEY. A Study of the Effect of Prophylactic Oral Sulfadiazine upon Infection in Soft Tissue Wounds Closed Secondarily, *Surg., Gynec. & Obst.,* 82:586-597, [May], 1946.

30. MELENEY, F. The Study of the Prevention of Infection in Contaminated Accidental Wounds, Compound Fractures and Burns, *Ann. Surg.,* 118:171, [Aug.], 1943.

31. FLOREY, H. W. and CAIRNS, H. A Preliminary Report to the War Office and the Medical Research Council on Investigations Concerning the Use of Penicillin in War Wounds, *Brit. M. J.,* [Dec. 11], 1943.

32. HOWES, E. L.   Local Chemotherapy of Wounds; Tissue Toxicity of Certain Anti-
    bacterial Substances, *Surg., Gynec. & Obst.*, 83:1-14, [July], 1946.

33. HOWES, E. L.   Prevention of Wound Infection by the Injection of Nontoxic Anti-
    bacterial Substances, *Ann. Surg.*, 124[No. 2]:268, 1946.

34. SMELO, L. S.   The Problem of Wound Healing. I. Effect of Local Agents, *Arch. Surg.*,
    33:493-514, [Sept.], 1933.

35. POWERS, J. H.   The Abuse of Rest as a Therapeutic Measure in Surgery. Early Post-
    operative Activity and Rehabilitation, *J.A.M.A.*, 125:1079, 1944.

36. JORDAN, EDWIN P.   *Surgical Use of Soap. Medical Uses of Soap*, J. B. Lippincott Co.,
    Phila., 1946.

37. TRAUB, E., NEWHALL, C. and FULLER, J.   *Surg., Gynec. & Obst.*, 79:205, [Aug.], 1944.

2

HEMORRHAGE AND SHOCK

John D. Stewart, M.D.

HEMORRHAGE

Physiologic Considerations. In the healthy adult the volume of the blood comprises about 8 per cent of body weight. There is considerable variation in different individuals, however, and figures ranging from 6 to 10 per cent of body weight have been obtained by the dye method of measurement.[1,21] Though blood volume may vary considerably in a group of normal individuals, in the same person the value tends to remain constant in health. It would be a mistake to consider the volume of the blood as a separate and distinct physiological entity which may be quantitatively reduced by hemorrhage or restored by blood transfusion. The fluid of the interstitial areas, approximating 15 per cent of body weight, and the fluid of fixed tissue cells, which is equal to about 45 per cent of body weight, is held in physicochemical equilibrium with the plasma. Reduction in the volume of the blood results in movement of fluid out of the interstitial and intracellular reservoirs, a buffering mechanism of the utmost importance.[2]

Reserves of red cells are withdrawn from the spleen and bone marrow, and plasma protein flows into the plasma as a part of the life-saving reaction instantly activated by hemorrhage. There is evidence that such loans of red cells, plasma protein, water and electrolytes are temporary and their replacement is a characteristic feature of the recovery from hemorrhage. The efficiency of the compensatory mechanisms in hemorrhage will depend on the state of health and nutrition of the individual, which may be termed physiological reserve, as well as on the extent and rate at which bleeding takes place. Though a healthy young adult may successfully withstand a sudden loss of one-third or more of his blood, this is not true of many patients upon whom the surgeon must operate.

Evidences of compensation for hemorrhage can be detected early by changes in the blood. The red cell count falls as interstitial fluid flows into the capillary bed and the plasma protein concentration declines. The leukocyte and platelet counts increase and the coagulability of the blood quickens. In severe hemorrhage the plasma potassium concentration rises as intracellular water and electrolyte contribute to the volume of the circulating plasma.[3] Hyperventilation of the lungs may cause an early alkalosis from loss of carbon dioxide, but as decline in blood flow and in the oxygenation of tissues persist, lactic acid accumulates in the blood and acidosis is detectable.[4]

It has been conclusively shown that a major feature of the protective adjustments to blood loss is sympathico-adrenal activation. Animals which have been ergotaminized or surgically sympathectomized are far more sensitive to hemorrhage than are normal animals. From 30 to 45 per cent of the blood can be removed in normal animals in 3 or 4 successive bleedings before the compensatory vasoconstrictor mechanism fails to raise the blood pressure, whereas after the administration of ergotamine or after sympathectomy compensation may be lacking following loss of only 13 to 15 per cent of the total blood volume.[5] By arteriolar constriction in nonvital areas the blood flow is maintained in the myocardium and brain. The fall of capillary blood pressure in the skin and splanchnic areas secondary to arteriolar vasoconstriction favors the attraction of fluid into the capillary bed by the colloid osmotic force of the plasma proteins. The heart rate speeds up and the lowered output of each contraction is offset by a greater rate, thus tending to preserve the normal cardiac output per minute. It has recently been shown that reflex vasodilatation in the deeper tissues of the body may be an early and transitory phenomenon in hemorrhage and may account for the sudden faintness.[6] The glucose concentration in the blood rises and provides a ready source of energy for critically mobilized vital organs.

The importance of arteriolar vasoconstriction and ischemic shunts in hemorrhage may be further illustrated by considering the effects of overheating the individual suffering from severe hemorrhage. If the limited amount of blood in circulation is diverted to the skin systolic blood pressure may fail immediately. Under these circumstances the physiological mechanism of heat control is placed in competition with the homeostatic device for maintaining oxygenation in vital tissues, and disaster may follow. This fact has obvious clinical implications.

An impressive feature in the bodily response to massive hemorrhage is increase in rate and depth of respiration. This may be so marked as to warrant the use of the descriptive term, air-hunger. Such hyperpnea is evidence of break in compensation, for it is due to anoxic stimulation of the respiratory centers in the medulla. It is therefore an unfavorable clinical sign, though quickened and deepened respiration in itself tends to speed up return flow of venous blood to the heart.

Protective physiological reactions to hemorrhage may be local, i.e. at the site of bleeding, as well as general. When a vessel is lacerated it contracts and the narrowed lumen allows less blood to escape. In the case of an artery which has been severed, contraction and shortening of the medial layer take place and the intima tends to curl up and plug the opening. A complete transection of the artery is more favorable to the success of these processes than is a tangential or axial wound, a point the surgeon should keep in mind. At the wound, clotting is facilitated by the liberation of tissue juice, particularly in lung or muscle. Rest may be afforded the wound by reflex muscle spasm and cessation of motion. The formation and fixation of a clot in the wounded artery is further promoted by reduction in systemic systolic and diastolic blood pressure.

After a severe nonfatal hemorrhage blood regeneration immediately becomes accelerated and the process may persist for weeks. Though blood volume may be brought back to normal within a few hours, deficits of red cells, hemoglobin and plasma protein require more time for correction. Increase in nucleated red cells is a characteristic finding during recovery from hemorrhage. Normocytic, normochromic anemia may be present, but in many clinical cases the presence of iron deficiency during recovery is evidenced by a hypochromic, microcytic type of anemia.

The critical danger in hemorrhage is tissue anoxia, particularly of brain and myocardium. Various degrees of failure in the functions of the central nervous system may be observed with varying degrees of hemorrhagic anoxia. There may be psychic disturbances, with disorientation and hallucinations, and at times maniacal excitement. Patients suffering from severe hemorrhage sometimes must be physically restrained, for they may be irresponsible and even show suicidal tendencies. Partial recovery from anoxia of the central nervous system may be manifested by temporary deafness or blindness, or by spasticity of muscle groups and irregularities in gait. Another complication of hemorrhage of considerable clinical importance, especially in the elderly and arteriosclerotic patient, is intravascular thrombosis in essential arteries of the brain, the heart or the kidneys. During the interval of hypotension and sluggish blood flow, clots may form at arteriosclerotic plaques in the intima and anuria, coronary occlusion or cerebral thrombosis may be evident a few hours or a few days afterwards.

Though much remains to be learned about the process of coagulation, considerable additions to knowledge of the subject have been made in recent years. Clotting is based on a series of enzymatic reactions which may be interrupted in a variety of ways. Prothrombin, one of the globulin fractions of the plasma formed in the liver, is converted by thromboplastin in the presence of ionized calcium to thrombin. Thrombin in turn rapidly converts fibrinogen into fibrin which contracts into a firm clot. The speed of these reactions is influenced by temperature and by concentration of the reacting substances. Thus clotting is delayed by cooling and is speeded by application of hot packs to the wound. Abnormal reduction in prothrombin concentration, as in obstructive jaundice, or lowering of the ionized calcium in vitro by addition of sodium citrate or potassium oxalate to blood retards coagulation. Increase in thromboplastin favors clotting, a point utilized surgically when muscle fragments are inserted in the bleeding wound, or when a dry gauze pack is applied. Blood drawn from a vein with a minimum of trauma and placed in a paraffinized sealed container clots only slowly owing to the fact that the platelets break down and free thromboplastin at greatly reduced rates under the circumstances.

Prothrombin deficiency is an important surgical problem and recent contributions from the laboratory have made it possible to prevent fatal postoperative hemorrhage in a hitherto baffling group of cases. In obstructive jaundice the bile salts essential for the proper absorption of vitamin K (and other fat-soluble vitamins) no longer reach the intestinal tract. Lacking vitamin K the liver no longer forms prothrombin in adequate amounts and the concentration in the plasma may fall to 10 per cent or less of normal. Fatal hemorrhage may occur unless vitamin K is supplied the liver by parenteral injection, by administration orally in water-soluble form, or by administration of bile salts and vitamin K orally. In external biliary fistula with prolonged diversion of the bile severe hypoprothrombinemia may develop for similar reasons. In advanced parenchymal disease of the liver, as in cirrhosis or acute yellow atrophy, deficiency of prothrombin may be based on impairment of liver function rather than failure in supply of materials. Hemorrhage and operative trauma lead to a transitory hypoprothrombinemia, and it has been shown that the prothrombin content of banked blood declines to a significant extent.

Further illustration of the clinical importance of the facts presently known about clotting can be seen in the surgical use of the anti-coagulants, heparin and dicumarol. Heparin, which is a carbohydrate substance, probably a compound of glycuronic acid, when added to blood in vitro or injected intravenously blocks the formation of thrombin. Its action in vivo is brief, however, and its effective use in combatting intravascular clotting requires that it be given by constant intravenous drip. Dicumarol, which is 3,3'-methylenebis-4-hydroxycoumarin, also prevents clotting in vivo, but this is accomplished through the action of the drug on the liver by which prothrombin production is inhibited. The drug acts more slowly and over a longer period than does heparin, and it can be taken by mouth. Its established effects are combatted by giving large doses of vitamin K parenterally (150 to 200 mg.) and by blood transfusion. Although such technique cannot be uniformly recommended it is possible to perform surgical operations on patients whose clotting time has been prolonged by heparin or dicumarol without undue bleeding in the wound. Apparently sufficient amounts of thromboplastin are liberated in the operative incision to nullify locally the effects of these anticoagulants. In this connection clinical experience has demonstrated that patients with hemophilia and thrombocytopenic purpura may be safely operated upon with the help of blood transfusions. Presumably the liberation of thromboplastin at the wound site in these diseases is also an effective aid to hemostasis.

With the development of a technique for measuring the amount of blood lost at operation, surgeons have shown that unexpectedly large amounts of blood may be lost during common surgical procedures. From 1 to 2 liters of blood may be lost during such operations as combined abdomino-perineal excision of the rectum, radical mastectomy, pulmonary lobectomy or pneumonectomy, craniotomy for brain tumors, prostatectomy or plastic procedures on the biliary ducts.[7-10] In a recent study average blood losses were noted for several standard surgical operations in good hands as follows: thyroidectomy —373 cc.; radical mastectomy—808 cc.; combined abdomino-perineal excision of the rectum—410 cc.; operations on the biliary tract—594 cc.; and gastric resection—599 cc.[10] It was pointed out that: (1) the amount of bleeding at operation is almost always greater than the surgeon suspects; and (2) replacement is most effective when whole blood is given as the loss occurs. Every surgeon undertaking major surgical procedures should familiarize himself with figures for blood loss during various operations, either as obtained from the literature, or, better still, from measurements on a series of his own cases.

In traumatic shock due to penetrating, lacerating or crushing wounds, large amounts of blood may be lost either by external hemorrhage, or as concealed bleeding into body cavities or tissue planes.[11,12] There is reason to believe that in this variety of traumatic shock hemorrhage is the most important etiological factor and blood replacement the essential therapy. This subject is dealt with more fully later in this chapter. In the severe hemoptysis of pulmonary tuberculosis, chronic bronchiectasis, lung abscess or occasionally in bronchogenic carcinoma several liters of blood may be lost. Massive hemorrhage into the gastrointestinal tract, as in peptic ulcer, gastric or cecal carcinoma, Meckel's diverticulitis, chronic gastritis or esophageal varices is a common clinical entity, the management of which often taxes diagnostic acumen and surgical skill. With hemorrhage into the upper gastrointestinal tract azotemia often occurs and the finding may be of some diagnostic value. The elevation of blood urea and nonprotein nitrogen is moderate (50 to 80 mg. per cent) and is probably due to such factors as reduced blood flow to the kidney, dehydration, and increased protein catabolism as blood is digested and absorbed from the alimentary canal.

Clinical Manifestations. The clinical picture of hemorrhage, which is best interpreted in the light of the physiological adjustments discussed above, is dependent on the amount and the rapidity of the bleeding and on the physiological reserve of the patient. In a sudden, severe, nonlethal hemorrhage there is a fall in systolic and diastolic blood pressure and narrowing of pulse pressure; there is usually a quickening of the pulse and the skin becomes cold, clammy and blanched. Thirst is present but water is unsatisfying and nausea or vomiting may balk efforts at drinking. Restlessness, excitement, delirium or coma may evidence anoxia of the brain. Respiration is faster and deeper and the volume of urine secreted is low. It is important to remember that this picture may be modified or masked by anesthesia. The break in compensation for gradual and uncorrected bleeding during surgical operation under general anesthesia may come suddenly, with rapid failure of blood pressure and speeding up of the heart rate. Likewise in traumatic shock the signs of hemorrhage may be obscured by associated conditions such as trauma to chest or abdomen or spreading infection or contamination of the peritoneal cavity. Repeated measurements of red cell count or hematocrit, or even determination of blood volume may be practical under such circumstances. As a rule, however, careful appraisement of the clinical signs and symptoms and search for signs of hemoperitoneum, hemothorax or extravasation into extremities will bring the diagnosis to light.

Treatment. Any discussion of the treatment of hemorrhage should be preceded by a consideration of prevention of hemorrhage. The proper use of the tourniquet and compression bandages as first-aid measures should be common knowledge. During surgical operations hemostasis is essential for clear exposure of the field, careful dissection, and accurate suturing. To a considerable extent the skill of a surgeon may be measured by his ability to control bleeding, for knowledge of anatomy, meticulousness and patience in technic, experience and directness of purpose are required. These factors cannot be overemphasized in the training of young surgeons.

In the local control of bleeding the actual and electric cauteries are sometimes of value. The high frequency current may be used for cutting or for coagulating, but the method is satisfactory only for smaller vessels. Secondary hemorrhage may result when the burn slough or coagulum separates. In operations such as thoracoplasty or radical mastectomy where many ties must otherwise be placed coagulation of smaller vessels by the diathermy apparatus saves much time. As a by-product in the preparation of albumin from human plasma, thrombin has recently come into use. As a 2 per cent aqueous solution, sterile and freshly prepared, this affords the surgeon a powerful coagulant, to be used as a spray, or applied to the bleeding point on pledgets of fibrin foam, absorbable cellulose or ordinary cotton or gauze.[13] Recently gelatin films have been tested clinically and experimentally with considerable success in controlling bleeding from large vessels and from the liver. In operations on the extremities, particularly on the hand, it is often essential to render the field bloodless by application of a tourniquet proximally at pressures of 200 to 250 mm. Hg. Ligation of the tributary artery is useful as a prophylactic measure in dealing with sloughing wounds or as a planned part of operation in certain vascular areas, especially in the case of the external carotid or its branches. Before resection of the jaw or tongue or, to forestall bleeding in malignant lesions in this region, ligation of the external carotid is a simple and effective procedure.

In the restoration of blood volume depleted by hemorrhage the urgent requirement is blood transfusion, and as mentioned above replacement ideally should keep apace with hemorrhage. The time factor is of the utmost importance as is the administration of a large enough volume of blood. From 1 to 3 liters will be required in many surgical patients, and in a critical situation transfusion through two veins simultaneously may be necessary to save the patient's life. Very generally nowadays citrated blood, containing 0.25 per cent sodium citrate, is used rather than unmodified blood. Unmodified blood must be drawn quickly into paraffinized containers and injected immediately into the recipient using surgical precautions, hence the method is inconvenient. Type-specific blood should be used preferably and tests for compatibility should be properly performed in each instance as a preliminary. If type O blood from the so-called "universal donor" is used it should have an agglutinin titer not greater than 1:16. In some instances autotransfusion is valuable. Following massive hemorrhage into the pleural or peritoneal cavities or during operations on the brain the blood may be aspirated under aseptic precautions, strained and re-infused into a vein. The theoretical objection that blood may become partially defibrinated and hemolyzed and consequently harmful under these conditions is not borne out by extensive clinical experience.

The plasma volume may be restored after hemorrhage by the infusion of plasma, albumin, gelatin and other colloid solutions. Though such solutions may be used as a temporary substitute when blood is not immediately available they do not take the place of blood transfusion. The critical danger in hemorrhage is tissue anoxia from reduced blood flow and loss of hemoglobin. Restoring the circulating blood volume at the cost of further dilution of hemoglobin values is misguided therapy, though it is conceivable that improvement in cardiac output under the circumstances may offset temporarily the reduction in oxygen capacity of the blood.

Oxygen therapy is valuable in the treatment of the state of hemorrhage. The basis for this is the increase in the amount of oxygen dissolved in the plasma. Oxygen in physical solution resulting from breathing 100 per cent oxygen is more freely diffusible into the tissues than is oxygen in combination with hemoglobin in red cells. Other aspects of the early treatment of hemorrhage include raising the foot of the bed, avoidance of either chilling or over-heating, promoting rest by local splinting and general sedation, and administration of 5 per cent glucose solution and 0.9 per cent sodium chloride solution. There is no evidence that vasoconstricting drugs such as ephedrine or adrenalin have any place in the treatment of hemorrhage.

In promoting recovery from the state of hemorrhage the general nutritional as well as the hematopoietic requirements of the patient must be considered. Iron should be given in dosage of 12 to 16 grains daily orally or parenterally. A high protein diet rich in the essential amino acids has been shown to speed regeneration of plasma protein and red cells, and liver, beef, eggs, milk and cheese are particularly good sources. A protein intake of 1 to 2 gm. per kilogram of body weight daily is desirable. Amino acid infusions are useful in supplying large amounts of biologically essential constituents of protein without disturbing blood volume or water distribution in the body. One liter of 5 per cent amino acids solution containing also 5 per cent glucose can be administered intravenously twice a day with good results. Adequate intake of calories (2500 to 3500 per day) and vitamins likewise are an essential consideration in the patient's dietary. Further blood transfusions are often indicated during the process of recovery from hemorrhage and the red cell count, hematocrit and plasma protein concentration should be determined every two or three days until the patient is well along in recovery.

SHOCK

Physiologic Considerations. In the state of traumatic shock interdependent, complicated and as yet imperfectly understood physiological reactions are brought into play. These reactions produce a characteristic clinical picture, but one which is nonspecific as to etiology. Despite the gaps in our knowledge of the fundamental mechanisms of traumatic shock certain principles stand out in its clinical management and may be listed as follows:

1. The diagnosis of the state of traumatic shock is readily made on clinical grounds.

2. The primary cause or causes should be recognized and treated as well as the physiological disturbances.

3. Reduction in cardiac output and effective circulating blood volume and tissue anoxia are the characteristic physiological disturbances, which urgently require correction.

4. The outcome is dependent on the severity of the trauma, the presence or absence of complications, the physiological reserve of the patient, and the rapidity with which proper treatment is carried out.

In the state of secondary shock, as distinct from neurogenic, transitory hypotension, there are present reduction in cardiac output and blood flow, fall in blood pressure, and peripheral evidence of arteriolar constriction. There is usually lowered basal metabolic rate and body temperature, rapid pulse, shallow respiration and sweating. Secondary shock may be seen in medical as well as surgical conditions and the syndrome may be classified on an etiological basis as follows:

1. Loss of propulsive force: This is cardiogenic shock as typified by coronary occlusion or severe cardiac arrhythmias.

2. Dilatation of the vascular bed: As seen in overwhelming invasive infections or in transection of the spinal cord loss of tonus in blood vessels may be the primary disturbance, followed by reduced venous return and cardiac output.

3. Mechanical interference with blood flow: Typical illustrations are volvulus of the intestine, cardiac tamponade, pulmonary embolism, portal or mesenteric thrombosis.

4. Primary reduction in blood volume: In this category come hemorrhagic shock in which blood volume has been depleted by loss of whole blood, burns or war-gas poisoning of skin or respiratory tract in which plasma has transuded through directly damaged capillaries, and dehydration.

The classification of secondary shock in this manner on the basis of principal causes is of value in that it emphasizes the varied nature of forces which produce a similar clinical picture. It follows that treatment will likewise vary. It is probably a fair assumption that reduction in cardiac output is present in secondary shock due to any of these causes, and that lowered blood volume is present in most instances. However, blood transfusion may be dangerous rather than beneficial in cardiogenic shock or pulmonary embolism, and though blood transfusion is helpful in intestinal strangulation, it is equally important to correct the mechanical defect by early surgical operation. In the state of secondary shock due to fulminating infections it is probably less important to treat the physiological disturbances than to treat the infection itself.[14] In the state of secondary shock due to losses from the circulation successful therapy must be based on knowledge of the nature of the losses. In hemorrhage whole blood is needed, in burns plasma, in dehydration water and sodium chloride. In many surgical patients the primary causes are present in combination and their recognition and treatment require all the diagnostic aids available in a well-equipped hospital. For example, in appendiceal perforation and peritonitis partial obstruction of the small intestine frequently supervenes. In this case loss of water and electro-lytes into the gastrointestinal tract produces dehydration, which intensifies the oligemia consequent on dilatation of the splanchnic capillary bed and transudation of fluid into the inflamed peritoneal areas.

In addition to primary shock-producing factors it is proper to speak of secondary or contributory causes. Any circumstances which tax further the homeostatic devices of the body or interfere with critical adjustments already in operation are to be considered in this connection. Environmental cold or heat, anoxia from crippling of the respiratory apparatus or from poor anes-thesia, fatigue, malnutrition or water-lack, severe pain or fright diminish the power of the body to withstand major trauma. Due consideration must be given to these contributory damaging forces in the treatment of shock, as noted below.

The term traumatic shock is used to denote the variety of secondary shock which is produced by external violence and should be applied to shock re-sulting from lacerating, penetrating, perforating or crushing wounds, burns and trauma of surgical operation. It is the type of shock with which the surgeon is particularly concerned and with which most of the subsequent discussion deals. From the foregoing remarks it will be seen that shock may be classified as (1) primary shock, which is neurogenic, transitory and based on vasodilatation, and (2) secondary or delayed shock. Traumatic shock is a variety of secondary shock, and is characterized by reduction in blood vol-ume, fall in cardiac output and venous return, lowering of the blood pres-sure, vasoconstriction and vascular shunts. Tissue anoxia supervenes first in less vital areas such as the skin, mucous membranes and splanchnic bed, but the protection afforded the heart and brain by compensatory mechanisms may be only temporary unless proper treatment is instituted. If the anoxia of the uncorrected condition persists serious and irreversible changes in me-tabolism occur and the state of "irreversible shock" appears as a prelude to death.

Clinical Manifestations. The diagnosis of traumatic shock is not difficult, though it is important to remember that one or more features of the typical clinical picture may be lacking. There is the evidence of trauma, there is reduction in systolic, diastolic and pulse pressure. The pulse is rapid and feeble, the skin is cold, moist and grayish, the respiration is shallow. The rectal temperature may be reduced, the patient is often restless, thirsty and nauseated. The mind is usually clear, though apathetic, and pain is not a prominent part of the syndrome. There is variation in this picture and in some cases the systolic pressure may be normal or even elevated temporarily, though the pulse be rapid.[11] Nevertheless reduction in systolic blood pres-sure remains as one of the most reliable clinical indices of the patient's condition. One of the striking aspects of the clinical picture is the instability of the precarious adjustments attained by the body, and the rapidity with which the patient's condition improves under treatment or grows worse. As previously pointed out anesthesia may alter the picture of shock, and in some cases of penetrating wounds the clinician may be caught off guard by concealed hemorrhage into body cavities, by tension pneumothorax or cardiac tamponade.

It should be the aim of the surgeon to recognize the presence of shock-producing factors wherever possible and by treating these to forestall clinical shock. The location and nature of the wound, the visible evidence of hemorrhage, the extent of the expected operative manipulation afford clues in this connection. Unfortunately no ready, practicable laboratory tests are available to measure the progress of the patient's condition toward the state of traumatic shock, and hence clinical judgment and experience must be relied upon in the management of the case.

In the presence of declared shock of traumatic origin certain laboratory findings are typical. The blood volume is found to be reduced to 40 or 50 per cent of normal, and the extent of depletion of blood volume is paralleled by the clinical signs of shock.[15] In the traumatic shock of penetrating, perforating, lacerating or crushing wounds oligemia with normal or reduced hematocrit is the rule, and this suggests that hemorrhage is the major underlying process. In the oligemia of severe burns there is rise of hematocrit, hemoconcentration and rise in viscosity of the blood. In traumatic shock the CO_2 content and chloride of the plasma fall, lactic acid, blood sugar, blood urea and amino acids rise. Leukocytosis is the rule and the red cell count may be either normal, increased or reduced depending on the cause of the oligemia. Basal metabolic rate is low and the secretion of urine is slowed. The glycogen content of the liver declines.

Considerable investigative energy has recently been devoted to the elucidation of the changes in intermediary metabolism in traumatic shock, particularly in relation to the state of irreversibility. There is some evidence at hand indicating that prolonged anoxia sets up a progressive decline in function of the liver, and that the process when started is irremediable. The factor of time in relation to therapy is again emphasized by this point.[16]

Treatment. The patient in traumatic shock should not be overheated. The time-honored custom of surrounding the patient with hot water bottles and covering him with blankets, or of warming him on a steam-heated table is not only useless but dangerous. An environmental temperature of 75° F. with the patient lightly covered is satisfactory. Constricting, damp, dirty or blood-soaked clothing should be entirely removed and with the minimum of manipulation. If the wound is on the extremity a tourniquet should be applied proximally, or if one is already present it should be loosened at half-hourly intervals and reapplied. The presence of a tourniquet which prevents arterial inflow into mangled tissues will facilitate the repair of oligemia by preventing further losses of blood during transfusion therapy. Where an extremity is hopelessly mangled and must be amputated the tourniquet may be left in place until the time of operation.

In the treatment of traumatic shock, and indeed in its prevention, chief interest centers on effective circulating blood volume.[17] Replacement therapy requires knowledge of the manner of depletion of the blood, as based on clinical experience and measurements of red cell count, hemoglobin and hematocrit. In traumatic shock due to crushing wounds, missile wounds, lacerating wounds, compound fractures or frank hemorrhage the blood picture is that of hemorrhagic oligemia. Blood volume is reduced by from 40 to 60 per cent, the red cell hematocrit is normal or low. The administration of whole blood by transfusion is an urgent requirement and takes priority over any other surgical measures except control of hemorrhage. It is sometimes desirable to use two veins at once and give blood at a rapid rate. It is a fallacious and dangerous practice to withhold blood on the thesis that elevation of the blood pressure to a normal value may result in further hemorrhage. It would be as sensible to treat the vomiting of intestinal obstruction by refraining from administering fluids parenterally to the patient. A common mistake in the management of wound shock is failure to appreciate the amount of blood or plasma required in replacement therapy. Experiences with the high-explosive casualties of World War II showed that from 1.5 to 4.0 liters of blood were needed to restore normal blood volume, and that even so deficits of hemoglobin and plasma protein were usually evident during the early stages of convalescence. Undoubtedly the same principle holds for traumatic shock of civilian practice. Whenever possible type-specific blood which has been tested directly for compatibility should be used. If type O blood must be used its agglutinin titer should have been demonstrated to be within safe limits (less than 1 to 16).

In wound shock (not due to burns) human plasma, preserved or reconstituted, and human albumin may be used to bolster a depleted plasma volume, but this is recommended only as a temporary emergency measure. The critical need is improvement in oxygenation of the tissues, and whole blood best meets the physiological requirements. From 1 to 3 liters of plasma, or a smaller volume of albumin solution (which is osmotically more active than plasma) will produce an increase in plasma volume at the cost of further reduction in hemoglobin concentration, and though blood pressure may be improved a dangerous and false sense of security is created. Under these circumstances in the early experience of World War II sudden death was not infrequently encountered in patients who seemed to be improving.

In the traumatic shock of severe burns the replacement needs are for plasma or albumin. Here plasma, and particularly the albumin component of the plasma proteins, has transuded through directly damaged capillaries. The hemoglobin, hematocrit, red cell count and viscosity have risen to a dangerous degree. Blood pattern as well as blood volume are corrected by the rapid administration of plasma. Large amounts, 1 to 3 liters, may be needed within the first 24 hours. Either the hematocrit or the gross extent of the burn may be used to calculate roughly, plasma requirements.[18] Replacement therapy should be controlled preferably, however, by measurement of hematocrit and red cell count every three or four hours during the first day. Later in convalescence after severe burns anemia is commonly present, but this is not a consideration in the immediate management of burn shock. Other colloid containing solutions, particularly those containing acacia, gelatin or even animal plasma, have been tested for therapeutic value, but their usefulness has not been established. Amino acids solutions, such as digests of casein or lactalbumin or synthetic mixtures have a place in the later management of traumatic shock. Regeneration of plasma and tissue protein are facilitated and nitrogen deficits and tissue wastage are reduced.

The circumstances of traumatic shock are apt to be dehydrating, whether as an accompaniment of wound shock or operative trauma. Consequently there is need for the administration of 0.9 per cent sodium chloride solution alternating with 5 per cent glucose solution after the primary oligemia has been relieved. One of the complications of wound shock treated by the proper transfusion of adequate amounts of blood is oliguria or anuria, and in a considerable proportion of such cases the complication is fatal. The renal lesion is predominantly tubular, but the cause is ill-understood. The importance of meeting the renal water and salt requirements is accentuated by this possible development early in the recovery period.

Oxygen therapy as provided by the administration of 100 per cent oxygen is theoretically beneficial in traumatic shock, and it has the support of clinical experience. Arterial oxygen unsaturation is not a feature of traumatic shock uncomplicated by thoracic lesions, but if the amount of oxygen in physical solution in the plasma can be increased, improvement in the supply readily available to the tissues follows. An oxygen tent, face mask or intranasal catheter may be used. From time to time alkali therapy has been proposed in the management of traumatic shock and it still has its enthusiastic advocates. As previously noted a mild acidosis can often be demonstrated which is presumably based on accumulation of organic acids in the plasma. It has not been satisfactorily shown, however, that alkali therapy through the administration of 2.5 per cent or 5 per cent sodium bicarbonate solution or sodium lactate solution is necessary or desirable. Neither has it been shown that alkalinization of the urine lessens the likelihood of renal damage.

There is small place for the use of vasoconstricting drugs in traumatic shock, for except in the unusual case of traumatic shock due to a wound which transects the cord arteriolar constriction is a constant and fundamental physiological reaction. Likewise, stimulants such as caffeine are of no particular value. A variety of drugs have been tested for value in traumatic shock with doubtful or negative results.[19] Morphine has the support of extensive clinical usage, and if the patient is restless, apprehensive or in pain its usefulness is unquestionable. It should not be given in doses large enough to depress the centers of the medulla. A point brought out in war experience was the importance of administering the morphine intravenously rather than subcutaneously or intramuscularly in severe traumatic shock.[20] Owing to sluggish blood flow absorption may be delayed, and the surgeon may be misled into giving a second quarter-grain dose. As circulation improves with blood replacement therapy an overwhelming amount of the drug may be absorbed in a short period of time. Fatalities have probably resulted from morphine poisoning in this manner.

Two extremely important questions confronting the surgeon treating patients with traumatic shock due to crushing, lacerating, penetrating or perforating wounds are: (1) how soon to go ahead with definitive surgical operation; and (2) what anesthetic to use? As regards the first question, blood replacement to the point of complete relief of oligemia and tissue anoxia is obviously the ideal before surgical operation is started. However, hemorrhage from internal wounds may continue, peritoneal contamination may progress, and further delay in definitive surgical operation, comes to be dangerous. A nice problem in surgical judgment results. No general rules can be offered, for the circumstances are endlessly variable. However, if systolic blood pressure has risen to above 80 and if the patient has received at least a liter of blood it is probably wise to begin operation. The administration of blood and oxygen should be vigorously continued during the operation, and afterward if necessary. Should the patient's blood pressure not rise to above 80 despite 1 or 2 liters of blood a presumption of continued bleeding is raised and hemostasis through operation becomes an obvious necessity.

The anesthesia chosen in traumatic shock should be that which allows the necessary operation to be done with the least harm to the patient. It should provide muscular relaxation, exposure of the field and control of respiration where these factors are essential, with the least anoxia and depression of the medullary centers. Cardiac depression, vasodilatation and inhibition of protective vascular shunts are undesirable. The anesthetic should not cause further damage to parenchymatous organs like the liver. In some instances procaine infiltration or field-block will serve, but often a general anesthetic is required. Spinal anesthesia has serious draw-backs. In general terms ether anesthesia as administered in a closed system with unobstructed air-way and with a high oxygen admixture is the method of choice. The short-acting barbiturates have been used to produce anesthesia intravenously in a large number of cases during the war, but the convenience and ease of the method are its outstanding advantages, rather than its specific applicability to the surgery of traumatic shock.

REFERENCES

1. GIBSON, J., 2ND and EVANS, W. A., JR. The Relation of Plasma and Total Blood Volume to Venous Pressure, Blood Velocity Rate, Physical Measurements, Age and Sex in 90 Normal Humans, *J. Clin. Investigation,* 16:317, [May], 1937.
2. ADOLPH, E. F., GERBASI, M. J. and LEPORE, M. J. The Rate of Entrance of Fluid into the Blood in Hemorrhage, *Am. J. Physiol.,* 104:502, 1933.
3. STEWART, J. D. and ROURKE, G. M. Intracellular Fluid Loss in Hemorrhage, *J. Clin. Investigation,* 15:697, 1936.
4. BENNETT, M. A. Changes in Acid-base Equilibrium of the Blood Caused by Hemorrhage, *J. Biol. Chem.,* 69:675, 1926.
5. SCHLOSSBERG, T. and MACSAWYER, M. E. Studies of Homeostasis in Normal, Sympathectomized and Ergotaminized Animals (The Effect of Hemorrhage), *Am. J. Physiol.,* 104:195, 1933.
6. BARCROFT, H., MCMICHAEL, J., EDHOLM, O. G. and SHARPEY-SCHAFER, E. P. Posthemorrhagic Fainting, *Lancet,* [April 15], 1944.
7. BUDDINGTON, W. T. and TAYLOR, G. W. The Loss of Blood in Certain Standard Operations for Malignant Disease, *New England J. Med.,* 218:285, 1938.

8. WHITE, J. C., WHITELAW, G. P., SWEET, W. H. and HURWITT, E. S.   Blood Loss in Neurosurgical Operations, *Ann. Surg.*, 107:287, 1938.

9. COLLER, F. A., CROOK, C. E. and IOB, V.   Blood Loss in Surgical Operations, *J.A.M.A.*, 126:1, 1944.

10. CROOK, C. E., IOB, V. and COLLER, F. A.   Correction of Blood Loss During Surgical Operations, *Surg., Gynec. & Obst.*, 82:417, [April], 1946.

11. STEWART, J. D. and WARNER, F.   Observations on the Severely Wounded in Forward Field Hospitals; with Special Reference to Wound Shock, *Ann. Surg.*, 122:129, 1945.

12. EMERSON, C. P., JR. and EBERT, R. V.   A Study of Shock in Battle Casualties. Measurement of the Blood Volume Changes Occurring in Response to Therapy, *Ann. Surg.*, 122:745, 1945.

13. INGRAHAM, F. D. and BAILEY, O. T.   Clinical Use of Products of Human Plasma Fractionation. III. The use of Products of Fibrinogen and Thrombin in Surgery, *J.A.M.A.*, 126:680, 1944.

14. STEWART, J. D.   Postoperative Shock Due to Hemolytic Streptococcus Wound Infection, *Surgery*, 9:204, 1941.

15. NOBLE, R. P. and GREGERSON, M. I.   Blood Volume in Clinical Shock. II. The Extent and Cause of Blood Volume Reduction in Traumatic, Hemorrhagic and Burn Shock, *J. Clin. Investigation*, 25:172, 1946.

16. FRANK, H. A., SELIGMAN, A. M. and FINE, J.   The Prevention of Irreversibility in Hemorrhagic Shock by Viviperfusion of the Liver, *J. Clin. Investigation*, 25:22, 1946.

17. PHEMISTER, D. B.   The Mechanism and Management of Surgical Shock, *J.A.M.A.*, 127:1109, 1945.

18. HARKINS, H. N., LAM, C. R. and ROMENCE, H.   Plasma Therapy in Severe Burns, *Surg., Gynec & Obst.*, 75:410, 1942.

19. FRANK, H. A., SELIGMAN, A. M. and FINE, J.   Treatment of Hemorrhagic Shock Irreversible to Replacement of Blood Volume Deficiency, *J. Clin. Investigation*, 24:435, 1945.

20. BEECHER, H. K.   Pain in Men Wounded in Battle, *Ann. Surg.*, 123:96, 1946.

21. STEWART, J. D. and ROURKE, G. M.   On the Measurement of Extracellular Fluid Volume with Thiocyanate and Body Fluid Analyses in 33 Normal Individuals, *J. Lab. & Clin. Med.*, 26:1383, 1941.

3

BURNS

CHARLES C. LUND, M.D. AND STANLEY M. LEVENSON, M.D.

INTRODUCTION

The high incidence of thermal injuries in the recent war has stimulated great interest in the problem of burns. Slowly but definitely, certain general principles have emerged, the understanding and appreciation of which are leading to a more rational handling of the burned patient. It is clearly recognized that for optimum care of the patient with burns of important size, the therapy of the local and general disturbances must be continually integrated from the time of injury to the end of convalescence. In this chapter the practical care of patients with extensive burns will be outlined without considering in detail the scientific background for these points. This latter aspect has been fully considered elsewhere.[1,2]

All patients with extensive burns must be cared for in a hospital, and preferably in a hospital which has made special provision for their care. All hospitals which receive an appreciable number of accident cases should be organized for the treatment of burns and large hospitals in industrial cities should have a burn service with definite wards and operating rooms set aside for these patients. The usefulness of this type of preparedness in the time of disaster was well demonstrated at the time of the Cocoanut Grove disaster in Boston in November 1942,[3] and at the circus fire in Hartford in 1944,[4] while its usefulness in day-to-day practice has been demonstrated for years at the Henry Ford Hospital in Detroit, and the Montreal General Hospital in Montreal. In addition to physicians trained in the handling of burn patients, there should be a sufficient number of experienced nurses to "special" severely burned patients, since without adequate nursing care the fatality rate is definitely increased and the morbidity markedly prolonged.

IMMEDIATE STUDY AND TREATMENT

Upon arrival at the hospital the patient should be taken immediately to the appropriate emergency room, placed on a sterile sheet, and, the clothing having been removed by adequately gowned and masked attendants, covered with another sterile sheet and blanket. The area and depth of burn should be carefully estimated and recorded.

At the present time the most widely used classification of burns according to depth is as follows: first degree, simple erythema; second degree, partial

51

destruction of skin, but without destruction of all the deep epithelial cells; and third degree, destruction of the full thickness of the skin (Fig. 21).

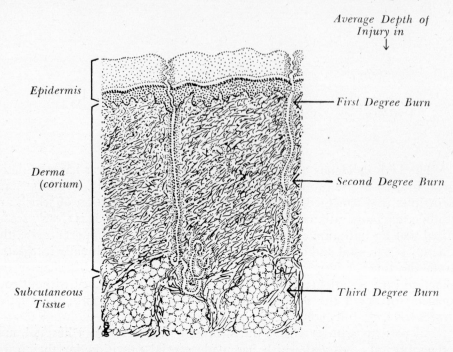

FIG. 21. Diagram of a cross section of normal skin showing the layers injured in the various types of burns. (From Cole, Warren H. and Elman, Robert, *Textbook of General Surgery.* Fifth edition, D. Appleton-Century Co., New York.)

At the occurrence of the burn it is frequently not possible to estimate correctly the depth of the injury. Many small blebs, some broken and some intact, with an external ooze of plasma, visible pink corium, and minimal subcutaneous edema indicate a second degree burn. A dry, dead white, brown or charred appearance with beginning subcutaneous edema indicates a third degree burn. The appearance of other burns is intermediate between those described and such burns cannot be classified until epithelization or granulation have become evident. Dingwall [5] and Patey and Scarff [6] have attempted to solve this difficult problem. The former has observed burns under ultraviolet light after intravenous sodium fluorescein injections, and the latter have studied serial microscopic sections of burns and the naked eye appearance after the application of Van Gieson's stain. Both these methods are promising but neither has been adequately evaluated.

Diagrams for charting areas burned are here reproduced from an article by Lund and Browder,[7] Fig. 22a and b).

In addition to estimating the area and depth of burn, note should be made of any possible respiratory damage or carbon monoxide poisoning. If the patient is conscious and in pain, but not intoxicated nor in shock, nor suffering from carbon monoxide exposure, nor respiratory tract damage,

BOSTON CITY HOSPITAL

Name..Age............Number..................

Burn Record. Ages 7½ to Adult. Date of Observation..

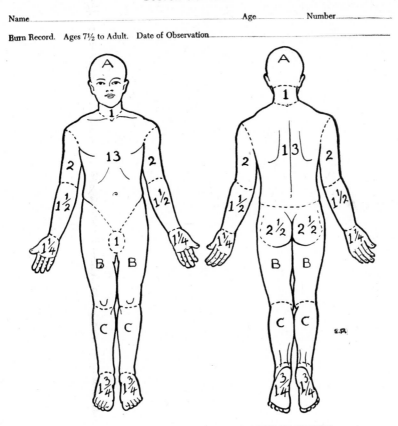

RELATIVE PERCENTAGES OF AREAS AFFECTED BY GROWTH

Area	Age	10	15	Adult
A = ½ of Head		5½	4½	3½
B = ½ of One Thigh		4¼	4½	4¾
C = ½ of One Leg		3	3¼	3½

% BURN BY AREAS

| Probable 3rd° Burn | Head.......... Neck.......... Body.......... Up. Arm.......... Forearm.......... Hands.......... |
| | Genitals.......... Buttocks.......... Thighs.......... Legs.......... Feet.......... |

| Total Burn | Head.......... Neck.......... Body.......... Up. Arm.......... Forearm.......... Hands.......... |
| | Genitals.......... Buttocks.......... Thighs.......... Legs.......... Feet.......... |

Sum of All Areas   Probably 3rd°..Total Burn..................................

FIG. 22a. Diagram for charting areas burned. Ages, 7½ to adult. (From Lund, C. C., et al., Surg., Gynec. & Obst., International Abst. Surg., 82(No. 6):443-478, June 1946. By permission of Surgery, Gynecology and Obstetrics.)

morphine in the usual doses should be given intravenously. The intravenous route is chosen because frequently the circulation is impaired following the burn and absorption of medication given subcutaneously or intramuscularly becomes unpredictable. If the complications listed are present, morphine should be avoided and demerol used.

BOSTON CITY HOSPITAL

Name.. Age................... Number...................

Burn Record. Ages—Birth—7½. Date of Observation...

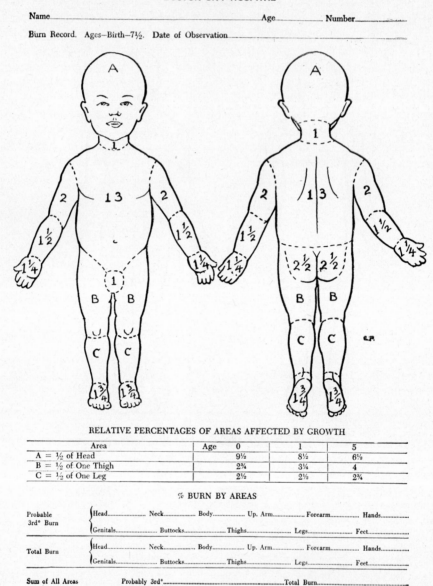

RELATIVE PERCENTAGES OF AREAS AFFECTED BY GROWTH

Area	Age	0	1	5
A = ½ of Head		9½	8½	6½
B = ½ of One Thigh		2¾	3¼	4
C = ½ of One Leg		2½	2½	2¾

% BURN BY AREAS

Probable 3rd° Burn	{Head.................... Neck................... Body.................... Up. Arm.................. Forearm.................. Hands..................	
	{Genitals.................... Buttocks.................... Thighs.................... Legs.................... Feet....................	
Total Burn	{Head.................... Neck................... Body.................... Up. Arm.................. Forearm.................. Hands..................	
	{Genitals.................... Buttocks.................... Thighs.................... Legs.................... Feet....................	

Sum of All Areas   Probably 3rd°..Total Burn...

FIG. 22b. Diagram for charting areas burned. Ages, birth to 7½. (From Lund, C. C., *et al., Surg., Gynec. & Obst., International Abst. Surg.,* 82(No. 6):443-478, June 1946. By permission of Surgery, Gynecology and Obstetrics.)

EARLY COMPLICATIONS OF BURNS

Shock is the most important early complication of extensive burns and unless combated immediately and vigorously, death will ensue. According to the present point of view, the most important etiologic factors are diminution of blood volume (chiefly the plasma fraction) and disturbances in electrolytes, plasma proteins and enzyme systems, both intracellular and extracellular. These factors have been discussed more fully in Chapter 2.

The clinical picture of burn shock has been adequately described by many writers. As with other forms of shock it is very simple to make the diagnosis in the final stages. However, the earlier periods of impending or mild shock are more difficult to diagnose. Since shock once established is much more difficult to treat than in its earlier stages, it is important to foresee impending shock so that prophylactic measures can be taken.

Careful estimation of the area and of the approximate depth of the burn is important to the anticipation of shock. Any patient with a burned area of 15 per cent or greater will probably suffer from shock unless adequately treated. Infants and elderly or feeble individuals may show failure of the circulation with burns of considerably less magnitude, such as 8 to 10 per cent body area.

Progressive hemoconcentration, falling plasma protein concentration, falling blood pressure, rising pulse and a lowering in urinary output are indications of impending shock. The significance and interpretation of these have been discussed elsewhere.[1] (Figs. 23 and 24).

PREVENTION AND TREATMENT OF BURN SHOCK

In the treatment of any form of shock any procedure that will increase the shock should be avoided insofar as possible and necessary shocking procedures, such as dressings, should be postponed until shock has been prevented or treated. Among the positive measures for the treatment of shock, those that restore and maintain the blood volume and correct the electrolyte and plasma protein disturbances are of paramount importance. Omission of these can in no way be compensated for by any of the adjuvant methods of treatment discussed later.

Intravenous saline had long been used as the primary replacement fluid in the therapy of burn shock because of its ready availability. To a lesser extent whole blood had also been used. It appeared, however, that when saline was used, the effect was frequently transient, and that plasma protein was "washed out." In regard to the use of whole blood, it had been felt that since hemoconcentration was already present in the severely burned patient, additional red blood cells would serve no useful purpose. Consequently when plasma became generally available in 1940 to 1942, it at first completely replaced these solutions. It was felt that the fluid lost from the vascular bed following burns was similar in composition to blood plasma, and it seemed logical to replace the lost fluid with plasma. However, although it has been demonstrated that burn shock may be prevented, or successfully treated in nearly all cases, if seen early, by plasma transfusions in adequate amounts, there have been in all reported series, a certain number of patients or animals in which shock could not be successfully treated in this manner. In addition, the subsequent appearance of secondary anemia and hypoproteinemia were

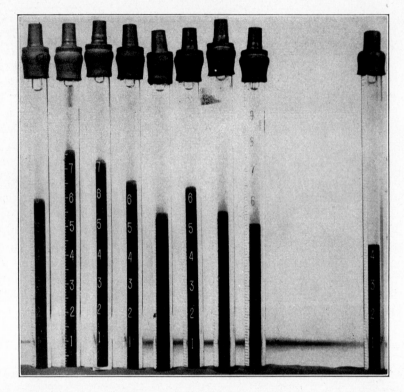

Fig. 23. Serial hematocrit determinations during first thirteen hours post-burn. Tube on right, normal control.

L. A., 20-year-old man with noncontributory history, sustained flame and electric burns and some damage to respiratory tract shortly before entry. Thirty-five per cent of body surface was involved in mixed second and third degree burns, chiefly the latter.

Examination on entry revealed well-developed and well-nourished man. The blood pressure was 130/70, pulse 100 and of good quality, and respirations 25. The hemoglobin was 141 per cent, and hematocrit 60 per cent.

During next 3 hours small amounts of water were administered orally, no other fluids being given. Patient gradually went into profound circulatory collapse, no blood pressure or pulse being obtainable for last half-hour of this period. The extremities were cold, clammy and cyanotic. There had been no output of urine. The hemoglobin had risen to 172 per cent, and hematocrit to 70 per cent. Administration of plasma was then begun, and during the next 2 hours systolic blood pressure was kept between 80 and 90 and was thereafter above 100. The pulse improved in quality, and extremities were no longer cold, clammy or cyanotic.

Plasma infusions were continued, total of 4000 cc. being given in first 13 hours. During this time the hematocrit fell gradually to 51 per cent. There were no further periods of circulatory failure.

important complications and the development of homologous serum jaundice in some cases a very serious one. In the past few years interest in the use of electrolyte solutions and whole blood has been revived, and at the present time replacement therapy is usually undertaken with a combination of whole blood, electrolyte solutions and plasma. The experimental, theoretical and clinical background for this has been discussed at length elsewhere.[8-12] With this method, it appears that not only is shock more effectively prevented and

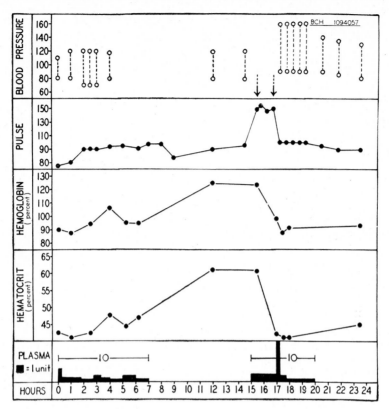

F<small>IG</small>. 24. Effect of plasma on burn shock (the vertical arrows mean that the blood pressure was not obtainable).

A 50-year-old white man with flame burns of 55 per cent of his body surface, chiefly third degree. Blood pressure, pulse, hematocrit and hemoglobin were normal on entry. Ten units (2500 cc.) of plasma were given in first 7 hours, during which time his burns were treated with tannic acid and silver nitrate. Hemoglobin, pulse, and blood pressure remained normal, and plasma infusion was stopped. Five hours later, hematocrit and hemoglobin were markedly elevated, but pulse and blood pressure were still normal. During next 2 hours patient became chilly, nauseated, and complained of feeling sick. Suddenly he became cold, pale and clammy. His pulse was very rapid and thready, and his blood pressure was unobtainable. The administration of 1100 cc. of plasma during next 90 minutes restored the hematocrit to normal, but had no effect on pulse and blood pressure. In the next 10 minutes 800 cc. of plasma were given into the femoral vein by the multiple syringe technic, with a return of pulse and blood pressure to normal. (From Lund. C. C., et al., Surg., Gynec. & Obst., International Abst. Surg., 82 (No. 6): 443-478, June 1946. By permission of Surgery, Gynecology and Obstetrics.)

treated, and kidney function better maintained, but that the early hypoproteinemia and secondary anemia are lessened.

The amount and rate of fluid replacement depends on many factors. First, the amount of fluid lost is roughly proportional to the area of surface burned. However, burns of certain areas, such as the face and genitalia, which are highly vascular and have loose subcutaneous tissue, are accompanied by particularly high fluid losses. Second, the rate of fluid loss is maximal in the first few hours after burn and then gradually decreases so that at the end of thirty-six to forty-eight hours, an equilibrium is reached between the amount of fluid lost and the amount returned to the blood stream from the interstitial spaces. Third, both clinical and laboratory data must be considered in determining the amount of fluid to be given. We have found that the best guides to the adequacy of therapy are the general clinical appearance of the patient and the urinary output. All patients with extensive burns should be placed on constant bladder drainage immediately after entry and an accurate hour-to-hour record of the urinary output kept during the first twenty-four to forty-eight hours. It has been shown that renal blood flow and urine output may be markedly reduced at a time when the peripheral pulse and blood pressure are normal, and before other definite signs of impending shock are seen.[13] When the urine output is good, one may feel sure that the general circulation is good. If, however, the urine output falls, one must anticipate early failure of the general circulation.

Since the maximal fluid loss occurs in the first few hours, it is during this time that the physician has the greatest opportunity to prevent shock. No unnecessary delays should be tolerated. When the usual peripheral veins are not available, there should be no hesitation about employing the femoral route or cutting down on a vein. The use of the femoral route was a life saving measure in the treatment of many patients at the Boston City Hospital where thousands of such punctures have been made for withdrawing blood or injecting various solutions intravenously without ill effects.[1] Cutting down on a vein is ordinarily not necessary but if no other route is possible it should be done without delay. By and large the fluid replacement should be roughly according to the following schedule which approximates the rate of fluid loss: One-half to be given in the first four to six hours, one-quarter in the next six hours, and the last quarter in the next twelve hours. Smaller amounts may be required in the next twenty-four hours in rare instances. If severe shock is already present at the time of beginning therapy, it is often necessary to administer the fluid very rapidly to improve the circulation. Caution must be used, of course, in infants, old people and in patients with heart disease. In the normal adult with a large burn, however, as much as 2000 ml. may be given in a period of an hour without danger of overloading the circulation.

Additional Therapeutic Factors. ALBUMIN. A few reports indicate that albumin is of value in the treatment of burn shock. At present it is prepared in a highly concentrated form (25 per cent), and can, if indicated, be administered without dilution. For emergency treatment of the patient who is not dehydrated it may well be of value. It has the advantage of a much greater osmotic effect than the same amount of protein in the form of plasma. However, it has the disadvantage of being a "pure" solution, that is, it does not contain other substances, such as prothrombin, which are also lost or depleted in shock. Additional electrolytes and water must be given to patients receiving albumin to replace the interstitial fluid which is drawn into the vascular system by the osmotic action of the albumin as well as that lost at the site of injury.

GLUCOSE. It has been demonstrated that additional glucose in the period following injury may help alleviate the derangement in carbohydrate and nitrogen metabolism. Consequently glucose should be given in substantial quantities, for example up to 200 grams in the first twenty-four hours.

VITAMINS. Experimental work in animals has indicated that the B-complex vitamins and ascorbic acid may have definite therapeutic effects on shock.[14,15] In addition, Levenson, Lund and associates [16,17] have found a great depletion of water-soluble vitamins during the shock of burns as well as in traumatic shock in humans. It appears logical to administer large doses of these vitamins during the early period.

POSITION. The circulation of the brain is improved by raising the foot of the bed even though by this maneuver the blood volume may not be materially altered. It is especially important to raise the foot of the bed during the first few minutes while more effective methods of treatment of shock are being started.

OXYGEN. There is no evidence that inhalation of 100 per cent oxygen alleviates tissue anoxia accompanying shock. Oxygen has been widely used clinically in the treatment of burn shock, but the only clear indication for its use is when the burn shock is complicated by respiratory tract injury.

EXTERNAL TEMPERATURE. It has been demonstrated that over-heating or under-cooling are both detrimental during shock.[18] An environmental temperature of about 24° C. appears to be optimal. It is important that in patients in shock with rectal temperatures below 34° C. or above 40° C., active measures should be taken to warm or cool them promptly, but these measures must be stopped when the temperature approaches normal.

SEDATION. Elman [19] has demonstrated that the mortality of burned dogs was increased when the usual doses of morphine or barbiturates were given. These findings and others of a similar nature, indicate that morphine and other sedatives should be used cautiously in patients with impending or actual burn shock, and, when used, the intravenous route is essential since the absorption of subcutaneous or intramuscular medication is unpredictable.[20] The action of anesthetics is also unpredictable and they are dangerous in burn shock. There is almost no occasion to use general anesthesia at the time of the first dressing in the opinion of the authors, because they have found no advantage from débridement or washing the burn (see below).

PRESSOR DRUGS. These drugs are at present considered to be of no value in the treatment of burn shock and may be definitely harmful.

ADRENAL CORTICAL EXTRACT. At the present time there is no evidence to indicate beneficial effects from adrenal cortical extract during the early phase following burns.

OUTLINE OF TREATMENT FOR SHOCK

When an extensively burned patient is admitted, intravenous fluid therapy should be begun at once. Usually electrolyte solutions are on hand immediately, whereas blood and plasma are not. It is suggested, therefore, that electrolyte solution be started first, and blood and plasma as soon as available.

We have used the following electrolyte glucose and vitamin solution almost exclusively the past three years:

Glucose	6.7 grams	1000 ml.
NaCl	5.6 grams	1000 ml.
NaHCO₃	2.5 grams	1000 ml.

This is made by adding to 1000 cc. 10 per cent glucose in isotonic saline, 500 cc. distilled water and 1 ampule (3.75 grams) sodium bicarbonate. To this is also added 1 gram ascorbic acid, 50 mg. thiamine, 50 mg. riboflavin and 500 mg. nicotinamide. The vitamin content is increased if the patient is intoxicated or in delirium tremors.

The choice between whole blood and plasma is made as follows: if the hemoconcentration is marked (above 60 per cent) and the patient is in severe shock or has serious cardiac disease, plasma is started first and whole blood begun later when the hemoconcentration and shock are controlled. In all other instances whole blood is begun immediately. Additional water should be given to provide for kidney function.

The amounts of electrolyte, water, whole blood and plasma to be given cannot be stated categorically. The therapy must be adjusted to fit the patient's individual requirements and response to treatment. As stressed before, the urinary output and the patient's general condition are the best guides as to adequacy of therapy. Abbott and Hirschfeld [10] have recommended the following approximate quantities (the electrolyte solution recommended by them is similar to the one described above without the added glucose and vitamins): 25 to 50 ml. whole blood for every per cent body burn or an amount equal to 2 to 6 per cent body weight. Electrolyte solution in amounts equal to 6 to 8 per cent of patient's body weight when area burned is 5 to 15 per cent; 8 to 12 per cent body weight for burns 15 to 35 per cent; and 12 to 14 per cent for burns 35 per cent or greater. We have used about the same total fluid but proportionally twice as much blood and one-half as much electrolyte.

COMMON COMPLICATIONS OF BURNS

Kidney Injury. Impairment of kidney function is the most important early complication of the severely burned patient. A complete discussion of kidney lesions in burns is presented by Goodpastor, *et al.*,[21] (Fig. 25). The important etiological factors of reduced renal function appear to be reduced renal blood flow and anoxemia secondary to impairment of the general circulation, acidosis, hemoglobinemia, and hemoglobinuria. Every effort must be made to prevent the occurrence of shock, or if shock is present, to combat it vigorously and immediately. By analogy with hemolytic blood transfusion reactions, prompt and continued alkalinization of the urine during the period of hemoglobinemia (usually forty-eight to seventy-two hours) is important. This can be accomplished initially by the intravenous injection of an ampule of sodium bicarbonate (3.75 grams) in addition to that already

dermal burns should not be delayed, and the separation of slough from deep burns should be hastened. At the present time pressure dressings [25] in conjunction with early débridement (chemical or surgical) seem to best meet these requirements, and have displaced to a large extent the escharotic treat-

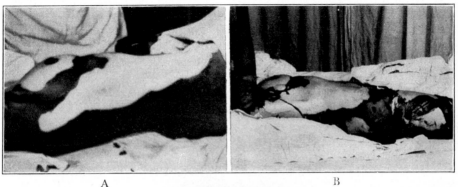

A   B

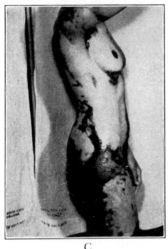

C

FIG. 27. Healing of a superficial first and second degree burn treated with petrolatum pressure dressing. (A) Appearance of burn on entry, after hot water scald. Superficial desquamation of epidermis; corium visible. (B) On the fifth day. Note the increased blistering that had occurred under one dressing. This is readily understandable since the dressing had been applied so soon after injury that all the pathologic changes had not yet appeared. This dressing had been removed unusually early in order to see the results of treatment. (C) Eleventh day. The burn is nearly healed and was healed on the fourteenth day. Pigment returned later. (From Clowes, G. H. A., Lund, C. C. and Levenson, S. M., *Ann. Surg.*, 118:769, Nov., 1943.)

ment (tannic acid, tannic acid and silver nitrate, and triple dye) which during the decade 1930 to 1939 had, in turn, replaced former methods of primary surface treatments. It should be stressed, however, that no fixed routine can be established for all cases and that the pressure dressing technique has definite drawbacks. Thus, in infants with weeping second degree burns it would be very desirable to have a nontoxic escharotic treatment which would stop the ooze. Chase [26] has recently described an agent which may prove to be of this type.

Technique of Application of Pressure Dressing. All dressings must be done under strict aseptic conditions. Until recently the custom of washing and débriding burns had not been challenged, but it has been shown in recent years that washing of burns is unnecessary when pressure dressings or casts are used. [1,27] Anesthesia should seldom or never be used for the first dressing of a burn. At that time a good firm and thoroughly satisfactory "pressure dressing" may be applied under light morphine sedation or in some cases with no sedation at all (Figs. 27, 28, 29, 30 and 31).

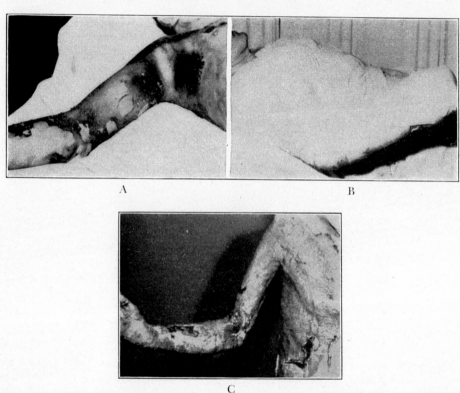

A B

C

Fig. 28. Third degree flame burn treated with dry gauze pressure dressing. (A) Before dressing the burn. Note edematous, brown, hard, charred appearance. (B) Pressure dressing in place. (C) Three weeks. Original dressing removed for first time. Note sloughing well advanced and granulations apparent.

Fine mesh gauze or rayon, dry or impregnated with a bland ointment such as petrolatum should be applied directly to the wound. Over this sufficient sterile gauze, absorbent cotton, cellucotton, or mechanics' waste should be placed so that even compression can be secured by means of a firm, wide bandage. If the padding is furnished in large rolls of material from 1 to 2 centimeters thick, 20 centimeters wide, and 4 meters long, it facilitates the application. It should be emphasized that to be maximally effective the dressing should be applied as soon as permitted by the general condition of the patient, since the greatest amount of swelling occurs in the first few hours after injury. Also, since the swelling is not limited to the burned areas, but occurs also in the immediately adjacent areas, these areas must be in-

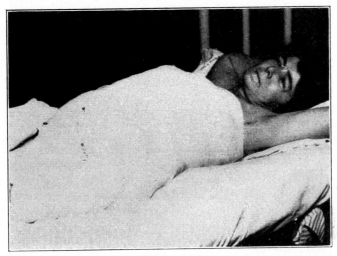

FIG. 29. Firm dressing over deep third degree burn of the trunk.

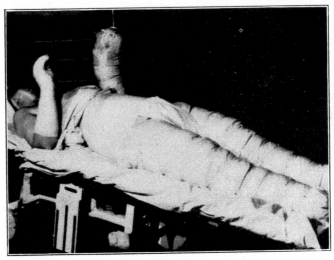

FIG. 30. Appearance of pressure dressing over deep second degree burns on legs, buttocks and left hand and forearm; cast on right forearm; fourteen days after application. Note that all are intact and in place.

corporated in the dressing. In burns of the extremities the dressing must extend distally to cover completely the hand and foot, even if these areas are not burned, otherwise the venous return will be obstructed, and as the back pressure builds up, the arterial blood supply will be impaired. Elevation of the extremity may help to prevent stasis and discomfort. In applying a pressure dressing the tension must be uniform, and care must be taken that no more pressure is used than is required. Serious harm, leading to long time stiffness of the fingers, or even to Volkmann's contracture may follow the improper application of a "pressure dressing" to a burn of the hand, forearm, or arm. The limb must never be wound circularly with long gauze bandages whether impregnated with petrolatum or not and whether thin or thick. Soft padding must be applied *very thickly* and *very loosely first*. Then this padding may be *firmly but gently and uniformly compressed* by circular elastic or elastic weave bandages.

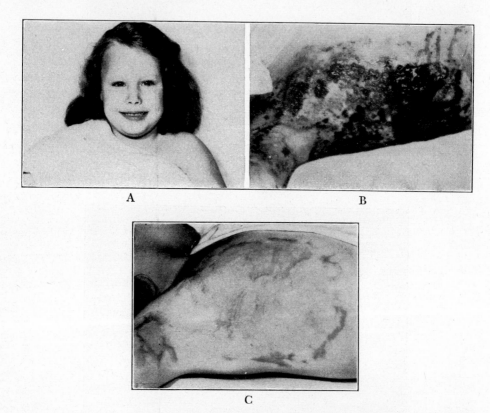

A B

C

Fig. 31. (A) Child with third degree burn of chest treated locally with dry gauze pressure dressings. Fourteenth day. Note obvious comfort. (B) Appearance of burn on fifteenth day. Note sloughing well advanced and granulations present. (C) Two months after injury. Burn grafted and healed.

In burns of the chest and abdomen a "pressure dressing" cannot be applied without interfering with the patient's respiration. Therefore, in this location a firm bulky occlusive dressing without pressure is used.

It is essential that the dressing be put on carefully and that sufficient adhesive tape be used to hold it firmly in place. Colebrook [28] has shown that the incidence of added infections in burns which were found to be imperfectly covered when redressed was ten times as high as that of the burn which had a perfect cover during the interval between dressings. Pressure dressings which remain dry on the outside prevent the entrance of additional organisms. If, however, the dressing becomes saturated, contamination is possible. This has been minimized by the incorporation of a cellophane membrane in the dressing.[29]

Technic of Application of Close Fitting Plaster Casts.[30,31] This type of dressing is recommended for burns of the extremities, particularly of the hands (Figs. 32 and 33), but it is not recommended for burns of the trunk, buttocks, head, or in burns of the extremities when the burn reaches within 3 inches of either the groin or the axilla. Under operating room conditions, one layer of sterile fine meshed gauze, dry, is applied to the entire area to be covered by plaster. This is covered with four layers only of sterile open mesh gauze layed on carefully without overlapping but not "bandaged" into place. Plaster slabs are then molded over the extremity, front and back. A thin layer of rolled plaster completes a nearly skin tight, light, well fitting plaster. The splint must be close fitting, but must be applied without compression at any point. As in the case of a "pressure dressing" it should extend proximally from 7 to 16 centimeters beyond the upper limit of the burn. It must extend distally to cover completely the hand and foot (including the tips of the fingers and toes) even if these areas are not burned; otherwise the circulation will be impaired. Hands should be put up in the position of function with a slight cock-up at the wrists and fingers in neutral position (half flexed). The extremities may be left elevated for the first 24 to 48 hours. It is all important that directions be followed exactly. There have been instances in which improperly made casts had to be removed to prevent gangrene.

The Use and Technic of Petrolatum Gauze Dressings. Allen and Koch[25] and others advise pressure dressings for burns of the face, head and neck. After using them on a number of patients we have given them up in treating these particular burns. Two reasons led to this decision. First, such dressings were always uncomfortable when used for serious burns and many patients complained of claustrophobia. Second, sufficient pressure could not be used to control the edema of the face or neck. We now use sterile petrolatum gauze strips applied without pressure and without bandage. These strips rub off from time-to-time and new ones are put on by a nurse. They are rectangular and approximately 8 by 16 centimeters. They are made of fine mesh cotton bandage material impregnated with petrolatum and sterilized. Other areas where pressure dressings are impractical are the genitalia and the anus. Petrolatum strips are also used here.

When this mode of treatment is used, the hazard of contamination is increased. However, this hazard is great in burns of these areas with any known treatment. It may be reduced by isolating the patient, by using sterile bed clothes, and careful aseptic nursing procedures.

Secondary Surface Treatments. The original "pressure dressings" or plaster should be left in place for two or three weeks except for very super-

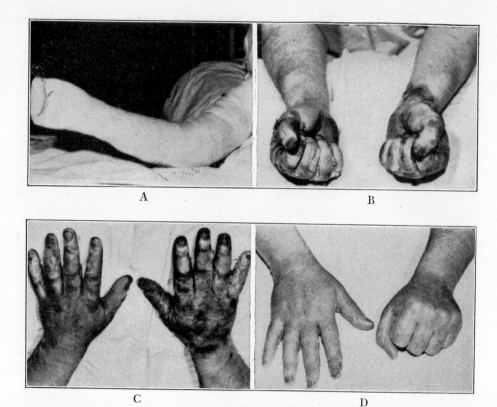

FIG. 32. (A) Second degree burn of hand and forearm treated with cast. Note slight dorsiflexion at wrist and neutral position of fingers. Left hand was also burned and similarly treated. (B and C) Eleventh day. Condition on removal of first casts. Note free flexion and extension. New casts applied. (D) Twenty-third day. Condition after removal of second casts and cleaning. Complete healing and complete return of function. (B, C and D, from Lund, Charles C. and Levenson, Stanley M., *J.A.M.A.*, 123:273, Oct. 2, 1943.)

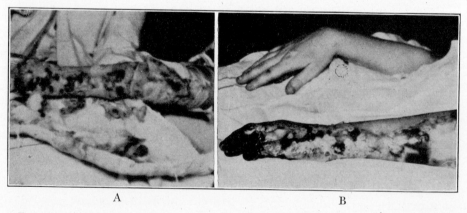

FIG. 33. (A) Third degree burn of hand and forearm. Thirteenth day. Cast and dry gauze removed. Petrolatum strips in place. Note small amount of exudate. (B) Thirteenth day. Petrolatum strips removed. Note minimal swelling and absence of spreading infection. (From Lund, Charles C. and Levenson, Stanley M., *J.A.M.A.*, 123:273, Oct. 2, 1943.)

ficial second degree burns that have in all probability healed prior to these times. Frequent changes of dressings, wet, dry or with ointments, traumatize the wound and increase the danger of bacterial contamination and the process of changing them is wearing to the patient. If the dressing becomes loose or slips, it should be repaired by adding more sterile material, new outside bandages and adhesive.

Changes of dressing should be made under aseptic conditions in an operating room. The patient should usually be prepared by a mild sedative. Anesthesia may be needed in severe, chronic cases at many late dressings. Cyclopropane is the anesthetic agent of choice. On removal of the dressing, the status of the wound is appraised and the further needs of the patient are estimated. Superficial second degree burns will usually be healed in two weeks, but deep second degree, mixed, and third degree burns will be covered with soft, foul slough, for 2 to 5 weeks. Purulent material and loose slough should be wiped off gently or débrided. As soon as large areas have become free of slough and if the granulations and the patient are both in good condition, grafts should be applied without waiting for the adjacent slough to separate. Methods to hasten the time of grafting by chemical (pyruvic acid) or surgical means are described below. The use of frequently changed wet saline or chlorinated soda dressings does not accomplish this efficiently, and in fact, may be harmful. At later stages, if necessary, after all grafting required has been done, daily tub baths and nonpressure dressings to the remaining small open areas should be carried out. If it is desired to irrigate areas localized to extremities, the technique described by Bunyan is useful.[32] He uses a transparent envelope with sealed inlet and outlet tubes.

SEPARATION OF DEAD TISSUE FROM DEEP BURNS. Skin grafting of deep burns should be carried out at the earliest possible time after injury (Fig. 34). There has been a great tendency, particularly among surgeons who treat burns only occasionally, to wait many months before doing any graft in order to allow nature to make its maximum efforts at healing. With such a laissez-faire policy, burns adjacent to the joints lead to crippling contractures and deformities and other burns develop unnecessarily thick and troublesome scars. In addition, until the epithelialization is complete, disturbances in nutrition, red blood cell formation and other important bodily functions persist. The technics of skin grafting are described elsewhere in this volume. We have found dermatome grafts backed with nylon the most satisfactory type,[33] (Fig. 35). Burns have been grafted in most clinics in the granulating stage. The time when the slough is completely separated is usually between the third and sixth weeks. Sloughs on small and more vascular areas, such as the face, separate more quickly than those on larger and less vascular areas.

Recently emphasis has been on methods which speed up the removal of dead tissue, and thus enable skin grafting to be done at an earlier date.

CHEMICAL DÉBRIDEMENT. Early separation of the slough has been encouraged by the application of various solutions such as the proteolytic enzymes, papain or pepsin, or by the application of pyruvic acid in a starch paste.[34] With the latter method, sloughs of deep second degree and third degree burns may be removed in from six to ten days without injury to any epithelium that may be present in the more superficial areas, or to the granulation tissue. Some very impressive results of its use in severe burns have been reported.

A   B

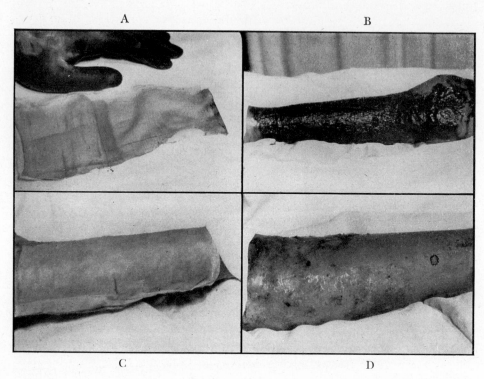

C   D

FIG. 35. (A) Cut dermatome graft with nylon backing. Note limpness of graft, yet normal tension of skin maintained. (B) Recipient site ready for grafting. (C) Graft in place. Note absence of sutures. (D) Graft three weeks postoperatively. Note the excellent "take." (From Green, R. W., Levenson, S. M. and Lund, C. C., *New England J. Med.*, 233:268-270, Aug. 30, 1945.)

PYRUVIC ACID TECHNIC.[34] Connor and Harvey describe their technic (Fig. 36) as follows: "The stock solution of pyruvic acid is made by adding 7 cc. of pyruvic acid CP to one liter of distilled water. The pH of the resulting solution should be 1.9.

"A content of from 8 to 10% of cornstarch is desirable in the pyruvic acid starch paste. The exact amount of starch necessary varies somewhat with different commercial brands, but the final consistency of the paste should be always semi-liquid permitting easy application. The preparation of the paste is the same whether a large or a small amount is made at one time. The desired volume of solution of pyruvic acid is separated into two portions, one (A) of about 20% of the total volume, and the other (B) of the remaining solution. Portion A is mixed without heating with a calculated amount of

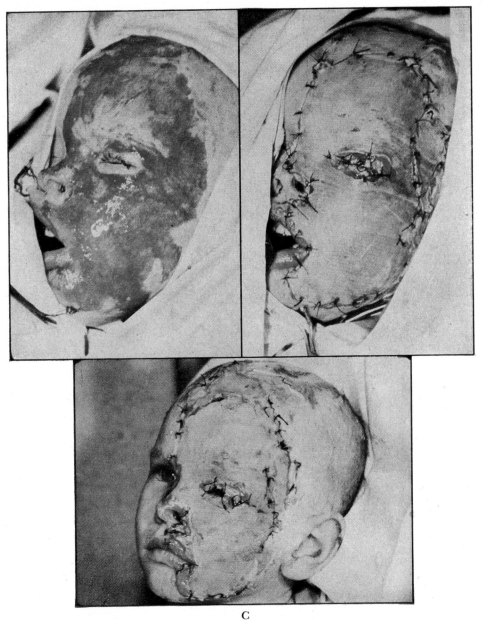

FIG. 34. (A) Third degree burn of face and scalp. Eighteenth day. Note area on face is granulating and free of slough, while slough still adherent on scalp. (B) Eighteenth day. Split-thickness skin graft applied. (C) Twenty-fifth day. Appearance at first post-operative dressing. Note almost complete "take" of graft. Further plastic work necessary.

cornstarch, 8 to 10% (of total volume, A and B) and thin cold starch paste obtained. Portion B is heated to just short of boiling. Portion B is then mixed with A, the cold starch paste, and stirred. If the total volume is greater than 400 cc. additional heating with constant stirring for about one minute may be necessary in order to produce an homogeneous relatively thick paste. This is then cooled by placing in a container in an ice bath. The paste thickens somewhat with cooling.

"In the use of this method, certain general points are of great importance and deserve emphasis: (1) the success of the method depends to a considerable degree upon the maintenance of a thick layer of active pyruvic acid paste in contact with the wound. A relatively large amount of paste should be applied to minimize neutralization by the wound fluids. The paste should be applied generally in a thick layer. For example, in the treatment of a burn involving the entire circumference of the leg from knee to ankle about 3,000 cc. of paste is advisable. This is most readily done by placing the paste on a thin layer of gauze on a sheet of appropriate size which is then applied with the paste next to the burn. An excessive amount of paste can be used with safety and an inadequate amount is relatively ineffective. After application, the inner dressing is covered with strips of vaseline gauze and some impermeable dressing so that it does not dry out. Over this a pressure dressing is applied. (2) Preliminary cleansing or débridement of the wound is unnecessary. (3) Blisters may or may not be opened. In any instance in which the presence of slough beneath the blisters is suspected, and this occasionally occurs, the blisters should be opened to expose the dead tissue. If this is not done, the treatment will be ineffective in this area. (4) Separation of the slough by this method proceeds from the margin of the wound. It is, therefore, highly advisable in large wounds to incise the slough with a scalpel in order to create more margin. This can be done without anesthesia. The incisions should be carried through the dead tissue in a linear manner." [34] In addition, loose slough should be excised at later dressing changes.

Pyruvic acid dressings must be done at fairly frequent intervals (2 to 3 days). This is one of the disadvantages of this method since each dressing change exposes the burned area to further contamination and is wearing on the patient and cannot be done without causing some pain. Such dressings are not as comfortable as pressure dressings because they are loose and do not splint the part.

Sulzberger et al.,[35] have studied the effects of pyruvic acid and other acids on the removal of slough from small experimental burns in man and have demonstrated that the action of pyruvic acid is apparently nonspecific and that essentially the same results could be secured with other acids e.g. 0.1 m. phosphoric. It was also demonstrated that certain forms of dry hydroscopic powders containing acids could be prepared, which on the addition of water would rapidly form suitable jells. These proved to be less irritating and almost as effective as pyruvic acid starch paste in removing slough and promoting healing of chemical and thermal burns.

SURGICAL EXCISION. Immediate excision and skin grafting has been carried out by several authors.[36] It is theoretically sound because after a deep burn is excised and the wound successfully grafted, the area is healed in a week or ten days. However, it has limited applicability because of the further physiologic upset caused by an extensive operation in a patient whose burn may already have caused shock. It is, therefore, indicated only in obviously deep burns of small area in which there is little likelihood of shock. Relatively few deep burns come in this category.

Delayed excision of skin grafting in extensively burned patients has been carried out recently in a number of cases by Cope *et al.*[37] It is their practice to wait at least until shock has been controlled before attempting excision. Large amounts of penicillin are given intramuscularly and locally through

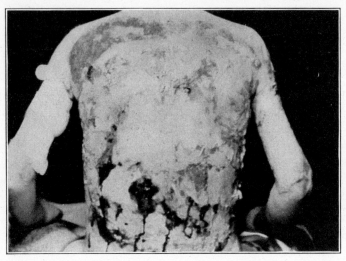

FIG. 37. One week after application of homografts to granulating third degree burn of back. Note good "take."

Dakin's tubes incorporated into a pressure dressing at the time of burn in an attempt to prevent infection. When the shock has been satisfactorily treated and the general condition of the patient is good, the burned area is excised down to normal appearing tissue and grafted at one operation, or grafted later within a few days. It was found that such grafts took very well if the excision was carried out within 48 hours after injury before infection had time to develop. However, the longer the excision of slough was delayed, the less probable was the success of the grafting. This was attributed to the fact that although penicillin was able to check invasive infection, it did not prevent bacteria from growing in the slough and infection from developing in the contiguous portion of the wound. It was therefore recommended that surgical excision and grafting be carried out as soon as the acute physiological upset is corrected. If the area of deep burn is very extreme, the procedure

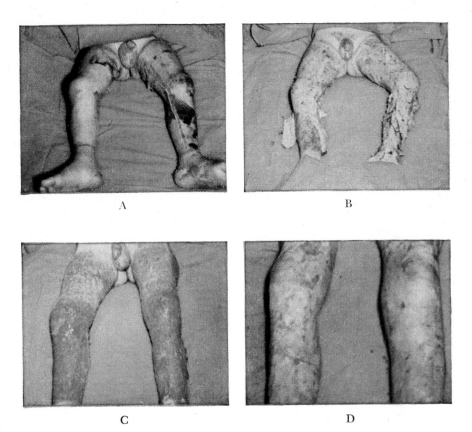

Fig. 36. (A) Appearance of third degree flame burns 3 days after injury. Initial surface treatment was a petrolatum pressure dressing. (B) Eight days after injury, 5 days pyruvic acid dressings. Much of the slough had already separated and most of the remainder of the slough was held in place only in soft strands. (C) Fifteen days after injury, 12 days of pyruvic acid dressings. Areas free of slough with healthy granulations present. (D) Twenty-seven days after injury, 24 days after the start of pyruvic acid dressings, and 12 days after first grafting. Note excellent takes of grafts. (From Conner, G. J. and Harvey, S. C., *Ann. Surg.*, 124:799-810, November 1946.)

must be done in stages, with a limit of about 10 per cent body area at any one operation. The results of these procedures have been excellent, and the method has great promise in the hands of surgical teams experienced in dermatome grafting operations and in the care of surgical shock. Blood transfusions to the amount of several liters may be needed at the time of, and immediately after, these operations. A similar procedure, begun at a later date, between the tenth and fourteenth days, has been followed by Ackman and his associates.[38] In their technic no parenteral chemotherapy is given but a sulfathiazole emulsion is used locally.

One of the difficulties in carrying out the principle of early surgical excision is the present impossibility of being able always to judge correctly the depth of the burn. This problem and methods to solve it have been discussed earlier.

HOMOGRAFTS. Homografting (Fig. 37), or the use of skin from someone other than the burned individual, has a limited but definite application in the care of the patient, particularly children, with extensive burns. With granulating areas covered, though only temporarily, the general condition of the individual can be made to improve enough so that by the time the grafts dissolve, autografting can be successfully carried out.

SCARS AND CONTRACTURES. Early skingrafting and intelligent physiotherapy as soon as feasible, will do much to eliminate contractures and scars which in the past have been important late complications of deep burns. The treatment of established scars is discussed elsewhere in this volume.

INFECTION

Infection is always a serious complication of extensive deep burns and frequently or rarely, according to the efficiency of treatment, a complication of burns of lesser severity.

The skin in superficial second degree burns retains most of the resistance that normal skin has against infection. If rest and avoidance of recontamination are provided, any bacteria growing on the surface soon die out as healing progresses. With deep burns the problem of infection is much more serious because deep burns are always infected from a few hours after the burn until healing is complete. Recent studies [39] have shown that in most instances the burns are infected with multiple species of organisms. The varieties of bacteria most commonly found are listed in Table I.

TABLE 1. *VARIETIES OF BACTERIA FOUND COMMONLY IN CULTURES FROM BURNS*

Staphylococcus hemolyticus, coagulase positive	Other streptococci
Streptococcus hemolyticus, (beta and gamma)	Other enterococci
Bacillus proteus	*Pneumococci*
Bacillus pyocyaneous	*Bacillus mucosus capsulatus*
Bacillus coli	*Bacillus welchii*
Diphtheroids	*Bacillus tetani*
Other staphylococci	Other *Clostridia*

Infection interferes with local healing, and intensifies the general bio-chemical and physiological derangements associated with burns. Its control, therefore, is one of the most important aims of therapy.

The hospital service should be organized to prevent what Clark [28] has termed, "added infection," that is, "infection of the burned surfaces with organisms not previously present. Added infection arises by the transfer of infective material from sources outside the patient. Clouds of pathogens are liberated during bed changes and when dressings are required. The clothing of doctors, nurses and visitors, especially those with throat infections, flies, drinking utensils, bed pans, thermometers, toys, and materials of occupational therapy are other sources of infection." As prophylactic measures the follow-ing procedures are useful: (1) The masking, gowning and scrubbing of all personnel coming in contact with the patient at the time when the burned areas are uncovered. This is most apt to be violated at the time of admission to the accident floor and rigorous attempts must be made to avoid this. (2) Only sterile materials must come in contact with the burn. (3) Adequate covering of the burned areas at all times. (4) Anti-dust measures and the elimination of flies. (5) Routine purification of the air of wards and operating rooms specifically set aside for the care of burn patients. (6) Segregation of infected cases in cubicles. (7) Exclusion of visitors or attendants with "colds."

Dressing. One of the chief drawbacks of the formerly popular tannic acid surface therapy of burns was the ready occurrence of infection at the edges and under the eschar. In contrast, the protection from external contamina-tions and the rest afforded by properly applied pressure dressings or casts are often sufficient to prevent spreading infections in even extensive deep burns. Also, early removal of slough and grafting have tended to lessen the seriousness of the infections.

Chemotherapeutic Agents. These agents have been widely used for the control of infection of burns. The sulfonamides have been used both locally and systemically but their efficiency in controlling the local infection of the burn has not been clearly demonstrated,[39] although Clark,[28] Ackman,[38] Andrus [40] and Howes,[41] feel that local chemotherapy with special prepara-tions has been of benefit. When one considers that there is usually a mixture of gram-positive and gram-negative organisms in the burned area, and, in addition, there is present considerable necrotic tissue and exudate, it is not surprising that there is no striking control by the sulfonamides. In addition, the most common infecting organism is the hemolytic *Staphylococcus aureus* which is highly resistant to the sulfonamides. In some instances it has been claimed that while the local infection is not controlled, spreading infection and blood stream invasion are prevented.[39]

The management of the sulfonamide chemotherapy in severely burned patients is complicated in the early stages by the presence of shock, impaired renal function and markedly acid urine. Consequently, if used locally, preparations should be used from which the sulfonamide is absorbed slowly and, if used systemically, extreme care must be exercised. Suitable local preparations have been described by Ackman [38] and Howes.[41] It must also be remembered that all deep burns will have an open wound harboring organisms until the last grafts have successfully healed and that this may take several months. As it is undesirable that any patient receive effective doses of sulfonamides for this length of time, it is recommended that no systemic sulfonamide treatment be used prophylactically but its use be restricted for some specific susceptible infectious complication.

Penicillin has been used locally and systemically in many cases of serious burn. Its chief advantages over sulfonamides are minimal toxicity, activity in the presence of pus, and greater effectiveness against hemolytic *Staphylococcus aureus*. When used locally in aqueous solution it has the great defect of rapid absorption from the wound. Attempts are being made to devise special ointment bases, such as carbowax, to delay absorption. With such a base some penicillin activity may be maintained for as long as 24 hours. Another serious defect is the presence in the wound of organisms not resistant to penicillin and the rapid destruction of penicillin by the action of penicillinases released by certain bacteria such as the colon bacillus. Penicillin has not eliminated local hemolytic staphylococcus infection but may eliminate the hemolytic streptococcus [42] and thus remove one of the important factors which prevent the taking of grafts. In addition, though the local hemolytic staphylococcal infection is not eliminated by penicillin therapy the invasive character of the infection is controlled. Consequently, it is recommended that penicillin be given intramuscularly in doses of 100,000 units every three hours in patients with deep burns, particularly in the period immediately preceding and following grafting. Recently some cases have been treated with penicillin from the start. Although fever is not eliminated there is a marked decrease in the odor of the dressings indicating that the usual infection may be in some way reduced.

Little work has been published to date on the use of streptomycin on burns. Theoretically it should be useful for short term use, in conjunction with penicillin, in cases where gram-negative organisms are also present in significant numbers. The development of "fastness" would probably preclude its long continued use.

NUTRITION

Loss of weight, often marked, has long been recognized as a serious complication in severely burned patients. Recent studies have indicated that protein and vitamin deficiencies are among the chief nutritional disturbances.[17,43] It appears that the protein deficiency results from a combination of reduced intake and excessive urinary and surface nitrogen losses. Since protein deficiency in man and in the experimental animal results in decreased resistance to shock and infection, delayed wound healing, including skin grafting, impaired gastrointestinal and liver function, progressive loss of weight, edema, prolonged convalescence and frequent complications, every possible means must be utilized to provide the seriously burned patient with good nutrition to prevent this. Otherwise even the best surgical technic cannot accomplish its purpose nor shorten the patient's period of convalescence and hasten his resumption of full activity. One can readily recognize the existence of protein depletion in an individual at a time when there is marked weakness, weight loss, hypoproteinemia and edema, but to wait for this stage to develop before a diagnosis of deficiency is made is analogous to waiting for an absent pulse and blood pressure before making the diagnosis of shock. Nutritional disturbances may never develop to the stage where gross anatomic changes occur, and yet it is certain that physiological functions are impaired early in the course of depletion. In the past clinicians have often set their sights on anatomical or pathological changes as indicative of deficiencies but institution of therapy at this time is entirely too late. The diagnosis of deficiency or impending deficiency must be made early if subsequent ill effects are to be avoided.

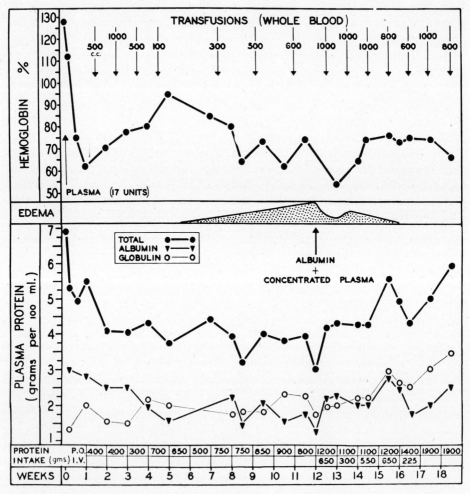

FIG. 39. Chart of patient in figure 38. Note (a) early protein deficiency gradually corrected after the twelfth week and (b) the large number of blood transfusions required to combat anemia.

A   B

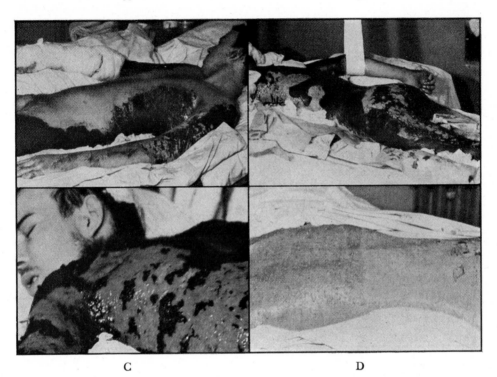

C   D

FIG. 38(A and B). Fourteen and twenty days after burn. Note extent of injury (55 per cent total, 45 per cent third degree) and good nutritional state. (C) Forty-four days after burn. Note drawn expression of face and edema of granulation tissue. (D) One hundred and thirty-seven days after burn. Improved appearance of granulations with disappearance of edema. Pin-point grafting begun. (From Levenson, S. M., *et al.*, *Surg. Gynec. & Obst.*, 80(No. 5):449-469, May 1945. By permission of Surgery, Gynecology and Obstetrics.)

E F

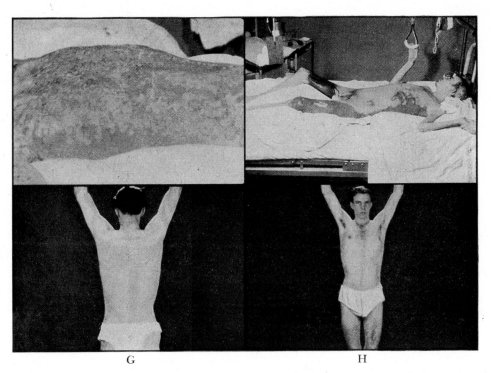

G H

FIG. 38(E). One hundred and forty-five days after burn. Note take and outgrowth of pin-point grafts. (F) One hundred and fifty-one days after burn. Note marked loss of weight (55 lbs.). Large decubitus ulcer over left femur. (G and H) Thirteen months after injury. All areas grafted and healed. Patient regained 35 lbs. weight and in good general condition. (F, G and H from Levenson, S. M., *et al., Surg. Gynec. & Obst.,* 80(No. 5):449-469, May 1945. By permission of Surgery, Gynecology and Obstetrics.)

There are many factors which must be considered in evaluating the state of protein nutrition of an individual. Among them are (1) dietary history; (2) the optimum, previous and observed weight of the patient; (3) the plasma and total blood volume; (4) the concentration of the total and various plasma protein fractions; (5) the hemoglobin concentration; (6) the nitrogen intake and nitrogen output; (7) estimation of the patient's strength, *e.g.*, by ergograph tests. It is not often possible to obtain all this data, and in most clinical work judgment must be based chiefly on a consideration of the nutritional history, an approximation of the patient's intake and probable nitrogen loss, serial determinations of the patient's weight and plasma protein concentration. Slight but persistent changes in weight are often the first indication of the patient's nutritional condition. The weights of these patients may be secured at each dressing change by putting the patient, covered with a sterile sheet, but with the dressings removed, on a weighed stretcher, each end of which is placed on a scale. By the large, a persistent and progressive loss in body weight is a fairly reliable guide as to the development of protein deficiency.

Large losses in weight may occur rapidly in seriously burned patients. Daily losses of 1 to 1½ pounds and overall losses totaling 50 pounds or more have been reported following major burns. It is imperative to anticipate the nutritional requirements and meet them before severe malnutrition occurs (Figs. 38 and 39).

The food provided must be an adequate metabolic mixture containing, in addition to adequate amounts of protein, sufficient calories, fat, carbohydrate, minerals, water and accessory food substances. As seen in Table 2, the minimum essential needs for protein, calories and vitamins are as great or greater than the need for these substances in any illness. This table is a tentative guide for adults and for children weighing 50 pounds and over. The values should be reduced by 25 per cent from 30 to 49 pounds, and by 50 per cent for patients weighing from 15 to 29 pounds. Under 15 pounds give 125 per cent, 150 per cent, 200 per cent and 300 per cent, respectively of normal protein and caloric requirements for well patients of this size, having also regard for the patients' age for 1 to 4, 5 to 9, 10 to 19 and 20 per cent burns and greater. Give 25 per cent of vitamins indicated for the area in Table 2 to these infants.

TABLE 2. *MINIMUM FOOD NEEDED DAILY BY PATIENTS WITH THIRD DEGREE BURNS, ACCORDING TO TOTAL AREA UNHEALED*

BURN AREA, PER CENT	PROTEIN, GM.	CALORIES	ASCORBIC ACID, GM.	THIAMINE, MG.	RIBO-FLAVIN, MG.	NICOTIN-AMIDE, MG.
20 +	300-400	5000	2.0	50	50	500
10-19	200	3500	1.0	25	25	200
5-9	125	3000	0.5	15	15	100
1-4	90	2500	0.5	10	10	50

Additional vitamins from liver and yeast are also important. Severely burned patients should be given up to 30 gm. of yeast a day and crude liver preparations in comparable amounts.

The principle of supplying adequate food to patients is simple and easy but the actual carrying out of the principle is often difficult. An "all out" effort must be made to maintain adequate nutrition. Whenever possible, nutritional losses or deficiency should be corrected by oral feeding. It is here that the roles of the dietitian and nurses are all important. They must see to it that the patient actually ingests the food that is ordered, for it is not enough that a high protein, high caloric, high vitamin diet has been ordered —it must be eaten. This is not an easy task, since the patient often has a poor appetite and must be cajoled patiently into eating. However, a surprisingly large amount of food will be taken by such patients provided attention is paid to the special likes and dislikes of the patient and an effort is made to serve well prepared appetizing meals when the patient is hungry rather than at stated intervals. Sedation interferes with appetite. Comfortable dressings are likewise essential in this respect.

Forcing the diet in a patient does not always result in a net gain. Nausea, vomiting, distention and diarrhea, singly or together, are limiting factors. In general, the sicker the patient, the less he is able to tolerate fat and the proportion of protein in the diet should be larger. It has been found that at least 25 per cent of the calories in the diet should come from protein and not over 15 per cent from fat. It is well to take a number of days to increase the food intake, since sudden increases are more likely to be followed by gastrointestinal symptoms, which can usually be avoided by more cautious increases.

Extensive research to devise recipes incorporating large amounts of protein is in progress at the Medical Nutrition Laboratory in Chicago.[44] Various food items of the day's menu are fortified with protein concentrates and hydrolysates. In this way the patient receives an increased amount of protein without the necessity of ingesting added bulk. Protein enriched products have been prepared which appear normal both for the eyes and taste buds and thereby are acceptable to the patients. These studies have been guided by the general principle that if it is desired to increase the consumption of a particular nutrient, success is likely to be achieved if the nutrient in question is added to many items in the daily diet without altering palatability. However, at times due to shortage of kitchen and ward help and nurses, the control of such diets is exceedingly difficult if the patient is on "ward care" and difficult even if special nurses are available. It will often be found that the most important dietary items presented to the patient are not consumed. When that happens frequently the patient will lose weight and strength rapidly. Under these conditions it has been found useful to place the major emphasis on high protein, high caloric, high vitamin, liquid supplements. The supplement is made the main diet, and the patient is allowed to eat any food desired at meal time but only if the supplement has been taken. A reasonably palatable simple mixture that contains all the food elements needed over long periods of time by the patient is the *sine qua non* of this procedure.

One of the simplest and most useful supplements is made by suspending 100 grams of skim milk powder in one quart of milk with suitable flavorings. This roughly doubles the protein content of milk, yielding a preparation containing about 65 grams of protein and 980 calories per quart. Most patients can take one to two quarts of this preparation readily. If more concentrated "drinks" are necessary, many of the oral or partially hydrolyzed protein preparations can be used. Many patients can tolerate larger quantities of these latter preparations than "whole protein." The most completely hydrolyzed preparations are not very palatable but can be taken by some patients. They are best given by gavage. Additional carbohydrate, fat, minerals, water and vitamins, crude as well as synthetic, are added to the "protein base" to make the preparation essentially "complete." These mixtures are made up daily by the dietitian and sent to the ward where they are stored in the refrigerator. One-twelfth of the mixture is brought to the patient every two hours, day and night, and the nurse watches him drink it. If the patient can do so he is allowed to anticipate some of the night feedings but never to postpone any. This oral liquid feeding regime has the unusual advantage that it makes the work easier for everybody concerned. It is easier for the patient to take, it is easier for the nurse to give, and it is much easier for the dietitian to furnish and record.

In the event that food cannot be given by mouth, either because of lack of appetite, pain or other similar factors, gavage feedings through an inlying gastric tube should be instituted. Once a gastric tube is in place, one is tempted to "pour" down at once large quantities of food. If this is done, marked gastrointestinal upsets will ensue. It is imperative to attain the desired number, concentration, and total quantity of gavage feedings by a gradual increase, over several days, in the amount and concentration of food administered. A suitable mixture for beginning gavage feedings consists of 200 cc. of an equal mixture of skim milk and water every two hours. We have found it most convenient to leave the gastric tube in place continuously, removing it only briefly for cleaning every third or fourth day. Mild sedation the first day will enable many patients to tolerate the tube feeding. Instead of supplying the mixture in intermittent doses, a drip apparatus may be used which, after a short period of training, can be regulated by the patient himself. Completely hydrolyzed protein preparations are very useful in gavage mixtures because of their high solubility and tolerance.

Forcing the diet orally is at times not beneficial to patients. Nausea, vomiting, distention and diarrhea are limiting factors. Under these conditions supplementation by the intravenous route is indicated. At the present time there is no suitable preparation of fat or fatty acids available for intravenous use. Water, salt, vitamins, carbohydrate, plasma proteins and amino acids can be given parenterally. It is preferable to give the carbohydrates as 15 or 20 per cent rather than as 5 or 10 per cent glucose solutions. The purpose is to increase the caloric intake without increasing the amount of fluid.

It is usually preferable to give the glucose along with or just before or after the administration of protein or amino acids in order to "spare" protein. Water soluble vitamins must also be given (with the intravenous fluids).

The high food intake must be continued at a sufficient level not only to maintain the patient in nutritional equilibrium but also to restore at a rapid rate all tissues that have been depleted. Recently testosterone pro- pionate has been used with considerable clinical success in the late stages of burns. The pain decreased, the granulations improved, the appetite in- creased, and weight was gained. The dose used was 10 milligrams per day, given intramuscularly.[1] Cognizance should be taken of the possible systemic changes brought about by this therapy when continued over long periods of time, particularly in females and young males.

Anemia. There is an acute hemolytic process starting immediately after an extensive deep burn and continuing for about 72 hours. The actual num- ber of red blood cells hemolyzed during this period is relatively small. How- ever, following this there is a chronic anemia which continues until healing is complete.

This anemia is progressive and its chronicity and severity are roughly proportional to the extent of the unhealed burn. In the early phase, this anemia is greater in patients treated with plasma during the shock phase than in patients treated with blood. Emerson and Ebert [45] recently demon- strated that pooled plasma and type O whole blood given to patients with types A, B, or AB blood may induce a persistent and severe hemolytic process. This can be avoided by the use of Witebsky substances.

The cause or causes of this anemia are poorly understood. Chronic hemo- lysis as evidenced by increased excretion of red cell breakdown products is suggested by Moore et al.[46]

Another factor in some is excess loss of blood in the dressings. This is particularly marked when the granulations are "poor" and edematous in patients in poor nutritional state. The protein deficiency in these patients may also lead to decreased hemoglobin formation. The bone marrow is ordinarily not markedly depressed.

The anemia does not respond to large intakes of iron, liver, protein, calories and vitamins. Blood transfusions are necessary at frequent intervals and in large amounts. It is important to keep the hemoglobin concentration at 85 per cent or above. To accomplish this may require as much as 1 liter or more of blood weekly during the patient's illness. If available, red blood cells suspended in saline solution are satisfactory for this purpose.

REFERENCES

1. LUND, C. C., GREEN, R. W., TAYLOR, F. H. L. and LEVENSON, S. M. Burns, Collective Review, *Internat. Abstr. Surg. (Surg., Gynec. & Obst.)*, 82:443-478, [July], 1946.
2. HARKINS, H. N. Present Status of the Problem of Thermal Burns, *Physiol. Rev.*, 25:531-572, [July], 1945.
3. COPE, O. Management of the Cocoanut Grove Burns at the Massachusetts General Hospital: Treatment of Surface Burns, *Ann. Surg.*, 117:885-893, [June], 1943.

4. WELLS, D. B. The Circus Disaster and the Hartford Hospital, *New Eng. J. Med.*, 232:613-616, [May 24], 1945.

5. DINGWALL, J. A., III. Clinical Test for Differentiating Second from Third Degree Burns, *Ann. Surg.*, 118:427-429, [Sept.], 1943.

6. PATEY, D. H. and SCARFF, R. W. Diagnosis of Depth of Skin Destruction in Burns and its Bearing on Treatment, *Brit. J. Surg.*, 32:32-35, [July], 1944.

7. LUND, C. C. and BROWDER, N. C. The Estimation of Areas of Burns, *Surg., Gynec. & Obst.*, 79:352-358, [Oct.], 1944.

8. MOYER, C. A., COLLER, F. A., IOB, V., VAUGHN, H. H. and MARTY, D. Metabolic Alterations Following Thermal Burns. IV. The Effect of Treatment with Whole Blood and an Electrolyte Solution Following an Experimental Burn, *Surgery*, 17:794-804, [June], 1945.

9. EVANS, E. I. and BIGGER, I. A. The Rationale of Whole Blood Therapy in Severe Burns, *Ann. Surg.*, 122:693-705, [Oct.], 1945.

10. ABBOTT, W. E. and HIRSHFELD, J. W. Present Concepts Concerning the Care of the Burned Patient, *Am. J. Surg.*, 74:296-301, [Sept.], 1947.

11. ROSENTHAL, S. M. Experimental Chemotherapy of Burns and Shock, Effects of Systemic Therapy on Early Mortality, *U. S. Pub. Health Rep.*, 58:513-522, [Mar. 26], 1943.

12. FOX, C. L. and KESTON, A. The Mechanism of Shock from Burns and Trauma Traced with Radiosodium, *Surg., Gynec. & Obst.*, 80:561-567, [June], 1945.

13. LAUSON, H. O., BRADLEY, S. E. and COURNAND, A. The Renal Circulation in Shock, *J. Clin. Invest.*, 23:381-402, [May], 1944.

14. GOVIER, W. M. Rationale for use of Vitamins in the Therapy of Shock and Anoxia, *J.A.M.A.*, 126:749-750, [Nov. 18], 1944.

15. PASQUALINI, C. C. D. Prevention of Shock by Vitamin C., *Revista de la San Militar Buenos Aires*, 45:551-678, [May], 1946.

16. LEVENSON, S. M., GREEN, R. W., TAYLOR, F. H. L., ROBINSON, P., PAIGE, R. W., JOHNSON, R. E. and LUND, C. C. Ascorbic Acid, Riboflavin, Thiamin and Nicotinic Acid in Relation to Severe Injury, Hemorrhage and Infection in the Human, *Ann. Surg.*, 124:840-856, [Nov.], 1946.

17. LUND, C. C., LEVENSON, S. M., GREEN, R. W., PAIGE, R. W., ROBINSON, P. E., ADAMS, M. H., MACDONALD, A. H., TAYLOR, F. H. L. and JOHNSON, R. E. Ascorbic Acid, Thiamin, Riboflavin, and Nicotinic Acid in Relation to Acute Burns in Man, *Arch. Surg.*, 55:557-583, [Nov.], 1947.

18. ELMAN, R., COX, W. M., JR., LISCHER, C. E. and MUELLER, A. J. Mortality in Severe Burns as Affected by Environmental Temperature, *Proc. Soc. Exper. Biol. & Med.*, 51:350-351, [Dec.], 1942.

19. ELMAN, R. Influence of Ether, Morphine and Nembutal on Mortality in Experimental Burns, *Ann. Surg.*, 120:211-213, [July], 1944.

20. BEECHER, H. K. Management of the Cocoanut Grove Burns at the Massachusetts General Hospital: Resuscitation and Sedation of Patients with Burns which Include the Airway: Some Problems of Immediate Therapy, *Ann. Surg.*, 117:823-825, [June], 1943.

21. GOODPASTOR, W. E., LEVENSON, S. M., TAGNON, H. J., LUND, C. C. and TAYLOR, F. H. L. A Clinical Pathologic Study of the Kidney in Patients with Thermal Burns, *Surg., Gynec. & Obst.*, 82:652-670, [July], 1946.

22. WALKER, J., JR. and SHEMKEN, H. Studies on the Toxemia Syndrome after Burns: II. Central Nervous System Changes as a Cause of Death, *Ann. Surg.*, 121:301-313, [Mar.], 1945.

23. AUB, J. C., PITMAN, H. and BRUES, A. M. Management of the Cocoanut Grove Burns at the Massachusetts General Hospital. The Pulmonary Complications: A Clinical Description, *Ann. Surg.*, 117:834-840, [June], 1943.

24. FINLAND, M., DAVIDSON, C. S. and LEVENSON, S. M. Clinical and Therapeutic Aspects

of the Conflagration Injuries to the Respiratory Tract Sustained by Victims of the Cocoanut Grove Disaster, *Medicine*, 25:215-283, [Sept.], 1946.

25. ALLEN, H. S. and KOCH, S. L.   Treatment of Patients with Severe Burns, *Surg., Gynec. & Obst.*, 74:914-924, [May], 1942.

26. CHASE, C. H.   A new Eschar Technique for Local Treatment of Burns, *Surg., Gynec. & Obst.*, 85:308-317, [Sept.], 1947.

27. COPE, O.   Care of Victims of the Cocoanut Grove Fire at the Massachusetts General Hospital, *New England J. Med.*, 229:138-147, [July 22], 1943.

28. CLARK, A. M., COLEBROOK, L., GIBSON, T. and THOMSON, M. L.   Penicillin and Propamidine in Burns. Elimination of Hemolytic Streptococci and Staphylococci, *Lancet*, I:606-609, [May 15], 1943.

29. OWENS, N.   Use of Pressure Dressings in the Treatment of Burns and Other Wounds, *S. Clin. N. Am.*, 23:1354-1366, [Oct.], 1943.

30. LEVENSON, S. M. and LUND, C. C.   The Treatment of Burns of the Extremities with Close Fitting Plaster of Paris Casts, *J.A.M.A.*, 123:272-277, [Oct.], 1943.

31. BARNES, J. M.   Treatment of Burns, *Brit. M. J.*, I:408-410, [April 3], 1943.

32. BUNYAN, J.   Envelope Method of Treating Burns, *Proc. Roy. Soc. Med.*, 34:65-70, [March], 1940.

33. GREEN, R. W., LEVENSON, S. M. and LUND, C. C.   Nylon Backing for Dermatome Grafts, *New England J. Med.*, 233:268-270, [Aug. 30], 1945.

34. CONNOR, G. J. and HARVEY, S. C.   The Pyruvic Acid Method in Deep Clinical Burns, *Ann. Surg.*, 124:799-810, [Nov.], 1946.

35. SULZBERGER, M. B., KANOF, A. and BAER, R. L.   Studies on Acid Débridement of Burns, *Ann. Surg.*, 125:418, [Nov.], 1947.

36. YOUNG, F. and FAVATA, D. V.   Fixation of Skin Grafts by Thrombin Plasma Adhesion, *Surgery*, 15:378-386, [March], 1944.

37. COPE, O., LANGOHR, J. L., MOORE, F. J. and WEBSTER, R. C., JR.   Expeditious Care of Full Thickness Burn Wounds by Surgical Excision and Grafting, *Ann. Surg.*, 125:1-22, [Jan.], 1947.

38. ACKMAN, D., GERRIE, J. W., PRITCHARD, J. E. and MILLS, E. S.   Report on Management of Burns using Occlusive Compression Dressings with Sulphathiazole Emulsion, *Ann. Surg.*, 119:161-177, [Feb.], 1944.

39. MELENEY, F. L.   A Statistical Analyses of a Study of the Prevention of Infection in Soft Part Wounds, Compound Fractures and Burns with Special Reference to the Sulfonamides, *Surg., Gynec. & Obst.*, 80:263-296, 1945.

40. ANDRUS, W. DE.W. and DINGWALL, J. A., III.   Further Experience with Treatment of Burns with Sulfonamide Impregnated Membranes, *Ann. Surg.*, 119:694-699, [May], 1944.

41. HOWES, E. J., JR.   Local Chemotherapy of Wounds. Tissue Toxicity of Certain Anti-Bacterial Substances, *Surg., Gynec. & Obst.*, 83:1-14, [July], 1946.

42. LEVENSON, S. M. and LUND, C. C.   Dermatome Skin Grafts for Burns in Patients Prepared with Dry Dressings and With and Without Penicillin, *New England J. Med.*, 233:607-612, [Nov. 22], 1945.

43. LEVENSON, S. M., DAVIDSON, C. S., LUND, C. C. and TAYLOR, F. H. L.   The Nutrition of Patients with Thermal Burns, *Surg., Gynec. & Obst.*, 80:449-469, [May], 1945.

44. SPINELLA, J.   Personal Communication.

45. EMERSON, C. P., JR. and EBERT, R. V.   A Clinical Study of Transfusion Reactions, *J. Clin. Invest.*, 25:627-638, [July], 1946.

46. MOORE, F. D., PEACOCK, W. C., BLAKELY, E. and COPE, O.   The Anemia of Thermal Burns, *Ann. Surg.*, 124:811-839, [Nov.], 1946.

4

PREOPERATIVE AND POSTOPERATIVE CARE

Robert Elman, M.D.

The scope of preoperative and postoperative care has expanded considerably during the past decade. Much of this has been stimulated by World War II. It has followed the obvious need for a more positive program of active therapy with the objective of further improving surgical results. Much of this improvement has greatly extended the field of surgery because many more patients previously considered inoperable are now a good risk even for extensive procedures. At the same time, improved methods have greatly reduced postoperative complications and made possible a more rapid and efficient restoration of the patient after operation by greatly shortening the period of disability.

In this chapter only the general features of preoperative and postoperative therapy will be considered, based largely upon abdominal operations. It is obvious that specific details will depend upon the part of the body to be explored and the type of operation to be carried out. These specific details will be described under each appropriate heading. However, many principles discussed in this chapter will apply to operation in all parts of the body.

GENERAL CONSIDERATIONS

It is necessary to consider first a number of general factors which greatly influence surgical convalescence [3] regardless of the operative procedure. These factors are closely related and affect each other in a reciprocal fashion, but will be discussed under the following three headings: nutritional, physical and psychogenic.

Nutritional Factors. Aside from the administration of water, electrolyte and glucose, the nutritional needs of the surgical patient have been long neglected. Yet it is obvious that malnutrition, present before operation or developing after operation, is of serious consequence. The harmful effects of nutritional deficiencies are now being recognized more and more.[4] Measures to prevent and combat them demand primary consideration in any plan of preoperative and postoperative care.

Under the term of nutrition one must consider the patient's needs for each of the six nutritional elements; these are water, electrolyte, carbohydrate, fat, protein, and vitamins. In this way it is possible to integrate under one designation the needs of the surgical patient not only for food itself, but also for such specific procedures as injections of saline, glucose, vitamins and amino acids, as well as whole blood and plasma transfusions. Many advantages recommend the inclusion of this therapy under nutrition. One of them is the fact that the various fluids, including whole blood and plasma, all contain elements which normally are met from the food we eat. Moreover, the basic physiological behavior of all fluids and food is the same, whether they are given through the oral or parenteral channel. Finally, the various elements are so intimately connected with each other that it is only by a sound understanding of their relationships that effective therapy can be carried out.

The objectives in the nutritional care of the surgical patient may be classified as: (a) the correction of deficits; and (b) the prevention of deficits. In many cases both objectives may be met through the oral channel by seeing that the patient ingests an adequate amount of the various elements which are missing or which are needed to maintain normal function. When gastrointestinal function is normal and the oral route can be used effectively, it is obviously the most convenient, the cheapest, the simplest, and usually the most efficient. On the other hand, the parenteral and particularly the intravenous route is often necessary, usually for one or both of the following reasons: (a) the deficit is so acute and the manifestations so severe that time becomes an important consideration and the missing elements must be given rapidly, usually directly into the blood stream; and (b) the gastrointestinal tract for one reason or another cannot or should not be used.

Even when the parenteral route is necessary it must always be employed for as short a period of time as possible. Intravenous injections are not only inconvenient and expensive, but not without potential danger. Although frequently life saving, they should be terminated as soon as the patient is able to take the needed elements by mouth.

THE ESSENTIAL NUTRITIONAL ELEMENTS. Of the six elements mentioned above, all but one (fat) may be listed as essential, at least for the short periods of time most patients are under surgical care. The probable amounts of each of the five essential nutritional elements required may be briefly listed as follows.

In the case of *water,* many liters may be required to correct acute deficits which occur in the simple dehydration which follows actual loss from vomiting, diarrhea, fistulae or excessive sweating. Up to 5 or more liters are often necessary in the average sized adult, dependent upon the severity of the loss. Water deprivation during complete starvation will also produce dehydration, but it will involve mostly intracellular water and be associated with loss of protein tissue. The amount of water lost may be quite large, but also requires protein for its restoration. For ordinary daily maintenance it is probable that 2000 cc. for an average sized adult is the minimum requirement, although as much as 3 liters can be used without difficulty. This water is needed to a considerable extent for efficient renal activity and for other purposes. The amount increases per unit of body weight in children and particularly in infants.

The exact amount of *electrolyte* required in surgical patients is known only as far as sodium chloride is concerned. Much less is known of the other salts. This is so because sodium chloride is the most important salt in the extracellular fluid. The behavior of this salt is fundamentally different than that of water because, unlike water, it is not utilized or consumed during metabolic activity. As long as there is no actual loss of sodium chloride as in vomiting, for example, the daily needs may be met with a few grams without physiological impairment. Because of the fact that excessive amounts may prove injurious, the general statement should be emphasized that sodium chloride is added to the intake of the surgical patient only when sodium chloride has been or is being lost from the body. For correction of salt losses, isotonic saline is used. Each liter contains 8.5 grams of sodium chloride. Because the fluid lost in vomiting, diarrhea, through fistulae and profuse sweating contains sodium chloride, several liters may be needed to correct the resultant dehydration.

The *energy* needs are best met by an adequate intake of carbohydrate and fat, lest protein be utilized for this purpose. For the average sized adult at rest in bed, 1600 calories per day are needed; more should be given in severe malnutrition, during fever and in other conditions. In well nourished individuals, much of the caloric need, perhaps three-fourths of it, may be temporarily and safely met by the patient's adipose tissue. A minimum of at least 100 grams of carbohydrate will be required to permit utilization of tissue fat and to obviate the loss of protein for caloric purposes. The energy needs in terms of body weight are much greater in childhood and infancy.

The need for *protein* is a little more complicated because of the fact that both acute and chronic deficits may be present or develop in surgical patients. For example, much protein tissue may have been lost because of protein starvation. Considerable protein tissue is destroyed after operation because of increased catabolic activity. Additional amounts may be lost in blood or plasma from wounds, ulcerating surfaces, inflammatory areas and into body cavities. For daily maintenance in a normal sized surgical patient not suffering excessive losses, it is probable that about 50 to 100 grams of protein a day are sufficient. Such an amount will not meet excessive acute losses nor will it rapidly correct chronic deficits. As much as 200 or 300 grams a day may be advisable in certain cases and as much as 500 grams a day have actually been administered. Protein may be given by mouth either in the form of whole protein or as hydrolyzed protein, the latter obviously sparing the need for digestion. Protein may also be injected intravenously, either as plasma or whole blood transfusions, which are especially valuable in correcting acute deficits in the blood proteins and red cells, or as amino acid and peptide mixtures (appropriate solutions of hydrolyzed protein) which are a means of providing parenteral protein food.

The *vitamin* needs of the surgical patient may be unusually great because surgical diseases and particularly operative procedures may increase greatly the requirements. For example, as much as a gram or more of vitamin C may be needed instead of the usual 100 mg. a day. The same is probably true of thiamine. Vitamin K will also be necessary in various types of hepatic disease. Because even large doses can be given either as a single pill or by a hypodermic injection, there is no practical problem in vitamin therapy. Indeed, it is probable that few surgical patients fail to get an adequate assortment of vitamins by mouth or by hypodermic, whether they need them or not.

SURGERY WITHOUT STARVATION. Attention to the nutritional needs of the surgical patient will permit extensive surgical procedures without starvation, which was frequent in the past and is still true at present. By means of methods now available, it is possible to meet a considerable part if not all of the nutritional requirements, regardless of whether the patient is able to eat or not. In this way, many of the untoward manifestations due to malnutrition may be partly or completely relieved or avoided. In planning a nutritional program, three general principles may be emphasized.

First of all, *nutritional care must begin at once.* If the patient is already malnourished at the time he is first seen, the problem is, of course, greater. While it may be difficult or impossible to restore the patient to a normal nutritional condition, treatment should be directed toward correcting as much of the deficit as is convenient. Too often, however, starvation occurs while the patient is under surgical care and this must be prevented by meticulous attention to the nutritional intake from the very beginning. If the surgeon awaits the development of severe nutritional deficiencies, the problem becomes greatly multiplied. Even one day of starvation must be considered as harmful.

A second practical consideration is the advisability of giving *preference to the protein requirements* by sacrificing when necessary a considerable amount of the caloric needs in sick yet fairly well nourished patients unable to take a full, well-balanced diet. This is based upon the relative dispensability of the patient's adipose tissue, which is a true store of body food and may be called upon to supply calories in times of emergency. Because about 80 per cent of the actual bulk of the diet is due to food meeting energy requirements, caloric restriction may be of considerable value. These considerations apply both to oral as well as parenteral administration.

A third consideration is one which is frequently overlooked, *i.e., food ordered but not eaten is of no nutritional value* to the patient. One may not assume that the patient has actually consumed the prepared diet; too often a barely tasted tray is removed by maids or orderlies who make no record thereof. Only close and continuous scrutiny will detect the discrepancy between what the surgeon has ordered the patient to eat, and what is really eaten. An actual study in a large convalescent hospital showed [15] that little more than a third of the protein needs were consumed.

Physical Factors. It is now recognized that prolonged rest and immobility after operation may be responsible for a number of postoperative complications. While rest is an important factor in promoting the healing process, this mechanism must be used judiciously and must not be taken to mean complete or indefinite immobility of the patient in the horizontal position. Such immobility may lead to decreased pulmonary ventilation and an increase in pulmonary complications; it tends to delay the return of normal function of the gastrointestinal and genitourinary tracts; it promotes the development of deep thrombosis in the legs and a consequent increase in the danger of embolism; it is responsible for impairment of neuromuscular and even peripheral circulatory function.

A planned program of movement must become a part of any modern postoperative régime. It begins with movements of the respiratory apparatus to promote aeration of the lungs. It involves a change from the horizontal to the upright position as early and as frequently as possible. It includes movement exercises in bed as well as the usual frequent change of position, and finally it means the termination of bed rest as soon as possible. The beneficial effects of early ambulation have been described by many, perhaps the most recent detailed study being that of Powers.[12] Contraindications to early ambulation are as follows: inflammatory lesions of the lower extremities, in which the dependency is harmful; intraperitoneal infections, particularly general peritonitis; severe circulatory impairment; and certain types of pulmonary disease.

Psychogenic Factors. To give adequate attention to the influence of mind over matter does not mean that the surgeon must become either a metaphysician or a neuropsychiatrist. It simply means that he must take a leaf out of the notebook of the general practitioner, whose great stock in trade was the fact that he *knew* his patients. In the case of the surgeon it may be impossible to know all about his patients, but this does not mean that he may limit his knowledge of a patient simply to the sex, age, and diagnosis. Such an impersonal and detached relationship of itself frequently permits the development of many psychogenic disturbances which in turn may impair the efficacy of surgical convalescence by leading to certain complications. It is axiomatic that the patient whose mind is at rest, who has few fears or apprehensions, and who has implicit faith in his surgeon, will overcome the effects of operation much more rapidly, will begin movement earlier, overcome anorexia earlier, and will return to full activity in a much shorter period of time. There have been but few studies by either surgeons or psychiatrists of the influence of psychogenic factors in surgical patients. One of the most stimulating has been that of Brooks.[1] Only a brief summary of his study has been published, and it is to be hoped that many further details will become available in the future.

The principal method used in psychotherapy is, in general, of course, a simple one. It consists of an adequate visit with the patient, which may be called an interview, the technic of which has been well discussed by Heath.[7] A useful interview requires a certain amount of time, but it is time that is well spent, not only before operation, but during the days after operation, before the patient leaves the hospital. Such an interview must be unhurried and must convey to the patient a real personal interest. Moreover, it must be a two-way procedure. The surgeon has a good deal to tell the patient in regard to the plans for operation and what is expected of the patient after operation. For example, many unpleasant procedures such as the passage of a nasal tube, will be better tolerated if the reasons for its use and the probable time of its removal are explained to the patient. A policy of early ambulation and of infrequent dressings may be misinterpreted by the patient or the family, unless the surgeon takes the time to discuss them before hand. But the interview should also be an opportunity for the patient to tell the surgeon of his fears, apprehensions, and any other important details he has on his mind. The presence of some members of the family may be advisable, although in some instances the absence of over-solicitous relatives may be a very important detail in evaluating the psychological situation. It is almost impossible to have a satisfactory visit while surrounded by a coterie of interns, residents and visiting doctors; the surgeon should not be accompanied by his "staff" during this interview. Very often talking with the family must be separate from that with the patient, particularly in the case of carcinoma.

The problem of what to tell the patient with cancer is not an easy one. Each case must be evaluated on the individual circumstances. It is the belief of the author that, as a general rule, patients should *not* be told that they have this disease unless a direct and unequivocal answer is demanded. On the other hand, some responsible member of the family should be told. Even in hopeless cases absolute dogmatism must be avoided, particularly as to the eventual duration of life. It has been the author's experience that most patients will accept any reasonable explanation of their illness and will not demand a definite answer in regard to the presence or absence of carcinoma. Various terms may be used by the surgeon to explain a malignant lesion. The justification for this pseudo-deception lies in the fact that it maintains the morale of most patients and gives them a hopeful attitude which in itself may be perfectly justified in case the carcinoma is adequately removed. This is important because of the almost universally hopeless reaction most patients have when confronted by the fact that they have carcinoma even though they are told that the entire tumor has been excised.

Attention to psychogenic factors is also important for still another reason. It gives the surgeon great psychotherapeutic opportunities not connected with the surgical lesion, often to the envy of his psychiatric colleagues. Many patients will accept important advice concerning their general health from the surgeon before they leave the hospital, when they will not do so from their own family physician. While many surgeons might refuse to accept this therapeutic opportunity, they should at least realize its possibilities. Indeed, the surgeon should consider himself as a part of the therapeutic team whose objective is to restore the patient not only to his previous condition of health, but, if possible, to a higher plane of physical and mental efficiency.

PREOPERATIVE PREPARATION

Preoperative preparation is of obvious importance in patients already ill for some time and therefore are poor operative risks. But even if the patient has been in good health, operation should never be carried out without at least a minimum of preoperative study. In discussing preoperative preparation, the following three headings will be used: diagnostic observations; special preparatory procedures; and routine preoperative orders.

Diagnostic Observations. A complete history, thorough physical and laboratory examinations are always important, but particularly so in surgical patients about to be operated upon. This responsibility of the surgeon in charge is often greatly aided by the interns' and even the nurses' routine observations. Thorough diagnostic study may avoid an unnecessary operation, particularly the tragedy of an ill-advised one; it may detect physical defects which may be important yet have nothing to do with the primary complaint. A number of examples may be cited. Thus, psychogenic factors may be detected which have a definite relation to manifestations of supposed surgical diseases; such information may clearly exclude a diagnosis of appendicitis, which seemed otherwise obvious. Evidence of an early pregnancy may be obtained in a patient about to have an abdominal operation for a suspected acute surgical lesion. Careful examination of abdominal pain and tenderness may show that they are located in the wall rather than in the peritoneal cavity. Finding pathogenic amoebae in the stool may explain the acute abdominal symptoms as a manifestation of amoebiasis and thus prevent an immediate abdominal operation which is known to be hazardous in this disease. An eruption characteristic of herpes zoster may be noted along the lower right costal margin and indicate that the diagnosis of acute cholecystitis was erroneous. Neurological changes may show that the patient's symptoms are due to a tabetic crisis rather than to a perforated ulcer.

The routine history and examination may reveal an upper respiratory infection, evidence of renal disease or diabetes, which may demand postponement of an operation of choice. A furuncle or other infection near the operative field may be found which may have a similar significance. On the other hand, the physical examination may reveal a carcinomatous lump in the breast of which the patient has been completely unaware. An important group of patients are those admitted soon after an accident which commonly involves multiple injuries, all of which must obviously be discovered and treated. These are a few examples illustrating the importance of maintaining a careful and thorough routine of diagnostic observations in all patients before operation.

Laboratory examinations are an important part of diagnosis and should include as routine, measurements of the red and white cell count and urinalysis. Unsuspected urinary infections, nephritis, diabetes, anemia, leukemia sometimes are often first made evident as a result of this routine. In a few cases additional laboratory examinations may be necessary, including blood chemical study; in surgical patients the following measurements may be of value: nonprotein nitrogen of the blood; fractional serum proteins; CO_2 combining power; and blood chlorides. In special cases involving disturbances in calcium metabolism, the phosphorus and calcium of the plasma may have to be measured. Other determinations may be indicated in special cases such as alkaline and acid phosphatase and tests of liver function.

In addition to the usual routine examinations, special procedures are sometimes necessary. If no urine can be passed or there is any evidence of retention of urine, the bladder may have to be catheterized. Catheterization may also be indicated in females who are menstruating or in whom considerable vaginal discharge is present, each of which tends to prevent the passage of uncontaminated urine. Lumbar puncture may also be indicated in special cases if there is any question about involvement of the central nervous system. X-ray examinations of various types are obviously indicated whenever necessary. Considerable judgment, of course, must be exercised in carrying out expensive and time-consuming diagnostic procedures lest many of them prove to be unnecessary. In general, however, if there is any doubt it is better to err on the side of finding a negative result than to miss important information which may decisively affect the need for an operation or the choice of anesthesia.

OPERATIVE RISK. Diagnostic observations are particularly important in estimating operative risk. Such information is useful to the surgeon not only in making a decision in regard to an operation of choice, but also in choosing the type of anesthetic when the procedure is urgent. For example, the existence of pregnancy may not contraindicate a necessary operation, but it should be known in order to take measures to insure against abortion following operation. While advanced age may permit a major operation with safety, it imposes certain requirements in regard to anesthesia, particularly the avoidance of depressing drugs and the use of local anesthesia when possible. Operation in the early years of life, on the other hand, offers no particular problem except for the fact that babies and young children have much greater metabolic activity and require larger amounts of fluid to maintain water balance.

The presence of organic disease such as hypertension, nephritis and heart disease may also influence the operative risk. In general, however, many major operations may be carried out in the presence of advanced conditions of this kind. Obviously the degree and seriousness of the disease in comparison with the urgency of the operation must be carefully evaluated. In the case of diabetes, preoperative preparation with insulin and glucose may greatly reduce the risk. Patients with liver disease can similarly be prepared and thus the risk of even major procedures greatly reduced. Sufficient time for adequate preparation is nearly always well spent.

Special Preoperative Procedures. To a considerable extent special preoperative procedures depend upon the type of operation to be carried out, the details of which will be found in chapters devoted to each particular operation. For example, gastric lavage is essential before operations on the stomach in the presence of gastric retention. The same is true of gastrointestinal decompression in the presence of certain simple mechanical obstructions of the intestines. Cleansing enemas before operations on the colon and gastrointestinal antisepsis with the unabsorbable sulfonamides may also be mentioned. In the case of a gangrenous infected extremity associated with severe systemic signs of toxemia, refrigeration may be indicated as a special procedure before operation. All of these procedures may often be carried out at the same time as nutritional and other deficits are being corrected.

CORRECTION OF DEFICITS. The hazard of operation will be greatly reduced if the patient is in a more or less normal biochemical status. Unfortunately, many patients, by the time they reach the surgeon, have suffered considerable loss of essential body constituents, some due to simple malnutrition, others from vomiting, hemorrhage or wound discharge. Many patients previously considered inoperable may be made relatively safe even for extensive procedures by recognizing and correcting such deficits. Insofar as many of these patients are unable to take fluids or food by mouth, the parenteral route will frequently be required. The length of time available for the correction of such deficits will obviously depend upon the urgency of the operation, a factor which has already been discussed.

The general features for the correction or prevention of deficits in surgical patients have already been described. It might be repeated here that, in general, the oral route should be employed whenever possible, *i.e.*, whenever the patient is able to take fluids and food by mouth and when sufficient time is available. On the other hand, speed is often an important consideration in the preparation of surgical patients and the parenteral, particularly the intravenous, route may be necessary. For example, anemia may be rapidly corrected by transfusions of whole blood or of red cells. This correction will be lasting, provided there is no further loss of red cells. Acute hypoproteinemia is similarly correctable. Depletion of vitamins, both acute and chronic, can also be rapidly replenished by the injection of an appropriate dose. In most cases, water and electrolyte dehydration may also be rapidly remedied by the administration of sufficient isotonic saline solution as such, or in 5 per cent or 10 per cent glucose.

Unlike the relative ease with which acute deficits may be corrected, the replacement of chronic nutritional deficits, particularly of protein, offer considerable difficulty, largely because of the tremendous amounts required. A severely malnourished patient may have lost several kilograms of protein tissue and this is not easy to replenish, particularly by the parenteral route. If the patient is able to eat, a high protein and caloric diet even up to a daily intake of several hundred grams of protein and 5000 calories is advisable and can be done even in the presence of extreme anorexia.[6,14] Even with a high intake, many weeks or months may be required to completely restore a severe deficiency. Hypoproteinemia of nutritional origin is particularly hard to correct, even with large plasma transfusions. This is true because plasma proteins represent but a small compartment (about 3 per cent) of the proteins in the body [13] and the depleted reserves elsewhere must be corrected at the same time. What probably happens after a plasma transfusion in a depleted patient is that the injected protein leaves the blood stream to be used elsewhere. In actual practice both plasma transfusions and protein by mouth are necessary to correct a severe protein deficiency. If the patient is unable to eat, an appropriate solution of hydrolyzed protein must be injected intravenously as a substitute for the ingestion of protein by mouth.

A good parenteral routine in the nutritional preparation of depleted patients unable to take anything by mouth is to inject 2 liters each containing 50 grams of glucose and 50 grams of hydrolyzed protein per day with a plasma or whole blood transfusion every second or third day. To this is added the necessary vitamins and whatever sodium chloride is being lost (as from gastric suction). In special cases acidosis or alkalosis may require special therapy. Naturally, the longer time available for preparation and the larger the intake, the more the deficit can be corrected. However, it is not really necessary to completely correct nutritional deficiencies; even partial correction of protein deficits has been shown to greatly improve the operability and reduce the risk of operative and postoperative complications. A monograph describing the details of parenteral alimentation is now available.[5]

Routine Preoperative Orders. Patients operated on early in the morning must, of course, be awakened in time for the usual routine preparatory procedures. However, this routine should be modified in patients whose operation is scheduled for later in the morning or for the afternoon. If the patient has been given a soporific and is sleeping soundly, there is no reason for awakening him only to have him wait 5 or 6 hours before the operation is to be carried out. Another frequent error in patients whose operation is scheduled for later in the day is the dehydration which results from the routine of ordering nothing by mouth after midnight. Deprivation of fluid and food for 6 to 8 hours is not harmful, but if the patient is to be operated upon in the afternoon, this deprivation may last 14 to 18 hours. In such a case, it is advisable to allow the patient in the morning to have either a liquid breakfast or to give an intravenous infusion of glucose solution, preferably containing hydrolyzed protein.

The night before operation, a soporific drug such as one of the barbiturates by mouth, is a useful routine in order to insure for the patient a good night's rest. A preoperative enema before operation is also advisable because the bowels are generally inactive for several days afterwards. Preoperative catharsis must be condemned because it has been shown to be harmful by increasing postoperative nausea, abdominal pain, vomiting and distention. The field of operation must be adequately prepared by careful shaving and cleansing of the skin over a wide area surrounding the proposed incision. Skin preparation must be especially thorough when the operation is to be carried out over exposed parts of the body such as the hands and feet. Several days may be utilized for this preparation, particularly in individuals with thick horny skin which may harbor many bacteria.

Preoperative anesthetic medication such as morphine, atropine or avertin depends upon the type of anesthesia to be used and is discussed under this heading.

ROUTINE POSTOPERATIVE CARE

Under ideal conditions postoperative care requires rather simple measures aimed at restoration of normal function as soon as possible. After a simple appendectomy or herniotomy, the patient should be able to lead a normal life almost immediately following operation. He begins to eat almost at once, moves about normally, has no pain, sleeps well, and requires very little if any medication. Indeed, in certain clinics patients have been sent home immediately after herniotomy, although such a program is potentially dangerous in view of the possibility of unexpected complications.

Barring complications, which are discussed separately, the routine care of the uneventful postoperative case may be described under the following headings.

Parenteral Fluid. If the effect of the anesthetic is such that the ingestion of fluids or food by mouth provokes nausea and vomiting, the parenteral route is obviously indicated. In adults, a liter of 5 per cent glucose in water, or preferably 5 per cent glucose and 5 per cent hydrolyzed protein is given the afternoon of the operation at a time when the patient is nauseated and cannot eat. This may be repeated the next day if nausea and vomiting persists and as long as the patient is unable to take an adequate amount of food by mouth. If the patient vomits considerably (*i.e.*, 1 liter or more) an additional injection of the same amount of isotonic saline should be given to correct for the loss of water and sodium chloride.

In many cases parenteral alimentation will be required for a longer period of time, particularly in the case of patients with peritoneal infection or patients in whom a gastrointestinal anastamosis has been carried out, particularly gastric resection. In these and other instances the surgeon wishes to keep the gastrointestinal tract completely at rest. In order to avoid starvation during this period, the parenteral route must be used and fluids injected should be as nutritionally complete as possible. A good routine in most cases is the injection of 1 liter in the morning and 1 liter in the afternoon of a solution containing 5 per cent glucose and 5 per cent hydrolyzed protein. This means that the patient will receive 2000 cc. of water, 100 grams of glucose, 100 grams of amino acids and 4 grams of sodium chloride per day, which with vitamins should be adequate. After extensive operation, as much as 1 gram of vitamin C per day should be given. Thiamine, riboflavin and niacin are also given, usually in one single injection once a day. Should there be abnormal loss of fluid either by vomiting, diarrhea, by drainage from fistulas or excessive sweating, isotonic saline must be added to this program to correct the loss, usually volume for volume. For example, if the patient loses 1 liter of gastrointestinal contents through an indwelling gastric catheter, the same amount of isotonic saline should be added to the other parenteral fluids. Other solutions may be indicated in special cases such as plasma where there is a large loss of plasma in the wound, peritoneum, etc., whole blood in case there is destruction or loss of red cells, sodium lactate or ammonium chloride solution in uncompensated acidosis and alkalosis respectively.

Resumption of Oral Intake. The resumption of a normal diet after operation should be done gradually, but as rapidly as possible. In simple cases such as an interval appendectomy, a full diet may be reached in 12 to 24 hours after operation. In the presence of peritonitis it will be necessary to await evidence that the infection has subsided. In the case of gastro-intestinal resection several days may be needed before secretory and motor function is restored sufficiently to permit the ingestion of fluid and food. In such cases, an indwelling gastric catheter placed at the time of operation furnishes a useful means with which to determine the exact time when oral fluids may be given. The tube is clamped before a test drink of water is given. The tube is opened after three hours and if no fluid returns and there is no epigastric distress, it is assumed that gastrointestinal function has returned and the tube is ready to be removed.

According to tradition, the patient, in resuming oral intake, is first given cracked ice, then water only, then a liquid diet without milk, milk is added followed by a soft and finally by a regular diet. This classification is need-lessly complicated, yet is not based on physiologic considerations. Many liquid foods become solid in the stomach and, of course, all solid foods eventually become liquid. The only reason for a division into solid and liquid food is the fact that many patients will not chew solids, but will take liquids without objection or difficulty. A more important and physiological factor is the presence or absence in the diet of food requiring digestion. Obviously, a food which can be absorbed directly requires less functional activity and should be used first. Based upon these considerations, the postoperative diets may be limited to 3, used in chronological order. They are as follows:

SIMPLE LIQUIDS. The first food given consists of simple solutions which require little or no digestion and can be absorbed directly. Common ex-amples are water, either plain or carbonated, tea, coffee without cream, strained fruit and vegetable juices, fat-free broths. These fluids contain only water, salts and glucose. Although broths are supposed to contain protein, actually there is usually so little that most of them are merely flavored saline solutions. These simple fluids are therefore all deficient in protein; the only way to provide a solution of protein food which can be similarly absorbed directly would be to administer an appropriate mixture of amino acids. This has been recommended in order to prevent protein deficiency without resort-ing to parenteral injections during the early postoperative period. If the usual simple fluids are used, protein starvation should be avoided by paren-teral injections of amino acids, as a solution of appropriately hydrolyzed protein.

FULL LIQUIDS. If the patient is able to digest protein, the fluids may be increased to include a sufficient amount thereof. Fluids which require diges-tion but are more or less complete nutritionally include milk, egg nogs, creamed soups, gruels, ice cream, custards. None of these foods require any mastication and therefore are advantageous in sick patients. Physiologically, however, these foods impose just as much digestive activity as solid foods. About 100 grams of protein a day should be provided.

If the patient has a serious protein deficiency or is losing excessive amounts of protein, the surgeon should increase the intake of protein. For this purpose a specially prepared high protein drink may be easily devised. A simple method is the addition of eggs, of skimmed milk powder, or of casein to milk. The following high protein formula has proved palatable and is extensively used at Barnes Hospital in various sick patients, unwilling or unable to ingest the usual diet of solid and liquid food:

Whole or skimmed milk	1 quart
Skimmed milk powder	135 grams
Casec (pure casein)	70 grams
Cocoa	20 grams
Sugar	20 grams

When mixed, this recipe makes a volume of 1600 cc., which contains 136 grams of protein. The caloric content is 1550 when made with whole milk, 1200 with skimmed milk.

THE NORMAL DIET. The patient should as soon as possible eat all solid foods present in the average well-balanced meal. This may prove difficult in many patients to whom the hospital diet does not appeal. Patients frequently will refuse to eat a well-balanced meal with the statement "I couldn't eat this even if I were well." Unfortunately, the objections of patients to hospital fare are frequently justified. Most hospitals buy good food and plan well-balanced diets, only to fail in the cooking and preparation of trays. The remedy is obvious, but not always easy. In view of the tremendous waste of food not eaten, it would seem economical as well as wise for other reasons to make more energetic attempts to improve hospital fare.

The Restoration of Normal Excretory Functions. In the simple cases, most patients require no especial aid in order to urinate or to defecate, particularly if they get out of bed soon after operation. Failure to void must be considered as a complication, and will be discussed under this heading later.

The use of an enema as routine to stimulate an early bowel movement is really unnecessary, inasmuch as most patients will defecate spontaneously within two or three days after operation. It is not absolutely necessary that the patient have a bowel movement immediately after operation and every day thereafter. Indeed, when the patient has received all fluids and food parenterally, little or no fecal matter is formed. The only problem after oral intake is resumed is the possibility of a fecal impaction, which is discussed as a complication.

Restoration of Mobility. The program for the restoration of normal movements should really start before operation with a detailed discussion with the patient. He is given full instructions in regard to movements in bed, breathing exercises and early termination of bed rest. The patient is reassured against any fears of dire consequences from such a program. This in itself will have a beneficial psychic effect and will make the actual carrying out of the program a good deal easier. As soon as the patient is awake from the anesthetic, frequent breathing exercises are started in order to restore full respiratory exchange as rapidly as possible. Calisthenic exercises including movements of the arms and legs at frequent intervals are also important. Early postoperative termination of bed rest, usually spoken of as early ambulation, when properly carried out in conjunction with body and breathing exercises, has been shown to minimize postoperative complications, especially pulmonary embolism and to lead to a more rapid restoration of appetite, strength and neuromuscular function, and in general to greatly shorten surgical convalescence. In spite of these proved advantages, early ambulation should not be used automatically and uncritically as a routine. Moreover, the following conditions contraindicate early ambulation: severe respiratory and cardiac disease, peritonitis, severe infections of the lower extremity, and insecure abdominal incisions. It is probable that early termination of bed rest should be started within the first 24 to 48 hours after operation, and must consist of the patient actually walking, bearing full weight. It is insufficient to merely allow the patient in a chair for 5 minutes and then permit him to remain immobile in bed during the rest of the day. If bed rest is not terminated soon after operation, it probably should be continued for the usual period of a week or 10 days. This belief is based upon the danger that, if the patient remains immobile in bed for 3 or 4 days and then gets up, a thrombus in the deep leg veins, which is likely to form during this period of immobility, will be encouraged to break off and thus increase rather than decrease the incidence of pulmonary embolism.

When the patient gets out of bed for the first time, the influence of example is often important. For this reason, patients on a postoperative ward will usually offer less difficulty. Seeing others carry out a proposed procedure is a very powerful incentive in most cases. The presence of the surgeon, particularly if he helps the patient during the important period when he first gets on his feet, is also effective. Once the patient gets up and walks about, it is usually not difficult to get him to repeat the procedure either the same day or for an increasing length of time on succeeding days. In many cases all that can be done at first is to permit the patient to walk from his bed to a chair and back again.

Patients who have started walking soon after operation are able to leave the hospital earlier than the usual fortnight. In most cases they may return to their home as soon as the sutures are removed or on the eighth or ninth day. If the patient is engaged in sedentary work he may wish to resume full activity by the fourteenth day after operation. For those whose work involves heavy lifting, full activity had better not be resumed for four weeks. Considerable individual variation is permissible, although it is probable that a much longer period is usually assigned to full convalescence than is necessary, particularly when full advantage is taken of the general methods described above.

Care of the Wound. The average clean abdominal wound which has been closed without drainage requires no dressing until the sixth or seventh day, when the skin stitches are to be removed. Occasionally, however, the dressings may have to be loosened if the patient complains of their being too tight. Only if a wound complication is suspected must the dressing be removed for inspection before this time. After removal of the stitches, dry dressing may be applied, which should be kept in place for another week.

After this, simple adhesive or elastoplast dressing may be applied for an additional week or two. This is particularly important if late keloid formation is to be minimized. This keloid is really due to a slow separation of the skin edges and is almost a normal phenomenon, at least in the case of abdominal incisions, and takes the form of a raised scar varying in width and thickness from one to several millimeters. It assumes a pink, sometimes a fiery red color, and may provoke some pain or itching in a few cases. Eventually this keloid diminishes in size, loses its red color and becomes quite inconspicuous. Many months, up to a year, however, may elapse before this occurs. These details should be explained to the patient beforehand lest he misinterpret their significance and become concerned that something has gone wrong with the wound.

When a drain has been placed in the wound, earlier, repeated dressings may be necessary. When the drain has been placed for purposes of allowing for the exit of capillary bleeding, it should be removed within 24 hours. If a loose cosmetic stitch has been placed at the site of the drain it should, of course, be tied at this time. If the drain has been placed for purposes of exteriorizing an infected or potentially infected area in the abdomen, it is usually left in place much longer, particularly if there is excessive discharge. In such a case, the wound may have to be dressed for purposes of cleanliness. In the absence of very much discharge, a dressing may be necessary in order to loosen the drain, usually within 3 or 4 days after operation, although this will depend upon the particular case and the wishes of the surgeon in charge. Complications of the wound will be discussed under another heading.

POSTOPERATIVE COMPLICATIONS

The prompt detection of postoperative complications requires continuous or repeated observation of the patient. An accurate record of the basic measurements (temperature, pulse and respiration) is a *sine quo non*. Frequent measurements of blood pressure, red and white blood cells and blood chemical changes are sometimes necessary. Simple bedside study of the patient is of obvious value. An alert, watchful intern and nursing staff may detect complications before they have become serious, at a time when therapy is apt to be much more effective.

All observations must be sufficiently detailed and carefully recorded beginning immediately after the patient leaves the operating room. Careful records are important not only for the use of relieving personnel, but also because it enables the surgeon to gain a graphic and chronologic picture of what has transpired previous to his visit. If patients do not have special nurses, a postoperative ward offers a convenient way of achieving this objective with a minimum of nursing personnel. In the following classification only the more common complications will be discussed, together with methods of prevention and cure.

Immediate Postanesthetic Complications. Recovery from general anesthesia may be uneventful, particularly if the patient has not had too much anesthesia and has been well aerated before leaving the operating room. In such a case the patient will promptly regain consciousness and present no particular complications. The anesthetist or a qualified nurse must be in constant attendance during this period, particularly to detect respiratory difficulties or circulatory impairment, and to institute resuscitation immediately. A transient fall in blood pressure is not uncommon and is usually neurogenic and returns spontaneously or following elevation of the foot of the bed or the injection of fluids intravenously. In a few instances extreme hyperactivity may be exhibited; such patients obviously require careful supervision and restraints.

Pain. Although pain may be entirely absent, it is commonly one of the earliest of postoperative complications. Although morphine is undoubtedly the best analgesic drug at our disposal, its routine use to combat pain must be condemned because of its depressant and other untoward effects. Morphine must be used only after adequate investigation as to the causes of pain, only in moderate doses, and promptly after the onset of pain. The effectiveness of morphine is greatly enhanced when used early or even prophylactically. Delay raises the pain threshold. The value of morphia increases up to a dose of 15 mg. (one-fourth grain) for a normal sized adult; larger doses above this level intensify the depressant effect, without significantly increasing analgesia.[16] Morphine in general should not be used in the aged, who, moreover, are apt to have much less pain than younger patients. It should also be remembered that the subjective sensation of pain is conditioned by the attitude of the patient. Careful study has shown that the pain threshold may be greatly lowered by fear and apprehension. In a few patients morphine fails to relieve pain or has unpleasant side effects; in such cases other narcotics should be used, such as dilaudid, demerol, pantopon.

Investigation as to the nature and causes of pain should precede medication. After abdominal operations pain is most commonly located in the incision and is largely due to trauma to nerves, deep sutures which have been tied around nerve filaments and the pressure of skin sutures which have been approximated tightly. Midline incisions and subcuticular sutures in the skin are less likely to be followed by such pain. Pain in the incision is always aggravated by severe inflammatory reactions. In most cases incisional pain disappears within 24 hours. In many cases simple measures will afford considerable relief such as gentle change of position, or loosening of tight dressings. When pain is cramp-like and more deeply seated, it occurs later and is often due to increased peristalsis, called "gas pains" and particularly associated with abdominal distention. Such pain will usually yield to gastric lavage or the passage of gas per rectum induced by rectal tube or a small enema. Cathartics are to be severely condemned. In certain patients abdominal pain in reality is due to *urinary retention* which must always be detected early by keeping a record of the patient's urination, and by percussing, if possible, the area of bladder dullness. Simple methods to encourage voiding should be used early and are usually effective: these include the upright position, warmth applied over the bladder area or perineum and a warm enema. Catheterization is sometimes necessary and, while inadvisable as a routine, should not be withheld if pain is severe and simple methods have proved ineffective.

Nausea and Vomiting. Early nausea and vomiting are nearly always transient and due to the effect of a general anesthetic agent, particularly ether. Trauma to the peritoneum in abdominal operations is also a factor. In sensitive patients, nausea and vomiting may persist for no detectable cause and present a difficult problem. Reassurance and nursing care are particularly important; gastric lavage may be indicated, particularly with the idea that gastric retention may be present. Keeping the gastrointestinal tract at rest, together with parenteral feeding for a period of 24 hours or more may permit resumption of oral feeding. In a few patients, solid foods will be tolerated better than liquids. Anything very much desired by the patient is less apt to produce nausea and vomiting. Patients allowed up out of bed early are less apt to suffer nausea and vomiting than those maintained in the horizontal position.

If vomiting is profuse, the loss of fluid leads to dehydration which in itself may provoke further nausea and vomiting. Such dehydration will obviously require the administration of sufficient amounts of isotonic saline, as discussed earlier. When vomiting occurs, an accurate record of intake and output is necessary in order to estimate the degree of dehydration. The secretion of only small amounts of concentrated urine is always significant. The development of acidosis or alkalosis during dehydration must always be kept in mind, in order that appropriate solutions may be used to combat this complication in case ordinary fluids prove inefficient. If nausea and vomiting continue for several days following adequate therapy, the existence of a serious complication should be suspected. These include intestinal obstruction, general peritonitis, and hepatic and renal insufficiency.

Distention. Abdominal distention may be due to a variety of causes including retention of urine, paralytic ileus, intestinal obstruction and acute dilatation of the stomach. *Acute dilatation of the stomach* is of particular importance in surgical patients because it is so readily relieved by gastric lavage, yet may prove serious if neglected. It may be accompanied by repeated regurgitation of small amounts of fluid. It is usually completely prevented by the use of an indwelling tube inserted at the time of operation as already described elsewhere.

General peritonitis may be the cause of abdominal distention but may develop insidiously with very few local or systemic signs, particularly in older individuals. The diagnosis of peritonitis must always be based upon the existence of a cause, which is usually a leak from an inadequately closed intestinal opening or anastamosis. Frequently it is mistaken for an over-distended bladder and may also simulate *intestinal obstruction*. Further details regarding peritonitis and intestinal obstruction will be found elsewhere in the text.

Lack of Sleep. Postoperative convalescence is often impaired by insomnia. Adequate sleep is just as important after operation as in health, but may require specific attention. Relief of pain is axiomatic, good nursing, absence of disturbing psychogenic factors, as already discussed, are also important. However, the surgeon must sometimes resort to pharmacological means. Barbiturates by mouth are commonly used and may be sufficient though they are depressants, especially in the aged. Much more effective and less harmful are chloral hydrate or paraldehyde; in using these drugs a sufficiently large dose must be given. For example, at least 10 to 20 cc. of paraldehyde is usually necessary in order to permit the patient to have a good night's rest, yet this dose is quite safe even in patients in poor general condition. Both chloral hydrate or paraldehyde may be readily given by rectum in patients unable to take fluid by mouth. It should be emphasized that morphine is seldom justified in the absence of severe pain, although occasionally it may be used as a last resort for its depressing effect on the cerebrum.

Failure to Urinate. Failure to urinate in a postoperative patient must always be viewed as an important complication. In most cases it is due to urinary retention, as already discussed. However, *oliguria* or *anuria* must always be suspected, particularly when there is no pain or distention, and when bladder dullness is absent. A definite diagnosis can be made certain when catheterization yields little or no urine. Anuria may be due to many causes, including actual disease of the kidney, functional or organic, obstruction to the ureters, or transient suppression of secretion, particularly due to dehydration. Correction of dehydration is obviously important either by the administration of adequate amounts of saline, plasma or whole blood. It is a mistake, however, to persist in giving parenteral fluids for anuria after dehydration has been corrected; such treatment soon leads to retention of fluid and edema. During periods of anuria the administration of protein nourishment, either by mouth or intravenously, has been condemned by many authorities because it increases the level of nitrogen in the blood. The opposite view is based upon the idea that protein starvation is more injurious than an increased retention of nitrogen. If anuria persists, uremia will supervene.

Aside from the correction of dehydration, anuria usually presents a serious problem in therapy. Correction of anemia, hypoproteinemia and the control of acidosis and alkalosis are of obvious importance. In many cases, however, correction of anuria is dependent upon a restoration of renal function and this in turn depends upon the nature of the primary cause, which may or may not be permanent.

Fecal Impaction. Fecal impaction after operation may in itself give rise to many abdominal complications, including distention, nausea and vomiting and even persistent fever. It is particularly apt to occur in elderly patients and in children. It can only be detected with certainty by rectal examination and will be frequently overlooked unless such an examination is made. A fecal impaction will not necessarily result in the absence of bowel movements, because many of these patients have frequent but small stools. They may have considerable rectal pain, or none at all. Fecal impaction must be treated promptly and by removal of the impaction. This may be achieved in the simple cases by an oil enema followed in several hours by a soapsuds enema. In severe cases, manual manipulation may be necessary to break up the impaction before giving the enema. In some cases instrumental removal may be necessary.

Pulmonary Complications. Postoperative pulmonary complications include a variety of lesions such as pneumonia, pleurisy, bronchitis, pulmonary embolism and massive or patchy atelectasis. Pulmonary complications are much more apt to occur in older patients, after operations in the upper abdomen, and following prolonged procedures and deep anesthesia. Obvious etiological factors are probably responsible in certain cases, such as aspiration into the lungs, particularly of gastric contents or pulmonary embolism from thrombosis in the leg veins. Undoubtedly, however, an important factor is the existence of incomplete pulmonary aeration and of anoxia at any period either during or after operation. The incidence of postoperative pulmonary complications, as reported by many observers, varies widely between about 2 and 3 per cent up to 10 and 20 per cent. The higher figures are undoubtedly due to easily preventable causes.

Early recognition of pulmonary complications is important and is based upon the development of rapid respirations, fever, chest pain, dyspnea, cyanosis and cough. When atelectasis is massive, *i.e.,* involves a lobe or a whole lung, characteristic physical signs such as absence of breath sounds on the affected side and a shift of the mediastinum to the involved side are diagnostic. The sudden development of respiratory difficulty followed by circulatory impairment always suggests embolism. Auscultation and percussion of the lungs are of obvious importance. Roentgenography may be very helpful in differential diagnosis.

The treatment of pulmonary complications should first of all be prophylactic. During the operation expert and individualized anesthesia plus gentle surgery are perhaps the greatest factors in reducing the incidence of pulmonary complications. Avoidance of anoxia, circulatory depression and, in general, large doses of the anesthetic agent, are all of obvious significance. In the case of general anesthesia, an early restoration of consciousness is important because it permits the early use of ambulation, of body movement and of pulmonary exercises which, as already mentioned, will increase vital capacity and pulmonary aeration and thus prevent many cases of patchy atelectasis, as well as other types of pulmonary disease. While the patient is unconscious, other means of inducing deep respirations may be used such as the frequent administration of high concentrations of carbon dioxide.[2] When pulmonary complications are suspected, particularly in obese, older individuals, chemotherapy with penicillin and even with the sulfonamide drugs may be justified as a prophylactic measure, beginning immediately after operation. The importance of ligation of the femoral vein in the prevention of pulmonary embolism is discussed elsewhere.

Once a definite pulmonary complication is present, treatment is largely medical, which in nearly all cases calls for the use of chemotherapy including either penicillin, sulfadiazine, or both. Evacuation of a bronchial plug in atelectasis is specific and often dramatically effective. It can sometimes be induced by rolling the patient from side to side and urging the patient to cough forcibly while supporting the abdominal wall. Aspiration of the bronchi by means of a catheter passed through the glottis may be indicated. Bronchoscopic removal of the obstructing plug may be necessary if simpler methods fail. Oxygen therapy is useful in combating anoxia, particularly when it is started early and combined with adequate respiratory interchange. Two excellent discussions of pulmonary complications in general,[2,11] and one on embolism [9] are recommended.

Thrombosis. Thrombosis following operation is most common in the lower extremities, particularly in the left femoral and saphenous vein. There are really two types of thrombosis, one of which is thrombophlebitis femoris, otherwise known as phlegmasia alba doldens, the so-called milk leg of pregnancy. The thrombus is usually hard, attached firmly to the vein and associated with considerable lymphatic obstruction and arterial spasm. Thrombophlebitis femoris calls for rest in bed, chemotherapy, elevation of the extremity. Much more serious and more insidious, however, is a type of thrombosis, sometimes called phlebothrombosis, in which the thrombosis is soft and loose and thus is much more likely to break off and lead to pulmonary embolism, which when extensive leads to immediate death or in some cases to a fatal outcome within several hours. The incidence of phlebothrombosis of the femoral vein following operation varies tremendously. Because it seems to be more prevalent in some clinics than in others has lead to the belief that geographic and climatic factors play a part in the etiology. The diagnosis of phlebothrombosis is not always easy; unexplained rise in fever and pain in the affected extremity along the veins, particularly in obese, older individuals, are suggestive.

The treatment of thrombosis in general must be based upon prophylaxis as much as possible, and there is considerable evidence that early ambulation will minimize its incidence. The use of anticoagulants as a prophylactic measure has been advocated, but it is certainly too drastic a measure to be used as routine. In selected cases in which thrombosis is to be feared or mild embolism has occurred it may be advisable.

As soon as phlebothrombosis is suspected, anticoagulant therapy has been advocated, to prevent further extension of the thrombus. Ligation of the affected femoral vein, however, is a much more important procedure, particularly as it is designed to, and will, lower the incidence of pulmonary embolism. An excellent discussion of postoperative thrombosis is that of Herman.[8]

Shock and Hemorrhage. Shock without hemorrhage is usually due to the existence of a large amount of damaged tissue in the wound and thus presents a much more complicated problem than shock which follows simple loss of blood. Hemorrhage as a postoperative complication is usually due to inadequate hemostasis during operation. Serious hemorrhage is usually seen from the uterine artery after pelvic operations, from the cystic artery following cholecystectomy, from the superior thyroid artery following thyroidectomy and the splenic artery following splenectomy. It is important to emphasize here that in the use of the silk technic such an accident is usually due to the fact that the ligature is tied too loosely, because of a desire to prevent the tie from breaking. Intestinal strangulation rarely occurs after operation but will also produce shock which may be difficult to differentiate from hemorrhage.

Recognition of surgical shock following operation may be complicated when a general anesthetic has been used and the patient is still under its influence. Knowledge of the details of the operative procedure, however, is of obvious importance. A reasonably certain diagnosis of hemorrhage may justify a second operation to ligate the bleeding vessel. The detailed treatment of shock has been described elsewhere.

Surgical shock may be mistaken for *cardiac failure,* a fortunately rare postoperative event which is apt to be manifested more by dyspnea and cyanosis and later by evidence of pulmonary edema rather than by circulatory impairment alone. The appearance of a fast and often irregular pulse, dilated rather than collapsed veins are also of importance in making a diagnosis of cardiac failure. It is obvious that the injection of large volumes of intravenous fluid may be disastrous in cardiac failure by provoking an immediate fatality due to cardiac dilatation. Indeed, venesection may sometimes be indicated. Appropriate supportive cardiac therapy should be given as indicated in the individual case.

Wound Complications. Complications in the wound include infection, disruption of the deeper layers or of the entire incision, sinuses or fistulas.

Wound infection is usually suspected by an unusual amount of pain or in some cases by asymptomatic fever. Under such conditions the wound should be inspected and if evidence of infection is found, one or more sutures should be removed to permit drainage. If redness only is found, local application of heat may be used in the attempt to prevent suppuration. Chemotherapy may be indicated, as discussed in Chapter 1.

Wound disruption involving the deeper layers may not be evident, yet may entrap a loop of small intestine and thus be responsible for signs of intestinal obstruction. More commonly, separation of the deep layers is only evident later when an incisional hernia develops. Complete disruption of the wound is likely to occur in patients who cough or vomit severely and repeatedly during the postoperative period. Other factors include deficiency of vitamin C and protein as well as inadequate wound closure. The first indication of a complete wound disruption may be the appearance of serous discharge in and through the dressing. On inspection the skin may be still partially healed, or the entire wound may be open and intestines escaping therefrom. Treatment of complete wound disruption, if very slight, may consist of adhesive strapping, but in most cases it is necessary to resuture the wound with through-and-through sutures embracing all of the layers of the abdominal wall. This is done under either local or intravenous pentothal anesthesia. If the patient is severely ill, sutures may be placed while the patient is in bed by infiltrating each side of the wound adequately with novocaine. It is very rare for peritonitis or herniation to follow an adequate secondary closure.

Deep silk or cotton sutures may produce minor wound complications often weeks or months after the patient leaves the hospital. A tiny abscess or sinus will form and persist until or unless the offending suture is discharged or removed. Removal is generally easy by means of a tiny mosquito clamp.

Fever. More than a degree of fever should not accompany even extensive operations in which no infection is already present. However, significant fever may normally follow release of a strangulated hernia or of an intussusception, due presumably to absorption of the products of tissue damage. Otherwise, postoperative fever should always be viewed with concern and an attempt made to determine its cause. In some cases the fever may be due to extensive tissue trauma or inflammation even without infection. Unexplained fever may indicate the development of thrombosis or pulmonary complications. The urinary tract must be searched for evidence of infection either in the kidney or in the bladder, particularly if catheterization has been frequent. The wound must be inspected in order to determine the possibility of a wound infection. In a few cases the cause of the fever may be impossible to determine; chemotherapy may be justified in these cases, although continued search should be made.

Malnutrition. The importance of maintaining the nutrition of the surgical patient has already been emphasized and there is really seldom any excuse for malnutrition which first develops as a postoperative complication. Malnutrition not only prolongs convalescence, but in itself leads to a number of unfortunate complications, of which *decubitus ulcer* is an important one. The nutrition of the postoperative patient must be considered as a responsibility of the surgeon, who must equip himself with a sufficient amount of knowledge in order to see that an adequate amount of food is consumed by the patient from the very beginning of treatment. In the treatment of decubitus ulcer a high nutritional intake plays an important role. Local treatment consists of cleanliness, débridement, and skin graft.

Miscellaneous. Under this heading a number of rare complications will be briefly mentioned. *Air embolism* may follow operations on the pleural cavity because of the access of air into the pulmonary vein, which carries it to the left heart and then to the brain. *Fat embolism* is due to the development of fat emboli in the blood stream, which plug pulmonary and cerebral capillaries. This remarkable and rare complication is more likely to occur after fractures, particularly of the long bones of the lower extremity. Symptoms consist of disturbances in the circulation and in respiration. Diagnosis can sometimes be made by finding the retinal vessels filled with fat, the appearance of fat in sputum, or in the urine. *Hiccup* may be transient and of little significance, except to be annoying to the patient. When persistent, it may be associated with serious complications such as general peritonitis, subdiaphragmatic abscess or uremia. Commonly, it responds to ordinary sedation or to gastric lavage, or to inhalation of CO_2 in high concentration, as for example, by rebreathing into and out of a paper bag for several minutes. *Parotitis,* usually unilateral, is now an infrequent complication and, when treated early, is readily controlled by penicillin therapy, inasmuch as the staphylococcus is usually the responsible organism. Radiotherapy has been used. When suppuration is present, incision and drainage is indicated. Oral hygiene and treatment by dehydration are the best preventive measures.

REFERENCES

1. BROOKS, B. *Ann. Surg.,* 119:289, 1944.
2. DRIPPS, R. D. and DEMING, M. VAN N. *Ann. Surg.,* 124:94, 1946.
3. ELMAN, R. and AKIN, J. T., JR. *Ann. Surg.,* 122:716, 1945.
4. ELMAN, R. *Ann. Surg.,* 120:350, 1944.
5. ELMAN, R. *Parenteral Alimentation,* P. B. Hoeber, Inc., New York, 1946.
6. GOODMAN, J. I. and GARVIN, R. O. *Gastroenterology,* 6:537, 1946.
7. HEATH, C. W. *New England J. Med.,* 234:251, 1946.
8. HERMAN, L. G. *Surg. Clin. N. Am.,* 25:1167, 1945.
9. LAM, C. R. and HOOKER, D. H. *Ann. Surg.,* 123:221, 1946.
10. MCCLURE, R. D. *Am. J. Surg.,* 70:1, 1945.
11. MCGRATH, E. J. *Surg. Clin. N. Am.,* 25:1190, 1945.
12. POWERS, J. H. *Bull. New York Acad. Med.,* 22:38, 1946.
13. SACHAR, L. A., HORVITZ, A. and ELMAN, R. *J. Exper. Med.,* 75:453, 1942.
14. SPENCE, H. Y., EVANS, E. I. and FORBES, J. C. *Ann. Surg.,* 124:131, 1946.
15. STEVENSON, J. A. L., et al. *J. Canad. Med. Soc.,* 2:345, 1945.
16. WOLFF, H. G., et al. *J. Clin. Investigation,* 19:659, 1940.

5

AMPUTATIONS

Francis M. McKeever, M.D.

Amputation is the operation of removal of all or part of an extremity. An amputation through a joint is called a disarticulation.

Successful management of patients requiring amputation requires a knowledge of the following subjects: (1) the indications for amputation; (2) the type of amputation suitable to the pathology present; (3) the relative functional value of the various sites of amputation; (4) the technical steps of the operation; (5) the preparation of the stump for use of a prosthesis; (6) selection of the prosthesis; and (7) education in the use of a prosthesis. The surgeon is responsible to his patient for all these aspects of his care. His responsibility does not cease with the removal of the stitches from the amputation stump.

Amputations are done to save life and to improve function. The usual indications for amputation to save life are: (1) uncontrollable infection; (2) severe irreparable trauma with severance of circulation distal to the site of trauma; (3) occlusive vascular disease with gangrene; and (4) malignant neoplasms of soft tissue or bone.

Amputation to improve function is indicated in deformities, either congenital or acquired, in which an artificial extremity will be more useful and less burdensome to the patient than the deformed and crippled limb. This indication is rare in the upper extremity. It is more frequently seen in the lower extremity for the reason that the functional value of lower extremity prostheses is vastly superior to the functional value of the upper extremity prostheses. Practically any remaining part of a hand, providing it has normal sensation, is superior to the best prosthesis available for the upper extremity, despite the degree of deformity. A hand completely devoid of sensation, due to irreparable nerve damage, is an indication for amputation because of the fact that it will constantly become abraded, ulcerated and infected. Total irreparable lesions of the brachial plexis are the common cause of such extreme disabilities of the hand.

Congenital deformities of the lower extremity in which misalignment and lack of length make ambulation painful and dependent on crutches may be an indication for amputation in adolescence or early adult life. The decision to amputate such an extremity should not be made in infancy or childhood, as the improvement associated with growth and the possibilities of reconstruction cannot always be foretold.

Ununited fractures of the bones of the lower extremity, in which there is a loss of large bone segments and in which bone grafts have failed or hold little chance of success because of extensive replacement of muscle by scar, the age of the patient, or concomitant irreparable nerve damage, may be an indication for amputation. On the other hand, an ununited fracture of the bones of the upper extremity is not reason for amputation. Even though union may be impossible to obtain, the normal hand on a flail arm or forearm cannot be equaled by any prosthesis.

Decisions making deformity an indication for operation are most frequently the result of a patient's experience. Not infrequently an economic aspect of a patient's life causes him to seek the removal of a crippled extremity so that he may function better in his sphere of activity.

PREOPERATIVE CARE OF THE PATIENT

The preparation of the patient for amputation is of great importance in reducing the mortality from this operation. A detailed knowledge of the patient's general condition is of extreme importance.

The individual who comes to amputation because of uncontrollable acute infection is by nature of the indication a desperately ill individual. The infection often has produced a rapidly progressive hemolytic anemia and protein depletion. Transfusion with whole blood prior to operation will often decrease the hazard of operation. The individual who comes to amputation because of a protracted chronic infection frequently has been depleted by chronic sepsis, and has had much parenchymatous damage and a weak myocardium. In such patients the restoration of protein balance and proper hydration before surgery will lessen the risk of the operation.

The individual who requires amputation because of acute trauma may be in severe shock from blood loss and tissue trauma. If this is so, shock should be overcome by supportive measures consisting of intravenous plasma or whole blood transfusion, before carrying out the amputation. Such patients may be suffering from internal injuries and should be thoroughly searched for all effects of trauma, such as cerebral concussion; hemothorax; ruptured hollow viscus, liver, or spleen, etc.

The individual with occlusive vascular disease and gangrene, in a high percentage of instances, is a patient whose margin of safety is narrow. The patient with arteriosclerosis obliterans frequently has a damaged myocardium. The individual with endarteritis obliterans may have the same process in the coronary arteries; and the patient who has plugged an artery with an embolus usually has a fibrillating myocardium. In addition, these patients have often experienced a long preoperative period of pain and narcotization during which depletion of their plasma protein has occurred and dehydration has ensued. The mortality from operation can be immensely reduced by the proper preparation of these patients for surgery.

Diabetes mellitus is a common background in occlusive vascular disease. The gangrenous tissue is often severely infected. The uninvolved tissues of the diabetic with a high blood sugar has little resistance to the progress of infection. Every medical measure *must be employed* to control the diabetes and to carry out the proper care of the diabetes subsequent to surgery. Antibiotics to combat infection should be employed preoperatively and post-operatively. Occasionally the presence of extensive gangrene renders insulin ineffective and makes it impossible to control the diabetes prior to operation. It may be necessary, in order to control the diabetes, to resort to amputation and remove the gangrenous area before the sugar metabolism will yield to insulin. Any neglect of preoperative and postoperative medical measures in diabetics with gangrene will result in a shockingly high mortality rate.

Gangrenous tissue frequently is infected with pathogenic gas bacilli. The value of the preoperative use of polyvalent gas bacillus antitoxin is questionable. It should be used postoperatively at the slightest indication of activity of pathogenic anaerobic bacilli.

With the availability of supportive measures, hasty amputation with disregard for the general condition of the patient is rarely justified.

Preparation of Skin. In those instances where the amputation is a clean surgical operation and the skin can be properly prepared without unduly disturbing the patient and without causing him unnecessary suffering, the extremity should be shaved and cleansed with soap and water and a fat solvent such as benzine. The fat solvent should be removed with ether and the skin coated with a skin antiseptic of high bacteriostatic quality and wrapped in sterile dressings, the day prior to the operation. Immediately preceding the operation, the sterile dressings should be removed and the operative field again coated with the skin antiseptic. The skin preparation should extend widely above the site of amputation and to the most distal part of the extremity below the site of amputation.

Often, because of extensive gangrene or infection, or because of acute trauma, this type of preoperative skin preparation is impractical and would cause the patient too much distress. Where distress would be caused the patient, the skin preparation prior to coming to the operating room should be dispensed with. In these instances the preoperative preparation should be carried out after anesthesia has been instituted. Under anesthesia a wide area of the extremity above and below the site of amputation can be shaved, washed thoroughly with soap and water, cleansed with a fat solvent and ether, and then coated with skin antiseptic. All potentially infected tissue should be thoroughly and snugly covered with drapes so that it will not be a constant source of contamination to the operator's gloves and the operative field.

CHOICE OF ANESTHESIA

Spinal anesthesia is a very satisfactory anesthetic for amputations of the lower extremities in most patients. Exceptions to this are patients in shock, impending shock, or recovering from shock. Spinal anesthesia may produce a marked fall in blood pressure through peripheral vascular dilation. Despite this, the skilled anesthetist may at times use a small, well controlled spinal anesthesia, and augment it with other agents, even in a patient recovering from shock.

The prevention of hypoxia is important in all anesthesia, but particularly so in the patient who comes to amputation because of occlusive vascular disease. These patients will not tolerate any degree of anoxia, and if inhalation anesthetic is used, it should be an agent which allows adequate oxygen content. The cardiac reserve of these individuals is easily overtaxed by mild degrees of hypoxia.

Patients undergoing amputations after prolonged sepsis may have extensive parenchymatous damage and anesthetic agents which have a toxic influence on parenchymatous organs must be avoided.

For amputations of the upper extremity, a form of inhalation anesthesia suitable to the individual patient is most satisfactory. Brachial block anesthesia can be used for amputations through the forearm, but it must be skillfully administered. Nerve block can be used successfully in amputations of the fingers or toes. If a finger is to be amputated at the metacarpophalangeal joint, and the tendons are to be cut off high in the wrist by pulling them down, local nerve block is not a satisfactory anesthetic.

PRINCIPLES OF SURGICAL TECHNIC

The operation of amputation requires the surgical treatment of all tissues of the body: skin, fascia, muscle, nerve, bone and blood vessels. The surgical technic of amputation has as its objective the production of a stump which has soft, flexible, nonadherent skin, and which has no redundant muscle. There should result no protruding bony prominences and the neuromas of all nerves should be well recessed and not subject to pressure. The general contour of the stump, the perfection of which is measured by the manner in which it uses a prosthesis, should be conical.

In order to prevent adherent skin, dissection of the skin flap in the subcutaneous plane must be avoided as much as possible (Fig. 40). Just enough freeing of the skin to permit a smooth closure should be carried out. This rarely needs to exceed 3 centimeters proximal to the distal end of the final skin flaps. The final skin flap is never cut at the initial incision. It is wisest and safest, when incising the skin, to err on the long side; and as a last step, to tailor the skin flap so that a smooth closure without tension and without redundancy results. In this way, wide undermining of the skin flap can be avoided, thus preserving a skin coverage which has normal mobility on its underlying fascia.

Fascia should, whenever possible, be closed over the bone end of an amputation stump. This should always be possible in a definitive closed amputation, but may not be possible in the secondary closure of a stump following an open amputation. Either fascia and skin, or skin alone, should be the only covering of the bone end. Muscle should never be used to cover the bone end. Its presence results in a redundant unattached sliding mass at the end of the stump which shrinks very slowly and ultimately turns to scarred avascular tissue. All muscle should be coned out, at least perpendicular to the bone end, and preferably with its periphery slightly proximal to the bone end. Even in the stump of vascular disease, the presence of excess muscle over the bone end in no way aids the skin circulation, as there are no perforating arteries between muscle and skin.

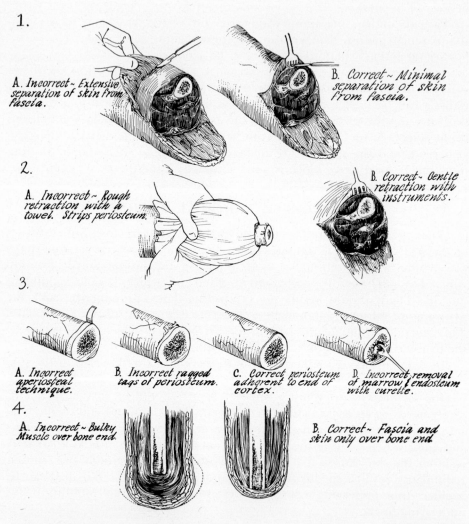

Fig. 40. Principles of surgical technic. (1A) Incorrect. Extensive dissection of skin from fascia. (1B) Correct. Minimal dissection of skin from fascia. (2A) Incorrect. Stripping of periosteum by rough massive retraction of muscles. (2B) Correct. Gentle retraction, periosteum not stripped. (3A) Incorrect. Aperiosteal technic. (3B) Incorrect. Tags of periosteum hanging from bone end. (3C) Correct. Periosteum cleanly incised and adherent to entire circumference of bone end. (3D) Incorrect. Curetting of marrow from bone end. (4A) Incorrect. Mass of muscle over bone end. (4B) Correct. Skin and fascia only, over bone end.

The bone end should be treated by cleanly incising the periosteum, leaving this membrane adherent to the very end of the cortex about the entire circumference of the bone. Extreme gentleness is necessary in handling the bone end, as the vascular periosteum strips easily and extensively with rough retraction. Every stripped or frayed tag of periosteum left in the stump is a potential spur, or myostic deposit. During the act of sawing the bone, the surrounding soft tissues should be protected from bone dust by covering them with moist sponges to catch the bone dust. The moist sponges should be removed when the bone section has been completed and the soft tissues should be thoroughly lavaged with warm saline solution.

Aperiosteal technic, which is the removal of a cuff of periosteum, varying in width from a quarter- to a half-inch, from the circumference of the end of the bone, is not advisable. Neither should the marrow or endosteum be scraped from the end of the bone with a curet. The removal of periosteum from the end of the bone deprives the uncovered bone of blood supply. In the presence of any infection, the ring of bone deprived of the periosteal blood supply will sequestrate. Even in the absence of all infection, in some instances, a ring sequestrum will form because of avascular necrosis of the bone end which has been deprived of the periosteum.

A nerve when sectioned, heals by the formation of a neuroma at its end, due to proliferation of the neuroglia. This neuroma, unless subjected to pressure or repeated blows, is not a source of discomfort. The sectioned end of a nerve in an amputation stump should be well recessed by cutting the nerve trunk high in the fascial plane. Gentle dissection up the fascial plane will permit cutting the nerve off high enough to recess it. It is not necessary to pull the nerve trunk down by forceful traction and then allow it to retract. Large nerve trunks should be ligated with a transfixion suture through their sheath, as they carry a large blood vessel.

The injection of chemicals, such as alcohol, into the nerve trunk does not prevent the formation of a neuroma. Neither does duck-bill closure of the nerve end. A recently advised method of burying the nerve ends in the medullary canal of the bone is inadvisable. If the nerve crosses a joint this may lead to traction on the nerve trunk, on motion of the joint.

Hemostasis is of utmost importance to the end result of an amputation. Large vessels should be ligated and transfixed, and all small muscle bleeders should be tied individually. The development of a moderate hematoma may delay recovery many weeks, produce extensive scarring, and even necessitate further surgery. To avoid the collection of blood under the flaps, even after careful hemostasis, it is well to drain the stump with a small rubber drain for forty-eight hours. Spinal anesthesia, which is frequently the anesthetic employed in lower extremity amputations, causes a drop in blood pressure and may lead to a false evaluation of hemostasis. It is well to know the patient's arterial tension before the wound is closed. If the patient's blood pressure is 20 to 30 millimeters below the preoperative pressure, it should be raised to normal by an injection of ephedrine before the flaps are closed. This will often make a field, that appeared dry, bleed profusely.

Suture material need not be heavy and coarse. Plain No. oo catgut, which causes little tissue irritation, is sufficiently strong for approximating tissue layers and for ligation of smaller vessels. Large arteries, such as the femoral, brachial, and popliteal arteries, should be ligated and transfixed with a slightly heavier suture, such as chromic No. 1 catgut. In open amputations which are severely infected and in which large arteries are present in the open stump, silk ligature may be advisable, as they will withstand the digestive action of inflammatory reaction. The use of small catgut in closing the tissue layers prevents the closure of tissues under tension. Regardless of the strength of suture material, tissues under tension will not remain approximated, as they will tear loose, even though the suture holds. Closure of amputation stumps under tension must be absolutely avoided.

USE OF TOURNIQUET

The use of a tourniquet, when possible, greatly facilitates an amputation and prevents blood loss to the patient. In amputations close to, or at the hip or shoulder, it is impossible to use a tourniquet, and bleeding should be controlled by primary isolation and ligation of the large vessels.

In patients with occlusive vascular disease, the use of a tourniquet in amputations is contraindicated. The pressure of the tourniquet may cause necrosis of poorly vascularized tissue. The use of a tourniquet also interferes with choosing the site of adequate vascularity of tissue for amputation. Bleeding in amputations for vascular disease can always be controlled by isolating and ligating the main vessels as the amputation proceeds. The smaller vessels bleed very little.

When a tourniquet is employed it must be removed after the ligation of the main vessels in order that the smaller vessels may be observed and ligated prior to closure of the stump. Failure to do this may result in a large hematoma in the stump. The removal of the tourniquet should be complete. A common error is to partially release the tourniquet, to a degree which does not stop arterial flow but does block venous return of blood. This results in unnecessary hemorrhage and blood loss to the patient, and can be avoided by making certain that the released tourniquet is producing absolutely no pressure on the skin.

OPEN AMPUTATION

By open amputation is meant an amputation in which the stump is left open so that the tissues may drain. No sutures are used to approximate any of the layers of tissue. The appearance of an open amputation stump is that of a cross section of the extremity. There are two types of open amputation: (1) the open circular amputation; and (2) the open flap amputation. The term "guillotine amputation," is often used to describe the open circular amputation, but is a poor term, as it gives a false idea of the technic of this procedure. "Flap guillotine" is a term used to describe the open flap amputation and is equally misleading. The term, "guillotine amputation," should be discarded.

Open amputation is indicated for any extremity which requires removal when infection is already established or in which the probability of contamination makes the chances for primary healing questionable. Thus, it is the operation of election for any extremity which must be removed because of a severe joint infection or an infected compound fracture; or for a severely traumatized extremity, in which amputation becomes necessary because of injury to the circulation or soft tissue. The patient recovering from severe shock will tolerate an open amputation, as it can be performed much more rapidly than a closed amputation, and with less additional shock. It is also indicated when operating conditions are inadequate, as under the circumstances of war. The open amputation is based on the sound surgical principle of drainage of infected, or potentially infected tissue. This is a surgical principle which has not been abrogated by the addition to the therapeutic armamentarium of the antibiotics, the sulfonamides and penicillin. This basic principle was impressively emphasized by the experiences of World War II. In the early days of the war, great reliance was placed on the antibiotics and with their use, wounds were closed. Despite the liberal use of sulfonamides, both the American and Canadian forces found out early in the African Campaign that drainage of potentially infected wounds was imperative and that violations of this basic surgical principle resulted in a great increase of morbidity and mortality.

The open circular amputation is a two-stage procedure. The first phase of this procedure is the operation for removal of the offending part of the extremity. It is accepted that a second, later operation, consisting of a closed reamputation at the site of election, or a plastic closure of the stump obtained from the open circular amputation, will be necessary at a later date to obtain the final result.

The technic of the first stage, or of the actual removal of the undesirable portion of the extremity, is aimed at producing a slightly concave, open cross section of the extremity, with the skin slightly longer than the superficial muscle and the deep muscle slightly shorter than its overlying muscle (Fig. 41).

Technic of Open Circular Amputation. A circular incision is made through the skin at the lowest level compatible with viable tissue and the skin is allowed to retract. The fascia is then incised in a circular manner at the level to which the skin has retracted. The superficial layer of muscle is then cut at the end of the fascia and permitted to retract. The deeper muscles are then sectioned at the line of retraction of the superficial muscles and allowed to retract. The periosteum is then cleanly incised in a circular manner at the level of deep muscle retraction and the bone cut through at this level. The nerves are cut short and allowed to retract into fascial planes. The larger nerves are transfixed and ligated just proximal to the point of section to guard against bleeding from their artery. Large vessels are transfixed and smaller vessels are tied with plain catgut. The entire cross section of the extremity is left open. The leg is not "chopped off, as if by a cleaver." This procedure, correctly carried out, produces a potentially inverted cone when traction is applied to the skin. It leaves no flaps to interfere with drainage or to trap infection.

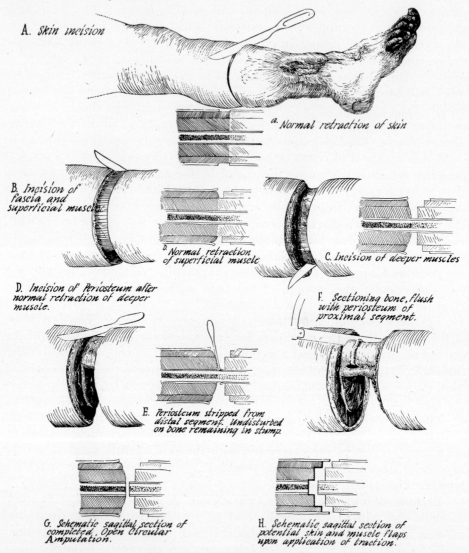

A. *Skin incision*

a. *Normal retraction of skin*

B. *Incision of fascia and superficial muscle*

b. *Normal retraction of superficial muscle*

C. *Incision of deeper muscles*

D. *Incision of Periosteum after normal retraction of deeper muscle.*

F. *Sectioning bone, flush with periosteum of proximal segment.*

E. *Periosteum stripped from distal segment. Undisturbed on bone remaining in stump.*

G. *Schematic sagittal section of completed, Open Circular Amputation.*

H. *Schematic sagittal section of potential skin and muscle flaps upon application of traction.*

FIG. 41. Technic of open circular amputation. (A) Skin incision; (a) Normal retraction of skin due to its elasticity. (B) Incision of fascia and superficial muscle at line of skin retraction; (b) Normal retraction of superficial muscle. (C) Deep muscle incised to bone at level of retraction of superficial muscle. (D) Incision of periosteum flush with level to which deep muscle has retracted. (E) Periosteum stripped from distal segment and left undisturbed on proximal segment. (F) Bone sawed through flush with periosteum attached to proximal segment. (G) Schematic sagittal section of completed open circular amputation. (H) Schematic sagittal section of potential skin and muscle flaps of open circular amputation upon application of traction.

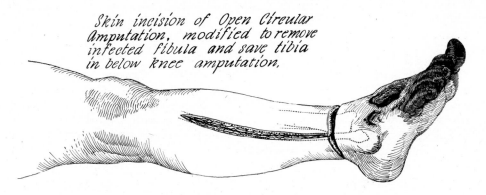

Skin incision of Open Circular Amputation, modified to remove infected fibula and save tibia in below knee amputation.

FIG. 42. Modification of skin in open circular amputation. Distal circular incision joined to longitudinal incision to permit removal of entire fibula.

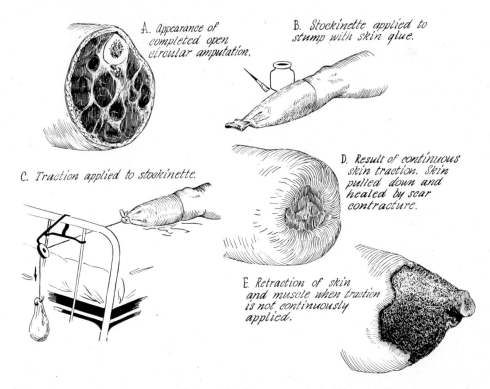

A. *Appearance of completed open circular amputation.*

B. *Stockinette applied to stump with skin glue.*

C. *Traction applied to stockinette.*

D. *Result of continuous skin traction. Skin pulled down and healed by scar contracture.*

E. *Retraction of skin and muscle when traction is not continuously applied.*

FIG. 43. Postoperative care of open circular amputation. (A) Immediate postoperative appearance of open circular amputation. (B) Stockinette applied with glue to skin for traction. (C) Traction pulling on stump through stockinette. (D) Appearance of stump of open circular amputation after traction has been continuously applied for six to eight weeks. Skin has come partly over end and the stump is closed by scar contracture. (E) Appearance of open circular amputation stump which has not had skin traction applied postoperatively. The skin and muscle have retracted from the bone, leaving denuded bone exposed at end.

For a compound fracture, or for an infected fracture, the site of the amputation is at the site of fracture. The incision of the skin need not always be transverse to the long axis of the leg. Its direction may be altered to meet circumstances. If necessary to preserve length, the incision may be at a diagonal to the long axis of the leg, or racquet shaped (Fig. 42). For example, to perform an open circular amputation for an old infected compound fracture of the tibia just above the ankle joint, and an osteomyelitis extending through the entire shaft of the fibula, with draining sinuses, a circular incision could be made just above the ankle. A longitudinal incision could then be extended up the lateral side of the leg in a racquet fashion, to permit removal of the entire fibula and drainage of the infected tissue. This would save a below the knee stump with a functioning knee joint. Any attempt to perform a closed amputation in these circumstances would necessitate a midthigh amputation with greatly increased disability and no assurance that the shortened stump would not become infected.

Meticulous attention to postoperative care is extremely important to the success of an open circular amputation (Fig. 43). Skin traction is absolutely essential after this type of operation. It must be applied immediately, before the patient leaves the operating table, and must be kept up continuously. This is easily accomplished by applying a suitable length of sterile stockinette over the lower 6 to 8 inches of the stump after it has been coated with skin glue, and using enough stockinette to project 12 inches beyond the end of the stump. Traction is applied by gathering up the overhanging length of stockinette and cinching a cord about it. Weights are then hung from the cord over a pulley. This traction in no way interferes with dressing the infected wound. The traction can be released and the stockinette rolled back for dressings. When traction is applied immediately after the completion of the operation, the potentialities of the concave cross section of the extremity are fully developed. The skin, owing to its elasticity, is gradually pulled down over the muscles, the bone end becomes covered by granulation tissue, and the skin margin closed by scar contracture.

If skin traction is not continuously applied, the potentially concave cross section of the leg becomes a greatly exaggerated convex cross section, with 2 to 3 inches of uncovered bone protruding, and a large collar of granulation tissue intervening between the constantly receding skin margin and the bare bone. Such a neglected stump requires a reamputation at a higher site with unwarranted sacrifice of ultimate length.

CLOSURE OF OPEN AMPUTATIONS

The second phase in preparing the open amputation for use of a prosthesis consists of an operative procedure to cover the end of the bone with healthy pliable skin which has good circulation and normal sensation. This closure is usually a simple matter. When there is an area of clean granulation tissue covering the bone end, and when there is no redness or edema of the skin margin the tissues will tolerate surgical closure. These conditions and maximum advance of the skin over the stump end can usually be effected by careful postoperative care, in six to eight weeks following the first operation.

Open circulation amputation in the arm and forearm, with proper postoperative care, will frequently produce a stump which is satisfactory for permanent use. The great laxity of the skin in the upper extremity, and the fact that the pressure exerted by an arm prosthesis is not so great, many times makes a secondary operation unnecessary.

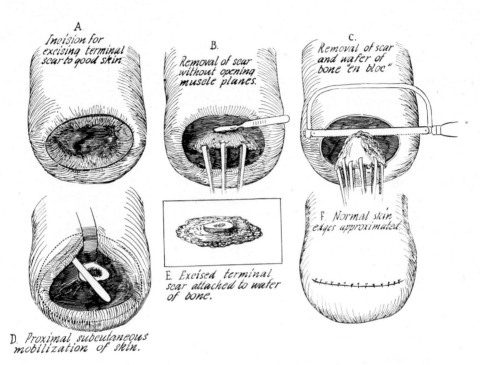

Fig. 44. Technic of closure of open circular amputation after maximum effect of traction has been obtained. (A) Scar on end completely excised to good skin. (B) Scar dissected free to its attachment to bone. (C) Wafter of bone sawed off with scar attached to its periphery. (D) Good skin undermined to permit enough laxity for closure. (E) Wafer of bone and scar which has been removed. (F) Edges of normal skin approximated with interrupted sutures.

Prior to the operative procedure of plastic closure, the stump should be elevated for a period long enough to obviate all dependent edema. Roentgenograms of the bone end should be obtained to determine whether sequestration is occurring. If a sequestrum is forming, closure should be delayed and the sequestrum removed at the proper time. A forming sequestrum can be removed prior to its complete separation by nipping through the line of granulation tissue activity with a bone cutter. This will save much time for the patient.

Plastic closure is usually a simple procedure (Fig. 44).

Technic of Plastic Closure. The scar at the end of the stump is excised to good skin and removed in one piece. If the scar surrounds and adheres to the bone end, the periosteum is incised cleanly about the circumference of the bone and a small wafer of bone cut through with the saw, removing the scar and wafer of bone as one piece. The skin is then separated proximally from the fascia enough to permit of approximation of the skin edges without tension. It may be necessary to undermine the skin for a distance of 7 to 12 centimeters about the entire circumference of the extremity. In many instances it is not necessary to remove any bone, and usually it is not necessary to uncover muscle or open fascial planes if postoperative care has been adequate. The muscle and fascia are always firmly attached to the distal portion of the bone and it is not necessary or advisable to free them and attempt resuture. In a few instances it will be necessary to cut out muscle and shorten bone to get adequate skin for coverage. In below the knee stumps, if the fibula projects, it should be cut off shorter than the tibia. Skin traction is often advisable after plastic closure until healing results, to obviate tension on the suture line.

Reamputation following the technic of a closed amputation can be carried out at the most ideal site possible, *if there is an abundance of stump and the length of the stump is longer than ideal.* For example, if the stump is just above the ankle, the reamputation can be carried out at the site of election in the middle third of the leg; or if a portion of the tarsus remains, a Syme amputation can be performed and closed by primary suture.

The incidence of complications in carrying out the secondary closure, or reamputation, of an open circular amputation is slight. In carrying out the definitive, or final operation, in one series of 2988 stumps in 2783 patients who had had an open circular amputation, a severe recrudescence of infection in the amputated extremity as manifested by cellulitis, abscess, high febrile reaction, and general sepsis, occurred in only twenty instances, or 0.66 per cent. No patient in the series died as a result of the definitive surgery on the open circular stump. Of these patients 5 per cent had some complication of their final surgery. The common complications were a mildly infected hematoma in the stump, without systemic reaction, or a marginal skin necrosis which required a minor skin plastic later. Most of the patients with the complication of hematoma, on its evacuation by the removal of a few stitches, recovered with a satisfactory stump and without further surgery.

OPEN FLAP AMPUTATION

Open flap amputation is carried out by cutting duck-bill flaps of skin fascia and muscle "en bloc" (Fig. 45). The muscle is incised on a diagonal, progressively more proximal than the skin. At the depth of the muscle incision, the bone is sectioned transversely to its long axis. Fascial and muscle planes are not separated. This type of open operation is most applicable to an extremity in which the bone is centered in a mass of muscle with an even distribution of the muscle bulk on all sides of the bone, such as the thigh, arm, or forearm. It does not lend itself well to the leg, in which the tibia is subcutaneous and most of the muscle is posterior to the bone. Open amputations through the hip joint and through the shoulder joint are always open flap amputations. Close to the torso, traction cannot be successfully applied. The duck-bill flaps are packed open until infection subsides sufficiently to

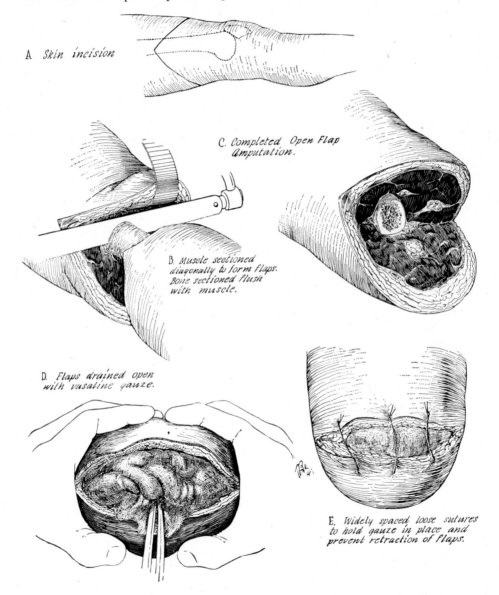

A. *Skin incision*

C. *Completed Open Flap Amputation.*

B. *Muscle sectioned diagonally to form flaps. Bone sectioned flush with muscle.*

D. *Flaps drained open with vasaline gauze.*

E. *Widely spaced loose sutures to hold gauze in place and prevent retraction of flaps.*

FIG. 45. Technic of open flap amputation: (A) Skin incision. (B) Skin-muscle flaps cut "en bloc" without separating planes. (C) Completed open flap amputation with duck-bill flaps of skin and muscle; bone sectioned transversely at level of muscle. (D) Flaps drained open with vaseline gauze. (E) Few loose stitches through skin to prevent vaseline gauze drain from falling out of flaps.

make closure safe. The flaps are then permitted to fall together, or an early secondary closure is done. The flaps easily trap infection. If recovery is uncomplicated in the open flap amputation, time is saved by accomplishing an earlier closure than is possible with the open circular amputation. The resultant stump, however, is very frequently a poor one, with redundant skin and muscle, and it will not suffice for a young, active man. Frequently late secondary operations are required to produce a well tailored stump that can be used hard. For the young, in whom perfection of stump is desired, the open circular type of operation which accepts a second definitive operation to produce the final result, is better than the open flap type of operation. For the aged, who will probably use the prosthesis infrequently and easily, and for whom repeated surgical incidences are not desirable, the open flap operation may at times be superior to the open circular operation.

USE OF SKIN GRAFTS IN AMPUTATIONS

Skin grafts are of little value in effecting closure of an open amputation and are unnecessary if the patient is given proper postoperative care by traction. If a pedicle graft is successfully attached, the skin has imperfect sensation and a small vascular margin of safety. On the lower extremity the flap will not tolerate the trauma of wearing a prosthesis well. The pedicle too often ulcerates and blisters under the trauma of the artificial limb socket. Repeated invalidism and ultimate reamputation at the request of the amputee is the final outcome. Rarely a pedicle graft to save enough of a forearm stump to avoid sacrifice of the elbow or to preserve part of a finger, may be justifiable. The wear and tear of the arm prosthesis is much less than that of a weight bearing artificial limb. Split grafts can be successfully applied early to an open circular amputation stump. *The employment of split grafts to produce early healing does not facilitate the final surgery but makes it more difficult.* The normal skin, instead of coming over the end, as it does with traction, recedes to the margin of the skin graft. When the final surgery is carried out there is a paucity of normal skin and the result is that useful bone length must be sacrificed. When a severely traumatized or burned extremity has widespread skin loss and there is much loss of plasma, early grafting may be the only means of restoring the patient to protein balance. Skin grafting of stumps for other than this reason is usually useless. If for any reason skin grafts are used, the donor site should not be any place on the extremity coming in contact with the prosthesis, as too often painful, irritable keloids result at the donor site, which interfere with the wearing of a prosthesis.

CLOSED AMPUTATION

Closed amputation is an amputation in which the tissues are cut and sutured in a manner which will effect healing of the tissues by first intention and will produce the ultimate desired stump. Closed amputation is indicated in any circumstance demanding an amputation, in which there is no danger from infection. There are several styles of closed amputation for almost every site where an amputation may be necessary. These various kinds of closed amputations are in many instances the product of an individual surgeon's personal taste. Their technic has been carried from book-to-book through the years. They bear no relationship to the practicability of the use of a prosthesis and the availability of the prosthesis. The usefulness of an amputation stump is dependent entirely on how well it uses a prosthesis and whether or not a suitable prosthesis is available to the amputee. Since at the present time the ideas of artificial limb makers vary in different parts of the world, a suitable amputation stump in the United States might not have a prosthesis available for it in another country. Other closed amputations are unsatisfactory from a functional viewpoint. Particularly is this true of many amputations through the foot, where muscle imbalance may be produced by the necessary ablation of antagonistic muscle groups. This muscle imbalance causes painful deformities, which makes the stump difficult to use.

The technic of those kinds of closed amputations which result in the best functional stump and which are most suitable to the prostheses available in the United States will be described in detail. Reference will be made to other closed amputations of less functional value and for which the securing of a prosthesis is more difficult.

CLOSED AMPUTATIONS OF THE LOWER EXTREMITIES

Amputation of Toes. Amputation of toes is not done for hammer toe deformity. The removal of one of the middle three lesser toes frequently allows the remaining toes to migrate medially or laterally, producing a more

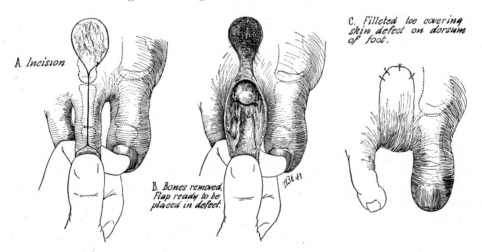

Fig. 46. Technic of filleting toe to save skin for use in filling skin defect. (A) Incision on dorsum of toe, excising scar and uncovering phalanges. (B) Bones and tendons totally removed. (C) Skin flap, representing skin of deboned toe turned back and sutured into defect.

troublesome deformity than that for which the amputation was done. Toe amputations are done for uncorrectable deformities which cause pain through pressure. Correction usually is impossible because of poor soft tissues which have resulted from healed infection. In circulatory disease with gangrene, more radical amputation than the removal of a toe is usually necessary to reach tissues with sufficient circulation to heal.

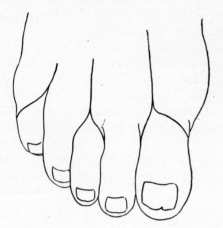

Incisions for disarticulation through Metatarso-phalangeal joints.

FIG. 47. Racquet incisions for disarticulation through metatarsophalangeal joints. On fifth toe, handle of racquet is to inner side of metatarsal bone. On great toe, handle of racquet is to outer side of metatarsal bone. This removes scar from pressure. For outer toes, handle of racquet is over shaft of metatarsals.

The most important of the toes is the great toe. It is the only single toe ever to be left on a foot. Any situation requiring the removal of the great toe and three of the minor toes had best be treated by eventually removing all toes. One remaining minor toe will become a source of trouble due to progressive deformity. It may be wise to temporarily preserve a toe so that the skin can be used on the dorsum of the foot (Fig. 46). By filleting (deboning) a toe, a piece of innervated skin approximating 3 centimeters square can be obtained to swing back over a skin defect on the dorsum of the foot.

Minor toes are not amputated through the two distal phalanges. They are either disarticulated through the metatarsophalangeal joint or amputated just distal to the bulge of the articular surface of the proximal phalanx. In amputating a minor toe the tendons are pulled down, cut off, and allowed to retract. The digital nerves are isolated and cut off high. If this is neglected, painful neuromas develop in the subcutaneous area and may require future surgery for removal. The digital vessels are ligated (Fig. 47). To disarticulate a toe, a racquet incision is made with the handle of the racquet on the dorsum of the foot. *The handle of the racquet should never be made on the sole of the foot,* as it will result in a painful scar on the weight bearing surface (Fig. 48). To amputate a toe through the proximal phalanx a long plantar flap is most desirable. The phalanx is best cut with a Gigli saw. Bone cutting forceps tend to crush and fragment the bone. The flaps are closed with interrupted sutures, loose enough so that no drain is needed.

The great toe is of considerable importance in producing a smooth gait. All possible length of this toe should be preserved. Stiffness in the interphalangeal joint, if not associated with a plantar flexion deformity, is not a source of disability and does not require amputation above this joint (Fig. 49). In amputation of the great toe at a level where the tendon of the extensor proprius hallucis tendon or the flexor hallucis longus tendon is cut, their ends should be either sutured to each other or individually

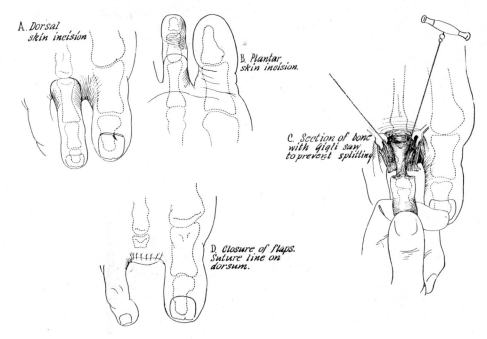

FIG. 48. Technic of amputation of toe through proximal phalanx. (A) Skin incision creating short dorsal flap. (B) Skin incision creating long plantar flap. (C) Bone sectioned with Gigli saw, not bone cutting forceps, which will fragment cortex. (D) Flaps approximated, suture line on dorsum away from pressure.

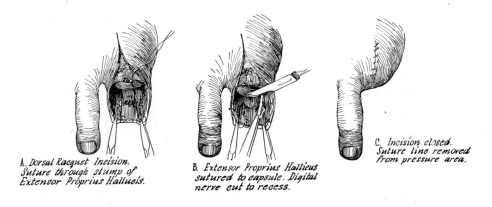

FIG. 49. Technic of disarticulation of great toe. (A) Racquet incision. Stumps of tendons of extensor proprius hallucis muscle and flexor hallucis longus muscle sutured to remains of capsule. (B) Digital nerve cut short to recess its neuroma. (C) Flaps approximated so that scar will fall away from pressure area.

sutured to the capsule of the joint or soft tissue, as they give effect to important muscles. To disarticulate the great toe at the metatarsophalangeal joint a racquet incision is used with the handle of the racquet on the dorsum of the foot, never on the sole or the medial border of the foot. In amputation distal to the metatarsophalangeal joint, a long plantar flap is advisable.

In amputation of the great toe through the distal phalanx, the pulp of the great toe should be used as a long plantar flap. The entire nail bed should be thoroughly removed. If part of the nail bed is left behind, a horny spike of nail may grow out and produce discomfort. Amputation at this point is occasionally the only way to relieve an intractable ingrowing toe nail and is termed "distal Syme amputation."

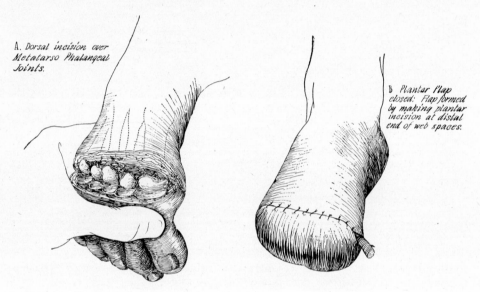

A. Dorsal incision over Metatarso Phalangeal Joints.

B Plantar flap closed: Flap formed by making plantar incision at distal end of web spaces.

FIG. 50. Technic of disarticulation of all toes. (A) Dorsal incision through skin and extensor tendons at level of metatarsophalangeal joints. Dorsal incision of joint capsules. (B) Plantar incision at level of distal end of web spaces, producing flap which removes scar from pressure by placing suture line near dorsum.

Removal of all the toes simultaneously, when indicated, is best accomplished by disarticulation through the metatarsophalangeal joints (Fig. 50). This can be done through a dorsal incision at the level of the metatarsophalangeal joints and a dorsal incision of the metatarsophalangeal joint capsules. A plantar incision at the level of the webs of the toes, which is nearly 3 centimeters distal to the joints, will leave adequate plantar flap to effect a closure with the scar away from the weight-bearing surface of the foot. *In all amputations in the foot, an effort should be made to have the scar site removed from pressure.*

Amputation through the Foot. There is a tendency on the part of surgeons, when amputation through the foot becomes necessary, to save all the bones possible, without regard for good skin coverage and good muscle

control of the stump. This is neither good nor conservative surgical judgment. A foot stump must have good skin coverage, otherwise repeated
ulceration and infection with disability and ultimate higher amputation
will result.

If muscle balance is lost in a foot stump, a progressive deforming force
results, which will ultimately produce a fixed deformity. A fixed deformity
makes weight bearing painful and
may make it impossible to wear a
shoe (Fig. 51). The gastrocnemius
soleus group is attached by the
tendo Achilles to the os calcis. Opposing the action of the calf group
is the anterior tibial muscle, which
attaches to the plantar surfaces of
the cuneiform bone and of the first
metatarsal bone. Additional antag-
onists to the strong calf muscles are
the extensor communis digitorum
and extensor proprius hallucis muscles. The main supinator of the foot
is the posterior tibial muscle. This
inserts on the medial and plantar
surfaces of the navicular and first
cuneiform bone. The principal
pronators of the foot are the
peroneus longus and brevis muscles. The former inserts on the
plantar surface of the cuneiform and
the first metatarsal bones. The latter
attaches to the tuberosity of the
fifth metatarsal.

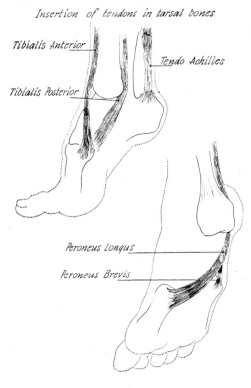

Insertion of tendons in tarsal bones.

Tibialis Anterior

Tendo Achilles

Tibialis Posterior

Peroneus Longus

Peroneus Brevis

FIG. 51. Schematic drawing of insertions
of muscles into tarsus. (A) Insertion of
gastrocnemius soleus group; posterior tibial
and anterior tibial muscles. (B) Insertion of
peroneus longus and peroneus brevis muscles.

Any amputation through the
foot proximal to the metatarsophalangeal joints sacrifices the
dorsiflexor power of the extensor
communis digitorum and extensor
proprius hallucis muscles. If only the action of these two muscles is lost,
a deformity does not ensue. If the amputation is proximal to the bases of
the metatarsals, an inversion deformity of the foot practically always results, even though the anterior tibial is still attached normally. This causes
a callus to form on the outer anterior side of the stump, which results
in great pain. If the amputation is through the tarsal bones proximal
to the insertion of the anterior tibial tendon, a severe fixed equino varus
deformity always results. Surgical attachment of the tendon of this muscle
and of the tendons of the other dorsiflexors cannot be done accurately
enough to balance the stump and practically always fails to obviate the

occurrence of the deformity. *The only satisfactory amputation through the foot is a transmetatarsal amputation.* This amputation leaves the anterior tibial, peroneus longus and brevis, and posterior tibial muscles normally attached.

TECHNIC OF TRANSMETATARSAL AMPUTATION. With the patient in the supine position, a transverse skin incision is made on the dorsum of the

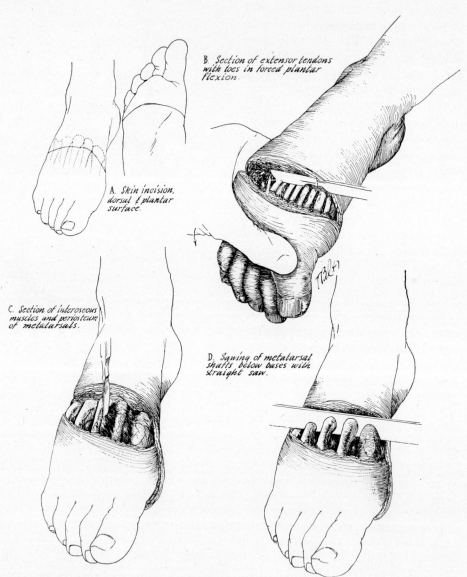

FIG. 52 (1). Technic of transmetatarsal amputation. (A) Skin incision just distal to bases of metatarsals on dorsum of foot with long plantar flap. (B) Sectioning of tendons at level of proximal skin incision. (C) Incision of periosteum and interosseus muscles. (D) Section of metatarsal bones with straight saw.

foot 3 centimeters distal to the base of the first metatarsal (Fig. 52). This incision is carried around the medial and lateral side of the foot to a level with the plantar surface of the first and fifth metatarsal bones. From this point the skin incision is extended distally parallel to the shafts of the first and fifth metatarsals, an adequate distance to form a sufficiently long plantar flap to suture without tension to the dorsal skin margin. The lateral skin incisions are then connected by a transverse incision on the plantar surface of the foot. The incision on the plantar surface of the foot is carried sharply through to the bones. It is wiser to err on the long side in forming the plantar flap, as it can always be trimmed shorter. The dorsal skin is reflected distally in the subcutaneous plane, a sufficient distance to expose the dorsum of the metatarsus. With the foot held in plantar flexion the extensor tendons

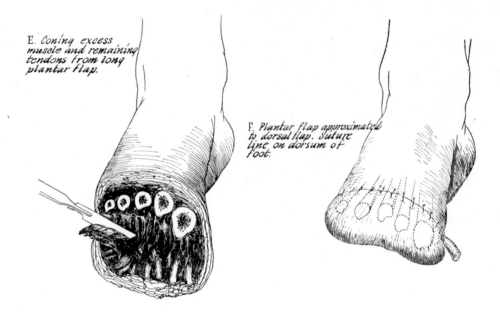

E. *Coning excess muscle and remaining tendons from long plantar flap.*

F. *Plantar flap approximated to dorsal flap. Suture line on dorsum of foot.*

FIG. 52(2). (E) Coning muscle and tendons out of long plantar flap. (F) Flaps approximated, suture line on dorsum of foot, away from pressure area.

of all the toes are sectioned transversely, at the level of the proximal skin edge. This causes them to retract. The periosteum of all the metatarsals is incised sharply on their dorsal, medial and lateral sides, cutting the intervening interosseus muscles with a sharp scalpel. All metatarsals are then sawed through simultaneously with a straight bladed saw at the incised periosteum. The portion of the foot distal to the saw line is gently depressed, and with a large scalpel beneath the metatarsals, the muscles and ligaments are cut extra-periosteally, close to the plantar surface of the metatarsals, until the transverse incision on the sole of the foot is met. This frees the portion of the foot to be discarded. The muscle and tendons are then coned from the plantar flap. Each digital nerve is isolated and cut high in the muscle plane and all digital vessels are individually ligated. Vessels are also present on the dorsum of the foot which require ligature, and any cutaneous nerve present in this area should be recessed. The margin of the plantar skin flap is then approximated with interrupted sutures, without redundancy or tension to the margin of the dorsal skin. The flap should have a drain beneath it for forty-eight hours.

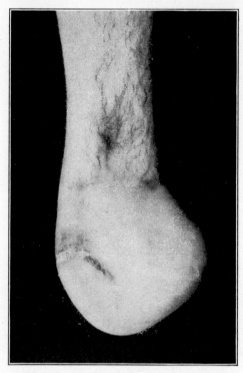

The foot is splinted for seven to ten days in a neutral position, by a posterior molded plaster splint extending from above the knee over the distal end of the stump. This prevents painful muscle cramps and protects the end of the stump if the patient rolls around in bed. Elevation of the extremity also facilitates healing.

Amputation through the foot proximal to the site of attachment of the dorsiflexor muscle destroys muscle balance of the stump (Fig. 53). For this reason the Chopart and Lisfranc amputation is not satisfactory. If amputation cannot be performed at the transmetatarsal level, a Syme amputation should be done. The Pirogoff amputation has no functional advantage over the Syme amputation. It is an osteoplastic procedure, requiring the union of two bones. This union may, and does, occur in a position of deformity. The additional length of the os calcis in the Pirogoff amputation also complicates the fitting of a prosthesis. This amputation might have justification for a field worker, who could not obtain a prosthesis (Fig. 54).

FIG. 53. Chopart foot stump. The anterior dorsiflexor muscle group have no attachment to tarsus. The remains of the foot is fixed in extreme equins, which is not a usable position. (From McKeever, *Surg., Gynec. & Obst.,* 82:495-511, May 1946. By permission of Surgery, Gynecology and Obstetrics.)

Syme Amputation. The Syme amputation is a closed amputation in which the weight bearing skin of the heel is turned over the flared end of the tibia and fibula, thus using skin and subcutaneous tissue which has been accustomed to weight bearing, for that purpose. It is an end-bearing stump; that is, a stump which takes the full weight of the body on the end of the stump, rather than distributing this weight through the sides and higher weight-bearing points.

For the male, the Syme amputation produces the best possible amputation stump in the lower limb, short of a well balanced foot stump (Fig. 55).

It has the advantages that the prosthesis does not extend above the knee and that even without the prosthesis the patient need not use crutches, or hop. Because of the length of the stump and because it is end bearing, an amputee with a Syme stump can walk about his home at night, and when swimming or golfing, can bathe and get around the shower without the necessity of carrying crutches with him.

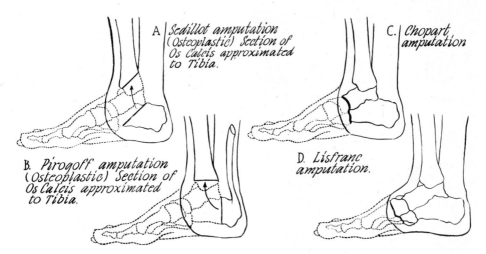

A | Sedillot amputation (Osteoplastic) Section of Os Calcis approximated to Tibia.

B. Pirogoff amputation (Osteoplastic) Section of Os Calcis approximated to Tibia.

C. | Chopart amputation

D. Lisfranc amputation.

FIG. 54. Amputations through tarsus which produce poor stumps, which are difficult to fit with prostheses. (A) Sedillot amputation, osteoplastic procedure, applying portion of os calcis to end of tibia. (B) Pirogoff amputation, osteoplastic procedure in which piece of os calcis must unite to tibia. (C) Chopart amputation, a stump with poor muscle balance. (D) Lisfranc amputation, a stump with poor muscle balance. (Dotted lines represent portion of foot removed.)

The Syme amputation is unsuitable for a woman. The prosthesis for this amputation is unsightly at the ankle, due to its bulkiness. From a cosmetic viewpoint, it is probable that a woman would be unhappy with this type of amputation, despite its superiority of function. The Syme amputation is contraindicated if there is any sign of circulatory inadequacy. If circulation is poor the heel flap will probably slough, and if it survives it will be painful on weight bearing.

The operative technic and the postoperative care of the Syme amputation are more exacting than in any other amputation. The vascular supply of the heel skin flap used to cover the end of the stump stems almost completely from the medial side of the ankle through a branch of the posterior tibial artery. *If the operation is carried out from the inside out, by disarticulating the ankle through the anterior part of the incision and the os calcis is enucleated subperiosteally,* the blood supply of the skin flap is never endangered and any chance of skin necrosis is obviated. If the foot is removed from the outside inward and the skin-fat flap of the heel is taken off the os calcis extraperiosteally, there is great danger that the blood supply to the flap will be damaged and that the heel skin will undergo necrosis (Fig. 56).

In the immediate postoperative period there is a tendency for the heel flap to slide to the inside of the stump and to assume a varus position, so that the pad of the heel is to the end of the tibia, like a side car on a motorcycle. This results in a useless stump, painful on the outer side, which cannot handle a prosthesis comfortably. This tendency of the heel flap to slide is easily overcome by maintaining it centered over the end of the tibia with adhesive straps, which are applied at the end of the operation and changed at intervals for a period of four weeks. At the end of this time the soft tissue pad is well bonded to the tibia and there is no further danger of medial displacement.

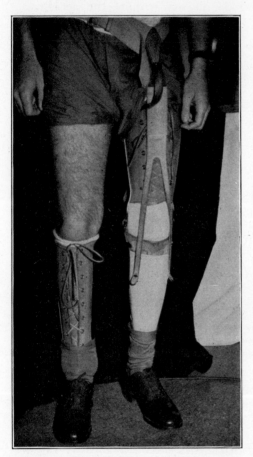

Fig. 55. Syme prosthesis on left leg. Does not extend above knee. Prosthesis on right leg is for six inches below the knee stump. (From McKeever, *Surg., Gynec. & Obst.,* 82:495-511, May 1946. By permission of Surgery, Gynecology and Obstetrics.)

TECHNIC OF THE SYME AMPUTATION. With the patient supine, the foot is elevated 4 inches from the operating table by placing a soft, stable pad under the middle of the calf. The foot is plantar flexed 10 to 20 degrees to permit palpation of the anterior ankle joint line. The skin is incised transversely, exactly over the anterior ankle joint line (Fig. 57). The skin incision is then carried diagonally posterior on both the medial and lateral side of the foot, passing 1 centimeter anterior to the tip of the internal malleolus of the tibia, and the same distance anterior to the tip of the external malleolus of the fibula. The incision is carried on both the medial and lateral side of the foot to the under surface of the heel, which it crosses transversely 1 centimeter posterior to the inner tubercle of the plantar surface of the os calcis. The incision on the plantar surface is carried vertically straight through skin and fat and the periosteum of the plantar surface of the heel bone. On the medial side, the incision is carried vertically through the tendons of the posterior tibial, flexor hallucis longus and flexor communis digitorum muscles, the posterior tibial nerve and artery, and the periosteum of the os calcis. On the lateral side it is carried vertically through the tendons of the peroneus longus and brevis muscle and the periosteum of the os calcis.

The foot is then forcefully plantar flexed with the left hand, and with the knife in the right hand, the tendons of the anterior tibial, the extensor proprius hallucis, and the extensor communis digitorum muscles are cut at the level of the distal end of the skin flap. The anterior tibial vessel is clamped as it is cut and the branches of the superficial peroneal nerve isolated and cut back high under the skin edge. The anterior joint capsule is incised transversely at the lower margin of the tibia. With the foot still forcefully held in plantar flexion, the deltoid ligament of the ankle on the medial side and the anterior astragalofibular (talofibular) ligament on the outer side of the ankle joint are sectioned from inside the ankle joint. This permits the astragalus to be completely dislocated by forceful plantar flexion of the foot and exposes the attachment of the tendo Achilles to the posterior tubercle of the os calcis. With a sharp periosteal elevator, working from the inside of the ankle joint and starting at the upper margin of the attachment of the tendo Achilles, the periosteum, which is a definite layer, is pushed off the sides and plantar surface of the os calcis to the point where the periosteum has been incised through the initial incision. When this point has been reached, the part of the foot to be sacrificed is free and can be discarded.

The incision at this stage presents the lower articular surface of the tibia and fibula and a distal posterior flap with heel skin, thick subcutaneous fat, a cup of periosteum continuous with the end of the tendo Achilles. On the lateral side, the stumps of the peroneus longus and brevis tendons may be visible. If they are, they are pulled down, cut with a knife, and permitted to retract. In the medial side of the flap the stumps of the tendons of the posterior tibial, flexor hallucis longus and flexor communis digitorum muscles may be visible. If so, they are pulled down, cut trans-

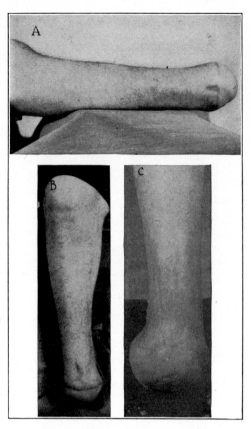

FIG. 56. (A) Lateral view of good Syme stump. Heel pad well centered. (B) Anteroposterior view of good Syme stump. Heel pad well centered under tibia. (C) Poor Syme stump. Heel pad displaced to medial side of tibia, end of fibula prominent. Will not tolerate prosthesis comfortably when heel pad is displaced to inner side. (From McKeever, *Surg., Gynec. & Obst.,* 82:495-511, May 1946. By permission of Surgery, Gynecology and Obstetrics.)

versely with a knife, and allowed to retract. In this side of the flap the end of the posterior tibial artery and any of its branches which are patent are isolated and ligated. The posterior tibial nerve is isolated, dissected upward in the subcutaneous tissue adequately to recess its neuroma, ligated and sectioned. In doing this, care must be exercised not to damage branches of the artery, which are the main blood supply of the flap.

The anterior skin flap and the sides of the flaps are gently retracted to expose the lower end of the tibia and fibula for a distance of 2 centimeters.

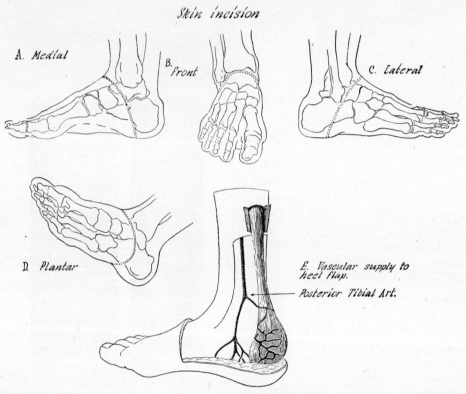

FIG. 57 (1). Technic of Syme amputation. (A) Skin incision, medial view. (B) Skin incision, front view. (C) Skin incision, lateral view. (D) Skin incision, plantar view. (E) Circulation to skin-fascia-flap, coming from posterior tibial artery, medial side of foot and extraperiosteal.

The periosteum of the fibula and tibia are incised sharply about the outer circumference of the joint and 1 centimeter proximal to the articular cartilage of the tibia. With a straight saw, a wafer of bone including the complete articular surface of the tibia, and about 1 centimeter of the cancellous end of the tibia is sawed through. The lower end of the fibula is sawed through transversely at the same level and in the same maneuver. This removal of the malleoli of the ankle joint is always below the inferior tibiofibular ligament so as not to result in a diastasis of the lower end of the tibia and fibula. Sectioned at this level there is a flare left, which is composed of the bound together ends of the tibia and fibula. Section of the bones above this flare results in an unsatisfactory stump, which will lack a bulbous end. As the posterior margin of the tibia is reached with the saw it must be moved gently. It is often wise to grasp the anterior margin of the piece of bone to be removed with a tenaculum, open the saw line gently, and sever the posterior periosteal attachments of the tibia with a scalpel.

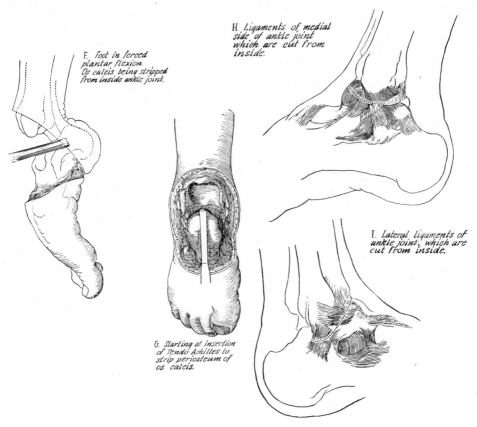

FIG. 57(2). (F) Astragalus dislocated by plantar flexion of foot. (G) Peeling os calcis out subperiosteally from inside. (H) Ligaments of medial side of ankle, which are cut from inside joint. (I) Ligaments of lateral side of ankle joint which are cut from inside joint.

When this is completed, the tourniquet is removed and all bleeding points clamped and ligated so that a very dry flap is obtained. Bone wax should not be used on the lower end of the tibia. The cancellous bone will ooze a little and then clot. If there is a spurter in the bone it can be crushed with a blunt instrument.

When hemostasis is satisfactory, the posterior flap of the heel skin is lifted up so that its distal margin approximates the distal margin of the anterior skin of the leg. The subcutaneous tissue is approximated with a few interrupted sutures of plain No. oo catgut and the skin with interrupted silk sutures, spaced to produce an accurate closure. When the proximal and distal flaps are approximated there will be a large dog ear at the medial and lateral end of the suture line. *These dog ears must be left and not trimmed to make a smooth closure.* Removing these dog ears endangers the blood supply by producing a narrow pedicle of skin between the heel flap and the leg skin, doing away with its broad base. A drain is placed in the

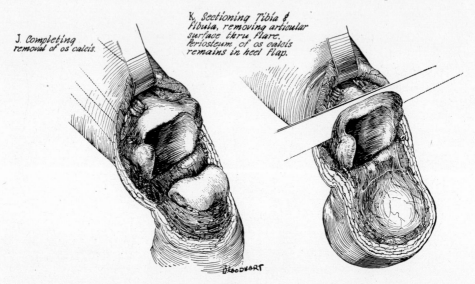

J. Completing removal of os calcis.

K. Sectioning Tibia & Fibula, removing articular surface thru flare. Periosteum of os calcis remains in heel flap.

Fig. 57(3). (J) Astragalus being peeled out of periosteum. (K) Foot completely amputated; periosteum of os calcis in posterior flap; articular cartilage of tibia and fibula being removed through flare.

medial or lateral dog ear, and left for forty-eight hours. It is well to suture the drain to the skin with one stitch through drain and skin. The incision is dressed with a small piece of vaseline gauze. The lower two-thirds of the leg and the heel pad are then coated generously with skin glue, avoiding the suture line, as sealing it off will prevent the escape of hematoma. The heel pad is then held accurately centered over the lower end of the tibia and fibula, both as to lateral and anteroposterior relationship. Strips of sterile canton flannel 1 inch wide and long enough to extend two-thirds of the way up the leg on two sides, are applied over the skin glue; one strip starting on the medial side, run across the heel pad, and up the lateral side; and the other strip started on the posterior aspect of the calf, run over the heel pad, and up the anterior aspect of the calf. A few dry dressings are then applied over the end of the stump. A tensor bandage is wrapped firmly in spiral fashion around the dressings and up the leg over the canton flannel strips. Further dressings of sheet wadding and pads are then applied for bulk and comfort. The canton flannel strips and tensor bandage must not be tight enough to shut off circulation, but must be firm enough to maintain the flap properly centered on the end of the bones. The calf group attached through the tendo Achilles tends to pull the flap medially and posteriorly.

This mode of fixation is changed as dressings are necessary or as it becomes soiled, but must be applied continuously until the skin-fat flap is bonded to the tibia and fibula. This requires four weeks, on the average.

Amputation through the Leg. The ideal length of bone in an amputation stump of the leg is 5 to 7 inches of tibia. For an individual over 6 feet in height, the tibial length should approach 7 inches. In an individual only

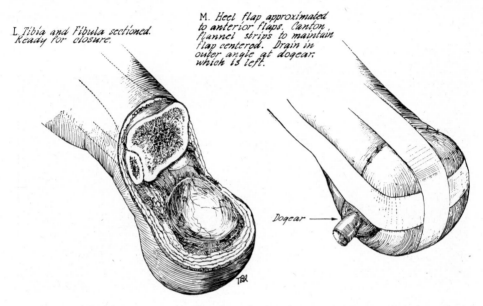

FIG. 57(4). (L) Stump completed and ready for closure. (M) Stump closed. Drain in medial angle of incision, next to dog-ear of skin which is not removed. Straps glued to skin holding flap centered over end of tibia and fibula.

slightly over 5 feet in height, 5 inches of tibia is sufficient. This bone length is best measured from the superior articular surface of the tibia, which is easily palpable at the joint line. The estimation of bone length should be done with a ruler and carefully marked. Sighting the length will result in errors up to an inch or more. The eye cannot be trusted. Leg stumps longer than this are difficult to fit with a prosthesis and may require a contour of the calf of the prosthesis which is disproportionate to the normal calf. Stumps longer than 5 to 7 inches also leave on the leg a portion of the tendinous part of the calf which is less well vascularized than the upper muscular portion. The presence of tissue which is below maximum vascularity leads to coldness, pain, and ulceration of the skin. Skin of this quality heals slowly from abrasions.

Leg stumps shorter than 5 inches are very useful and the inability to amputate at a level which produces this length stump does not indicate an above the knee amputation. Providing it can be covered with good skin, any length of stump which can be seen to project when the knee is flexed, should be saved. A stump which projects as little as 1 inch when the knee is flexed to a right angle is of value to the patient as a motor for moving the prosthesis through the motion of the normal knee. Although a patient with such an abbreviated below the knee stump will have to wear the same type of prosthesis as an above the knee amputee, he will use his prosthesis better than an above the knee amputee and will have greater security and control in going down inclines. A patient with a stump which projects 3 inches below the thigh when the knee is flexed will be able to do well with the ordinary below the knee prosthesis and will not need an ischial bearing prosthesis.

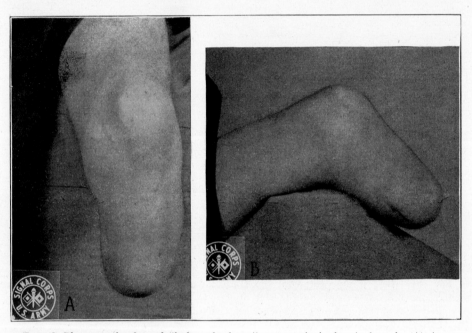

Fig. 58. Photograph of good "below the knee" stump, six inches in length. (A) Antero-posterior view. (B) Lateral view scar posterior to bone end; stump conical. (From Mc-Keever, *Surg., Gynec. & Obst.,* 82:495-511, May 1946. By permission of Surgery, Gynecology and Obstetrics.)

Fitting of short below the knee stumps with a prosthesis is difficult and trying. Despite this, the knee should never be sacrificed when the stump can be seen to project with the tibia flexed to a right angle on the femur, if there is good circulation in the stump and if the stump can be covered with normal skin.

The fibula should never project beyond or to the same level as the tibia. In a leg stump the fibula must always be cut shorter than the tibia. The end of the fibula in the ideal stump should be 3 centimeters above the end of the tibia (Fig. 58). If it projects beyond or reaches to the level of the end of the tibia it is pressed on by the socket of the prosthesis and the superior tibiofibular articulation, a diarthrodial joint with little motion is sprung. This results in pain. The pressure over a projecting fibula often results in a painful bursa. In leg stumps short of the ideal length, shortening of the fibula relative to the tibia may lead to the presence of such a short section of fibula that it projects laterally and is unstable. In these circumstances the entire fibula should be removed. Removal of the entire fibula may produce enough laxity of skin to permit of satisfactory closure of an otherwise inadequate skin flap. In these circumstances, removal of the entire remains of the fibula is indicated, even though its absence does make the fitting with a prosthesis more difficult. Removal of the head of the fibula does not produce instability of a disabling degree in the knee joint of an amputee.

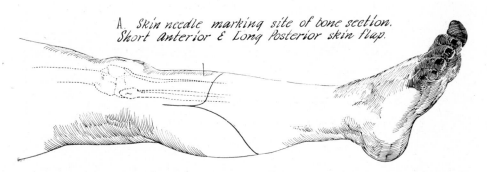

A. Skin needle marking site of bone section. Short anterior & Long Posterior skin flap.

FIG. 59 (1). Technic of below the knee amputation. (A) Skin incision, needle marking level of bone section.

A leg stump is not an end-bearing stump. The weight is distributed in the socket of the prosthesis through the tibial tuberosities, the head of the fibula, the tibial tubercle, and the entire circumference of the stump. In the socket of the prosthesis, the skin is tensed by upward traction. It is desirable to have the terminal scar fall just behind the posterior surface of the tibia, so that it will not adhere to the end of the bone. However, stump length should not be sacrificed to place the terminal scar at any certain position.

TECHNIC OF AMPUTATION THROUGH THE LEG. With the patient supine, the thigh is supported on a rest or pad, with the hip flexed 45 degrees. The prone position is advocated by some surgeons in performing below the knee amputations. In this position the knee can be flexed easily to make the end of the stump upright. It is a tiresome position for the elderly patient and adds to the difficulties of anesthesia. Unless a surgeon is doing amputations frequently, the anatomy is presented from an unusual angle and errors in cutting flaps can happen. For the surgeon doing an occasional amputation, the supine position is better. This elevates the leg 10 to 12 inches from the surface of the operating table and makes it possible to freely flex and extend the knee (Fig. 59). The desired length of tibia, 5 to 7 inches, dependent on the height of the patient, is measured from the superior-articular surface of the tibia with a ruler or steel tape. The desired length of bone is accurately marked by inserting a skin needle through the skin, well into the muscles on the medial side of the tibia. The needle is left in place for a marker until the bone is cut. The skin flaps are cut by incising the skin and

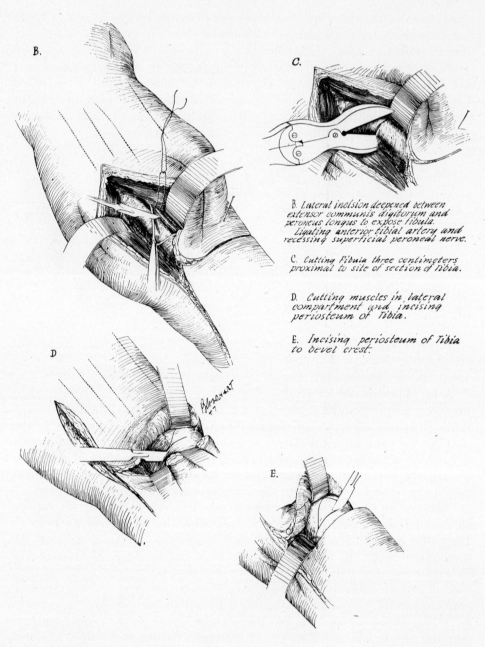

B.

C.

B. *Lateral incision deepened between extensor communis digitorum and peroneus longus to expose fibula. Ligating anterior tibial artery and recessing superficial peroneal nerve.*

C. *Cutting fibula three centimeters proximal to site of section of tibia.*

D. *Cutting muscles in lateral compartment and incising periosteum of Tibia.*

E. *Incising periosteum of Tibia to bevel crest.*

D.

E.

FIG. 59(2). (B) Fibula exposed through lateral incision. (C) Cutting fibula with double action bone cutting forceps. (D) Exposing tibia by cutting muscles of lateral compartment transversely at level of bone section. (E) Sharp incision of periosteum of tibia, cutting flap for bevel.

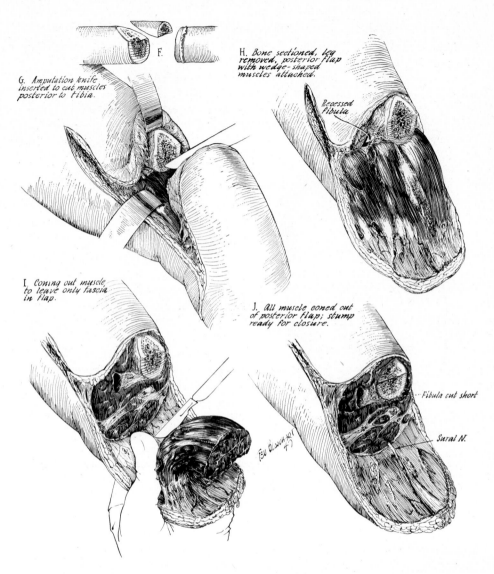

FIG. 59(3). (F) Schematic drawing of section and bevel of tibia. (G) Cutting posterior muscle with amputation knife after complete section of tibia. (H) Amputated portion of leg removed; wedge of muscle in posterior flap. (I) Coning out muscle vertical to bone to leave only fascia in posterior flap. (J) All muscle coned out of posterior flap. Ready for closure of stump.

subcutaneous tissue in U-shaped flaps with broad bases, which meet on the lateral side just anterior to the fibula and on the medial side of the leg at a corresponding level. The anterior flap should project 6 to 8 centimeters below the needle which marks the point where the tibia is to be sectioned. The length of this flap will depend on the thickness of the tibia. The posterior skin flap should be twice as long as the anterior flap, 12 to 16 centimeters. At the point on the lateral and medial side of the leg where the curve of the anterior and posterior flaps meet, a horizontal incision is carried through the skin and superficial fascia proximally for 5 to 7 centimeters. The enveloping fascia of the leg, over the front of the tibia and lateral compartment of the leg is thin and sometimes indefinite. This fascia is incised, following the contour of the anterior skin flap. The cut anterior flap, consisting of skin, subcutaneous tissue, and enveloping fascia, is turned upward to a point 4 centimeters proximal to the point at which the tibia has been marked by the needle to be sectioned. Care is taken not to separate skin from fascia. The fascia in the lateral incision is incised and raised adequately to expose the opposed edges of the extensor communis digitorum and the peroneus longus muscles. This junction is opened through the length of the lateral incision, the plane of cleavage developed, and the muscle belly of the extensor communis digitorum pulled forward with a smooth retractor, exposing the anterior sharp edge of the fibula and the interosseus membrane. The superficial peroneal nerve and anterior tibial artery are visible in the incision and are grasped with snaps and cut. The anterior tibial artery is ligated. The circumference of the fibula is exposed extraperiosteally by sharp dissection, cutting away the interosseus membrane and the origin of the peroneal muscles. The periosteum of the fibula is incised sharply, about the circumference of the bone at the point 3 centimeters proximal to the site at which the tibia is to be sectioned. Distal to this periosteal incision, the periosteum is pushed off the fibula for an inch with an elevator. The proximal periosteum is not disturbed. The fibula is then cut at the end of the adherent periosteum with a powerful double action bone cutting forceps. To do this cleanly without fragmenting the fibula, it is necessary to first nip into the bone. Attempts at cutting the fibula in one bite will result in splintering of the cortex.

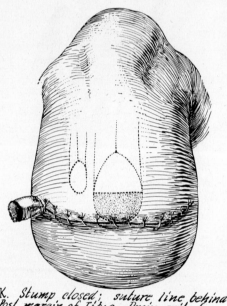

K. Stump closed; suture line behind Post. margin of Tibia. Drain exits from Fibular fossa.

FIG. 59(4). (K) Stump closed. Suture line posterior to bone; drain from lateral angle of suture line into fibular fossa.

The muscles of the lateral compartment are incised transversely at the level at which the tibia is to be sectioned. The periosteum of the tibia is then incised with a sharp scalpel about its circumference, at the point of section. A tongue of periosteum with the point proximal and the base distal is cut on the front of the anterior half of the crest of the tibia, tapering the crest for 2 centimeters. With a sharp elevator, the periosteum is pushed off the tibia distal to the line of incision, but not disturbed proximally. The tibia is then cut with a straight saw immediately adjacent to the adherent proximal periosteum while the incised muscles are gently retracted. The taper on the crest is first cut with the saw to a point beyond the expected transverse section. The tibia is then sawed through transversely at the selected level. As the posterior cortex is cut through it is necessary to support the part of the leg to be removed, to prevent splintering of the tibia and stripping periosteum. The distal segment of the leg is dropped slightly, opening a V at the point the tibia is sectioned. The muscles posterior to the tibia are cut into with a scalpel through this V. An amputation knife is then passed through the calf muscles and behind the fibula just anterior to the cut margins of the posterior skin flap at the level of the bone section and moved distally, cutting the gastrocnemius-soleus muscles and fascia diagonally from before, backward along the margins of the posterior skin flap, to the end of the flap. When this maneuver is complete the portion of the leg to be discarded is free and is removed.

The posterior flap, containing a triangular wedge of muscle, is then supported on a moist sponge in the palm of the left hand. The base of the triangular mass of muscle is cut across transversely, or slightly convexly, so that the distal end of the muscle will eventually be 1 to 2 centimeters proximal to the end of the tibia. The muscle is cut through until the thick, shiny posterior enveloping fascia is seen, and then peeled distally off the fascia. The muscle separates nicely from the fascia without shreds. When this is accomplished, the sural nerve is seen coming out of the muscle and perforating the fascia. This nerve is pulled through its foramen in the fascia, followed up into the muscle, ligated, and recessed.

The superficial peroneal nerve which has previously been identified in the fibular incision is ligated and recessed. The posterior tibial nerve is isolated, its sheath transfixed, and the nerve ligated well up in its fascial plane, so that its resulting neuroma will be recessed.

The posterior tibial artery and veins are isolated and ligated by transfixion with No. 1 chromic catgut. The peroneal vessels, which lie just medial to the fibula, and posterior to the interosseus membrane, are identified and ligated by transfixion. The anterior tibial vessels were previously ligated. If a tourniquet has been used, it is released completely, making sure there is no obstruction to venous backflow. All bleeding vessels, muscular branches, are individually ligated. Time is spent to obtain a dry field. Large veins are encountered in the subcutaneous tissue of the posterior flap, which should be carefully tied.

The skin is then separated for a centimeter or two from the fascia. The fascia of the posterior flap is pulled up and sutured to the fascia of the anterior flap, after tailoring it to fit without tension or redundancy. Plain No. 00 catgut is large enough for this. A rubber drain is placed beneath the fascia in the lateral aspect of the suture line so that it drains the muscular fossa around the shortened fibula. The skin is cut to fit smoothly without tension or redundancy and approximated with interrupted sutures of fine silk. The drain is sutured to the skin with one suture, cut long for identification, so that the drain will not fall out of the stump. Closure should be adequate to produce good approximation but not so tight that blood cannot escape.

The suture line is covered with vaseline gauze, copious dressings are applied, and the stump wrapped with sterile sheet wadding to the groin. A tensor bandage is wrapped snugly over the sheet wadding to midthigh. A posterior molded plaster splint is applied from the gluteal fold to the end of the stump and turned up and over the distal end of the stump to afford protection. The knee is placed in 15 to 20 degrees of flexion. Splinting prevents muscle spasm.

If the amputation is done just below the tuberosities of the tibia to preserve a very short stump, there will be no muscle to remove from the stump. Posteriorly the loose areolar tissue of the popliteal space is met between the small gastrocnemius heads. The peroneal nerve will be encountered in its entirety and should be mobilized and sectioned well up behind the femur. This can be accomplished by retraction without disturbing the contour of the skin flaps. At this area only skin and subcutaneous tissue are available to cover the bone end.

Amputation through the Thigh. The ideal site for amputation through the thigh is through the supracondylar area of the femur. Amputation at a level just below the point at which the femur begins to flare for the condyles produces a stump which is conical, which has a long, well controlled bone lever, and which has a broad base for end bearing. Section of the femur at this level also leaves room enough for a knee mechanism in the prosthesis, without making the calf of the prosthesis short. British surgeons do not favor amputation at this level. They condemn all end-bearing stumps and they fit all thigh stumps with a prosthesis which has a brake mechanism in the knee. The knee joint in use in British prostheses takes up more room than amputation at this site provides, without necessitating a disproportion between the thigh and calf pieces, which causes the knee of the prosthesis to project beyond the normal knee when the amputee is sitting down. As the length of femur in a thigh stump decreases above the supracondylar area, the difficulty of using a prosthesis increases. With the stump produced by removal of the entire femur, as in a disarticulation of the hip, the use of a prosthesis is so difficult that many people prefer to use crutches rather than to tolerate the cumbersome artificial leg. If an amputation through the thigh cannot be done as low as the supracondylar level, all possible length of the femur should be saved.

There are two types of supracondylar amputations for producing an end bearing thigh stump. These are: (1) tendoplastic amputation, in which the patella is removed and the tendinous portion of the quadriceps muscle pulled over the end of the femur; and (2) Gritti-Stokes amputation, in which the patella is placed at the end of the sectioned femur. These operations both produce excellent end bearing stumps and as far as function is concerned, there is little choice between them. The Gritti-Stokes operation will, in a certain number of instances, result in an unsatisfactory stump, despite the best of technic. It is an osteoplastic procedure, requiring the union of two bones to be successful. Even a mild infection may cause a failure of union of the patella to the femur, or an osteomyelitis of both the patella and femur (Fig. 60). Because of potentially infected tissue, the Gritti-Stokes type

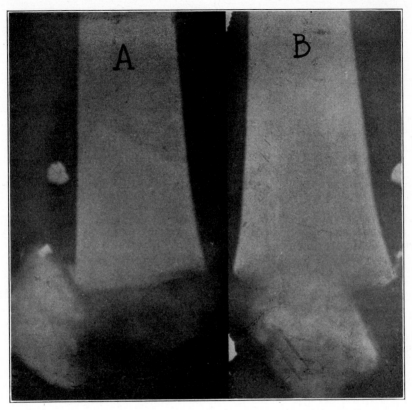

FIG. 60. Roentgenograms of Gritti-Stokes stump, which, due to infection, has resulted in osteomyelitis of tibia and patella with non-union. (A) Lateral view. (B) Anteroposterior view. (From McKeever, *Surg., Gynec. & Obst.*, 82:495-511, May 1946. By permission of Surgery, Gynecology and Obstetrics.)

of amputation is not often applicable to the reamputation or closure of open amputations. Even though the best of technic is employed in carrying out the Gritti-Stokes amputation, the patella will, in a few instances, be pulled off the center of the end of the femur and a nonunion, or a union in a position of deformity, will result.

TECHNIC OF SUPRACONDYLAR TENDOPLASTIC AMPUTATION. The patient is placed in a supine position on the operating table. The skin incision is planned to place the scar at the junction of the posterior aspect of the thigh and the end, so that it will not be subject to irritation from weight bearing (Fig. 61). This is accomplished by cutting a long anterior and short posterior flap. The skin incision is started on the medial side of the thigh, 5 to 7 centimeters above the adductor tubercle of the femur and about 2 centimeters anterior to it. This bony landmark is easily palpable. The incision through skin and subcutaneous tissue is extended distally to the level

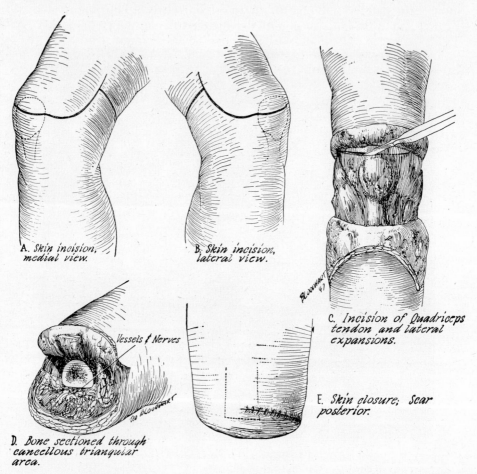

A. *Skin incision, medial view.*

B. *Skin incision, lateral view.*

C. *Incision of Quadriceps tendon and lateral expansions.*

Vessels *&* Nerves

D. *Bone sectioned through cancellous triangular area.*

E. *Skin closure; Scar posterior.*

Fig. 61. Technic of supracondylar tendoplastic amputation. (A) Skin incision, medial view. (B) Skin incision, lateral view. (C) Skin flap turned back, incision of quadriceps tendons and lateral expansions. (D) Bone sectioned through triangular cancellous bone. (E) Stump closed. Suture line on posterior circumference to remove scar from pressure.

of the superior margin of the patella and then transversely across the upper third of the patella and extended vertically for 7 centimeters up the lateral aspect of the thigh, at the same level as the medial incision, producing an incision in the shape of a U with a broad base. The posterior flap is cut by incising the skin and subcutaneous tissue across the back of the thigh from the proximal end of the anterior flap incision on the medial side of the leg, to the proximal end of the lateral incision, with a distal convexity of 4 centimeters, so that a short skin flap is produced posteriorly. The skin and subcutaneous tissue of the anterior flap are elevated enough to expose the attachment of the quadriceps tendon into the patella. The quadriceps tendon is cut through cleanly at its attachment to the patella and the lateral and medial fascial and muscle expansions of the quadriceps are cut through to bone on the same contour as the distal margin of the skin flap. This creates an anterior flap which comprises skin, subcutaneous tissue, quadriceps tendon, fascial expansions, and some muscle laterally and medially. The skin distal to the flap in the posterior incision is reflected so that the fascia on the posterior aspect of the leg can be cut slightly longer than the skin. The fascia is then incised to the bone along the contour of the distal end of the skin flap, and about 1 centimeter longer than the skin. The hamstring muscles are cut and allowed to retract, and the incision is carried through to bone. The anterior and posterior flaps are gently retracted and the periosteum of the femur sharply incised about the circumference of the bone at the level of bone section. The bone is sawed through just below the beginning of the flare of the condyles so that its end will present a triangular shape rather than a circular shape. The cut end of the bone should have cancellous structure and not show marrow cavity. Preservation of the slight flare of the lower end of the femur for a broad base is important. The synovial membrane of the quadriceps pouch is present between the anterior flap and the front of the femur. By lifting the flap this membrane can be removed, using a scissors for a spreader and opening it in the cleavage plane between the synovial membrane and the under surface of the tendon and muscle. The margin of the bone end is smoothed with a fine rasp if necessary, while the soft tissues are protected with moist saline sponges.

The thigh is elevated and in the areolar tissue posterior to the femur the femoral vessels are isolated and ligated by transfixion suture. As these are large caliber vessels, chromic No. 1 catgut is used. The sciatic nerve is isolated and ligated with a plain No. oo catgut suture, transfixed through its sheath, after developing it up its fascial plane for a distance adequate to recess its neuroma. At this level the sciatic nerve may have already divided into its peroneal and tibial branches. If this is the case, each branch is treated individually, in the same manner. If a tourniquet has been used, it is completely removed, making certain that venous return has not been blocked. All bleeding points are individually ligated with plain No. oo catgut to obtain dry flaps. The anterior flap is then allowed to fall backward and the fascia and tendon of this flap are sutured to the posterior fascia with interrupted sutures of plain No. oo catgut. A small rubber drain is placed beneath the fascia and brought out at the outer angle of the suture line. The skin and subcutaneous tissue are freed from the fascia of each flap just enough to permit of a smooth closure of the skin, without tension or redundancy. The skin edges are approximated with interrupted sutures of fine silk. The drain is sutured to the skin with one suture, cut long for identification. The suture line is covered with vaseline gauze. Dressings are applied to the end of the stump. The lower two-thirds of the stump and dressings are wrapped in sterile sheet wadding and a tensor bandage applied over the sheet wadding for mild compression. The stump is kept elevated on pillows during the immediate postoperative period.

In patients with vascular disease it is desirable to perform this amputation without a tourniquet. The large vessels may be isolated and clamped through the medial incision by cutting the sartorius, gracilis, semimembranous and semitendinous muscles transversely just above the tibia. This gives free access to the popliteal space and with easy retraction, the large vessels can be identified and controlled in the first step of the operation. The hamstring muscle flap can be shortened before closing the flaps if necessary.

TECHNIC OF GRITTI-STOKES AMPUTATION. The patient is placed in the supine position on the operating table. The adductor tubercle of the femur is palpated (Fig. 62). The skin incision is started 3 centimeters above the adductor tubercle and carried horizontally on the side of the thigh to the level of the articular surface of the femur. It is then swung in a broad curve across the middle of the patellar ligament and extended proximally on the outer side of the extremity to the level at which the incision started on the inner side of the thigh. The posterior flap is cut by connecting the proximal ends of this incision, by an incision crossing the posterior half of the thigh, with a convexity downward of 3 centimeters. The skin is allowed to retract normally. The anterior flap is deepened by cutting through the patellar ligament and the fascial expansions of the quadriceps covering the knee joint. These structures are incised at the level of the skin incision, following the same contour as the skin incision. This creates an anterior flap consisting of skin, subcutaneous tissue, patellar ligament, patella, fascial expansions of the quadriceps, and synovial membrane of knee joint. The posterior incision is deepened to the bone by cutting through the tendons of the inner hamstring muscles and the adductor muscle insertion on the medial side, through the tendons of the outer hamstrings on the lateral side, and through the adipose tissue, vessels and nerves in the popliteal space. The anterior and posterior flaps are then gently retracted to expose the site of section of the femur, which is just below the beginning of the flare of the condyles, so that the femur, when cut, will show a triangular end filled with cancellous bone. The periosteum is incised circularly at this level. The femur is cut through transversely to its long axis at the line of incision of the periosteum. This permits removal of the amputated portion of the extremity. The articular surface of the patella is then turned to the outside by folding the anterior flap back on itself. The patella is steadied by a tenaculum, or bone holding clamp with narrow jaws. A wafer of bone, including all the articular cartilage of the patella, is cut off with a thin flat bladed saw, leaving at least the anterior half of the patella in the patellar ligament. This section of the patella leaves a cancellous bony surface on its inner face. The removal of the cartilage from the patella is done better with a saw than with a chisel. The tissues are then thoroughly irrigated with warm saline to remove any bone dust. The synovial membrane of the quadriceps pouch is removed by spreading a scissors in the cleavage plane between it and the fascia. The femoral vessels which are posterior to the femur are isolated and ligated by transfixion with a ligature of chromic No. 1 catgut. The sciatic nerve, which at this level may have already divided into its peroneal and

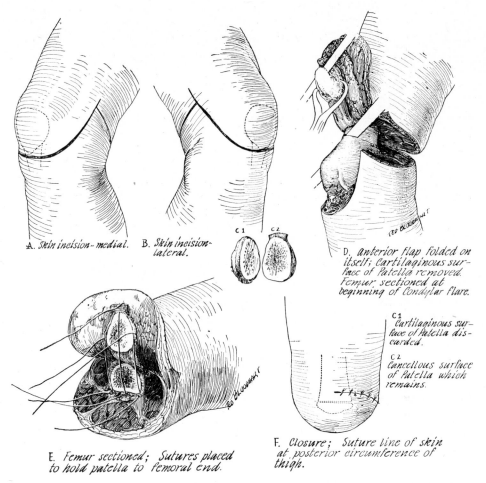

A. *Skin incision - medial.* B. *Skin incision - lateral.*

C 1 C 2

D. *anterior flap folded on itself; Cartilaginous surface of Patella removed. Femur sectioned at beginning of Condylar Flare.*

C 1 *Cartilaginous surface of Patella discarded.*

C 2 *Cancellous surface of Patella which remains.*

E. *Femur sectioned; Sutures placed to hold patella to femoral end.*

F. *Closure; Suture line of skin at posterior circumference of thigh.*

FIG. 62. Technic of Gritti-Stokes amputation. (A) Skin incision, medial view. (B) Skin incision, lateral view. (C1) Cartilaginous surface of patella, which is discarded. (C2) Cancellous portion of patella, which is left in tendon to approximate to femoral end. (D) Anterior flap folded back on itself, cartilaginous portion of patella being removed with saw. (E) Cancellous surface of patella ready for approximation to triangular end of femur. (F) Stump closed, patella centered under femur. Suture line posterior, to remove scar from pressure.

tibial branches, is isolated. The sheath of the nerve is transfixed, the nerve ligated with plain No. 00 catgut, in a recessed position. The nerve trunk is sectioned with a knife at a point below the ligature so that its neuroma will be well covered by soft tissue.

The tourniquet is removed and all bleeding points in the flaps ligated with plain No. 00 catgut ties, spending time to be sure the flaps are dry.

The patella, with its under surface completely denuded of cartilage, is let fall back over the end of the femur. If the femur has been cut to the right length, the patella fits snugly and flush on the end of the femur. If the under surface of the patella has to be forced against the end of the femur, the femur is too long and should be sectioned again at a slightly proximal level, which it is estimated will permit a flush junction of the two raw bony surfaces without tension or slack in the quadriceps tendon. When there is slack in the quadriceps tendon, the femur has been cut too short.

The projecting tag of the patellar ligament is then sutured with a few interrupted chromic No. 1 catgut sutures to the periosteum on the posterior side of the femur. On the posterior lateral and medial aspect of the patella there is fascia projecting, which can be anchored with interrupted sutures to periosteum. The patella should be securely anchored under the center of the femur. Usually three to four well placed sutures will accomplish this anchorage. If, through rough handling, the periosteum has been lost, drill holes may be made through the cortex of the femur and sutures passed through these drill holes for anchorage. The success of this operation depends on firm, accurate anchorage of the patella, so that union to the femoral end in good position may result.

The remaining free margin of the fascia lateral to the patellar ligament is sutured with interrupted sutures of plain No. 00 catgut to the fascia of the posterior flap. A drain is placed beneath the fascia to exit from the outer angle of the suture line. The skin margins of each flap are elevated from the fascia just enough to permit of tailoring them for an accurate closure with the resultant suture line at the level of the posterior half of the circumference of the thigh. The skin margins are then approximated with interrupted sutures of fine silk. The drain is sutured through the skin with one suture cut long, for identification. The suture line is covered with vaseline gauze and dressings are applied. The lower two-thirds of the thigh stump is wrapped with sterile sheet wadding and a tensor bandage applied over the sheet wadding. The stump is elevated on pillows with the hip flexed, during the immediate postoperative days.

TECHNIC OF AMPUTATION THROUGH THE FEMUR ABOVE THE SUPRA-CONDYLAR LEVEL. Thigh stumps above the supracondylar level are not end-bearing stumps. In any stump above the supracondylar area, weight is borne on the ischial tuberosity and through the sides of the stump. The skin flaps are fashioned to place the scar posterior to the end of the femur so that it will not adhere to the bone end. The femur lies anterior to the center of the thigh.

The patient is placed in the supine position on the operating table. A mark is made on the skin at the site of the contemplated level of the bone section (Fig. 63). Anterior and posterior skin flaps are planned, with the anterior flap longer than the posterior flap. The flaps are fashioned so that the line of closure will meet 2 centimeters behind the posterior margin of the sectioned femur. The junction of the upper end of each flap is 3 centimeters proximal to the point at which the bone is to be sectioned. After defining these points, the skin and subcutaneous tissue is incised, placing the junction of the flaps in the center of the lateral and medial surfaces of the thigh, 3 centimeters proximal to the point of bone section. The fascia is then incised around the contour of the skin incision at the level of the skin incision. In planning the flaps it is well to err on the long side. The skin and fascia of the posterior flap is then elevated proximally to the point where the

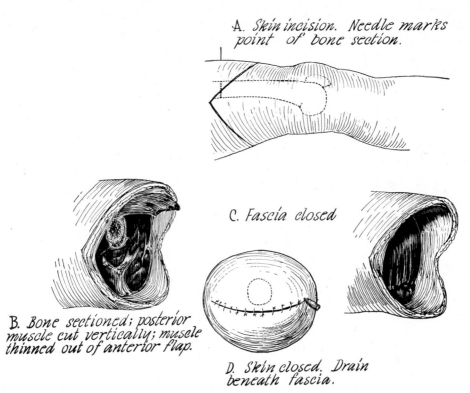

A. Skin incision. Needle marks point of bone section.

C. Fascia closed

B. Bone sectioned; posterior muscle cut vertically; muscle thinned out of anterior flap.

D. Skin closed. Drain beneath fascia.

Fig. 63. Technic of amputation through thigh above supracondylar level. (A) Skin incision, needle marking point of bone section. (B) Muscle coned out of posterior flap, muscle thinned on anterior flap. (C) Fascia closed over bone end. (D) Stump closed, suture line posterior to bone end, drain in outer angle of suture line.

bone is to be sectioned. At the angle of junction of the flaps the muscles are cut through to bone in a V fashion along the margins of the skin flaps with a scalpel to the level of the anterior and posterior surfaces of the femur. A long amputation knife is then thrust through the thigh at the angle of the V in the incised muscle anterior to the femur, taking care not to make a perforation in the medial side of the anterior skin flap. After the knife emerges from the medial side of the muscles it is moved distally and anteriorly along the margins of the skin flap with a back and forth motion. This cuts a wedge of muscle, fascia and skin, en bloc, with its base proximal. The free posterior skin flap is then retracted proximally to protect it. The long amputation knife is thrust through the incised muscle posterior to the femur at the point the bone is to be sectioned, with its dull edge bearing on the posterior surface of the femur. The posterior muscle mass is then cut from front to back, transversely at the level of bone section. If the amputation is done without a tourniquet, the muscles should not be sectioned with a long amputation knife. When the amputation is carried out without tourniquet, the femoral vessels can be exposed and clamped through the medial arm of the incision. The muscles should then be cut gradually with a scalpel, allowed to retract as they are cut, and the bleeding controlled by clamping vessels as they are encountered. The sectioned muscles are then covered with moist sponges and gently retracted to expose the point of bone section. The periosteum of the femur is then incised sharply about its circumference and transverse to the long axis of the bone. The distal periosteum is pushed off for a distance of 2 centimeters with an elevator, care being taken not to disturb the proximal periosteum. The bone is then cut through with a straight saw at the level of adherent periosteum. When this has been accomplished, the amputated portion of the leg is free and is removed. The extremity is ready to be prepared for closure.

The tissues of the stump are thoroughly lavaged with warm saline. The muscle in the anterior flap is thinned and removed from the point at which the anterior flap will fall over the front of the femur to the end of the flap, so that there will be no muscle closed over the end of the bone. If necessary, the circumference of the end of the femur is smoothed with a fine rasp, while the muscles are protected with moist sponges.

The large vessels, the femoral and profunda femoris artery and veins, are isolated and ligated with a transfixion ligature of chromic No. 1 catgut. The position of the femoral vessels will shift at the different levels of amputation. In the lower third of the thigh these vessels are posterior to the femur. As the hip is approached, they become progressively more medial and anterior, following Hunter's canal, beneath the sartorius muscle to the femoral triangle. In the middle third of the thigh there is a vessel worthy of ligature near the linea aspera of the femur.

The sciatic nerve is isolated and freed for 3 to 4 centimeters in its fascial plane. Its sheath is transfixed and the nerve ligated with plain No. oo catgut. The nerve is then sectioned with a knife below the ligature, high in the fascial plane, so that its neuroma will be recessed.

The tourniquet is removed and all bleeding vessels are isolated and ligated with plain No. oo catgut. There are many rather large muscular branches of the great arteries which bleed freely and time should be spent obtaining a dry field to avoid hematoma formation. Washing with warm saline will show up bleeding points.

When good hemostasis has been accomplished, the fascia of the anterior flap is neatly sutured to the fascia of the posterior flap with interrupted sutures of plain No. oo catgut. A drain which exits from the outer angle of the suture line is placed beneath the fascia. The skin margin is separated for a centimeter or two from the fascia and correctly tailored to permit of a smooth closure without tension or redundancy. The skin edges are sutured with interrupted sutures of fine silk. The drain is sutured through the skin with one suture of silk cut long, for identification.

Vaseline gauze is placed over the suture line. Dressings with an absorbent pad are applied. The stump is wrapped to the groin with sterile sheet wadding. A tensor bandage is applied and made secure with adhesive tape strips extending on to the skin of the abdomen, the buttock, and the hip above the trochanter, so that it will not slip off. If the stump is above the middle of the femur it is well to extend the bandage around the lower abdomen and back in a spica fashion. A well padded splint is applied on the posterior surface from just below the ribs to the end of the stump and the stump bandaged to the splint. Splinting the stump prevents severe flexor muscle spasm and adds to the comfort of the patient.

Amputation through the Hip. Amputation through the hip is usually indicated because of malignancy high in the femur or thigh, chronic uncontrollable infection in the region of the hip, or severe trauma to the upper third of the thigh with damage to major blood vessels. This is a formidable operative procedure because of potential blood loss and shock, and should never be undertaken without first having typed the patient for transfusion and having compatible blood available in the operating room. The use of a tourniquet in this amputation is not practical, as its presence interferes with the operation.

Amputation through the hip is done at three levels: (1) through the hip joint; (2) through the neck of the femur; and (3) at the level of the trochanters of the femur. Amputation at the level of the trochanters leaves the most satisfactory stump. Even though the bone length is very short, a patient with a transtrochanteric or subtrochanteric amputation is often able to get along with a saucer socket in a thigh prosthesis and a wide pelvic band, whereas the patient disarticulated through the hip requires a tilting table prosthesis with a large cuplike saddle. The prosthesis for a disarticulated hip is so cumbersome that the patient often discards it in favor of crutches. Even though function is a consideration, bone length should never take precedence over a complete ablation of pathology. Residual pathology may result in a total failure of the amputation and even loss of life.

The principal problem in amputation through the hip joint is the control of hemorrhage. If the pathology which makes the amputation necessary is so crowded against the pelvis, or its presence has resulted in the development of such an extensive collateral circulation that control of hemorrhage may be difficult at the time of operation, the common iliac artery should be ligated as a preliminary to the amputation. This can be done through an incision lateral to the rectus abdominus muscle by exposing the vessel retroperitoneally, without opening the abdominal cavity. Preliminary ligation of the common iliac vessels gives complete control of the blood supply to the area of operation, and does not interfere with the circulation of the skin flaps. The time consumed by this preliminary ligation is compensated for by the lack of blood loss and the facility and speed with which the extremity can be removed.

TECHNIC OF DISARTICULATION OF THE HIP. It is well to have two assistants for this operation; one to manipulate the extremity and the other
to retract tissues and expose the operative field. The patient is placed in
the supine position on the operating table. The side on which the extremity
to be removed is located should be elevated from the surface of the operating
table by tilting the patient 45 degrees on the opposite side and fixing him
stably in this position with a sand bag or triangular rest under the back and
shoulders. The patient is draped so that the lower half of the abdomen and

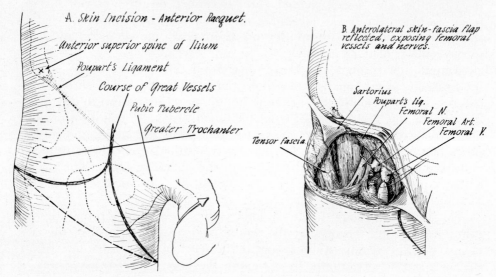

FIG. 64(1). Technic of disarticulation of hip. (A) Skin incision, anterior racquet,
creating anteromedial and posterolateral flap. (B) Anterolateral position of skin flap
reflected, femoral artery and vein ligated and sectioned to control hemorrhage.

the anterior five-sixths of the iliac crest are exposed and the genitals well
covered. The skin flaps are planned so that the suture line will be on the
anterolateral side of the stump. This site removes the scar from the pressure
of the prosthesis, on which the patient sits. It also has the advantage that
the incision is away from the anus, so that in the healing period contamination is unlikely. A racquet incision is used. The handle of the racquet is on
the anteromedial aspect of the hip, over the femoral vessels (Fig. 64). The
handle of the racquet begins 6 to 7 centimeters above Poupart's ligament on
the abdominal wall, follows the course of the femoral vessels to a point 8
centimeters below Poupart's ligament, where it is curved outward over the
anterior and lateral aspect of the thigh to cross the prominence of the great
trochanter. It is continued around the posterior aspect of the thigh with a
gentle distal sweep 5 centimeters below the gluteal fold. The skin incision
is brought to the inner aspect of the thigh 10 centimeters below the pubic
tubercle. From the inner aspect of the thigh it is curved gently proximally
to meet the handle of the racquet. The vertical portion of the incision over
the femoral vessels and part of the lateral curve of the incision is first made

through the skin. The skin and fascia are incised over Scarpa's triangle and laterally almost to the trochanter. The lateral skin fascia flap is elevated proximally to expose the tendinous origin of the sartorius and rectus femoris muscles. The femoral artery and vein are separated and the origin of the profunda femoris artery from the common femoral artery located. The common femoral artery is then ligated above the origin of the profunda femoris with chromic No. 1 catgut. Two ligatures are placed above the site

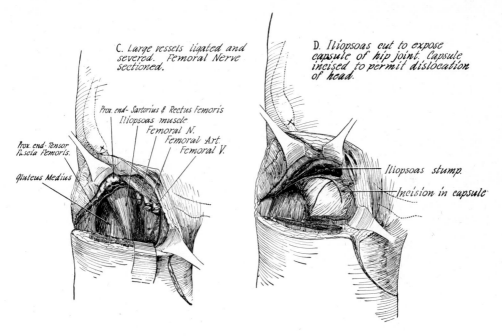

C. *Large vessels ligated and severed. Femoral Nerve sectioned.*

D. *Iliopsoas cut to expose capsule of hip joint. Capsule incised to permit dislocation of head.*

Prox. end- Sartorius & Rectus Femoris
Iliopsoas muscle
Femoral N.
Femoral Art.
Femoral V.

Prox. end- Tensor Fascia Femoris.

Gluteus Medius

Iliopsoas stump.

Incision in capsule

FIG. 64(2). (C) Stumps of ligated vessels and femoral nerve. (D) Iliopsoas exposed after section of sartorius, rectus and tensor fascia femoris muscles.

at which the vessel is to be sectioned and one ligature below. The femoral artery is then divided. The femoral vein is treated similarly, the ligatures being tied after the leg has been elevated in order to drain as much blood as possible from the extremity. The distal ends of the artery and vein are freed enough so that they can be easily retracted out of the way to protect them. The femoral nerve which lies lateral to the artery is freed, ligated under the edge of Poupart's ligament, above its ramification, and its stump placed in a recessed position under the inguinal ligament so that its neuroma will be well covered. If the common femoral artery is ligated below the origin of the profunda femoris, large bleeders will be encountered later and this error should be avoided. When this preliminary control of the major vessels has been completed the remainder of the incision is made through the skin and superficial fascia. The skin and superficial fascia on the lateral side of the thigh are mobilized 5 centimeters above the tip of the trochanter and on the posterior surface of the thigh, up to the ischial tuberosity. The rectus femoris, the sartorius, and the tensor fascia femoris muscles are divided transversely through their tendinous and fascial origins and allowed to retract distally. This exposes the psoas muscle, which lies over the hip joint capsule. The extremity is then adducted and the gluteus medius and minimus, and fascial end of the gluteus maximus muscles which attach to the greater trochanter are sectioned through their tendinous expansions.

With the severed muscles well retracted, the psoas muscle is cut transversely, exposing the capsule of the hip joint. The circumflex arteries lie

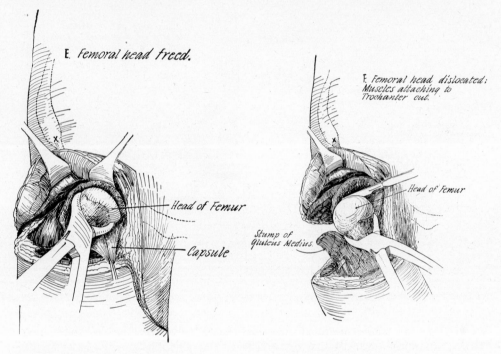

E. *femoral head freed.*

F. *femoral head dislocated: Muscles attaching to Trochanter cut.*

Head of Femur

Head of Femur

Stump of Gluteus Medius.

Capsule

Fig. 64(3). (E) Capsule opened, head of femur dislocated. (F) Muscles attached to greater trochanter sectioned at insertion, posterior capsule being freed.

under the psoas. If the femoral artery has been ligated above the origin of the profunda these vessels will not be a source of severe hemorrhage, but will bleed enough to require attention. If the profunda is patent they will bleed profusely. The hip joint capsule which is now visible is cut widely around the margin of the acetabulum and distally along the upper surface of the neck of the femur in a T fashion. The hip is flexed, adducted, and externally rotated, dislocating the head of the femur. In this maneuver, the leg, with the knee bent 90 degrees, is used as a lever. After the hip has been extended, the neck of the femur is grasped with a long handled bone holding forceps and lifted forward. The posterior capsule is then completely cut with a scalpel. This allows further anterior displacement of the head and neck of the femur. The posterior structures, consisting of the gemelli, pyriformis, and obturator internus muscles, which attach to the posterior aspect of the trochanter; the sciatic nerve, and a portion of the gluteus maximus, are cut from the inside out. The sciatic nerve is clamped as it is cut to control its vessel.

This frees all attachments of the extremity except the adductor muscles. The removal of the limb is completed by cutting a muscle flap from the adductor muscles. This muscle flap is tapered from above downward to the distal edge of the medial skin flap. In cutting the medial flap the obturator vessels will be encountered. These vessels should be controlled as they are cut, after removal of the extremity. The sciatic nerve is sectioned high, fixing

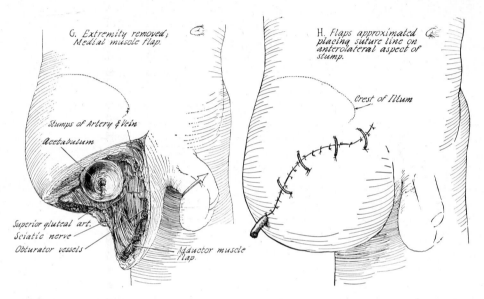

Fig. 64(4). (G) Extremity removed; long medial muscle flap. (H) Flaps closed. Drain in inferior angle of suture line.

its sheath with a suture of plain No. oo catgut and ligating its stump to control the artery. All individual bleeding vessels in the flaps are clamped and tied with a plain No. oo catgut.

The fascia of the posteromedial flap is approximated to the fascia of the anterolateral flap with interrupted sutures of chromic No. 1 catgut. This causes the flap of adductor muscle to fall over and into the acetabulum. The edge of the flap can be sutured to the remains of the capsule about the acetabulum. The skin is then mobilized and trimmed so that its edges can be sutured to effect a neat closure without redundancy or tension. The skin edges are approximated with interrupted sutures of silk. Retention sutures of heavy dermol over rubber should be used at intervals of 2 inches in the closure of the skin, as there is a tendency to separation. The skin closure is considerably facilitated by using three or four large towel clips to hold the skin flaps together while closing them with sutures. A drain is placed beneath the fascia up to the acetabulum from the inferior angle of the suture line and sutured to the skin with one suture cut long for identification. The suture line is covered with vaseline gauze. Copious dressings are applied and tensor bandages wound around the stump and abdomen.

TECHNIC OF TRANSCERVICAL AMPUTATION. The technic of amputation through the neck of the fumur differs from disarticulation of the hip only in that after the anterior capsule is cut, the head of the femur is not dislocated. Instead, the capsule is cut only enough so that a Gigli saw can be passed around the neck of the femur inside the capsule. The neck of the femur is then sectioned just below the head. The neck of the femur is then pulled forward with a long handled bone holding forceps and the posterior capsule cut below the head, which remains in the acetabulum. After this, the completion of the operation is the same as in a disarticulation of the hip.

TECHNIC OF AMPUTATION THROUGH THE TROCHANTERIC AREA. This amputation is done through the same type of racquet incision as the disarticulation of the hip, with the same preliminary control of the large vessels. The lateral skin flap, however, is cut longer on the side and in the back, crossing the femur 5 to 10 centimeters below the prominence of the trochanter. The sartorius, rectus femoris, tensor fascia femoris, and iliopsoas are cut across at the same level that the bone is to be sectioned. The gluteus medius, minimus, and maximus are not detached from the trochanter. The muscles attaching to the posterior aspect of the trochanter are not severed. The femur is sectioned by passing a Gigli saw from medial to lateral side behind it, and sawing from back to front. The proximal end of the distal portion of the femur is lifted forward with a long handled bone forceps and the posterior structures, consisting of the sciatic nerve and the hamstring and adductor muscles, are cut from before backward at the level of the bone section, with a long amputating knife. After proper recessing of the nerves and control of bleeders in the flaps, the fascia and skin are approximated to close the stump. The suture line falls in the same general area and direction as it does in a disarticulation of the hip.

Inter-innomino Abdominal Amputation (Transiliac Amputation). Inter-innomino abdominal amputation is an amputation in which the innominate bone from the symphysis to the sacro-iliac joint, with its attached limb, is removed. The removal of the extremity is carried out between the inner surface of the innominate bone and the peritoneum. Only large muscle flaps are left to support the pelvic contents. This operation is a massive surgical procedure, requiring extensive supportive treatment during and after the operation. The procedure is rarely indicated and rarely justified. Neoplasms of the innominate bone may be an indication. This amputation is mentioned as a rare necessity and its technic will not be described.

CLOSED AMPUTATION OF THE UPPER EXTREMITY

The loss of a major portion of an upper extremity produces greater economic displacement than any single amputation of the lower extremity. Individuals without a hand are, with but few exceptions, excluded from employment which requires meeting the public. Neither the steel hook nor the gloved artificial hand is pleasing to a discriminating clientele. In some states an individual with an artificial arm cannot obtain a license to operate a motor vehicle. Compensation laws often make the individual without a hand unemployable because of increased liability.

The general attitude of surgeons toward amputation of the arm is "to save all possible." This is a good attitude but it should be applied with discrimination, as certain arm stumps are more satisfactory from the functional viewpoint than others.

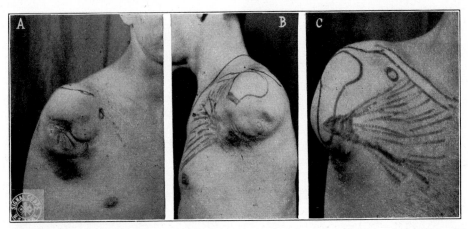

Fig. 65. Humeral stumps of no functional value. (A) Disarticulation of shoulder. (B) Amputation through neck of humerus. (C) Amputation of humerus at level of pectoral insertion. Retention of prosthesis on these short stumps is difficult and apparatus cumbersome. (From McKeever, *J. Bone & Joint Surg.*, 26(No. 4):626-671 and 706, 1944.)

Certain amputation stumps of the upper extremity have absolutely no functional value, and even offer very difficult cosmetic problems. Foremost among these is the stump resulting from the disfiguring intrascapulothoracic amputation. This amputation gives to the upper torso of the individual an unsightly sloping contour from the neck to the costal margin. The only attempt at a prosthesis which is of any use, is a pad to enlarge the shoulder and fill out the coat (Fig. 65).

No amputation through the arm above the level of the humeral insertion of the pectoralis major muscle has any functional value worthy of consideration. This does not mean that the head of the humerus should be removed unnecessarily, as its presence tends to round out the shoulder, and from a cosmetic viewpoint, is desirable. When only an inch or two of the humerus remains, if the pectoral attachment has been lost, the end of the short piece of humerus is pulled by the shoulder rotators into abduction and forward flexion. Amputations immediately below the pectoral attachment are also of little value in motivating a prosthesis. At this level, the remaining piece of the humerus stays opposed to the thoracic wall and only a flicker of forward and backward motion of the stump is possible. This is of no practical value in moving an artificial arm. The skin and pectoral muscle belly forming the anterior axillary fold interfere with the fitting of a prosthesis. To hold a prosthesis in place on these high humeral amputations, an elaborate, uncomfortable harness is necessary (Fig. 66). Because of the cumbersome, uncomfortable harness, the weight of the prosthesis, and the uselessness of the artificial extremity, most patients soon discard the mechanical extremity and go about with an empty sleeve.

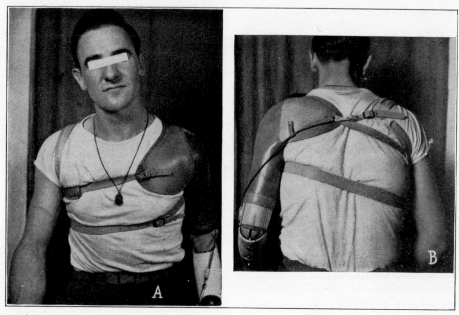

FIG. 66. Photograph of extensive harness necessary to retain prosthesis on humeral stump above pectoral insertion. (A) Front view. (B) Back view. (From McKeever, *J. Bone & Joint Surg.*, 26(No. 4):626-671 and 706, 1944.)

The shortest bone length of the humerus that will motivate an artificial arm sufficiently well to make its use attractive to the amputee, is 2 to 3 inches below the pectoral insertion. This necessitates that a total of 5 to 6 inches of the humerus be present. Even though this length of humerus remains, a rather extensive shoulder harness is still a necessity and the mechanical hand or hook can only be operated well with the elbow in the extended position.

The importance of saving the elbow joint, when possible, cannot be too greatly emphasized. The functional value of the elbow to the upper extremity stump is even greater than that of the knee to the lower extremity stump. Without an elbow joint under voluntary control, the arm amputee is restricted to a few positions of the forearm, controlled by a mechanical lock, which he must unlock with the other hand to release. In close quarters, even with a long humeral stump, he may have to place the forearm in one of the few available positions, with the other hand. This difficulty is obviated to a large degree by even a relatively short forearm stump. An elbow joint may be of value even though it does not have complete motion and even though the condition of the humerus is not normal. Since the arm is not a weight-bearing extremity, a fibrous union of the humerus may be adequate for excellent use of an elbow and forearm stump, as the corset of a prosthesis will help to stabilize the humerus. No hasty sacrifice of the elbow joint or unnecessary reconstruction, which through long immobilization might lead to stiffness of the elbow, should be undertaken when there is a chance that it will jeopardize function. An elbow which has been resected may work well in a prosthesis and this method of mobilizing a stiff elbow joint should be tried before the elbow is discarded.

Amputation through the Fingers and Metacarpals. These two sites of amputation are considered together because of the fact that the best result from both the viewpoint of function and cosmesis may be served by removing part of a metacarpal bone with the digit, which requires amputation. In general, as much of a finger as possible should be preserved, providing the portion remaining functions well and does not interfere with the function of the remaining fingers. One finger, stiff in extension at the proximal interphalangeal joint, may prevent a good closure to the palm of the normal fingers, and one finger, stiff in flexion at the proximal interphalangeal joint, may prevent complete extension of the normal fingers.

For individuals who do work requiring firm grip, breadth of the palm and integrity of the palmar arch are desirable. For these individuals, metacarpal bones should be preserved, even though they may be prominent, and even though the hand is not as graceful as a hand tapered by their removal. Individuals whose station in life places the cosmetic effect ahead of the function of grip may be better off with a metacarpal removed. In instances in which the index or middle finger, or both, have been removed, the ability to grasp fine or small objects may be enhanced by removing parts of one or both metacarpal bones to form a more open web between the thumb and the fourth finger. All amputations of fingers must be planned with a view to the use to which the hand is to be put. What may be a good amputation in the hand for a blacksmith may be a poor amputation for a watchmaker or a croupier.

Amputation of fingers can be done under nerve block, infiltrating the digital nerves in the web spaces lateral to the shafts of the metacarpals. However, to adequately handle tendons, when it is desired to section them high, the patient should be asleep and relaxed. A small rubber catheter clamped with a hemostat at the base of the finger serves excellently as a tourniquet. Palmar skin is desirable as a covering for the end of the stump.

TECHNIC OF AMPUTATION OF FINGER THROUGH PHALANX OR INTERPHALANGEAL JOINT. With a tourniquet applied at the base of the finger, a palmar flap adequate in length to come beyond the dorsal aspect of the phalanx is cut by starting a lateral incision one-half centimeter proximal to the site of bone section, opposite the center of the phalanx. The phalanx lies in the dorsal third of the finger so that the lateral incision is dorsal to the center of the digit. This incision is carried through the skin and subcutaneous

tissue distally an adequate distance to cut a palmar flap which will extend
beyond the dorsal surface of the cut phalanx (Fig. 67). The incision is then
curved abruptly across the palmar surface of the finger and carried proximally on the opposite side of the finger to a point corresponding to the
start of the incision. The skin and subcutaneous tissue on the dorsum of the
finger are then incised transversely at the point of contemplated bone section

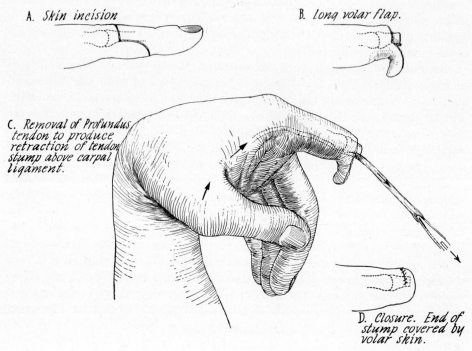

A. *Skin incision*

B. *long volar flap.*

C. *Removal of Profundus
tendon to produce
retraction of tendon
stump above carpal
ligament.*

D. *Closure. End of
stump covered by
volar skin.*

Fig. 67. Technic of amputation of finger through phalanx. (A) Skin incision. (B)
Long volar flap. (C) Removal of profundus tendon to produce retraction of tendon
stump above carpal ligament. (D) Closure. End of stump covered by volar skin.

to connect the two lateral incisions. The skin and subcutaneous tissue on
the dorsum are reflected proximally to a point one-half centimeter above the
point of bone section. The extensor tendon is cut through at the level of bone
section and permitted to retract. The palmar incision is deepened to expose
the flexor tendon. The skin and subcutaneous tissue are reflected proximally.
The flexor tendon is secured with a hemostat and cut transversely below the
clamp. After incision of the vinculum the tendon drops away from the
phalanx. This exposes the phalanx, which is incised about its circumference
through its periosteum. The bone is then sectioned with a Gigli saw from
palmar to dorsal surface. Cutting the phalanx with a bone cutting forceps or
rongeur will splinter the shaft. If necessary, the end of the bone is smoothed
with a fine rasp. The digital nerves which lie laterally are isolated, ligated
high with plain No. oo catgut, and cut off below the ligature with a knife.
With a mosquito forceps, the ligated end of the nerve is tucked high up in

the soft tissues to completely recess its neuroma. Neuromas on the digital nerves close under the skin flap are very painful and require removal. The digital vessels are ligated with plain No. oo catgut. After removal of the catheter tourniquet all other bleeding points are individually tied to obtain dry flaps. The flexor tendons are then pulled down forcefully with the wrist and metacarpophalangeal joint in palmar flexion, and cut transversely with a knife at the end of the sectioned phalanx. This causes the flexor tendon which no longer has a finger to motivate, to retract above the transverse carpal ligament so that its end will not adhere in the finger or palm and act as a checkrein to the tendons of the remaining fingers. This maneuver cannot be done under local anesthesia and pentothal will be necessary to accomplish sufficient stretch of the flexor muscle. Neither can it be done with a tourniquet around the base of the finger. The skin and subcutaneous tissue flaps are tailored to make a neat closure without dog ears, and the skin edges are approximated with interrupted sutures of fine silk, without tension or redundancy. A drain is not necessary. The suture line is covered with vaseline gauze and a dressing bulky enough to act as a partial splint is applied.

If the amputation is carried out by disarticulation at the distal interphalangeal or proximal interphalangeal joint, the procedure is the same except that the bone to be removed is separated by cutting through the capsule of the joint. The articular cartilage is then eraded from the distal end of the remaining phalanx. Flaps are cut, nerves and tendons are treated exactly as when bone is sectioned, and closure is in the same manner (Fig. 68).

TECHNIC OF AMPUTATION THROUGH DISTAL PHALANX. Amputation through the distal phalanx is done in the same manner, with a long palmar flap. Thoroughness must be exercised to totally ablate the nail bed. If any of the matrix of the nail is left, a troublesome horny spike will form, which may require removal. The tendon of the flexor profundus digitorum attaches to the base of the distal phalanx. When the distal phalanx is totally removed by disarticulation this tendon should be cut off short, as it has no further function and its presence can only interfere with the motion in the remaining fingers (Fig. 69).

TECHNIC OF DISARTICULATION THROUGH METACARPOPHALANGEAL JOINT. Disarticulation through the metacarpophalangeal joints is done through a racquet incision. The handle of the racquet is on the dorsal surface of the hand, never on the palmar surface. For removal of the middle and ring finger the handle of the racquet can be centered over the shaft of the metacarpal bone. In disarticulating the index finger the handle of the racquet should be to the ulnar side of the shaft of the second metacarpal bone so that the scar will be removed from pressure. In disarticulating the fifth finger the handle of the racquet should be to the radial side of the shaft of the fifth metacarpal bone for the same reason. The distal end of the racquet handle is carried 1 centimeter distal to the metacarpophalangeal joint. The circular portion of the racquet is made by cutting around the sides of the finger and across the palmar surface, 1 centimeter distal to the proximal flexion crease of the finger. It is to be remembered that the palmar side of the web of the finger is distal to the metacarpal head by approximately 2 centimeters. The tendons, nerves, vessels, and articular cartilage of the metacarpal head are treated in exactly the same manner as previously described. The incision is closed by approximating the subcutaneous tissue with interrupted sutures of plain No. oo catgut and the skin with interrupted sutures of fine silk. The suture line is covered with vaseline gauze and dressings applied. There is no large muscle mass to ooze and it is not necessary to drain the incision.

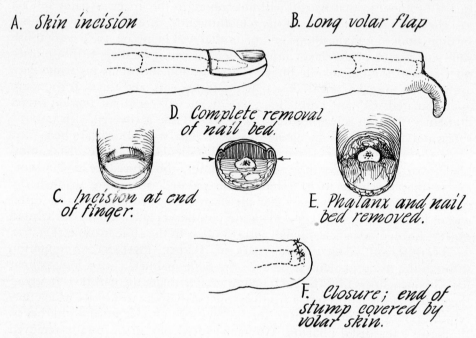

FIG. 68. Technic of amputation through distal phalanx. (A) Skin incision. (B) Long volar flap. (C) Incision at end of finger. (D) Complete removal of nail bed. (E) Portion of phalanx and nail bed completely removed. (F) Closure. Suture line on dorsum; end of stump covered by volar skin.

If it is desired to remove a portion of a metacarpal bone this can be done through the handle portion of the racquet incision, which can be extended as far proximally on the dorsum of the hand as is necessary for good exposure. If it is elected to remove the second metacarpal bone, it should be sectioned near the base. If the shaft is left in its entirety in this location it will project and be subject to pressure and abrasions. If for any reason both the second and third metacarpals are to be removed, the bone section should be near the bases to deepen the web between the thumb and the fourth finger. If only the fifth metacarpal bone is to be removed, as much of its length as possible should be preserved, as it gives a better appearing and more useful hand. Removal of either the third or fourth metacarpal bone alone should be avoided. Their removal disturbs the intrinsic muscle function and causes the fingers, when flexed, to deviate toward the defect left by the absent bone.

Amputation of the Thumb. Under all circumstances, even those which are most discouraging, the greatest conservatism should be observed re-

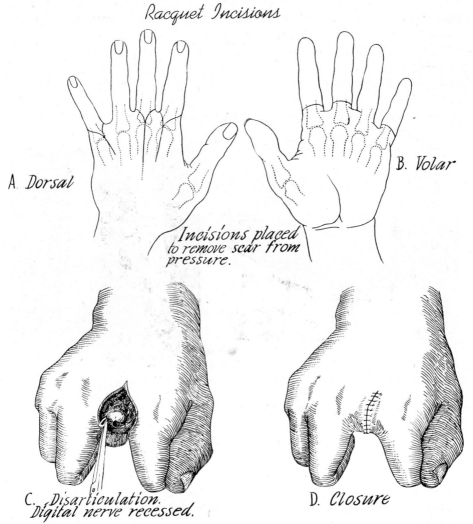

Racquet Incisions

A. *Dorsal*

B. *Volar*

Incisions placed to remove scar from pressure.

C. *Disarticulation. Digital nerve recessed.*

D. *Closure*

F<small>IG</small>. 69. Technic of disarticulation through metacarpophalangeal joint. (A) Racquet incision; dorsal view. Incisions placed to remove scar from pressure. (B) Racquet incision; palmar view. (C) Finger disarticulated; metacarpal head in view. Digital nerve being recessed. (D) Closure. Suture line on dorsal surface and in interdigital space, away from pressure.

garding amputation of the thumb. All length possible should be saved in the thumb. A palmar flap is desirable to cover the end of a thumb stump, but under no circumstances should useful bone length be sacrificed to obtain such a flap. It is justifiable to resort to a pedicle graft by attaching the end of the thumb to the abdominal skin to preserve length. An effort should always be made to maintain the thumb in the position of opposition if stiffness is likely to result from the trauma or disease requiring partial amputation, and not to permit it to ankylose at the side of the metacarpus where the fingers cannot be opposed to it. What appears to be a hopelessly damaged thumb may, with conservative treatment, after the lapse of time, turn out to be very useful, even though deformed in appearance. The only early justification for removal of the thumb is total circulatory loss or gangrene.

Neoplasty, the formation of a new thumb by tube skin grafts and implantation of bone grafts, is a surgical feat which can be accomplished. It is a time consuming, multiple-stage operative procedure. The result obtained rarely compensates the patient for the time spent, and the expense incurred.

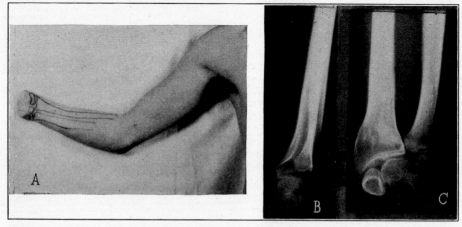

FIG. 70. Amputation stump containing carpal bones. (A) Photograph. (B) Roentgenogram, lateral view. (C) Roentgenogram, anteroposterior view. (From McKeever, *J. Bone & Joint Surg.*, 26(No. 4):626-671 and 706, 1944.)

Amputation at the Carpometacarpal Articulation. The stump which contains the proximal or proximal and distal rows of carpal bones is a very useful and satisfactory stump from the functional viewpoint. From the cosmetic aspect it has a few disadvantages. This amputation results in a good stump because of necessity it is covered by soft tissue with a good blood supply, the palmar skin of the heel and upper half of the hand. The inferior radio-ulnar joint is stable and painless and there are no unpadded bony prominences. The length of the stump containing carpal bones, together with the slight voluntary flexibility of the distal end, due to the remaining attachments of the wrist flexor and extensor muscles, make it of considerable aid to the patient without a prosthesis. The stump can be used satisfactorily for a stabilizer in such activities as driving a car, tying shoelaces, tying a necktie, buttoning a coat, etc. This stump also requires a great deal less harness to maintain a prosthesis in place and to powerfully motivate it than do amputations higher in the forearm (Figs. 70 and 71).

TECHNIC OF CARPOMETACARPAL AMPUTATION. This amputation will usually be indicated as the result of devastating trauma to the metacarpal area of the hand and thumb so that an exact skin incision for cutting flaps cannot be described. An effort should be made to get as long a palmar flap as possible so that the end of the stump will be covered by the highly vascularized, tough skin of the palm. If this cannot be obtained, a dorsal flap can be used. The tendons of the flexor sublimis and flexor profundus muscles and thumb flexors are pulled down and cut off so that they will retract above the carpal canal. The median and ulnar nerves are isolated. The former is ligated with a suture of plain No. oo catgut transfixing its sheath and is sec-

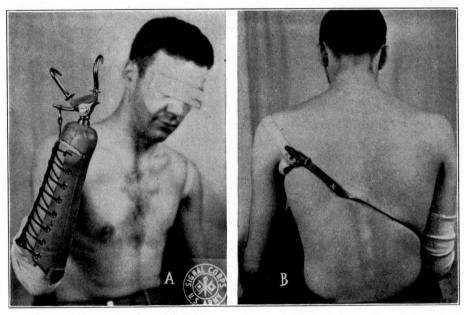

FIG. 71. Photograph of prosthesis on amputation stump containing carpal bones. No elbow joint and no corset above elbow is necessary. (A) Front view. (B) Back view. (From McKeever, *J. Bone & Joint Surg.*, 26(No. 4):626-671 and 706, 1944.)

tioned transversely and tucked up under the transverse carpal ligament. The ulnar nerve is treated in the same way and tucked up beyond the pisiform bone to recess its neuroma. The ulnar, radial, and interosseus vessels are ligated. The extensor tendons at the level of the lower end of the radius are permitted to retract. The bony stump is fashioned. If the metacarpal bones are so badly damaged that they are useless to their bases, or if there is inadequate skin flap to cover more than the carpus, the metacarpals are disarticulated at their bases by cutting the ligaments. If portions of the second, third, fourth and fifth metacarpals are usable, they can be left in the stump. A single long projecting metacarpal should not be left unless the thumb is present. The presence of a single metacarpal will complicate the fitting of a prosthesis and add nothing to function. *The thumb should never be sacrificed to obtain this kind of stump.*

All bleeding points are separately ligated. The long palmar flap, if it has been possible to obtain one, is lifted over the end of the carpal bones and the subcutaneous tissue sutured with interrupted sutures of plain No. oo catgut to the subcutaneous tissue of the dorsal flap. The skin edges are approximated with interrupted sutures of fine silk, with the suture line on the dorsum of the stump. The suture line is covered with vaseline gauze; dressings applied; the stump bandaged with sterile sheet wadding to the upper third of the forearm; and a tensor bandage applied. It is well to insert a drain in one angle of the suture line.

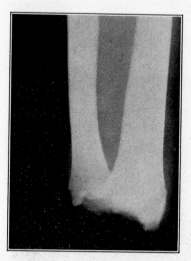

FIG. 72. Roentgenogram of disarticulation through wrist. This is unsatisfactory stump because of poor circulation and prominent radial and ulnar styloid processes, which become abraded. (From McKeever, *J. Bone & Joint Surg.*, 26(No. 4): 626-671 and 706, 1944.)

Disarticulation through the Wrist. Disarticulation through the wrist joint does not produce a satisfactory stump and is not a good amputation (Fig. 72). It has no more functional value than a stump in the middle third of the forearm. In addition, the inferior radio-ulnar joint may be very painful on pronation and supination of the stump. The loss of the carpal abutments and attachments causes a loss of stability in this joint which results in pain on motion. The prominent subcutaneous styloid processes of the radius and ulna are prone to become abraded in the prosthesis, and the stump end is likely to be sensitive. The lower third of the forearm is an area which is almost totally tendinous and has only the radial, ulnar, and interosseus arteries transversing the area to supply the hand, so that the stump is likely to be cold and cyanotic.

Amputation through the Forearm. The ideal forearm stump is one through the junction of the lower and middle thirds of the forearm (Fig. 73). This level leaves enough bone length for a firm grip on the cuff of the prosthesis by the stump. This length of stump also allows 2 to 3 inches of the volar surface of the forearm, below the elbow to be unencumbered by the sleeve of the prosthesis. This eliminates interference to flexion by the prosthesis cuff impinging on the front of the arm at the anticubital area. This level is also just above the point at which the forearm becomes tendinous and avascular. Such a stump has an excellent blood supply, is warm, and its skin will tolerate well the friction of a prosthesis cuff. The forearm stump at the junction of the middle and lower third of the forearm preserves the motions of pronation and supination, which are being utilized in modern forearm prostheses to great advantage. Forearm stumps shorter than this are very useful, but as the length between the end of the stump and the insertion of the tendon of the biceps brachii muscle into the radius decreases, the necessity for covering the greater portion of the stump's volar surface is increased, and flexion of the elbow may be interfered with by the encasement of the prosthesis. In the lower third of the forearm where the muscles have become tendinous, there is inadequate circulation, as only main arterial trunks transverse this area. Stumps through this area are cold and many times the skin covering them has a cyanotic hue. Chronic ulceration of the skin is not uncommon in stumps through the lower one-third of the forearm, due to the reduced blood supply. The difference in temperature at these two levels is readily detectable in amputation stumps by palpation with the hand.

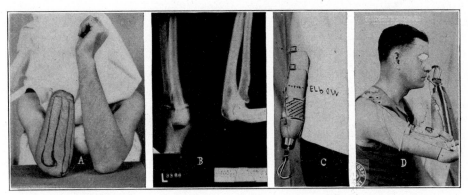

Fig. 73. Ideal forearm stump, junction of middle and lower third of forearm; stump is well vascularized and provides adequate lever for hard use of prosthesis. (A) Photograph. (B) Roentgenogram. (C) Prosthesis on stump. Socket does not encroach on anticubital space. (D) Prosthesis in full flexion. (From McKeever, *J. Bone & Joint Surg.*, 26(No. 4): 626-671 and 706, 1944.)

The short stump of the forearm need contain only a piece of the ulna, and conditions demanding removal of the upper end of the radius do not interfere with active flexion of the elbow since the brachialis muscle attaches to the ulna. Removal of the remaining portion of the radius may at times be a valuable adjunct in obtaining enough skin for closure of a very short forearm stump.

The forearm stump takes pressure on the sides and is not end-bearing. The flaps are planned to put the scar on the end and to have it run horizontal and not vertical to the plane of the radius and ulna. If the scar falls vertically across the interosseus space it will retract into this space, producing a dimpled end.

TECHNIC OF AMPUTATION THROUGH THE JUNCTION OF THE MIDDLE AND LOWER THIRDS OF THE FOREARM. A tourniquet is used on the arm. The patient is placed in the supine position on the operating table with the arm outstretched on an arm board so that the elbow can be freely flexed. A straight skin needle is placed in the skin and muscles on the dorsal surface of the forearm at the point the bone section is planned (Fig. 74). Volar and dorsal flaps are planned, not lateral flaps. The radius and ulna at this level lie more to the dorsum of the forearm than to the volar side. Skin flaps of equal length are cut. Equal flaps, because of the radius and ulna being more dorsal than volar, remove the scar from the bone ends. With the elbow

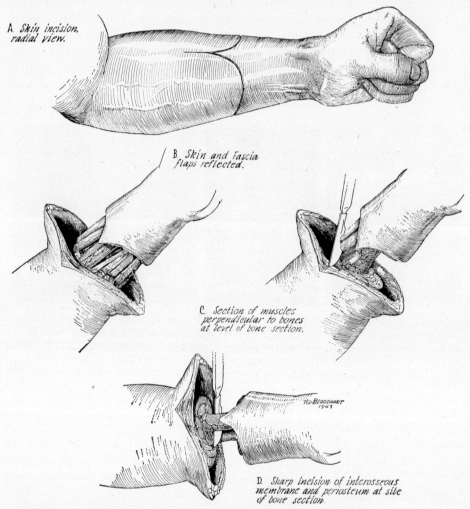

FIG. 74(1). Technic of amputation through junction of middle and lower thirds of forearm. (A) Skin incision, radial view. (B) Skin-fascia flaps reflected. (C) Muscles incised perpendicular to bones at level of bone section. (D) Sharp incision of interosseus membrane and periosteum at site of bone section.

flexed, an incision is made through the skin and fascia on the side of the arm, starting 2 centimeters above the point of bone section. The incision is carried distally 3 to 5 cm. from the point of bone section at the level of the volar surface of the radius, the length of the flap depending on the thickness of the forearm. The skin incision is then curved quite abruptly to cross the dorsal surface of the forearm. After crossing the dorsal half of the circumference of the forearm, the incision is curved abruptly to the volar surface of the ulna, which it parallels proximally to a point 2 centimeters proximal to the point of bone section. At the point where the incision curves abruptly, a similar incision is similarly curved abruptly to cross the volar surface of the forearm from the radial side and connected to the incision, paralleling the ulna. These incisions are carried through both skin and the enveloping fascia of the forearm. The skin and fascial flaps are turned back slightly beyond the point of bone section. The muscles and musculotendinous junctions are cut through vertically at the point of bone section with a sharp knife. The distal muscles are retracted and interosseus membrane is cut

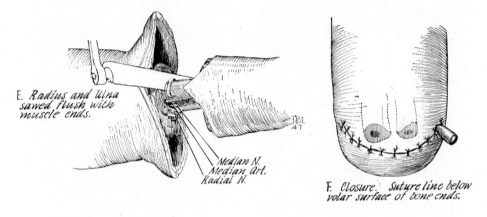

E. *Radius and Ulna sawed flush with muscle ends.*

Median N.
Median Art.
Radial N.

F. *Closure. Suture line below volar surface of bone ends.*

FIG. 74(2). (E) Radius and ulna sawed through flush with muscle ends. (F) Closure. Suture line below volar surface of bone ends.

through sharply at the level of bone section, incising the periosteum on the contiguous sides of the radius and ulna. The periosteum of the radius and ulna are then completely and cleanly incised about the remains of their circumference. With a periosteal elevator, 2 centimeters of periosteum is pushed off the radius and ulna distal to the incision, not disturbing the proximal periosteum. The muscle masses are covered with moist sponges. With a straight saw the radius and ulna are sawed through flush with the proximal periosteum. This permits the removal of the amputated portion. With the muscle masses covered with moist sponges, the bone edges are smoothed with a bone rasp, if necessary.

The ulnar artery, which lies on the ulnar side of the arm under the flexor carpi ulnaris muscle and which is accompanied by the ulnar nerve, is isolated and ligated with a transfixion suture of plain No. oo catgut. The ulnar nerve is ligated high under the muscle with a plain No. oo catgut suture and recessed so that its neuroma will be covered. The radial artery, which lies volar to the radius and under the medial edge of the brachioradialis muscle is isolated and ligated with a transfixion suture of plain No. oo catgut. No nerve accompanies the radial artery. The median nerve, which lies in the center of the volar surface of the forearm, under the flexor sublimis digitorum is next isolated. Its sheath is transfixed with a plain No. oo catgut suture and the nerve ligated well above the end of the stump, so that its neuroma will be well recessed. There is another good sized artery near the interosseus membrane on the volar surface which should be separately ligatured. The tourniquet is removed and all bleeding vessels tied separately with plain No. oo catgut ties. The skin and fascia flaps are then tailored so that on closure there will be no tension or redundancy, and so that the terminal scar will be volar to the bones. The fascia is approximated with interrupted sutures of plain No. oo catgut. A drain is placed under the fascia and carried

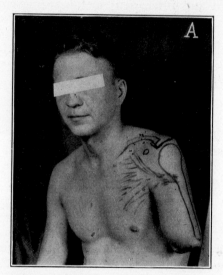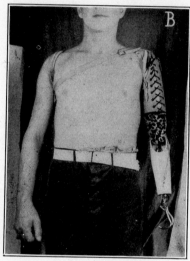

FIG. 75. (A) Photograph of ideal humeral stump. (B) Prosthesis on upper arm stump. Stippled area is space required for elbow block and mechanism. (From McKeever, *J. Bone & Joint Surg.*, 26 (No. 4):626-671 and 706, 1944.)

out through an angle of the suture line. The skin is approximated with interrupted sutures of fine silk. The drain is sutured to the skin with one suture cut long, for identification, so that it will not fall out. The suture line is covered with vaseline gauze, sterile sheet wadding is bandaged around the stump and arm, and a tensor bandage is applied over this. A molded plaster splint is then applied over the arm and forearm stump on their posterior aspect, with the elbow flexed at a right angle. The plaster splint is turned up over the end of the stump for protection.

Amputation through the Arm. The best site for an amputation through the humerus and the bone length which is most effective in using a prosthesis, is the level immediately above the beginning of the flare of the condyles of the humerus (Fig. 75). This removes 5 to 7 centimeters of bone above the articular surface of the humerus. This site of amputation results in a humeral stump that is well controlled by muscles; that can be abducted, flexed and extended; and that has sufficient strength and a strong enough grip on the prosthesis to make its use attractive. The long lever enables the amputee to develop a trick swinging motion, by means of which the forearm of the prosthesis can be flexed on the arm without raising it with the other hand, as is frequently necessary with the shorter humeral stumps. This long stump also gives stability to the prosthesis, so that the mechanical hand or hook can be operated more effectively in many more positions. This site is superior to a disarticulation through the elbow. It allows room for the mechanism of the elbow block, without placing the elbow at a lower level than the remaining normal arm and does not require a disproportionate forearm in the prosthesis. The absence of the condyles and the loss of the distal 5 to 7 centimeters of the humerus does not detract enough from the functional value of the humeral lever to offset the cosmetic and mechanical difficulties in the prosthesis, caused by the presence of the condyles.

TECHNIC OF AMPUTATION AT THE CONDYLES OF THE HUMERUS. The patient is placed in the supine position, with the arm abducted at the shoulder and extended on an arm board. A tourniquet is placed high on the arm, adjacent to the axilla. With the elbow flexed 40 to 60 degrees, a straight skin needle is inserted into the skin and muscles on the lateral side of the arm, and left projecting from the skin, to mark the point of bone section, which is just at the point where the humeral condyles begin to flare. With the elbow flexed moderately the bony landmarks are much easier to palpate than with the elbow fully extended (Fig. 76). Anterior and posterior skin flaps of equal length are planned. Since the humerus at this level lies nearer the extensor than the flexor surface of the arm, flaps of equal length will bring the terminal scar anterior to the bone end so that it will not become adherent. An incision is started 2 centimeters above the point of bone section on the lateral side of the middle of the arm, just anterior to the humerus. This incision is carried through the skin and enveloping fascia distally, a distance of 3 to 5 centimeters, and then curved abruptly across the flexor surface of the extremity to the center of the medial side of the arm. The incision then is abruptly curved so that it is parallel with the anterior border of the humerus and extended proximally on the medial side of the arm to a point 2 centimeters above the point of contemplated bone section. From the point where the vertical incisions are curved, an incision is made across the extensor aspect of the arm, cutting a flap of length equal to the anterior flap. These incisions are both carried through the enveloping fascia of the arm. The skin and fascial flaps are dissected proximally as a unit to a point 1 centimeter proximal to the point of bone section. With these flaps retracted, a curved flap of the tendinous portion of the biceps brachii muscle is cut with a scalpel. This flap of tendon is reflected proximally to the level of contemplated bone section. The brachialis and the origin of the brachioradialis muscles are then cut across vertical to the long axis of the humerus at the level of bone section. On the extensor surface of the arm the tendinous portion of the triceps muscle is cut in a curved flap which is slightly shorter than the skin flap. This is reflected proximally to the level of bone section. All muscle fibers are removed from this flap so that there will be no redundant muscle at the end of the stump. The tissues distal to the incision are retracted. The periosteum of the humerus is sharply incised about its entire circumference at the level where the proximal muscles are attached. The periosteum is pushed off the humerus for 2 centimeters distally, not dis-

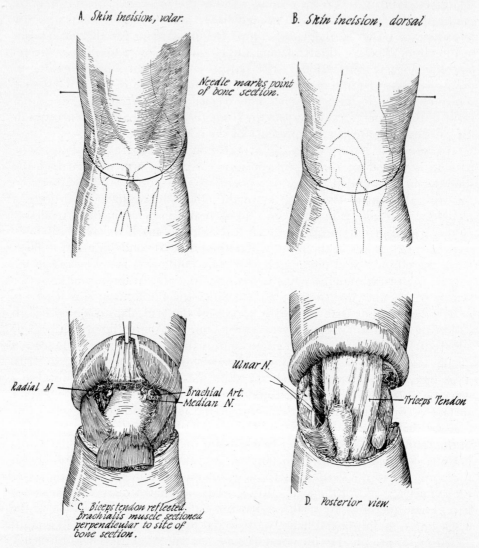

A. *Skin incision, volar.*

B. *Skin incision, dorsal*

Needle marks point of bone section.

Radial N.

Brachial Art.
Median N.

Ulnar N.

Triceps Tendon

C. *Biceps tendon reflected. Brachialis muscle sectioned perpendicular to site of bone section.*

D. *Posterior view.*

FIG. 76(1). Technic of amputation through humerus at level of flare of condyles. (A) Skin incision, volar view. (B) Skin incision, dorsal view. (C) Biceps tendon reflected, brachialis muscle cut perpendicular to site of bone section. (D) Posterior view. Tendon of triceps and ulnar nerve visible.

turbing the proximal periosteum. The humerus is then sawed through flush with the periosteum. This permits removal of the part to be amputated. If necessary, the edge of the distal end of the humerus is smoothed with a fine rasp. The brachial artery and vein which lie on the medial side anterior to the humerus in the plane between the biceps and brachialis are isolated and ligated with a transfixion suture of chromic No. 1 catgut. Accompanying these vessels is the median nerve which is developed up the fascial plane. The sheath of the nerve is transfixed high with a suture of plain No. oo catgut. The nerve is then cut off high under the biceps below the suture so that its neuroma will be well recessed. On the lateral side of the stump just at the level of the front of the humerus between the brachioradialis and the brachialis muscle, the radial nerve is isolated, developed up its fascial plane,

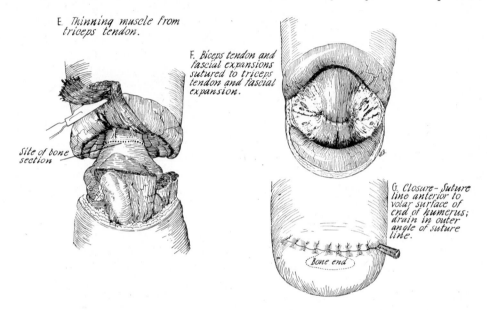

E. Thinning muscle from triceps tendon.

F. Biceps tendon and fascial expansions sutured to triceps tendon and fascial expansion.

Site of bone section

G. Closure- Suture line anterior to volar surface of end of humerus; drain in outer angle of suture line.

Bone end

FIG. 76(2). (E) Thinning muscle from triceps tendon. (F) Biceps tendon and fascial expansions sutured to triceps tendon and fascial expansions. (G) Closure. Suture line anterior to volar surface of end of humerus. Drain in outer angle of suture line.

its sheath transfixed with a suture of plain No. oo catgut, and the nerve ligated. It is then cut off high in the fascial plane just below the ligature so that its neuroma will be well recessed. About the center of the anterior muscle flap between the biceps and the brachialis is the lateral antebrachial cutaneous nerve, a small nerve which should be treated in the same way. On the medial side of the arm at the level of the posterior aspect of the humerus on the medial border of the triceps close to the skin is the ulnar nerve which is transfixed and cut off high to recess its neuroma. Just beneath the skin, in the region of the lateral intramuscular septum is another fairly large cutaneous nerve which it is well to recess. The basilic vein on the medial side of the arm should also be ligated. The tourniquet is completely released and all smaller vessels ligated individually with plain No. oo catgut. The tendinous flaps are then tailored to make a neat closure without tension or redundancy. The tendons of the biceps and triceps are approximated with interrupted sutures of plain No. oo catgut. A drain is placed beneath the approximated tendons, emerging from the outer angle of the suture line. The skin edge is then freed just sufficiently to permit it to be trimmed for a smooth closure, and the edges are approximated with interrupted sutures of fine silk. The drain is sutured through the skin with one suture cut long for identification. Vaseline gauze is placed over the suture line and dressings applied. Sterile sheet wadding is wrapped about the lower half of the stump and a tensor bandage applied over this, for gentle pressure. The bandage is taped to the upper arm with adhesive strips crossing over the end of the stump in a cruciate fashion. The arm stump is supported postoperatively on a pillow.

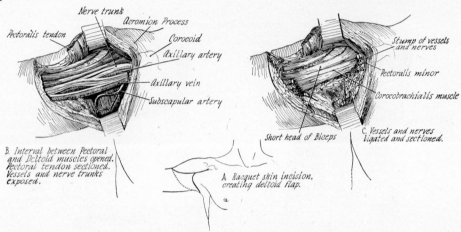

FIG. 77(1). Technic of disarticulation of the shoulder. (A) Skin incision; handle of racquet follows deltoid-pectoral interval. (B) Axillary artery and vein and nerve trunks isolated. (C) Axillary artery and vein ligated, nerve trunks sectioned, and proximal ends ligated.

Amputation through the Shoulder. This is an extensive surgical procedure and may result in considerable blood loss with shock. The use of a tourniquet in this operation is not practical. Prior to carrying out this operation the patient should be typed for transfusion and blood of the proper type should be available in the operating room. Amputation through the shoulder is done either as: (1) a disarticulation of the shoulder joint; (2) an amputation through the neck of the humerus, leaving the humeral head in the stump. If the humeral head can be left in the stump without leaving behind pathology, the cosmetic result is better than if it is removed. The humeral head should never be left in the stump at the risk of incomplete ablation of the pathological tissue.

TECHNIC OF AMPUTATION THROUGH THE SHOULDER. The patient is placed in the supine position on the operating table and tipped 35 degrees on the side opposite to the involved extremity by placing sand bags or a triangular rest under the thorax. Drapes are applied so that the top of the shoulder to the root of the neck, the upper half of the anterior thoracic wall, the axilla, and the vertebral margin of the scapula are visible and available.

The arm is draped so that the shoulder girdle can be easily manipulated and the elbow flexed. It is well to have two assistants for this operation, one to manipulate the arm, and the other to retract tissues for exposure (Fig. 77).

A racquet incision is used and the large vessels, the brachial artery and vein, and the cephalic vein are ligated in the first step of the operation to control the main source of hemorrhage. The handle portion of the racquet incision is made first. This portion of the incision extends from a point 3

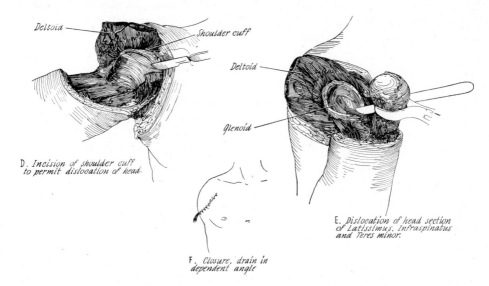

FIG. 77(2). (D) Capsule of shoulder incised to mobilize head of humerus. (E) Head of humerus freed; latissimus dorsi teres major and remaining muscles which hold humerus to thorax, sectioned. (F) Closure. Glenoid covered by deltoid flap. Drain in dependent angle of suture line.

centimeters above the coracoid process distally to the point where the anterior axillary fold meets the arm, and is over the interval between the deltoid and pectoralis major muscles. At the anterior axillary fold it is curved with a distal convexity to cross over the deltoid. This incision is best made with the shoulder abducted 70 degrees and externally rotated. The incision is carried through skin and fascia and the interval between the deltoid and pectoralis major muscles is opened. Along the margin of the pectoralis major the cephalic vein is encountered. This vein is ligated with plain No. oo catgut and divided. The tendon of the pectoralis major muscle is then sectioned with a knife close to the humerus, while the arm is in abduction and external rotation. The pectoralis major muscle is then retracted distally and the deltoid superiorly. The axillary artery and vein are separated from the median ulnar and radial nerves. The axillary artery is then clamped near the border of the pectoralis minor muscles. Two ligatures of chromic No. 1 catgut are placed above the clamp and one ligature of chromic No. 1 catgut below the clamp. The artery is then cut between the clamp and the lower ligature. The axillary vein is then treated in the same manner and cut. If the acromiothoracic trunk which perforates the pectoralis minor muscle can be exposed it is ligated. This will lessen posterior bleeding in the later stages of the amputation. The median, ulnar, radial, and musculocutaneous nerves are then pulled down separately and ligated separately with plain No. oo catgut. They are sectioned with a knife below the ligature and their ligated stumps are recessed under the pectoralis minor muscle so that their neuromas will be hidden. Having completed control of the main blood supply the skin incision is completed by carrying it across the deltoid to the posterior axillary fold and thence across the axilla on the lateral axillary wall of the arm to meet the handle of the racquet, thus completing the incision. This incision is carried through skin, subcutaneous tissue, and fascia. The incision through the deltoid is carried to bone and the deltoid flap turned upward to the acromion, exposing the cuff of the shoulder capsule. In turning up the deltoid flap the circumflex artery may be encountered and should be ligated. With the deltoid flap retracted, the arm is externally rotated and the capsule of the shoulder is incised, cutting the tendon of the subscapularis. The arm is internally rotated, cutting the posterior-superior part of the capsule of the shoulder joint and the tendons of the supraspinatus and infraspinatus muscles. The cut margin of the capsule is retracted distally and the long head of the biceps cut near the superior margin of the glenoid. This permits the head of the humerus to be dislocated cephalically and grasped with a large bone holding forceps. The capsule on the inferior aspect of the shoulder joint is then cut with a knife through the cephalic opening. With a large bone holding forceps maintaining the humeral head out of the way, the short head of the biceps muscle, the coracobrachialis, and the long head of the triceps muscle, are cut close to their origin on the coracoid process and the inferior rim of the glenoid. The latissimus dorsi and teres major are cut close to their insertion into the humerus, which permits the arm to be removed. All vessels are individually ligated until good hemostasis is obtained. If the tendons of the pectoralis major muscle, of the subscapularis and of the latissimus dorsi and teres major muscles are long enough, they are sutured to the capsule projecting from the margin of the glenoid with interrupted chromic No. 1 catgut. All ragged margins of capsule are removed. The flap of the deltoid is then permitted to drop over the glenoid and trimmed to fit the defect in the lateral thoracic wall. The fascia is approximated with interrupted sutures of plain No. oo catgut. A drain is placed at the dependent angle of the suture line beneath the muscle. The skin margins are elevated sufficiently to tailor them for a neat closure, and trimmed. The skin edges are then approximated with interrupted sutures of fine silk. The drain is sewed with one suture cut long, for identification, to the skin. The suture line is covered with vaseline gauze. Dressings are applied and a bandage applied over the stump, top of the shoulder, around the thorax, and under the opposite axilla, with tensor bandages to exert gentle pressure over the deltoid flap.

TECHNIC OF AMPUTATION OF SHOULDER THROUGH THE SURGICAL NECK OF THE HUMERUS. Amputation through the neck of the humerus is carried out through the same incision as disarticulation of the shoulder. The pectoral deltoid interval is developed, the vessels and nerves isolated and disposed of, and the deltoid flap elevated exactly as in a disarticulation of the shoulder. When this has been accomplished the capsule of the shoulder joint and the attachment of the rotator muscles to the tuberosities of the humerus are not disturbed.

Instead, with a blunt dissector and by rotation of the arm, the muscles are freed extraperiosteally, never subperiosteally, for a distance of 3 centimeters around the sides and the medial aspect of the neck of the humerus. A curved hemostat or large aneurysm needle is passed around the humerus and a Gigli saw pulled through from the medial to lateral side. The humerus is then cut through the neck with a Gigli saw. The proximal end of the distal fragment of the humerus is then grasped with a bone holding forceps and gently pulled out while the muscles are cut away from the lateral and medial side of the upper end of the distal fragment for a distance of 2 to 3 centimeters. This is done extraperiosteally. With the distal fragment of the humerus retracted out of the way, the remaining muscles holding the humerus to the torso, the tendon of the long head of the biceps, the coracobrachialis, the short head of the biceps, the triceps, teres major, and latissimus dorsi, are sectioned at the level of the lower end of the head fragment. This completes the removal of the extremity. Closure of the wound and dressings are exactly as in a disarticulation through the shoulder.

Intrascapular Thoracic Amputation. This amputation removes the scapula, the outer two-thirds of the clavicle, and the entire upper extremity. It is rarely indicated and is a massive surgical procedure, requiring supportive treatment. The end result is severe disfigurement, sloping the individual from the neck to the costal margin. No functional prosthesis is applicable to the stump, which is the upper rib cage. The indication is usually malignancy in the region of the shoulder which has invaded the axilla and in which disarticulation of the shoulder is inadequate. The technic of this operation will not be described.

EARLY POSTOPERATIVE CARE

In any amputation which has been done through or adjacent to tissues which have previously been infected, the administration of antibiotics should be resumed immediately after surgery. Either penicillin or sulfadiazine should be administered on schedule until it is evident by the patient's postoperative course that there is going to be no recrudescence of infection. Usually the administration of one or the other for 5 to 7 days after operation is adequate.

Morphine in doses large enough to keep the patient comfortable should be used in the first forty-eight to seventy-two hours. In elderly patients this may be inadvisable, due to its depressant effect. During this period there may be severe muscle spasm, which is prevented to a large degree by splinting, and there may be severe "phantom pains," the patient feeling burning or vice-like clamping in the foot or hand which has been removed. Reassurance that this phantom pain will subside should be given. Morphine must be used judiciously in the care of amputees. After the first few days the pain should be handled by codeine or aspirin. As a group, due to the psychological shock of the loss of an extremity, amputees are more likely to succumb to the use of narcotics. Any evidence of a desire by the patient for the continuance of the use of narcotics beyond a justifiable period should be frankly dealt with, explaining their dangers and keeping them from the patient.

If there has been considerable blood loss at operation, or marked sweating, blood substitutes, depending on the severity of the state, should be administered. Intravenous glucose may be adequate. In severe depletion, plasma or whole blood may be indicated.

Elevation of the fresh stump adds greatly to the comfort of the patient and promotes healing by preventing dependent edema of tissues. This can be easily accomplished by keeping the leg stump elevated on pillows. Early ambulation is not advisable in amputation of the lower extremity; in fact, it is contraindicated. The dependency leads to swelling and edema, which impedes healing, and dependence may even cause ecchymosis of tissues, due to increased venous pressure. In arm amputations, early ambulation is practical. The arm can be kept elevated on an aeroplane splint which prevents swelling and edema.

If a drain has been inserted at operation it should be removed at the end of forty-eight hours. At this time if there is a localized collection of blood, the removal of an occasional stitch may be indicated. It adds greatly to the comfort of the patient to remove the initial dressing at forty-eight hours, as it has often adhered by dried blood, and pulls on the stitches.

Stitches are not removed early in amputations. There is a great tendency for the healing incision to spread and a narrow scar is desirable as an end result. On the average, ten to twelve days is about the length of time stitches are left in place. If a nonirritating skin suture has been used, they may at times be left in as long as fourteen to eighteen days with advantage to the patient.

EARLY POSTOPERATIVE COMPLICATIONS

Despite the greatest of care, *hemorrhage* to a severe degree may occur in an amputation stump. This may be manifested by soaking of the dressings with blood, a rapid pulse, and impending shock. At other times the hemorrhage may be entirely retained within the flaps where it will produce great tension. Under these circumstances severe unrelenting pain may be the only symptom. Hemorrhage usually occurs and manifests itself in the first twenty-four hours, but can occur rarely as late as the tenth postoperative day.

If the degree of shock is severe the patient should be given a transfusion. Under appropriate anesthesia and aseptic surgical conditions the stump should be completely opened, the hematoma and clots washed from the tissues, and the bleeding vessel, or vessels, isolated and securely ligated. It is usually not one of the large main vessels, but a moderate size muscular branch which causes the hemorrhage. The stump should be again closed in layers, as at the time of the initial operation after obtaining complete and thorough hemostasis.

If the hemorrhage is of small size and is entirely retained within the flaps, in a number of instances pressure bandages along with elevation and morphine, will control the situation. However, if there is a large collection of blood it is wisest to open the stump in the operating room and wash out the clots. Enormous hematomas delay healing and lead to a large indurated mass at the end of the stump. Tension from the hemorrhage may also embarrass the circulation of the skin flaps. Under no circumstances should the stump be opened without anesthesia, or in the dressing room with inadequate facilities for asepsis. If it is decided to be necessary to open the stump, the procedure should be done in the operating room under anesthesia, with the same precautions and preparation as the initial amputation.

Hematomata of small size in an amputation stump are more common postoperatively than massive hemorrhage. Small hematomata can usually be evacuated by taking out a suture or two and inserting a sterile instrument into the area in which the blood has collected. This does not interfere with the ultimate healing of the scar. After the hematoma has emptied itself the edges of the incision can be pulled together with butterfly straps of adhesive. Minor collections of blood do not interfere with the final outcome and they do not demand that the entire stump end be opened. However, every effort should be made to avoid a hematoma of any size by spending time to tie individual muscle bleeders at the operation.

Tension on the skin flaps may be evident at the first dressing, when the drain is removed. Due to swelling and edema, what appeared in the operating room to be skin flaps of perfect length, may be pulling on the suture line, and the outline of the bone end may be evident through the skin. This tension is readily relieved by traction. Skin traction should be immediately applied, just as in an open amputation, and continued until solid healing of the incision has resulted.

Infection may abruptly and suddenly manifest itself in the first twelve to twenty-four hours postoperatively by marked hyperpyrexia, rapid pulse, and severe toxemia. The stump may exhibit an extensive cellulitis with brawny induration of the skin and massive edema of the entire remaining portion of the extremity. This swelling in some instances may extend from the leg to the abdomen, or from the forearm to the thorax. These manifestations of infection, which are usually the result of a very virulent streptococcus or staphylococcus, demand that the stump be immediately and completely opened and that the amputation be treated as an open amputation. Appropriate antibiotic therapy and other adequate supportive measures are indicated. Extensive necrosis of the flaps may result from a virulent infection of this type. In these times of prophylactic antibiotic therapy such infections fortunately are rare.

Since many amputations are in tissue adjacent to previously infected areas which have healed, mild infections are not uncommon. The presence of even small hematomata favor the development of abscesses. Many abscesses can be aborted by the early evacuation of small hematoma. Most localized abscesses under flaps can also be satisfactorily treated by the removal of a suture or two, which permits them to drain. Taping the edges together after they have emptied will usually result in sound healing without further surgery and eliminate the necessity of a later skin plastic operation.

Gas bacillus infections occasionally result as a complication of amputations. Crepitus in the soft tissues should make one suspicious of virulent gas forming anaerobes. Gangrenous tissue with an open lesion harbors *Clostridii welchii* in a high percentage of patients; consequently, in amputations in occlusive vascular disease with gangrene, gas gangrene is a potential hazard. Virulent gas bacillus infection was reported by Macey and Bickel in one series of amputations done for occlusive vascular disease to be a complication in 4 per cent of patients. The presence of crepitus, with any signs of toxemia such as increase in pulse rate and fever, is an indication to open the stump widely and give the patient adequate doses of polyvalent perfringens antitoxin and roentgenotherapy over the infected area. Either penicillin or sulfadiazine should also be administered to patients with gas bacillus infection, as streptococci are usually present and invasive in this type of infection, as well as *Clostridium welchii.* Muscles which undergo necrosis may have to be excised surgically and it may even be necessary to perform an open amputation at a higher level.

Tetanus, if it should occur, requires appropriate treatment with massive doses of tetanus antitoxin and sedatives. This complication should be rare. A patient who has suffered trauma of the severity which might result in amputation should have received a prophylactic injection of tetanus antitoxin in the period immediately following the injury. In instances in which there has been high probability of contamination of wounds with tetanus and long intervals have intervened between the injury and the amputation, it is advisable to give a prophylactic dose of tetanus antitoxin before the amputation, even though an initial prophylactic dose of antitoxin may have been administered. If the patient has had a previous dose of tetanus antitoxin he will be sensitive to horse serum and it will be necessary that the antitoxin be administered in fractionated doses to avoid an anaphylactic reaction. Individuals who have been immunized with tetanus toxoid, if it has been six months since their last booster dose, should receive a booster dose of toxoid before operation. Tetanus toxoid is the ideal agent for prevention of tetanus, but requires that the individual have been immunized before the accident or condition indicating amputation has occurred. Reactions of any type to tetanus toxoid are practically nonexistent. In World War II, all soldiers were immunized with toxoid, and tetanus was unknown in the American Army. Tetanus has occurred after the use of a single dose of tetanus antitoxin given prophylactically, so that if there is any well founded suspicion of its possibility, three prophylactic doses of antitoxin of 1500 units each should be given at weekly intervals, following the injury requiring amputation.

Thrombophlebitis is not a common complication of amputation. When it does occur its manifestations are the same as under any other circumstances in a similar locale and the therapeutic indications are the same.

Necrosis of skin flaps at their terminal ends occurs occasionally, due to thrombosis in the veins of the skin. This usually is of minor extent and is followed by dry gangrene of a small portion of the terminal end of the skin flap up to the suture line. When of slight degree, removing the gangrenous area and approximating the trimmed edges with adhesive strips will bring about satisfactory healing without further surgery. Skin traction may also be of value in treating this complication.

Infiltration of the skin by blood may occur when only skin and not fascia covers the end of the stump. This causes an area of skin to assume a deep purple color as in any ecchymosis. It should not be mistaken for gangrene of the flap. It will recover without loss of skin and no treatment is necessary.

PREPARATION OF THE STUMP FOR USE OF PROSTHESIS

The ultimate aim of any amputation is to produce a stump which will use a prosthesis satisfactorily and effectively, so that the individual deprived of part of an extremity will approach normal function. In order that a stump use a prosthesis as well as possible, it is necessary that it be: (1) of proper shape and length; (2) that it undergo shrinkage; (3) that the skin of the stump be flexible and the scar nonadherent; (4) that the joints in the stump be free of contractures and have as nearly normal range of motion as possible; and (5) that the strength of the muscles moving the joints in the stump be well developed.

The proper shape and length of the stump result from a well planned and executed operation. It is not always possible for the surgeon to effect a stump of the ideal length, but it is possible to create the conditions for a stump of proper shape by proper treatment of the bone end, by coning out excess muscle and by removing redundant skin.

All amputation stumps, during the first six months after they are healed, undergo a degree of shrinkage in circumference. This is due to disappearance of swelling and edema, as the circulatory status of the stump returns to normal and to the atrophy of all soft tissues, more especially of the muscle in the stump, which no longer has to carry out its previous function. This shrinkage in most instances progresses rapidly during the first three to five months, and after this progresses only very gradually for the next year or two. If a prosthesis is obtained prior to three months after healing of the stump and without shrinking the stump, it is likely that changes will have to be made in the socket of the prosthesis at such a rapid rate that the leg will be in the shop most of the time. This is an expensive and trying experience. Shrinkage of the stump should be brought about to a large degree before the amputee is sent for his permanent prosthesis.

Shrinkage of the stump is most effectively brought about by use of the stump in walking, and by bandaging the stump when it is not being used for walking. Bandaging of the stump to produce pressure can be instituted as soon as the sutures are removed and the skin is healed. This is best done with an elastic type of bandage 3 to 4 inches wide and long enough to completely encase the stump well above the joint at its distal end. For a below the knee stump there should be a bandage of sufficient length so that it will encase the leg above the knee for 4 to 6 inches; and for a midthigh amputation the bandages should be adequate to have a few wraps around the abdomen, otherwise the bandages are liable to slide off the conical stump (Fig. 78). Narrow bandages are prone to roll on themselves and act as con-

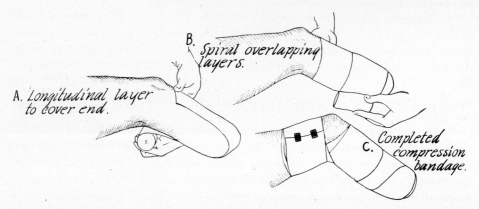

FIG. 78. Technic of applying tensor bandage to stump to produce shrinkage. (A) Longitudinal layer to cover end. (B) Spiral overlapping layers. (C) Completed compression bandage.

stricting cords, producing edema below them. These bandages are wrapped around the stump in a manner planned to exert constant gentle pressure from the end of the stump to the first joint. This requires that the end of the stump be covered by the tensor bandage, which is accomplished by running folds of the bandage vertically on the front and back of the stump, over its end. These vertical layers of tensed bandage are held in place by circular layers over them, which start at the distal end of the stump and progress proximally, exerting even pressure all the way up the stump and covering all the stump with wide overlaps. If the edges are not widely overlapped, skin will bulge through between the bandage and result in constriction. The bandage is changed frequently during the day as it slips and loosens. The bandages tend to lose their elasticity and when this occurs new bandages should be obtained. If the end of the stump is not compressed and encased by the bandages it will bulge through and a section of soft tissue at the lower end becomes choked with resulting chronic edema and induration.

The most effective measure in expediting shrinkage of the soft tissues is the use of the stump in weight bearing. This can be accomplished by constructing a simple prosthesis, in which the socket is made by constructing a mold of the stump from plaster bandages (Fig. 79). After the mold has hardened, a peg of adequate length is attached to it with more plaster. This

peg can be a single pole or can be the lower portion of a crutch. Webbing straps to go over the shoulder or about the waist are then riveted or attached with more plaster to the upper end of the plaster socket. Where leather workers are available, an adjustable socket can be made of leather. In Army amputation centers a provisional leg of fiber, in which the socket could be taken up or changed, with joints like a permanent prosthesis, was used. This is an excellent method but requires skilled mechanics and is expensive. The plaster peg leg or pylon can be fab-
ricated anywhere, at very little ex-
pense, and suffices well.

Adherent scars on any part of an amputation stump to be covered by, or pulled on by the socket of a prosthesis, are undesirable, due to the fact that they are painful, break down, and ulcerate. Care in the sur-
gery of amputations and avoidance of separating skin and fascia widely, minimize the chances of adherent scars. Most adherent scars can be mobilized by massage. If for any reason they do result, massage has a definite place in freeing adherent scars, but is of negligible value in hastening shrinkage of the stump. If there are no adherent scars, massage has no place in the treatment of an amputation stump.

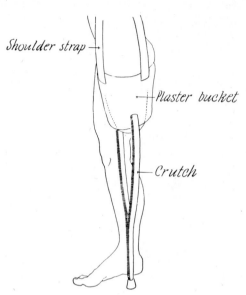

Fig. 79. Simple plaster pylon. Made from plaster bandages, crutch and webbing straps.

Contractures in amputation stumps are rather common. They frequently develop in the preoperative period of invalidism, due to the patient's desire to prevent pain and the surgeon's failure to realize that soft tissue contractures develop in a short period of time if a position is assumed and main-
tained constantly. The individual with an injury in the arm or forearm, to avoid pain, will maintain the shoulder adducted with the arm to the side. The patient with injury or disease in the lower extremity is frequently confined to bed with the leg elevated on pillows or in a splint, with the hip and knee flexed. Even after an amputation, patients are too often left for an in-
definite period of time to assume these positions, which induce contractures.

The flexion contracture of the hip joint is the most serious detriment to the best use of a prosthesis and is most frequently unrecognized (Fig. 80). This contracture results from shortening of the lateral or abductor muscles of the thigh. When the stump is abducted it is not apparent; when the stump is adducted it may be very obvious. This deformity, when present, can be demonstrated by placing the patient in the supine position and flexing the opposite thigh on the abdomen to flatten the patient's back. With the amputee in this position the stump is brought to the adducted position.

When an abduction-flexion contracture is present the posterior surface of the stump will not rest on the examining table, but will be flexed at the hip. This deformity makes it obligatory for the patient, when standing, with the feet a normal distance apart, either to bend forward at the hips and thus succumb to gravity, or to arch his back to compensate for the flexion, in order that he may have his head over his feet. The patient with an abduction-flexion contracture of the hip usually walks swinging the artificial leg widely and with an unsightly gait. In trying to compensate for the flexion the patient also increases the lordosis of the lumbar spine, which leads to backache

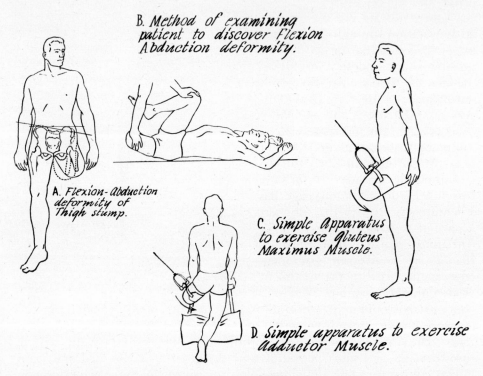

FIG. 80. Flexion-abduction deformity of thigh stump. (A) Deformity and tilt of pelvis when corrected. (B) Method of examining for deformity. (C) Apparatus for exercising gluteus maximus. (D) Same apparatus employed to develop adductor muscles.

and early hypertrophic arthritic changes in the articulations of the lumbar vertebra.

The fitting of a prosthesis to a thigh stump with an abduction-flexion contracture is difficult. The inability of the stump to extend to the normal position at the hip must be compensated for in the construction of the socket and thigh piece of the prosthesis. It is this deformity which usually causes the socket to press on the adductor tendons and pubis, with great discomfort to the patient. In very short thigh stumps, the abduction-flexion contracture cannot be relieved and the socket of the prosthesis must be constructed to accommodate for its presence.

In all thigh stumps which preserve half the length of the femur, this contracture can be released by stretching exercises and the development of the muscles which prevent it. The development of these contractures can also be obviated by the simple expedient of having the patient lie periodically on his stomach and actively contract the gluteal muscles, instead of sitting in bed with the hip flexed on pillows for twenty-four hours a day during the preoperative and postoperative period. Any contracture of this type which does not yield to some degree rather rapidly, under stretching, should be investigated with x-rays of the hip joint to determine whether or not there is intra-articular pathology.

Flexion contractures of the knee occur frequently in below the knee amputations and when present to over 10 degrees are a serious impediment to walking. The partially flexed knee lets the patient down. They are best prevented, and this is easily done, by having the patient contract the quadriceps, moving the patella upward, straightening the knee. This also helps to prevent atrophy of the quadriceps muscle. When present, this contracture usually yields readily to passive stretching of the hamstring muscles and the capsular structures, by the physical therapist. A more resistant contracture may require wedging casts to relieve it. Rarely, the operation of posterior capsulectomy may reclaim a severely flexed knee joint.

In the upper extremity, the frozen shoulder, with the humerus bound to the side, is easily prevented by keeping the injured or amputated extremity on an aeroplane splint in 90 degrees of abduction. This is also a very great adjuvant to healing, as it obviates the dependent edema and bogginess in the tissues. Simply having the patient elevate the arm to touch the top of the bed several times daily, which requires carrying the shoulder through abduction and external rotation, is a valuable prophylactic measure to prevent the frozen shoulder. A contracture of the shoulder will yield, just as any adhesive bursitis, to passive stretching of the contracted pectoral muscles and active exercise of the deltoid and rotator muscles. No amputation stump can be expected to use a prosthesis with maximum efficiency until all contractures are released.

Muscular development of certain muscle groups is necessary for the best use of each prosthesis. No muscle can be expected to work efficiently against a contracture. All contractures must be overcome in order that maximum muscular development be achieved. Too often, after the invalidism which has brought about the amputation, the muscles needed to properly motivate the prosthesis are weak and atrophied.

To efficiently use an artificial leg in the above the knee amputation, the gluteus maximus muscle which extends the hip and the adductor muscles of the thigh which pull the thigh toward the midline, must be strong and well developed. Special exercises against resistance to strengthen these muscle groups should be instituted as soon as the stump is healed from surgery. This can be done by having the patient carry out extension and adduction of the hip while a nurse resists this motion with her hand. A simple apparatus can be assembled with a pulley, rope, flannel sling, and some weights. The pulley attached to the foot of the bed will serve for the patient to lift weights while standing on the good foot. It does not take a masseuse to carry out this training. In the absence of a well coordinated physical medicine department, the surgeon who removes the extremity should instruct the patient in these exercises and see that they are carried out by the patient to the point of good muscular development. Otherwise he has completed his job no more than has the surgeon who removes an eye and leaves an unsuitable socket for the artificial eye.

The patient with a below the knee stump, in addition to having good musculature to extend and adduct the hip, must have good muscles to extend the knee. Exercises to develop the quadriceps femoris should be started early and continued until there is good strength in this muscle group.

Powerful abdominal muscles, to flatten the pelvis in the erect posture, are a great aid in the use of the prosthesis to an individual with an amputation above the knee. Active exercises to strengthen the abdominal musculature should be persisted in by the patient. Too often the amputee is permitted to loaf around and acquire a pendulous fat abdomen, which adds to his burdens and increases his difficulties in the use of a prosthesis.

The arm amputee must have a good deltoid. If he has an elbow joint, he must have a good biceps brachii muscle to flex the arm prosthesis and a good pronator teres in the long forearm stump to take advantage of this motion in the newer type of arm prosthesis.

SELECTION OF PROSTHESES

A surgeon is not a leg fitter. Leg fitting is a craft which requires long experience and great skill in which a surgeon does not have the time or the opportunity to become proficient. However, every surgeon who takes care of amputees should have a knowledge of the fundamentals of prostheses. The surgeon has a knowledge of the tissues which are to use the prosthesis, which the leg fitter does not have. The surgeon must be able to tell the leg fitter the type of prosthesis which is best for the individual patient, and after the prosthesis is delivered to the patient, know whether or not it fits satisfactorily and meets the requirement of his stump.

Many different materials are used in the construction of artificial limbs. The requirements of materials to be used in the construction of artificial limbs are: (1) that they offer maximum strength and durability with minimum weight; (2) that they be amenable to shaping; (3) that they be non-irritating to skin; (4) that they have low conductivity for heat; and (5) that they not acquire an offensive odor from body secretions.

A wood which most nearly meets all these requirements is willow. A good deal of skill and time is necessary in working willow, and willow limbs are expensive. The willow can be made very thin and is strengthened by a covering of rawhide. The leg maker skilled in handling willow can shape its socket to handle the most irregular stump. Willow limbs today, except for expense, are still the best prostheses.

A metal which has proven most satisfactory for use in artificial limbs is duraluminum, which is an alloy of aluminum. Limbs made of this metal are far lighter than those made of any other material, and when lack of weight is important, as in very large prostheses, as for a hip disarticulation or a high thigh stump, or in elderly, weak individuals, metal should be used. Metal limbs have the disadvantage that specially equipped shops are necessary for their adjustment and realignment.

A fiber which is a product of rag pulp, is also used in artificial extremities. It is slightly heavier for the same prosthesis than either willow or metal. It is, however, easily adjustable. Fiber limbs have a riveted seam which allows for changes in the circumference of the thigh and skin piece. Much less skill is needed to handle fiber than willow and much less equipment is necessary for adjustments than with duraluminum. Fiber prostheses are less costly than those of metal or willow.

Plastics and plywood have been experimented with extensively during and since World War II for the construction of artificial extremities. While the most suitable plastic has not as yet been arrived at, it is not improbable that the ideal material for the construction of prostheses may be found in this field.

Leather is unsuitable for use in the construction of the main portion of artificial limbs. It does not hold its shape and without great thickness and weight has no strength. It absorbs body secretions and becomes offensive. Leather may be used to cover parts which do not come in contact with the stump, such as the foot, and for straps and belts which can be easily changed when they lose shape or become offensive.

LOWER EXTREMITY PROSTHESES

The essential elements of a lower leg prosthesis are: (1) the thigh and shin pieces; (2) the foot; (3) the joints; (4) the socket; and (5) the suspension apparatus. The thigh and shin pieces are constructed of either willow, metal, fiber, or plastic. Their shape should conform as nearly as possible to the normal limb. This is particularly true of the shin piece if the prosthesis is to be worn by a woman (Fig. 81).

The foot must be durable, light and noiseless. The best combination of materials for the foot is wood and sponge rubber covered with thin leather. The fore part of the foot is split and separated from the posterior part of the foot by a rubber bumper to give smoothness to the gait. Rubber is properly placed on the sole and heel to relieve shock in walking. Some feet on the market have lateral motion in them, but this is neither a necessary nor a desirable feature.

Joints are made of metal. Their construction must be good to avoid noise and possess durability. Complicated mechanisms in joints are as a rule neither desirable nor necessary. A simple U type of joint for the ankle has been proven by time to be the most satisfactory. The range of motion in the ankle joint is rarely more than 20 degrees of plantar flexion.

The knee joint connects the shin piece and the thigh piece. There are two types of knee joint: the single axis knee joint and the polycentric knee joint. The single axis knee joint consists of a tapered bolt passing through a hole in the knee block, in which there are bushings of leather or metal. Friction is used in this joint to slow the motion of the shin piece on the thigh piece. Some knee joints have an accurately adjustable braking mechanism in them and are called Brake Knee Joints. The knee joint also contains a back check mechanism to prevent the shin from extending beyond 185 degrees on the thigh. There may also be a controlling apparatus in the knee to regulate extension.

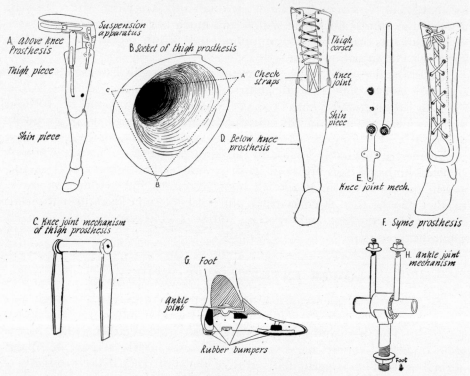

FIG. 81. Prostheses. (A) Above the knee prosthesis. (B) Socket for thigh stump. (C) Single axis knee joint. (D) Below the knee prosthesis. (E) Outside knee joint mechanism for below the knee prosthesis. (G) Foot. (H) Ankle joint mechanism.

The polycentric knee joint is a complicated mechanism, the purpose of which is to have the shin piece rotate around the thigh piece as the tibia rotates around the femur, as it flexes. While theoretically, this simulation of the normal knee is desirable; practically, it is not necessary, and the polycentric knee joint has no advantage over the single, fixed axis knee joint.

In a prosthesis to be used on a below the knee stump without ischial weight bearing, side joints such as are employed in a brace are used. Ball bearing construction is desirable in these side joints. Braking, friction, and extensor control are not necessary, as the stump does this.

Hip joints are not used except in appliances for very short stumps resulting from amputations near or through the hip. This type of joint has a locking device in it which is under control of the patient.

The socket is the element of the prosthesis requiring the greatest skill and experience to construct. It is that portion of the prosthesis into which the stump fits and through which the stump motivates the prosthesis. Irregularities or defects in the fit of the socket will abrade and injure the stump. It is made separately and then attached firmly to the thigh or shin piece so that proper alignment can be obtained and so that changes can be made without discarding the entire prosthesis. Willow wood and metal are most frequently used for sockets, the latter is used for metal legs. Leather is not satisfactory for sockets, as it is unhygienic. The shin piece and socket in a below the knee prosthesis of willow wood are all one piece. The socket must put the weight at the points which can tolerate it best, and not distribute it evenly. In Germany, suction sockets for thigh amputees have been used and they are now being experimented with in this country.

The suspension apparatus is the mechanism by which the prosthesis is kept from sliding off the conical stump. This is accomplished in the above the knee prosthesis either by suspenders going over the shoulders which are attached to the thigh piece, or by a pelvic band attached to the thigh piece. The pelvic band is constructed of metal and leather and encircles the patient's waist at the level of the iliac spines. This is attached, by an extension arm which has a ball bearing outside joint in it, to the thigh piece. The pelvic band suspension gives the patient better control and unity with the prosthesis and a better gait.

Prostheses for thigh amputations above the supracondylar level are ischial bearing prostheses. That is, the weight of the body is borne for the most part on the tuberosity of the ischium and not on the end of the stump. A small amount of bearing is taken by the sides of the stump but the bulk of the weight falls on the ischial tuberosity. The patient actually sits in the socket, which is rigid at the ischial tuberosity and is triangular in shape to fit the upper part of the thigh. The prosthesis is suspended on a pelvic band, which prevents it from rotating and from slipping distally on the stump.

Prostheses for amputations through the thigh at the supracondylar level of the femur, the end bearing tendoplastic amputation, and the Gritti-Stokes amputation take the major portion of the body weight on the end of the stump and a lesser portion on the sides of the conical stump. A long leather mold, made from an accurate model of the stump, is used for the socket. This leather socket is attached to the shin piece by a knee joint with outside joints. Hyperextension of the knee is prevented by check straps extending from the posterior aspect of the thigh socket to the shin. Under ideal circumstances, no suspension apparatus is necessary. Occasionally this type of stump will not tolerate unrestricted end bearing. This situation may be met by extending the leather socket to take some ischial bearing. If no end bearing can be tolerated, a total ischial bearing socket can be used as in a typical prosthesis for shorter thigh stumps.

Prostheses for below the knee stumps bear weight on the internal tuberosity of the tibia, the head of the fibula, the crest of the tibia, and the sides of the stump. The prosthesis is kept on the patient or suspended by a thigh corset which extends from above the knee, variable lengths up the thigh. This corset laces in front. This maintains the prosthesis in place due to the bulge of the femoral condyles. For below the knee stumps which are very short, it may be necessary to incorporate partial or "soft" ischial bearing in the leather lacer by running it in a flare under the ischial tuberosity. Even total ischial bearing may at times be necessary. For a sensitive below the knee stump which breaks down or ulcerates from weight bearing, total or partial ischial bearing may relieve the difficulty. As below the knee stumps move slightly like a piston in the socket, vents are always put in the shin piece to obviate noise.

Prostheses for the Syme stump take weight on the end. This prosthesis consists of a laced leather socket made from a mold of the stump. The cuff laces in the front and is set in vertical metal extensions from the ankle. The cuff extends to the tibial tuberosities. The bulbous end of the stump holds the molded cuff and is all the suspension necessary. This prosthesis has of necessity a bulky ankle, and is unsuitable for a woman.

Prostheses for amputation through the metatarsal area require only a plate with a sponge rubber tip to fill the shoe.

Amputations of toes require, at the most, only padding in the end of the shoe to keep the tip from curling up.

There are prostheses for the Chopart and Lisfranc type of amputation, but they are bulky and cumbersome and as unsatisfactory as are the stumps.

Alignment of the prosthesis is as important as the fit of the socket. The aligning of a lower extremity prosthesis takes skill, experience, study of the individual, and in many instances, trial and error methods. There are, however, general principles of alignment which the surgeon should thoroughly understand.

The most difficult artificial leg to align is the above the knee prosthesis, which must operate without the aid of the quadriceps extensor apparatus. In the use of this leg the act of progression is performed by flexing the trunk on the remains of the thigh. This throws the center of gravity forward, thus supplying a propulsive force. Most of the weight is borne on the ischial tuberosity. The socket must be so shaped that there is room for the adductor tendons and so that it permits of no pressure in this area on the inner side of the thigh. The socket should come well up in the perineum and fit snugly over the greater trochanter. Any pressure in the pubic area is very uncomfortable. The joint in the suspension apparatus, that is, the movable section of the bar between the pelvic band and the thigh piece, must not be over the greater trochanter, but should be well anterior to it. The reason for this is that the axis of motion in the hip joint is not the neck of the femur, but runs from forward and outward to backward and inward, coinciding with the center of the acetabulum. This axis varies greatly from individual to individual, and often many trials are necessary to get the joint in the position of best function. If this joint is improperly placed, the prosthesis will rotate on the stump at each step and the joint will break easily.

When a flexion deformity is present in the thigh stump and cannot be relieved this deformity must be allowed for in the construction of the socket by increasing the anterior bowing beyond normal.

In the above the knee prosthesis the knee joint is placed so that the axis of its center bolt is posterior to the true center of the knee. The center bolt may be at the junction of the posterior and middle third of the knee joint. This, when the foot is properly placed, causes the center of gravity of the amputee in walking, to fall anterior to the center of the knee joint.

The foot and ankle must be in proper relation to the other joints of the prosthesis. The foot of the artificial limb should be in the same degree of valgus on the shin piece, or "toe out" to the same degree, as the normal foot. This position increases stability. The ankle joint should be placed well forward on the shin piece, usually at the junction of the anterior one-fourth of the shin and the posterior three-fourths. The foot should be so regulated by the bumpers that it is in 5 degrees of plantar flexion and dorsiflexion beyond 90 degrees is impossible. Twenty to thirty degrees of plantar flexion should be allowed by the ankle. The ankle joint should be as near to the center of the foot as possible. This alignment of the joint in the pelvic suspension, knee joint, foot and ankle, gives easiest control of the prosthesis, with the greatest stability and smoothest gait. With a reasonably long stump, an amputee can do well without an extension apparatus in the knee.

The socket of the prosthesis for the below the knee stump bears weight on the tibial tuberosities, the head of the fibula, and the tibial tubercle. The presence of the head of the fibula keeps the prosthesis from rotating and the fibula should not be removed unless it projects laterally, as it frequently does in a very short stump. The popliteal space will not stand any pressure. The posterior aspect of the socket should run well up on the gastrocnemius in the middle of the space and have depressions laterally and medially for the hamstring tendons. If the socket is not constructed this way the soft tissues bulge, and pressure results on the vessels, which chokes the stump. The side joints of the artificial knee should be placed so that their axis is posterior to the center of the knee. They should also be above the tibio-femoral articulation at the level of the center of the patella. If they are not in this position, the stump will ride up and out of the socket on flexion. The thigh corset should be long, coming high on the inside and over the greater trochanter on the outside. The bars extending up from the joint must fit the thigh well. The corset should be cut out in back of the popliteal space so that it does not pinch on flexion, and in front should extend to the patella. The foot and ankle should be aligned as previously described for the above the knee prosthesis.

An end-bearing thigh prosthesis is simply a well fitting socket for the long stump attached through an outside knee joint to a shin piece on the same principles as the below the knee prosthesis.

The Syme prosthesis has only an ankle joint and foot. The foot must be thinner than for other prostheses, but the same principles of alignment, modified by space requirements, apply for the ankle joint and foot.

The length of a lower leg prosthesis should be that which most nearly levels the pelvis of the patient and gives him the most effortless gait. The length should be such that when the amputee is standing, bearing full weight on the prosthesis and the normal leg, the anterior-superior iliac spines are in the same horizontal plane. This can always be achieved in the prosthesis for an amputation below the knee and in most prostheses for above the knee amputations, unless the stump is very short. In extremely asthenic, or aged individuals, it may be necessary to make the prosthesis slightly shorter than the normal leg. This discrepancy in length between prosthesis and normal leg should not exceed 1 inch.

If an individual is to wear two artificial legs it may be wise to make his total standing height a few inches lower than his stature prior to amputation. This lowers his center of gravity and makes balance easier. Two to four inches can be deleted from the stature of a person of average height without making an obvious disproportion between legs and torso.

Certain individuals, because of the underlying pathology, which by its manifestation in the extremity made the amputation necessary, will be unable to use a prosthesis. A patient who has lost an extremity because of embolic occlusion of an artery, may have a cardiac status which would contraindicate the effort required to master the use of an artificial leg. Individuals of this type may be better off using crutches for the small amount of activity they will pursue. Aged patients who have come to amputation because of arteriosclerosis obliterans may have severe cerebral manifestations of this condition and be generally asthenic. Their remaining days may be more satisfactorily spent in a wheel chair than in attempting to use an artificial leg. These problems must be decided by the surgeon. Such patients should not be sent to the limb maker, who has no way of determining their capacity for successful use of a limb.

UPPER EXTREMITY PROSTHESES

Prostheses for the upper extremity do not substitute as well for the lost part as do prostheses for the lower extremity. There is little or no cosmetic demand on the lower extremity prosthesis as it is almost completely covered by conventional attire. The upper extremity prosthesis, on the other hand, to be ideal, should be cosmetically attractive as well as functionally satisfactory. The cosmetic and functional elements cannot be combined in a single prosthesis to be used at all times. As the functional value of an arm prosthesis is increased, the cosmetic value is decreased.

The essential parts of an upper extremity prosthesis are: (1) the suspension apparatus; (2) socket; (3) joints, elbow and wrist; (4) power apparatus; and (5) prehensile apparatus.

The same factors apply to materials for use in construction of the artificial arm as for the artificial leg. Since the artificial arm is not a weight-bearing prosthesis, it is not subjected to as great stress and strain and can be lighter than the leg.

The suspension apparatus consists of a leather harness which goes over the shoulder and around the chest to keep the appliance on the arm. The shorter the stump, the more harness is necessary. In upper arm amputations, at or above the level of the pectoral insertion, so much harness is necessary to hold a prosthesis on the very short stump that the patient usually will not tolerate it and goes without a prosthesis.

The socket for an artificial arm does not have to bear weight. It is merely a sleeve into which to put the stump. It must fit well so as not to abrade, but its fabrication does not require nearly the skill required to make a weight-bearing socket.

The joints of the upper extremity prosthesis do not have nearly the stress and strain to tolerate that they do in the lower extremity prosthesis. The alignment of the elbow joint should simulate the normal elbow; that is, it should be placed with the outer joint slightly higher than the inner joint, so that the forearm will be in slight valgus on the arm, preserving a carrying angle. If this is not done, an object carried with the extended elbow, such as a suitcase, will strike the leg. If the forearm stump is very short, flexion of the elbow will be blocked as the upper edge of the socket will strike the antecubital space, due to the short area for grasp of the stump. This can be overcome by setting the forearm piece on the socket at an angle of moderate flexion.

The wrist joint makes no attempt to simulate the motions of the normal wrist joint. It is simply a rotation apparatus that can be set at different angles on a circle in a fixed position, in order that the direction of the prehensile apparatus can be altered. It also has a chuck, or screw socket, in its end so that the type of prehensile apparatus can be easily and quickly changed.

The prehensile apparatus and elbow of the artificial arm are motivated from the opposite shoulder of the patient. A loop encircles the opposite shoulder and axilla, from which runs a power line across the patient's back and over the arm and forearm portion of the prosthesis, through eyelets to the prehensile apparatus. By contracting the pectorals and the muscles which move the scapula, the opposite shoulder is moved forward and backward. This opens and closes the prehensile apparatus. Rawhide thongs were in years past used for the cord, but at present encased wire such as is used to control automobile carburetors is being used. This eliminates much power loss due to friction.

Newer types of prostheses are using pronation and supination, when the forearm is present, both to rotate and to open and close the prehensile apparatus. This is accomplished by compound gears.

In the conventional type of prostheses available today for the upper arm amputee with an artificial elbow joint, the elbow has to be flexed through the cord, moved by the opposite shoulder, or by a trick swinging motion. The joint locks in a few positions of flexion. When locked in a position of flexion, it is released by unlocking with the other hand or by striking the lock against the side of the body to release the joint. Efforts are under way at present to develop an electrically motivated elbow joint for upper arm prostheses.

The prehensile apparatus of the artificial arm has only the function of pinch and of hook. Grasp similar to that produced by closing all the fingers and thumb is not present. Tactile sensation of all types is absent, so that it is a poor substitute for the normal hand, or for even part of a hand. The prehensile apparatus of most use is the split hook. This is a metal appliance shaped like a hook, which has two halves, opposing each other. It is hinged with a scissors action, and maintained closed by a spring action. By moving the opposite shoulder the halved hook can be opened. It will then close of its own power, to hold, by pinch action, whatever is between the halves. When closed, the hook can be used to carry and to lift. Although the hook is not pleasing in appearance, it enables an individual to do many things. With will power enough, a person who has even two forearm amputations can become a very useful citizen if he will master the use of the hooks. For agricultural work, or occupations which require repetitive actions such as using a pitchfork, wheelbarrow, hoe, etc., the Bowler hook is superior to the split hook. This appliance has an adjustable loop instead of a halved hook. It permits a round handle to slide back and forth through the loop.

The mechanical hand for general use is far inferior to the split hook. The only motion possible in the mechanical hand is opposition of the thumb to the fingers. The thumb is opened by the opposite shoulder and closed by a spring action. In most hands the grip is poor, and certainly from a cosmetic viewpoint, the glove which is worn on the hand is conspicuous and calls attention to the disability.

The most effective attitude toward a prosthesis, and one which the arm amputee must acquire before he will make progress toward normalcy, is that the arm prosthesis at best is a "tool holding device." This principle has been used for a long time in Canadian and British arm prostheses, and recently has appeared in American-made prostheses. By using a chuck at the end of the prosthesis, and making different tools to meet different demands, the scope of usefulness of the prosthesis can be greatly widened. Each amputee has his own individual problems, and his own approach to these problems. A device suited to any need can be slipped easily into a chuck at the end of such a prosthesis.

To some individuals and to some occupations, the cosmetic aspect of the prosthesis is the most important consideration. Recent developments in plastics and latex have given rise to possibilities along cosmetic lines. In individual instances, certain fairly lifelike hands have been produced. However, cosmetic hands of this quality at present are not an article of general distribution and their production requires the time and talent of a craftsman with artistic ability and training. Such prostheses, at their best, will not stand close scrutiny, and will only pass for the normal hand in a crowd or in

sports when so inclined. An individual with one below the knee amputation can do practically anything a two-legged individual does. With interest and effort he may develop a gait that is hard to discern from the normal. An individual with one leg amputated through the thigh can also become extremely proficient.

Individuals with two below the knee stumps can accomplish much and can and should walk without canes. Individuals with two legs amputated through the thighs with stumps of reasonable length, can walk with two canes.

Every amputee should have instructions in operating a motor vehicle. Appliances which are easily attached to all cars have been developed and are readily obtainable. The amputee should also be encouraged to develop the ability to "hop" on the remaining foot, as this will stand him in good stead many times.

In order for the amputee to steadily improve in the use of the prosthesis, he must understand the muscle groups which are essential to the use of the prosthesis. Exercises to develop and maintain at good strength the adductors of the thigh, the extensors of the hip, and the extensors of the knee, should be carried out by the patient. He should also be taught to contract the abdominal muscles and flatten the pelvis in standing and walking. Much agility can be added to the gait by controlling the tilt of the pelvis through the abdominal and gluteal muscles.

The reeducation of the upper extremity amputee is, in one sense, easier than that of the lower extremity amputee; and in another sense, much more difficult. The single arm amputee acquires great "one-handedness" spontaneously. Complex use of the prosthesis requires long practice. By the time a single arm amputee is fitted with an artificial extremity he will usually have acquired considerable skill with the remaining hand, even though it is his minor hand which remains. Patients learn to write a legible hand rather rapidly with the remaining hand. They also learn to shave and to handle their personal needs with one hand quickly. Simple modification in clothes, such as substituting snaps for buttons, and ready tied neckties, are items the patient should have called to his attention. The patient, after acquiring the prosthesis can practice such things as eating by having imitation pieces of meat made of plasticine to cut with a knife and fork. Skill in using power tools and other complicated devices can be acquired. The one-armed individual may become proficient at such detailed work as tying flies, handling small tools, radio work, etc., by practice and the modification of tools to his handicap. His accomplishments are limited only by his will to improve.

An individual who has lost both arms below the elbow can become a very useful economic unit. An individual who has lost both arms above the elbow is severely handicapped but can still care for himself. It is hoped that the application of modern mechanical knowledge to prostheses will open new fields to this most severely handicapped of amputees.

CARE OF THE STUMP

The amputee must also be educated in the care of the stump. Proper hygiene is necessary to the health of the stump. The stump itself should be bathed daily with a nonirritating soap and thoroughly dried, when the prosthesis has been removed after the day's use. If there are any skin creases they should be thoroughly cleansed. Greasy ointments should be kept away from the stump, as they macerate skin. Alcohol applications, or other dessicating and astringent solutions, if used constantly and repeatedly, will irritate the skin, particularly in aged people. The skin can be improved by exposure to air and by tanning with sunlight.

An amputee should always use a stump sock when wearing a prosthesis. This sock should be of pure virgin wool and should be changed daily. These socks should be washed with pure white, nonmedicated soap, in lukewarm water. All soap should be rinsed out of the sock with lukewarm water. The sock should be applied to the stump smoothly and without wrinkles. A patient may use more than one sock to accommodate for shrinkage in the stump.

Excellent care should be taken of the remaining foot, particularly if the amputee has occlusive vascular disease. Ingrowing nails, abrasions due to ill-fitting shoes, and undue exposure to moisture or cold should be avoided.

LATE AFFECTIONS OF AMPUTATION STUMPS

An ulcer frequently develops on an amputation stump. A stump ulcer is most often induced by a socket in the prosthesis which fits poorly and produces pressure or abrades the skin of the stump. If the stump has normal circulation the ulcer will heal rather promptly on discontinuing the use of the prosthesis and will not recur after it is soundly healed, if the faulty socket is rectified. If the circulation of the stump is markedly deficient it may be impossible to keep the ulcer healed as long as any attempt is made to use the prosthesis. If the circulation of the stump is impaired to this degree the skin will be cyanotic and cold and the underlying tissues indurated. When this condition exists, reamputation at a level of circulatory adequacy may be necessary to permit the use of a prosthesis. This may mean sacrificing a knee joint. Sympathectomy is inadvisable if the circulatory deficiency is on the basis of occlusive vascular disease and it has little chance of benefitting the stump if the impaired blood supply is a local ischemia due to extensive deep fibrosis.

Inclusion cysts of the skin occur in amputation stumps, due to the sealing over of the orifice of a sebaceous gland. They frequently are infected. When present, they should be completely excised, removing all of the cyst wall, so that there will be no recurrence. If the cyst is acutely infected, complete excision should be delayed until drainage has been instituted and the infection has subsided.

Bursa occur in amputation stumps over bony prominences. A bursa is the reactive metaplasia of connective tissue to constant irritation. Frequently a readjustment of pressure areas in the socket will cause the bursa to disappear. Excision of a bursa, if over a bony prominence such as a bony spur at the tip of an end-bearing stump, will accomplish nothing. The bursa will promptly recur. If it becomes necessary to remove a bursa surgically, the bony prominence beneath the bursa, which is the cause of pressure, must be removed; otherwise a useless operation has been performed.

Bony spurs occur on the ends of bones in amputation stumps almost in direct proportion to the care which is exercised in handling the periosteal covering of the bone at the time of amputation. If the periosteum is stripped from the bone end and tags of periosteum are left hanging from this bone end, bony spurs are sure to eventuate. Extensive hematoma in stumps may become calcified and result in myositic deposits in the soft tissues. Spurs, when present in an area and to a degree that they produce a painful pressure site and interfere with the wearing of a prosthesis, should be removed surgically. *The mere presence of a bony spur in a roentgenogram is not an indication for its surgical removal.* The spur must be so located and of adequate size to produce painful pressure before it is treated surgically. Removal of a spur which is not the cause of discomfort is meddlesome surgery.

A spur should never be removed in its early stage of formation. When the tissues are opened in the formative stage of a spur, they are brawny and gritty around the developing spur. Operation during this period of calcification disseminates bone forming elements throughout the tissues, with the result that a spur of a larger size forms than would have resulted had the stump been left alone. Before surgical removal of the spur is undertaken, the roentgenogram should show that the spur is mature, completely ossified bone, and the tissues over the spur should be soft and pliable.

In the surgical removal of a spur, no subperiosteal dissection or blunt pushing of the tissues from the bone should be done. The muscle and scar over the spur and distal end of the bone should be sharply incised with a scalpel and a reasonable margin of muscle left attached around the entire circumference of the spur. The periosteum should be sharply incised at the point of removal and the bone cleanly sectioned. Periosteum should be adherent about the entire end of the bone remaining in the stump. If any periosteal tags are left, new spurs will form.

A neuroma occupying a superficial position in an amputation stump may be a cause of discomfort. Every sectioned nerve heals by the formation of a neuroma, despite thermal or chemical means to prevent their formation. It is the normal reaction to trauma of the tissues which make up a nerve trunk. If the healed bulbous end of a nerve is properly recessed in its fascial plane at the time of amputation so that it is well covered by muscle, it will cause no trouble.

The only indication for surgical removal of a neuroma is a superficial location, which would cause it to be subjected to pressure, thus producing pain. This pressure may come either from the prosthesis or as a result of the bare stump resting on or striking a hard surface. Tapping the superficial neuroma will produce a "shock-like" sensation. The removal of neuromata for the treatment of any phase of the "painful phantom limb syndrome" will result in failure.

Sequestra occur in the bone of an amputation stump, either as a result of infection or as a result of aseptic necrosis from circulatory loss. Their location is generally at the terminal end of the bone. They often are "ring shaped," consisting of a small portion of the total circumference of the bone. Eventually their presence is obvious in a roentgenogram, but it may be weeks after the occurrence of an abscess before the sequestrum can be seen on the x-ray plate. Any persistent sinus should make one suspicious that sequestration is occurring in the bone.

Healing will not result until the sequestrum extrudes itself or is removed surgically. Many times simple removal of the dead piece of bone will result in prompt healing. If drainage has persisted over an extended period of time there may be much scar in the end of the stump. When the condition is present a block removal of the sinus, scar, sequestrum, and adjacent portion of bone may be advisable. Following such a procedure the stump should be treated as an open amputation with traction.

Phantom limb is a term applied to the phenomenon by which the amputee is conscious of his absent limb. The sensations of which the patient is aware in his absent extremity may be painful to the degree of torture, or they may be painless, merely being an awareness of the amputated extremity. The sensations are always felt in the distal portions of the extremity. In the upper extremity, they occur in the fingers, palm or wrist; in the lower extremity, in the toes, arch, instep or ankle.

A certain degree of phantom limb sensation seems to be almost physiological, and this fact should be appreciated. Every individual with an amputation stump has a phantom limb. Rarely does an individual with an amputation stump have a "painful phantom limb." This phantom sensation has a fairly constant life history. It is present as a complaint in the days immediately following an amputation and is often more pronounced when the amputation has resulted from crushing trauma or is followed by extensive suppuration.

As inflammation and induration recede and healing progresses, the patient becomes less conscious of the phantom pains. He will tell you that he is aware of his lost foot or hand, but that it does not particularly annoy him. After the phantom has become less articulate and the patient has learned to live with it, any surgical procedure on the stump will temporarily aggravate the phantom sensations. This will happen, even though the surgical procedure in no way involves the nerve ends in the stump. Simple excision of a minor skin scar may result in a severe exacerbation of phantom pains. As healing of the skin progresses, the unpleasant aspect of the phantom again subsides.

When the patient gets a prosthesis and uses it successfully, the phantom phenomenon rapidly assumes a less troublesome role in his scheme of life. After using a prosthesis, many patients will proffer the information that the

phantom is a help to them. It gives them some inkling of the location of
the hand or foot of their prosthesis, and what position it is assuming. This
is the usual history of the phantom phenomenon.

The rare patient with the abnormal "painful phantom limb" must be
distinguished from the common group, which has the normal residual. Although rare, this type of patient is not difficult to distinguish. The distinction can at times be made by the patient's scars. Too often such a patient
displays scars, marking the site of removal of neuromas and section of nerve
trunks at various levels in his stump. At the base of the stump the well
healed scar of a surgical attack on the sympathetic nervous system may be
present. In addition to these healed surgical incisions, he may also present
the pigmented marks of the morphine needle. The permanent cure of a
truly "painful phantom limb" by any surgery is extremely dubious. Certainly there is no rationale for the excision of neuromas or for peripheral
nerve section in the treatment of this complication of amputation. Neither
does sympathetic nerve interruption have any great number of successes to
recommend it. Prefrontal lobotomy and excision of a portion of the pre-
motor area of the cerebral cortex have been employed in a few instances, but
up to the present, there is no very convincing proof of the effectiveness of
either operation.

Probably the only successful treatment of this baffling syndrome is its
prevention. Unfortunately, this cannot always be done by the surgeon, since
it is an impossibility for him to control the future environment of his patients. However, in the early care of the amputee, he can use narcotics
judiciously and promptly take all surgical measures to reduce and shorten
extensive suppuration and tissue necrosis. It is almost universal that the
syndrome of "painful phantom limb" is linked with morphine or alcohol,
and with poor adjustment of an individual to his environment. To date, no
known surgical procedure offers a permanent cure for these unfortunate
individuals.

"The following case history is illustrative of the complex nature of
these patients:

"A paratrooper lost his right arm in combat. He was a wiry little individual who had a great record for valor. His arm was knocked off by an
88 mm. shell, and a companion applied a tourniquet. Following this, he
continued in combat for a short time, until he was wounded in the thigh.

"On admission to the hospital in the United States he was cheerful,
hard to keep track of, and was all over the building. He had no complaints
about his arm. He always seemed to enjoy talking about combat and his
own personal exploits. His amputation stump was revised and he was fitted
with an artificial limb, which he used with great dexterity despite a very
short stump.

"After using his prosthesis for about six weeks, he announced that he
was returning to duty. This was most unusual, but it seemed that while on
leave from the hospital he had gone to a paratroop base, where he con-

tacted some friend in authority, who asked for his return to duty. While on leave he had also made some jumps.

"A few months after leaving the hospital for duty he returned, complaining bitterly, and constantly, that the fingers of his hand were clenched in the palm and that the nails were cutting the flesh and burning like fire; he could not sleep and paced the floor; the typical picture of the 'painful phantom limb syndrome.'

"On questioning this patient about the onset of the trouble, he related the following story: After going to duty he did well and had no trouble. He had joined a paratroop battalion. After training with them he had finally talked his superior officers into sending him overseas again with the combatants. He arrived at the port of embarkation. Here he was given a medical examination. The examining medical officer put his hand on the prosthesis and, as he did so, said, 'You can't go overseas with a wooden arm.' The patient amputee said that at that instant he became infuriated, that the fingers of his amputated extremity dug into the palm of the absent hand with excruciating pain, and that if his arm had been his own he would have slugged the damn medic. This pain pattern had persisted since this disappointment.

"The patient insisted his pains were due to palpable neuromas in the stump. At his insistence, and with great skepticism, these neuromas were removed. His complaints continued unabated. Then one day, about two months after the removal of the neuromas, out of a clear sky, he came to the medical officer in the ward with a telegram in his hand and announced that he was cured. He stated emphatically that he had no discomfort in his stump and no phantom sensation. To demonstrate his recovery he waved his prosthesis around and tipped a table off the floor with it. It had been impossible prior to this, to get the patient to wear the prosthesis. The telegram which he had received was an order from a relief organization for him to go overseas for duty with them in the zone of activity." *

This case history is well worth remembering. It does not infer that knowledge concerning the "painful phantom limb syndrome" is complete and that there may not come, in the future, some organic approach to this distressing problem. At present, however, the "painful phantom limb syndrome" should be listed as a condition not relieved by surgical treatment. A careful analysis of all patients suffering from this syndrome will reveal one or all of the following factors to play a prominent role, viz., drugs, alcohol, or severe maladjustment and frustration.

REFERENCES

1. KIRK, N. T. *Amputations*, The W. F. Prior Co., Inc., Hagerstown, Md., 1942.
2. KIRK, N. T. Amputation Stumps of the Lower Extremity, *J. Bone & Joint Surg.*, N. S. 15:101-111, [Jan.], 1933.

* McKeever, F. M., *Surg., Gynec. & Obst.*, 82:495-511, May 1946. By permission of Surgery, Gynecology and Obstetrics.

3. KIRK, N. T. and MCKEEVER, F. M.   Guillotine Amputation, *J.A.M.A.*, 124:1027-1030, [April 8], 1944.

4. MCKEEVER, F. M.   Controversial Points in Amputation Surgery, *Surg., Gynec. & Obst.*, [May], 1946.

5. MACEY, H. B. and BICKEL, W. H.   Amputations of the Lower Extremities in Occlusive Arterial Disease; a Ten-year Review, *Surg., Gynec. & Obst.*, 74:821-827, [Apr.], 1942.

6. GHORMLEY, R. K.   *Amputation in Occlusive Arterial Disease. Peripheral Vascular Diseases*, ALLEN, BARKER, HINES, W. B. Saunders Co., Phila., 1946.

7. MCKEEVER, F. M.   Upper Extremity Amputations and Prostheses, *J. Bone & Joint Surg.*, 26[No. 4]:662-671, [Oct.], 1944.

8. SLOCUM, D. B. and PRATT, D. R.   The Principles of Amputations of the Fingers and Hand, *J. Bone & Joint Surg.*, 26[No. 3]:535-546, [July], 1944.

9. WHITE, J. C.   Pain After Amputations and Its Treatment, *J.A.M.A.*, 124[No. 15]: 1031-1045, [April 8], 1944.

10. THOMAS, A. and HADDAN, C. M.   *Amputation Prosthesis*, J. B. Lippincott Co., Phila., 1945.

6

THE FACE, MOUTH AND JAWS

JAMES BARRETT BROWN, M.D. AND FRANK McDOWELL, M.D.

FACIAL INJURIES

Severe blows about the face may produce extensive fractures with only contusions on the surface, and widespread soft tissue lacerations may not be complicated by fractures. However, the two occur together so often that the care of the soft parts and of the bone cannot be separated and careful consideration of the possible occurrence of fractures should be made in all patients. If it is assumed that fractures can be considered and cared for after swelling has occurred and subsided, the best chance for correct bone replacement is missed. If the true picture is recognized, simple procedures for bone replacement and fixation usually suffice. Special splints are seldom required although it is important to have someone on hand who understands the dental requirements because one of the most important functions to maintain is mastication, and this requires that the teeth occlude naturally.

The number of complications possible makes the problem in severe injuries difficult, and one should be alert to make as complete a diagnosis as possible and have his findings recorded either before or at the time of operation. If tissue has been completely lost, this is of great importance in the final outcome and the extent should be noted. Skull fracture and brain injury, damage to the cervical spine and lesions of the orbit and the eye itself are very frequent and always should be looked for, recorded and treated as indicated.

Final union in upper jaw fractures may never be solid because of the thin plates of bone present or because of infection. In the lower jaw there is usually solid union but the fracture line may remain visible in the x-ray.

X-ray Examination. It is not necessary to rush these patients to the x-ray room, because manipulation might be contraindicated if there were skull or cervical spine damage. However, when safe for the patient, complete views of all involved regions should be taken.

For the lower jaw, complete views of both sides including both condyles should be taken, because multiple fractures may be missed even at operation.

Roentgenograms of the facial bones should be taken, but are apt to be somewhat disappointing due to the superimposition of shadows in this area.

The heavier ridges of bone show quite well in the antral and vertico-submental positions, but there may be many comminutions of the maxilla, ethmoid, nasal and other thin bones that are entirely missed on the x-ray plate. Therefore, this condition has to be searched for at the time of operation.

When to Do Primary Repair. The primary repair should be done as soon as the patient's general condition permits and in the first twenty hours if possible, before swelling, organization of clots, and infection have occurred. If seen after this initial period and there is the necessity of manipulation through contaminated clots and edematous tissue, it is sometimes better to just approximate the soft parts and await the subsidence of swelling before replacing the bone fragments. However, the replacement of bone fragments rarely should be delayed longer than seven to ten days, because the fixation of small, comminuted chips after this time may make their accurate realignment impossible. Shock and neurological damage may necessitate delay and an intoxicated patient should not have his jaws wired together.

Type of Anesthesia. In many of these patients nerve blocks, especially deep injections of the branches of the fifth nerve (Figs. 82 and 83), are the most satisfactory for anesthesia. Occasionally field blocks or local infiltration suffice. These may or may not be combined with a basal anesthetic such as avertin. General anesthesia is to be avoided when possible, but is often necessary, especially in children.

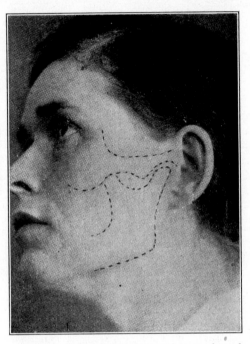

FIG. 82. Deep injection of second and third divisions of trigeminal nerve. Above bony landmarks are located by palpation, and a lumbar puncture needle is inserted between the coronoid and condyle just beneath the zygomatic arch. It is directed toward the same point on the other side of the face and inserted until it strikes the pterygoid plate. (From Brown, *Surg., Gynec. & Obst.,* Dec. 1931. By permission of Surgery, Gynecology and Obstetrics.)

When used, the endotracheal method is almost always employed, though occasionally endopharyngeal insufflation is sufficient in very small children. Intravenous anesthetics may create serious airway problems.

General Operative Procedures. In extensive injuries, it is often best to wait until the patient is in the operating room before manipulating the tissues simply to find out the extent of damage. There should be determination and recording of the loss or tearing of all the features and the extent of detachment of bones. The steps necessary to carry out the repair should then be determined and systematized into a definite, orderly procedure.

Cleaning of these facial wounds is extremely important and should be done with soap and water followed by ether and saline irrigations so that local antiseptics are seldom necessary. The decision of when to clean and when to anesthetize is somewhat difficult. It is often best to clean as far as possible with the patient enduring it, and then get the local or block an-

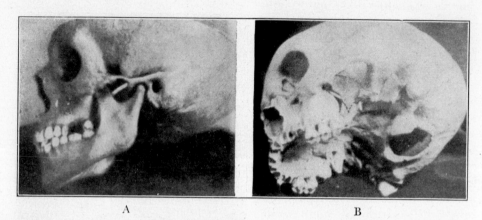

A   B

FIG. 83. (A) Straw shows approximate relation of needle to bony landmarks. After striking pterygoid plate, needle is partially withdrawn and inserted in a more upward direction until it strikes the angle between it and the great wing of the sphenoid. (B) By partially withdrawing and reinserting the needle, it is worked forward in this angle until it drops off the plate into the sphenomaxillary fissure, where 3 cc. of 2 per cent novocaine (containing ½ drop of epinephrine) is injected to anesthetize the second division. Similarly, the needle is worked backward along the angle until it just drops off near the foramen ovale where the same amount of novocaine is injected to anesthetize the third division. (Ten minutes may be required for the solution to infiltrate the nerves. It is important not to go posteriorly or deep more than ½ to 1 cm. from the plate, and to aspirate to be certain the needle is not in a blood vessel.) (From Brown, *Surg., Gynec. & Obst.*, Dec. 1931. By permission of Surgery, Gynecology and Obstetrics.)

esthetic in, or proceed with the induction of general anesthesia if it is necessary and safe to do so. Oil ground into abrasions is difficult to remove and may require scrubbing with a brush and the use of solvents such as ether or benzine. Bits of glass from rear vision mirrors or from completely broken shatterproof glass are especially apt to be overlooked and for this reason it is well, if possible, to find out whether or not any glass was broken at the time of the accident.

Meticulous cleaning should constitute almost the entire débridement. The usual plan of wide excision of all torn edges should not be practised in the face. Very ragged edges may be smoothed by minimal clean excision, remembering that the loss of even 1/16 of an inch in a child's eyelid or ala may be deforming. Extreme conservatism should also be the rule in dealing with loose bone chips, as it is probably better to leave in some bone frag-

ments that might die, than to needlessly discard any good supporting fragments that might live.

BONE REPLACEMENT. If the nasal airway is occluded, it can be reestablished by carefully introducing a long speculum and dilating it and then
slipping a good-sized rubber tube through the meatus on each side; other
bone replacements should then be done, such as elevation of orbits and the
nose.

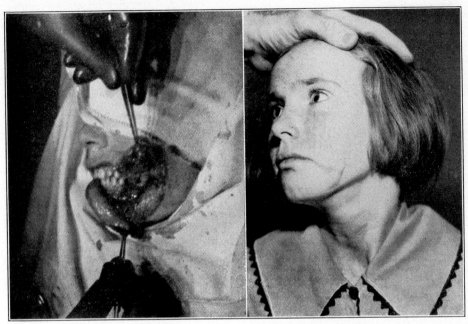

FIG. 84. Cheek torn open from an automobile door handle catching in angle of mouth.
The known points are the junction of the skin and vermilion on the upper and lower
flaps. These are united first. The lateral points of the upper and lower flaps are then
united, and the remaining areas successively bisected with ooo white silk subcuticular
sutures and ooo black silk skin sutures put in not more than 1 to 2 mm. from the edges.
Mucosa carefully closed in same manner. Stay sutures put in from inside to avoid any
wide suture marks on the face.

If the lower jaw is fractured, attention may be given to it at this time.
If the patient is under general anesthesia, the individual dental wires may
be placed, but the jaws should not be wired together until he is awake and
has ceased vomiting.

The care of the various types of facial fractures will be considered under
separate paragraphs, but it is usually best to complete as much of the bone
replacement as possible before diverting attention to the soft tissue repair.

SUTURE OF SOFT TISSUES. For suturing the soft parts, new cleaning can
be done and fresh instruments used if the mouth secretions can now be
avoided. Surface key sutures may be used for the known points and these
may have to be deep, but should never be wide, as wide suture marks can

never be completely obliterated. Between these, buried No. 000 white silk sutures should be used to completely approximate all wound edges unless the skin edges are so thin that these cannot be put in. The remaining surface sutures are then placed not more than 1 or 2 mm. from the wound edges to obtain the final fine adjustment. No. 000 black silk usually suffices and may be removed in one to four days. Stay sutures may be put in from the inside of the cheek or nose. If they are needed on the outside, they should always be tied over a gauze pad to prevent cutting across the wound and leaving a permanent scar.

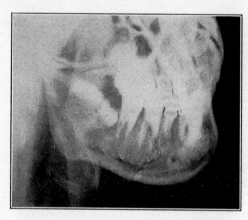

FIG. 85. Ordinary Gilmer interdental wiring suffices for most fractures of the mandible. No. 24 stainless steel wire is anchored around individual teeth; strands on opposing teeth are then twisted together to immobilize the jaw in occlusion. Above illustration shows importance of leaving in posterior molar teeth which may be in fracture lines or loose. They often serve as splints to hold the other fragments in position.

In complicated tears (Fig. 84) a correct replacement may be difficult, but a start is made at some known point such as the nostril border, or the edge of an eyebrow. If none can be figured out, closure may be started in the center of the wound, and the remaining areas bisected successively until complete closure is obtained. If the final adjustment is not satisfactory, one should not be reticent in completely opening and resuturing it. Triangular or trap-door flaps should be adjusted with particular care to avoid late deformity, especially about the lids, nose, and mouth.

Small drains may be placed advantageously, ordinary rubber bands sufficing for small wounds. If the immediate covering of the wound is of fine mesh grease gauze, it may be removed later with minimal trauma to the wound edges and sutures. A firm pressure dressing of mechanic's waste or marine sponges should be applied overall to minimize hemorrhage and swelling and, thereby, infection. The dressing should be regarded as a part of the operation and should be carried out with the same meticulous attention to detail.

Fractures of the Lower Jaw. The treatment varies according to the site of the fracture, but complicated appliances can be dispensed with in almost all instances. The keynote of the treatment, as in all other fractures, is accurate reduction of the fragments followed by immobilization. The patient's sensations may be of great assistance in telling when his natural occlusion has been reestablished. No attempt to improve upon the patient's former occlusion should be made in the treatment of these fractures.

In the majority of fractures in older children or adults with good teeth, immobilization may be accomplished by ordinary Gilmer interdental wiring from the four lower premolar teeth to the corresponding upper premolar teeth (Fig. 85). In addition, it is a good plan to have at least one set of interdental wires posterior and one set anterior to the fracture site if possible. The tooth in the fracture line should usually be left in place during the period of immobilization, even if it is a little loose. This is especially true of molar teeth, which often prevent the tendency to upward displacement of the posterior fragment in this area (Fig. 85).

Symphysis fractures usually require a dental arch or band in addition to the above, to prevent the tendency to "rocker motion" of the fragments. The method of Risdon is an excellent one in caring for these fractures (Fig. 86).

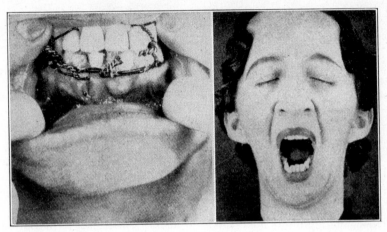

Fig. 86. Method of Risdon in applying an anterior arch by putting long wires on the posterior teeth, bringing them around in front, fastening them together, and then anchoring individual teeth to this arch with finer wires. Besides this support, which is used mainly for symphysis fractures, fixation to the upper jaw with the teeth in normal occlusion is done. (From Brown, *Surg., Gynec. & Obst.*, 68:564-573, 1939. By permission of Surgery, Gynecology and Obstetrics.)

Fractures of the condyles are frequently amenable to attempts at closed reduction followed by ordinary interdental wiring. It is usually not necessary to consider open reduction or primary excision, unless the condyle is completely out of the glenoid, notwithstanding many statements which have been made to the contrary.

Edentulous jaws may require circumferential wiring of the mandible to the patient's dental plate or to his upper teeth, direct wiring of the bone fragments, or internal fixation with Kirschner wires.

If the soft tissues have been torn off the jaw exposing the fracture site, it is usually most expedient to do direct wiring of the fragments (Fig. 87).

A small dependent drain should be placed directly up to the fracture site, unless one is reasonably certain that it is not compounded into a tooth socket.

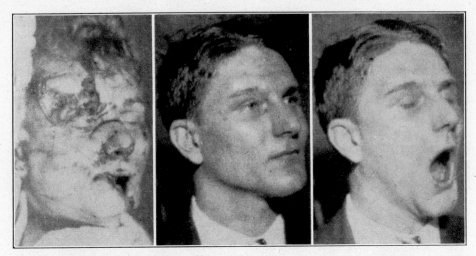

Fig. 87. Extremely widespread soft tissue injury plus complete separation through the symphysis. Direct wiring of symphysis fracture through the open wound plus careful closure of soft tissues. Complete restoration in 1 operation which was done a few hours after the accident. (From Brown, *Surg., Gynec. & Obst.,* 68:564-573, 1939. By permission of Surgery, Gynecology and Obstetrics.)

Internal Fixation of Mandibular Fractures with Kirschner Wires. Internal fixation with Kirschner wires is the simplest and most positive fixation for many fractures of the mandible in which one or both fragments are edentulous. The method requires two surgeons and an electric power drill (or a drill attachment on an electric bone saw). One surgeon reduces the fracture, lines the fragments up, and holds them in position while the other one drills the wire longitudinally along the bone, across the fracture site, and well into the other fragment. The wire point should be sharp and the drill run at not too high speed to avoid any heat necrosis of the bone.

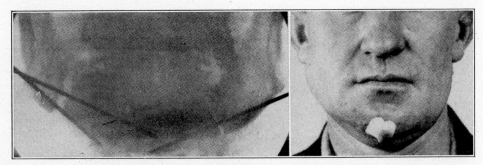

Fig. 88. Internal Kirschner wire fixation of fractures in front of both angles in a man with very few teeth. Long posterior fragment on right side edentulous and one on left side contains just one tooth. Interdental wires also were left on a few days. Patient returned to work within 10 days and solid union was obtained. (From Brown and McDowell, *Surg., Gynec. & Obst.,* 75:361-368, 1942. By permission of Surgery, Gynecology and Obstetrics.)

A B

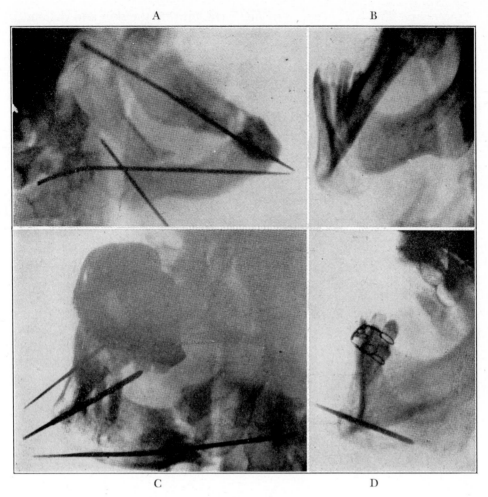

C D

Fig. 89. (A) Bilateral fracture in a totally edentulous jaw. Patient was able to put the upper and lower dental plates in and eat soft foods after the first week, though the lower plate was painful if left in continuously. Returned to work in 2½ weeks. (B) Angle and mental foramen fractures in an almost edentulous jaw. (C) and (D) Fixation of an almost edentulous jaw in an insane man, which was solid enough to hold without any cooperation. (From Brown and McDowell, *Surg., Gynec. & Obst.*, 75:361-368, 1942. By permission of Surgery, Gynecology and Obstetrics.)

A single wire suffices for most fractures, but if the fixation does not seem to be solid enough, some auxiliary method of fixation may be used, or a second wire may be put through above the first one in a totally edentulous jaw (Figs. 88 and 89). When teeth are present, and a single wire is used, it is usually possible to keep it below the nerve canal and any tooth roots.

The whole procedure is done in the operating room with all possible sterile precautions and dependent drainage of the fracture site is instituted if necessary. The wire is cut off about 1 cm. outside the skin and the end is kept covered with a small dressing until it is removed, usually four to eight weeks later.

Displacement of Bones of the Upper Jaw. *Transverse facial fractures* occur usually from heavy blows dispersed over the face. There may be a level of separation at the frontal-zygomatic suture line and at the glabella on both sides; there may be one through the wall of the antrum that may extend all the way around and involve the pterygoid region; and frequently there is a complete separation entirely around just above the dental arch. The whole face may sag down and become noticeably elongated, and the dental arch may be completely loose to the patient's own sensation and on moving it with examining fingers (Figs. 90 and 91).

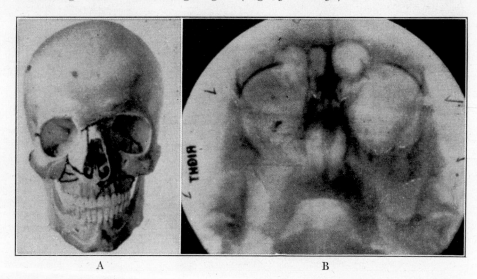

A   B

Fig. 90. (A) Diagram of frequent separations of the upper jaw and facial bones, to which should be added a horizontal fracture all the way around on both sides just above the alveolus. (B) Multiple comminutions of the facial bones, some of the areas having been scratched in for clearness. Separation of the zygomatic-frontal suture lines, crumpling of the zygomatic arches and comminution about the orbital borders and antrum. (From Brown, *Surg., Gynec. & Obst.,* 68:564-573, 1939. By permission of Surgery, Gynecology and Obstetrics.)

Nasal, septal, and palate fractures frequently occur along with the above separation, and these small thin bones may be comminuted into multiple pieces. The nasal structure, including the cartilages, may be completely crumpled, and there may be one or more complete lacerations through the palate caused by the disrupted bone cutting through; the nasal passages may be completely occluded also (Fig. 92).

THE ZYGOMATIC BONE AND ORBIT. The zygomatic bone (malar or cheek bone) frequently receives the blow but is itself seldom broken. Instead, it is torn loose from its moorings at the frontal, zygomatic process of the temporal bone, and the maxilla. The main displacement will be according to the direction of the force; if from the front, the zygomatic process will be crumpled back and broken by the zygoma itself; if from the side, the ascending ramus of the zygoma may be tipped in and impinge on the orbital space. In nearly all loosening of this bone, the antral wall crumples, and if it should sag down too much, the orbit becomes elongated and the globe may descend so much that binocular vision is impaired (Fig. 93). Blindness may result from section of the nerve by a loose thin piece of bone and from intraocular or direct ocular damage. The extra-ocular muscles and nerves may also be torn. The lacrymal apparatus may be impinged on if the frontal process of the maxilla is driven in.

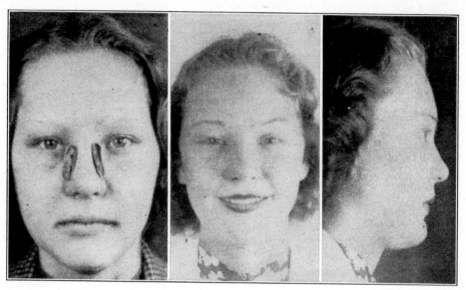

FIG. 91. Early and late postoperative views of patient who had nose flattened backward until level with cheeks, and multiple comminuted fractures of other bones in the middle third of the face. The nasal bones were dug out of the face and held out forward by a double wire sling anchored on either side over lead plates as shown. Symphysis fracture held by Risdon arch and interdental wiring (cf. Fig. 86). Upper jaw fracture maintained in occlusion by interdental wiring. Orbital floor held up and cavity of maxillary sinus reestablished by iodoform gauze packing in the latter. (From Brown, *Surg., Gynec. & Obst.*, 68:564-573, 1939. By permission of Surgery, Gynecology and Obstetrics.)

Inner canthus displacement occurs if the nose with the frontal processes of the maxilla is crushed backward, there being an actual chiseling open of the front of the face. This deformity is as important as any other in which to accomplish an early repair, because, if left until fixation occurs, the canthi probably never will be sunken in normally again (Fig. 92).

Nasal flatness goes along with the canthus displacement and the two are corrected together by withdrawing the depressed tissue and bones, molding them into their normal positions, and frequently holding them there with through-and-through silver wire sutures inserted under the separated frontal processes and held on the outside of the nose over lead plates (Fig. 91).

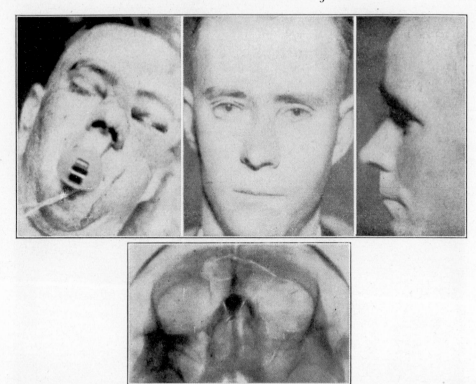

FIG. 92. Comminution of the facial and frontal bones with involvement of the frontal sinuses, displacement of the inner canthi, and flattening of the nose. Patient seen a few hours after the accident and restoration done immediately, that is, replacement of the comminuted fragments, rubber tube left in the frontal sinus to drain into the nose, fragments of the nose held up and inner canthi replaced by through-and-through wire sling, placed through the fracture lines of the frontal processes and held over lateral lead plates on the outside of the nose. Restoration of the nasal bridge and normal direction and situation of the inner canthi in one operation. (From Brown, *Surg., Gynec. & Obst.*, 68:564-573, 1939. By permission of Surgery, Gynecology and Obstetrics.)

The general rule for repair is simply to replace these fragments and maintain them in position with the least manipulation possible. This replacement amounts to an open reduction, and access to the orbital border can be gained by a short incision in the buccal fornix, then into the antrum through the fracture line that is almost always present. The depressed border can then be elevated into position with a Kelly clamp. This bone may be locked in place, but, if there is much comminution, the whole number of fragments, including the anterior and lateral walls of the antrum, may be "mulched" in position and held with an iodoform pack in the antrum, with the end left just through the opening in the fornix.

Qualifications of Treatment. A detailed account of the care of all the fractures and other complications cannot be included here, but in the indi-

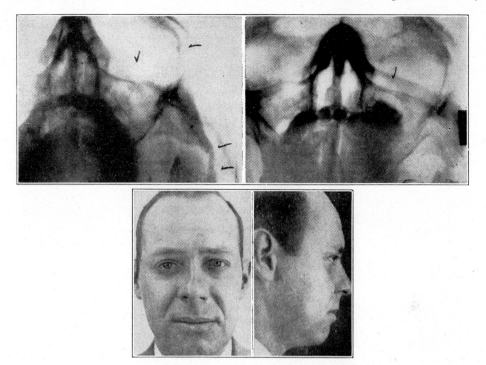

FIG. 93. Depressed orbital border with zygoma torn loose from its moorings and zygomatic arch crumpled. Incision made through buccal fornix underneath upper lip, antrum entered through fracture line in its anterior face, Kelly forcep inserted and orbital floor pried up into place. Antrum packed with iodoform gauze for one week. Photographs show late result with restoration of binocular vision. There had also been extensive tearing of the ear and nose. (From Brown, *Surg., Gynec. & Obst.,* 68:564-573, 1939. By permission of Surgery, Gynecology and Obstetrics.)

vidual patient all parts have to be considered and it is not possible to consider bone or soft tissue repair entirely alone. A few further noteworthy subjects are as follows:

Where wide areas of soft tissue have been lost, as good a closure as possible should be made, with an accurate notation of the estimated loss for future reference in repair. If necessary, simple closure of skin to mucosa can be done.

If orbital borders are left down too long there may be such derangement of the ocular muscles that binocular vision may never be attained, even though the globe is later raised.

Late lip scars often become so hard that it may be thought that a foreign body has been left; this is apparently due to the glands that are present, and occasionally is relieved by radiation.

If the late deformities are studied, the requirements of early care may be made more clear. Wide suturing, infection, misplacement of flaps, failure to accurately replace bone fragments, and keloid formation seem to account for most deformities. However, some secondary repairs are necessary in almost all extensive injuries, and this possibility should always be considered from the start with the patient or some responsible relative.

THE TREATMENT OF FACIAL PARALYSIS

The facial nerve may be interrupted intra-cranially (*e.g.* in removal of eighth nerve tumors), in the fallopian canal (*e.g.* mastoiditis or mastoidectomy), in the face after it has divided into several branches (*e.g.* in lacerations or from removal of parotid tumors), or it may be congenitally absent. When divided intracranially, anastomosis with the hypoglossal nerve may be considered. When divided in the fallopian canal, resuturing or free nerve grafts may be considered. However, when the individual branches have been cut, in the face, or when the nerve is congenitally absent, support of the paralyzed face with transplanted strips of fascia lata seems the best procedure; this operation may also be used in conjunction with the nerve operations for intracranial or canal injuries, or may be used after them if the nerve operations do not work as well as desired.

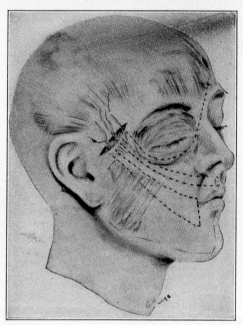

FIG. 94. Pathways of the subcutaneous fascial loops. The two lower loops are the ones commonly employed, the upper strip being used only when it is impossible to correct the lagophthalmos by a canthoplasty or other local operation on the lids. (From Brown and McDowell, *J.A.M.A.*, 135:18-20, 1947.)

The Operation. Endotracheal anesthesia is employed with the tube coming out of the opposite corner of the mouth. Strips of fascia lata about 1 cm. wide are obtained in the longest lengths possible from the iliotibial band, by use of the Masson or other stripper. The temporal incision is made in the hair-bearing area and is carried down to the temporalis fascia. A small stab opening is made in the middle of the upper lip and another one in the lower lip 1 to 2 cm. inside the angle of the mouth and 1 cm. below the vermilion. The first strip is then passed subcutaneously from the temporal wound down through the face, out the upper lip stab opening, and back up to the temple by a different route so that it forms a loop and encircles a good deal of soft tissue in the lip. Another strip is passed similarly down to the stab opening in the lower lip and back, care being taken again to avoid puncturing the buccal mucosa. The fascia may be carried through the face by a special fascia needle, or by an ordinary long sack-sewing needle (Figs. 94 and 95).

After being placed, the loops are worked back and forth a little to take out any slack and the temporalis fascia is opened about 1 inch above the coronoid to expose the muscle fibers. Using a heavy full curved fascia needle, one end of each strip is passed around a good segment of muscle and tied to the other end by a surgeon's knot. The knots are pulled taut with the mouth in considerable over-correction and then fixed by several interrupted wire stitches through the knots and by sewing the ends of the strips down. A pressure dressing is applied to cover the eye, ear and entire side of the face and helps materially in getting smooth early healing.

Postoperative Care. The pressure dressing is left on four or five days (if the eye is comfortable) and then replaced by a smaller one. Chewing is limited for the first week, but is gradually resumed as any tenderness in the temple subsides. The overcorrection disappears within about ten days and after two or three weeks, the patient may practice biting down in front of a mirror until he can produce some lateral movement of the mouth. He notes how this is done and then strives to increase the extent of the movement. A little later he may try

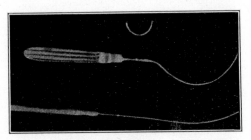

FIG. 95. Three needles ordinarily used for placing the fascial strips. From above downward; Gallie needle used for anchoring the strips in the temporal muscle; semicircular needle used for placing strip in lower lid; long needle used for placing the main strips in the face. The two needles were devised by Dr. R. Douglas Sanders and are made of bent heavy Kirschner wires with a large eye cut through near the tip and a handle attached on the other end. (From Brown and McDowell, *J.A.M.A.*, 135:18-20, 1947.)

to balance the movement with a small smile on the normal side (Figs. 96 and 97), and meanwhile should practice repressing massive movements on the normal side. This latter point is emphasized, as almost any patient with a facial paralysis will try so hard to move the paralyzed side that he forms the habit of throwing exaggerated movements into the normal side. He must learn that balance in the face is more important than the actual range of motion and always strive for this balance. As a starting point, he may consciously try to remain a little "glum" and then work from this point forward as he learns better to control his expressions. Sudden large laughs can never be balanced adequately in these patients, and may reveal a paralysis which is otherwise pretty well controlled.

Variations in the Operation. Preserved fascia, kangaroo tendon, and wire have been used, but it is thought that autogenous fascia is superior to any foreign material and it is easy to obtain.

Additional loops may be put in to the prominence of the cheek, around the mouth, or to the angle, but the two simple slings described usually suffice.

The anchorage above may be to the temporal fascia or to the zygomatic arch, rather than to the muscle, but this does not permit any movement of the face or even enough to take any slack out of the loops if they stretch or slip a little.

Older persons with paralysis of long duration may have considerable excess skin. This may be excised by a unilateral "face-lifting" operation as a separate procedure. It is a little safer to do it before the fascial transplant, but the amount to be excised can be estimated better afterwards. Younger individuals, or those with paralysis of lesser duration, will usually tighten up the stretched skin spontaneously during the first few postoperative months.

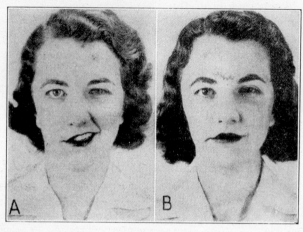

FIG. 96. Congenital paralysis of twenty years duration. Result of single operation (fascial transplant). (From Brown and McDowell, *J.A.M.A.*, 135:18-20, 1947.)

The Eyelids and Forehead. The paralyzed upper lid seldom requires any treatment (unless combined with third nerve paralysis) but the sagging lower lid may create a large palpebral fissure, apparent or actual exophthalmos, and a "staring expression." The general elevation of the face usually helps this and nothing else is required in some cases. If this is not sufficient, a small external canthoplasty may be done, excising a full thickness wedge of the lower lid near the outer canthus. Occasionally, it is worthwhile to put a thin fascial strip horizontally through the lower lid near the tarsal border, anchoring it externally to the temporal fascia above, and medially to the opposite frontalis muscle or fascia (Fig. 94). These operations do a lot to prevent irritation to the globe, but it is always advisable for these patients to avoid excessive exposure to strong, cold winds or to dust.

No known operation will restore movement to the forehead. However, if the brow is heavy and low, it may be elevated by excising an ellipse of skin in the hairline just above, undermining and sliding that side of the forehead up. A separate strip of fascia may be put in, from high in the temporal region, through the brow and then carried high up on the opposite side and anchored.

The amount of movement obtained varies from little to a noticeable amount, the majority having a small range of definitive motion which is of value in expression. The cause of this variation is not entirely understood, though some individuals seem to have much thicker and more active muscles than others. An occasional patient will have the fascial loops "freeze" to all of the surrounding tissues throughout their length and this almost precludes movement, but leaves a balanced face in repose which is still worthwhile. The patient's own efforts and general morale have a good deal of influence on the final result in many cases.

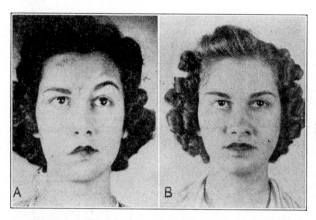

Fig. 97. Total paralysis resulting from removal of malignant parotid tumor. All of the branches were individually severed in the parotid area. After one operation (fascial transplant) the patient appears quite normal in repose and with a small smile. (From Brown and McDowell, *J.A.M.A.*, 135:18-20, 1947.)

The point of initial overcorrection might be mentioned again, as we have never had to loosen any of these loops secondarily (even when the mouth was pulled far over to the paralyzed side) though we have had to tighten a few and insert additional loops in a few later. The single operation suffices in nearly all patients, and it is not entirely clear why an occasional one will need secondary tightening. It may be due to: (a) stretching of the fascia (or not using wide enough strips); (b) the loops cutting through some soft tissue above or below (the reason for encompassing as much soft tissue at either end as possible); or (c) persistent overactivity on the normal side.

The most dramatic results are obtained in total paralysis, but worthwhile results have been obtained in partial paralysis (where nerve operations would be contraindicated). However, the closer these latter are to normal, the less is to be expected from any operative procedure, as the net gain will be less.

The chief disadvantages of the operation are: (a) the occasional necessity of secondary adjustments outlined above, and (b) that in common with all other operations, it does not restore completely normal movements to the permanently paralyzed face.

Advantages that might be listed are: (a) its simplicity and directness; (b) early definitive results; (c) no resulting annoying tics or mass actions and little possibility of complete failure; (d) it can be used later when nerve operations have not been as successful as anticipated or desired; (e) can be used in conjunction with nerve operations; (f) can be used in practically all patients, regardless of etiology or duration; and (g) does not produce any additional disability or visible scars.

TREATMENT OF TUMORS OF THE FACE

Excision of Skin Tumors. Small warts, moles, fibromas, papillomas, keratoses, and even carcinomas (Fig. 98), are often best removed with the fine electric cautery (the Ziegler type employed by the opthalmologists with a fine platinum wire tip that heats white hot is useful for this purpose;

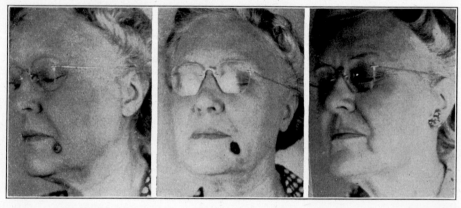

FIG. 98. Basal cell carcinoma excised with fine "white-hot" electric cautery, cutting through the normal skin all around the lesion and then cutting through the normal fat under the tumor. Specimen, with small margin of normal tissue, removed in one piece. Wound granulates up and heals by secondary intention in about 3 weeks. (Middle photograph was taken immediately after excision, to show width and depth of removal.)

the radio-frequency machines may destroy an unnecessary amount of tissue and one must guard against sparks jumping to the cornea or elsewhere).

Novocaine is injected under and around the lesion and tension is made in all directions by an assistant's fingers to stretch the skin taut. The cautery wire is used as a bloodless knife, cutting all around the lesion down into healthy, subcutaneous fat and then staying within the layer of fat while cutting across beneath the lesion. The wound granulates up and heals by secondary intention, usually requiring two to three weeks. A small dressing is kept on it during this time.

Larger lesions can be excised elliptically in the known lines of skin tension with the knife and closed by undermining and suturing, using interrupted ooo white silk sutures subcutaneously and in the derma and interrupted ooo black silk sutures in the skin, put in not more than 1 to 2 mm. from the wound margin. The suture line is covered with fine mesh grease gauze and a pressure dressing applied when possible. Sutures may be removed in from two to five days if the wound is supported after that with adhesive strips, fine mesh collodion gauze, or some combination of these.

The defects from sharp excision cannot be closed by direct suturing when they are large, or when such a procedure would pull on or distort some adjacent feature. In such instances, one may try to devise a satisfactory closure by rotation of local flaps, or it may be necessary to use free skin grafts. Small to medium grafts of good texture and color can often be obtained from the clavicular area; larger grafts from the lower abdomen and inguinal area; or very thick split grafts from the lower anterior chest wall. Each patient requires individual selection of the best donor area.

Radiation therapy is sometimes used for basal cell carcinomas, especially the larger ones when located away from the nasal cartilages or the eyes, and can be used for some squamous carcinomas. A word of caution is necessary in treating the latter in patients with "sailor's" or "farmer's" skin (atrophy, telangiectases, and keratoses from long exposure to sun). Any radiation which is scattered elsewhere on such a skin may accelerate the degenerative processes in it.

Excision of Subcutaneous Tumors of the Face. Lipomas, dermoid cysts, deep fibromas, and other benign subcutaneous tumors are excised through an incision made in one of the known lines of skin tension. Any spurting vessels are grasped with a fine mosquito forceps and tied with ooo white silk; oozing is controlled by prolonged pressure with 1:5,000 adrenalin sponges or hot saline packs. Hematomas are one of the major causes of postoperative infections or irregular healing in the face, and are prevented by complete hemostasis before closing the skin and a good pressure dressing afterwards.

The resultant subcutaneous defect is filled in by mobilizing little flaps of fat from either side of the wound and suturing them in place with interrupted ooo white silk. The same sutures are used to approximate the derma, and tiny interrupted ooo black silk sutures are used for the skin, putting them on a very fine, half curved, cutting needle such as the ⅝-inch Lane cleft palate needle.

Small sebaceous cysts can sometimes be removed by making a tiny opening with a stab blade knife and teasing out the entire lining with a chalazion curet.

Larger sebaceous cysts will nearly always have at least a tiny area of skin attachment. This area must be surrounded by a small elliptical incision so as to remove the attached skin with the cysts. Infected sebaceous cysts are always drained preliminarily and excised when entirely quiescent. It is sometimes best to drain noninfected cysts when large, squeezing or curetting all the sebaceous material out of them, and allowing them to heal. This may reduce them to about one-fourth their former size, rendering the subsequent excision of them easier and producing a smaller scar.

Treatment of Hemangiomas of the Face. Hemangiomas of the face may be divided into three types; arterial, venous, and port-wine stains.

The arterial hemangiomas are bright red, growing tumors appearing in the skin of new-born or very young babies. They destroy the skin as they grow and rapidly increase in thickness so that they are elevated. While it is true that some of these tumors may disappear spontaneously after a few years, they may destroy or disfigure features in the meantime so that they generally should be treated, with some exceptions being made when they can be closely observed and seem to be retrogressing.

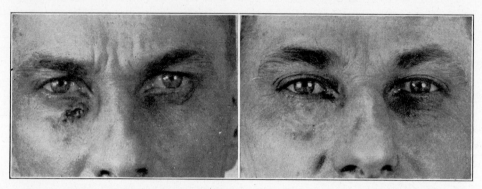

FIG. 99. Wide surgical excision of basal cell carcinoma of lower eyelid and immediate closure of wound with thick split-skin graft. Any attempt to suture this wound, or healing by secondary intention, would have produced a marked ectropion. Any possible radiation effect on the eye is avoided.

The small ones of only a few millimeters in diameter are usually best destroyed with the fine, white hot, electric cautery (after anesthetizing the area with novocaine). Larger ones on a flat surface (such as the forehead) which are only a few millimeters thick may be treated with surface radium, using about 25 mg. hrs./sq. cm. and shielding it with $\frac{1}{2}$ mm. lead and 1 mm. rubber. Any additional treatments should not be applied in less than six weeks and should be reduced in amount. It is not necessary for the tumor to entirely disappear in six weeks, and if definite signs of retrogression are present any secondary treatment is postponed until it seems stationary or there are signs of renewed activity of the lesion.

Thicker ones, or lesions appearing on moving or curved areas (such as the lips or eyelids) are often best treated with interstitial gold radon seed, using $\frac{1}{8}$ mc. or $\frac{1}{4}$ mc. seed implanted about 1 cm. apart. The smaller seed should be used in thin areas such as the nose, eyelids, or lips or on the more rapidly growing, brighter, tumors covered with very thin epithelium. The larger seed can be used on the remainder, but should be spaced just a little farther apart. It is seldom necessary to repeat the treatment on any one area (Fig. 100).

Port-wine stains are more of a congenital anomaly in the number of capillaries within the derma, than tumors and they are not sensitive to radiation. They are purely a cosmetic problem, but a very serious one. Small ones can sometimes be excised and closed by undermining the edges and suturing, or by local rotation of flaps, or by multiple partial excision. Larger ones will often require excision and resurfacing of the area with full thickness or very thick split skin grafts. Some experimental work is being done in injecting permanent pigments within the derma in these lesions, but no definite recommendations concerning this can be made yet.

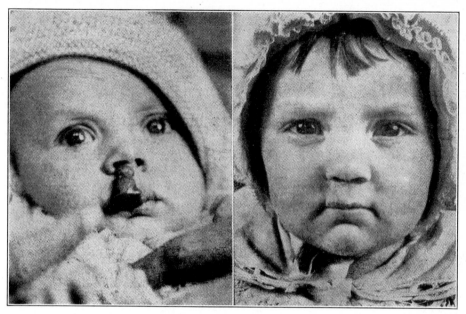

FIG. 100. Growing, destructive, "arterial" hemangioma of lip in baby treated with interstitial radon seed. This type of tumor may entirely destroy a feature if left alone. (From Brown and Byars, *Am. J. Surg.*, 39(No. 2):452-457, 1938.)

Venous (or Cavernous) hemangiomas are subcutaneous collections of dilated veins which are compressible, are distended when dependent, and collapsed when elevated. Many of them probably contain arterial leaks. Their color varies with their proximity to the surface—lesions which have thinned out the overlying skin may be blue. Excision is the best treatment when applicable, but may be difficult for large ones in the cheek (because of danger to the facial nerve branches) and in some other locations. When excision seems contraindicated, injection with 5 per cent sodium morrhuate solution or some other endothelial sclerosing agent may be helpful. The solution should always be injected within the lumen of the vein and not more than 2 to 3 cc. should be used each time, even in adults.

Excision of Parotid Tumors. The common tumor of the parotid gland is the mixed tumor. More than three-fourths of them are benign and well encapsulated when they first come to the surgeon, and they would not present much of a problem except for the scars incident to their removal and especially the very real danger to the branches of the facial nerve during the excision. One of the commonest causes of facial paralysis is the removal of parotid tumors, by inexperienced surgeons.

The mixed tumor is a firm, rounded mass, freely movable under the skin and over the ramus, but attached to the parotid tissue. It is not tender and the skin over it is not reddened. Stenson's duct will be open on probing, and the saliva from it will be clear. Sialograms are of little value in the

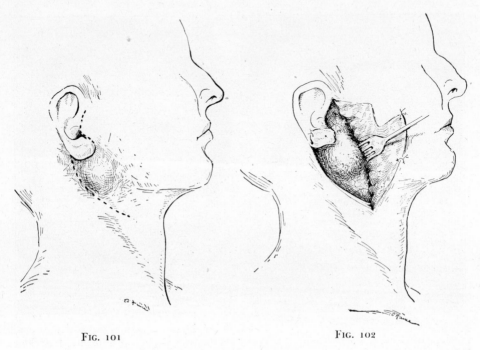

FIG. 101   FIG. 102

FIG. 101. Line of incision for removal of parotid tumor. The lower end can be carried farther forward for larger tumors.

FIG. 102. Skin flap undermined and reflected forward to expose the tumor and adjacent parotid. The lobe of the ear can be detached from the parotid and fastened up to the helix when necessary for exposure.

diagnosis. The tumor must be differentiated from sebaceous cysts, which will usually have some skin attachment, and from enlarged lymph nodes in the tail of the parotid. The presence of other enlarged lymph nodes, or of squamous carcinoma in a location which drains to this area will help in the diagnosis. It must be differentiated from suppurative parotitis (with or without stone) in which pus will be draining from Stenson's duct, and from epidemic parotitis (mumps) in which the gland will be tender, the enlargement of short duration, and often redness around the opening of Stenson's duct. Lipomas in the area will be soft, and hemangiomas compressible. Unilateral hypertrophy of the masseter muscle may be difficult to differentiate, but the swelling will usually be soft when the jaw is relaxed and hard when it is clenched.

Malignancy of a mixed tumor can be diagnosed preoperatively when there is paralysis of any of the branches of the facial nerve, fixation to the skin, mandible, or mastoid, or enlarged hard nodes in the upper carotid sheath below the tumor, or lung metastases.

The excision is best done under general endotracheal anesthesia and it is essential that the entire face be exposed during the entire operation.

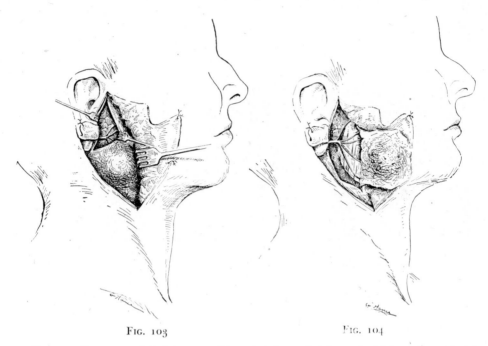

FIG. 103   FIG. 104

FIG. 103. Exposure of facial nerve. Dissection is carried inward right on the anterior surface of the tragal cartilage to expose the facial nerve trunk at the inner border of the mastoid process about 1 cm. above its tip. The field must be "bone dry" at all times. A nasal speculum and small suction tip are often helpful in providing exposure at this stage. As soon as the trunk is identified, it is followed a short distance forward until it branches, and then each branch is followed beyond the limits of the tumor.

FIG. 104. After the facial nerve branches are isolated and retracted out of the way, the parotid tumor is removed with much or all of the surrounding parotid tissue.

The principal danger is the possibility of damage to any of the branches of the facial nerve and this must be kept in mind throughout the operation.

The incision is made just inside the tragus of the ear, down between the lobe of the ear and the face, back up behind the ear, and then down and forward in one of the horizontal creases in the upper neck (Fig. 101). The skin flap thus outlined is then completely undermined and reflected forward to expose the entire parotid area. The lobe of the ear is detached from the parotid and sutured up out of the way if necessary. The entire field is then made completely dry by tying off any spurting vessels with ooo white silk and stopping any oozing with pressure with 1:5000 adrenalin sponges (Fig. 102).

If the tumor is not large and any portion of it seems quite superficial, it may be possible to remove it without doing a nerve dissection. In doing this, a sharp-nosed straight mosquito forceps without teeth is used for the dissection, pushing in the tip a few millimeters and spreading the blades in a direction that is always parallel to any of the nerve branches in the area (it is essential to be completely familiar with the detailed anatomy of the facial nerve for this operation). While a trusted assistant watches the face, any vertical fibrous septa thus encountered are very lightly squeezed with the forceps and divided if there is no twitching. It is essential that the most experienced assistant watch the face throughout the operation, and that

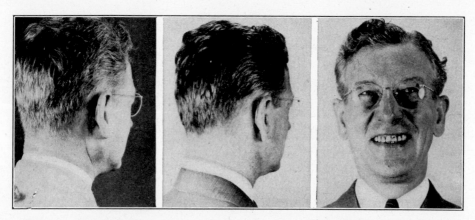

FIG. 105. Removal of medium-sized parotid tumor which, however, went in quite deep and required a complete nerve dissection. All branches of nerve preserved and resultant scar is almost invisible.

the field be kept completely dry at all times. The initial dissection is done horizontally over the most superficial part of the tumor, and then carried by degrees all around the tumor, staying just a millimeter or two outside the capsule at all times and taking care not to puncture it.

If the tumor is large, or deep seated, a nerve dissection is essential preliminary to the actual removal. To expose the main trunk of the nerve, the dissection is carried down on the anterior surface of the tragal cartilage, staying right on the surface of the cartilage to avoid any bleeding. The trunk will be found emerging horizontally, deep to the parotid, from the inner surface of the mastoid process and about 1 cm. above its tip (Fig. 103). Small deep retractors, or a nasal speculum, may be used to gain exposure at this stage. The field is frequently washed out with saline to keep it from becoming even slightly blood-stained. The dissection is done entirely by spreading until the main trunk is identified. If there is any question, it can be lightly tapped and the whole face will twitch. The trunk is then followed distally until it branches, and each branch followed out individually until it is dissected free from the gland and the tumor. After all branches have been dissected out and retracted out of the way, the tumor may be removed with a generous amount of parotid adherent to it (Fig. 104). If there is any suspicion that it is malignant, the entire parotid may be removed. If it is known to be malignant beforehand, of course, the facial nerve is disregarded and the entire parotid is excised with the definite understanding with the patient that facial paralysis will be produced, and a neck dissection may be done at the same time.

After removal, the wound is thoroughly irrigated with saline, the ear lobe sutured back in place if it was detached, and the skin flap replaced and closed with fine interrupted ooo black silk sutures around a small rubber dam drain placed to the tumor bed. A large pressure dressing is applied over the whole area, and the drain and sutures removed about the fifth day (Fig. 105).

REPAIR OF SINGLE CLEFT LIPS

Types of Operations. *V-excision of the cleft* and bringing the edges together is the most simple type of repair for single cleft lips (Fig. 106A). This plan has been used by many surgeons, with good results, particularly in partial clefts. One objection to it is the straight-line scar which may contract to produce a notch or "whistling deformity." Another objection is that the lip which is produced comes straight down (as seen in the profile view) from the nostril floor to the vermilion.

The normal lip curves forward (in profile) just above the vermilion border. This "break" normally occurs about two-thirds or three-fourths of the way down the lip and a repair which reproduces this "kick-out" of the vermilion and the skin just above it will more closely resemble a normal lip (Fig. 106B, J). To do this, one needs to use a design which will give an extra amount of tissue in this region and to close the tissues firmly up toward the top of the fornix on the inside.

The essentials of the plan are that: (1) a V-excision operation is marked out first; and (2) then instead of completing this operation, a small flap is designed on the cleft side to turn down and across to the central side. This saves tissue, fills out the lower border, and (when careful mucosal closure is done) leaves a protruding lip.

At the primary operation, it is of major importance to obtain: (1) a symmetrical alar level; (2) a good alar direction toward the columella; (3) satisfactory nostril floor; (4) a normal nostril curve, that is—across the tip; (5) a straight columella; (6) a full lip border in advance of the lower lip with a normal concavity from above downward (this might be called a flexion crease); and (7) a full vermilion without a notched "whistling deformity." It is necessary to get primary healing, but this is usually not difficult if care is taken in the accurate apposition of raw surfaces and in avoiding tension by the wide mobilization of surrounding facial tissues.

Anesthesia. Ether vapor seems to be the safest sedative for babies. If both infraorbital nerves are blocked by injecting 2 per cent novocaine around the region of the foramina, much less ether will be needed. The vapor is blown through a long, curved, sterile metal tube which is held about 1 or 2 inches from the mouth. The anesthetists are encouraged to give just enough so that the baby will remain reasonably still, but not enough to abolish the cough reflex, and it is better to err on the light side. An assistant uses a sucker from time to time to keep the mouth clear of blood. The operator sits above the head of the patient, thus seeing the face upside-down throughout the opera-

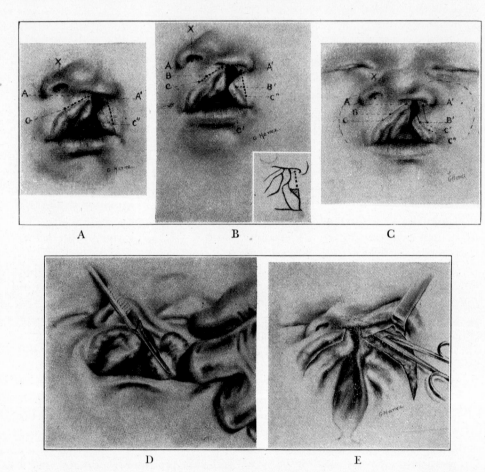

Fig. 106(1). Operation for primary closure of single cleft lip. See text for explanation. (From Brown, J. B. and McDowell, F., *Surg., Gynec. & Obst.,* 80:12-26, 1945. By permission of Surgery, Gynecology and Obstetrics.)

tion. Intratracheal gas-ether is used when the patients are old enough (in adults, local anesthesia usually suffices).

The marking is done with care after due consideration of all of the elements of deformity in the individual patient. Time spent at this stage will save operative time later because a good design can be followed throughout the operation without change. A mechanical drawing pen and 5 per cent alcoholic methylene blue are used, puncturing in the dots, scratching in the lines, and wiping off any excess dye with an alcohol sponge.

Marking out the V-excision Operation. To mark point A, the columellar side of the lip is pushed over into the cleft until the columella is straight and in the midline (Fig. 106A). A is then punctured near the mucocutaneous junction on the level of the base of the columella. (It may be put in on this line while it is still in its diagonal position.) Point X is punctured in the floor of the other nostril in a position corresponding to A.

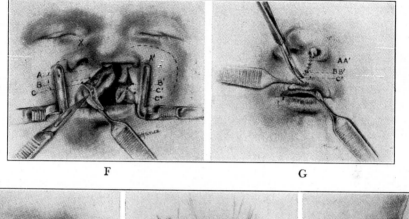

F   G

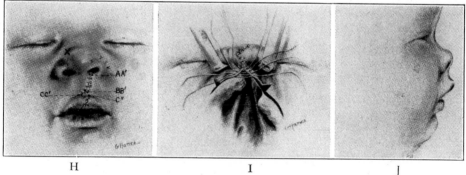

H   I   J

Fig. 106(2). Operation for primary closure of single cleft lip. See text for explanation. (From Brown, J. B. and McDowell, F., *Surg., Gynec. & Obst.*, 80:12-26, 1945. By permission of Surgery, Gynecology and Obstetrics.)

The relationship of X to the curve around the base of the normal ala is noted. A' is then placed in the same relation to the base of the ala on the cleft side. If it is difficult to determine the grooves between the ala and cheek and lip, these landmarks can usually be brought out by temporarily pushing the lip medially over into the cleft.

C is on the mucocutaneous line, at the medial end of the full thickness of vermilion. This point, where the vermilion first begins to thin out, can be best ascertained by looking at the lip from above. At times it is almost over to the philtrum on the normal side.

C" is on the mucocutaneous line, the same distance from A' that C is from A. A small caliper is useful for measuring these distances.

To do the V-excision operation, lines are drawn from A to C and A' to C", the edges of the cleft are excised accordingly and fitted together. This operation is not used except in a few partial clefts and in a few secondary operations. It is the easiest design to carry out.

Marking out the Flap Operation. The V-excision operation is marked out first (Fig. 106B, C). C′ is then located on the mucocutaneous junction at the highest point where the vermilion on the alar side is still of full thickness. This point, where the vermilion first begins to thin out, is again most easily seen from above the patient (Fig. 106B).

B′ is on the line A′—C″ and equidistant from C′ and C″. The isosceles triangle C″—B′—C′ is the Mirault flap and is the additional amount of lip which is saved by this operation. B′ is usually about one-third or one-fourth of the way up from C″.

B is on the mucocutaneous line and the same distance from C that B′ is from C′.

Discussion of Marking. Any error in placing A′ should be on the low side. The lower the mark, the higher the cleft nostril will be and this is the reverse of the common deformity.

An additional check can be had by measuring the distance from X vertically down to the mucocutaneous junction. A—C should not be greater than this distance, or the lip will be too long, a common error.

Both C and C′ should be opposite good thick vermilion. This is one of the instances in which two halves cannot be satisfactorily joined to make a whole, and if either of these points is opposite thin vermilion, a "whistling" defect is almost certain to result. However, if either of the points is placed too far laterally, an unnecessary amount of lip will be sacrificed.

Due to the curvature of the surface of the lip, one is measuring "air distances" rather than "ground distances" in locating all of these points. This would seem to be a source of error, but in practice these inequalities usually cancel each other.

The Operation. After one is satisfied with the marking, the lines A—B—C and A′—B′—C′ are lightly incised with a knife (Fig. 106D-J). The mucosa is also divided from the skin above A up in the nostril. The incision on the other side from C′ is carried upward into the nostril along the mucocutaneous junction. A rectangular skin flap is thus outlined between C′ and A′ and may be used later, if necessary, to form the nostril floor by rotating it 180 degrees up into place (Fig. 106C).

MOBILIZING THE LIP AND NOSE. An incision is made in the buccal fornix on the cleft side, extending from the molar region forward to the cleft (Fig. 106D). The soft tissues of the cheek are elevated carefully from the bone up toward the orbital border. This freeing of the cheek should allow that side of the lip to be brought easily across the cleft and the nostril to be rotated into its proper position. If tightness of the lining of the nose prevents this, it may be necessary to make a small vertical incision in front of the anterior end of the inferior turbinate (Fig. 106E). After the lip and ala are freely mobilized, small scissors are introduced through the buccal fornix and the skin of the nose is elevated throughout the lower half and over across the midline toward the normal side (Fig. 106E). This tends to minimize "corrugation" of the lining when the nostril is rotated inward and up to its new position, and possibly helps establish a columellar-alar angle instead of the straight line that is present here in wide clefts. The undermined cheek is packed temporarily with one-fourth strength adrenalin on gauze.

Similar mobilization of the lip (but not the nose) is done on the opposite side, though it is usually not so extensive. If the nose is badly deviated, it may be necessary to elevate the base of the normal ala up out of the pyriform recess with a small periosteal elevator. Sometimes it may also be necessary to make a small cut across the base of the septum underneath the lip. When mobilization is complete, the two sides of the lip can be brought together with practically no tension.

EXCISING THE CLEFT. The lines A'—B'—C' are now cut through the full thickness of the lip, care being taken to keep the level of the cut on the mucosal surface identical with the skin. After the incisions have been made, any tiny line of skin attached to the vermilion near C should be carefully excised (Fig. 106F).

In designing and fitting the two sides together, it is better to work with them as though working in wood, than as though they were rubber and could be pulled, stretched and molded into position. All incisions should be sharp, clear cut, definitive ones, and when the lip is opened as in swinging the triangular flap down, the cut at the angle should be complete so that the angle can fit up snugly against B on the columellar side.

At no time during the whole operation is it desirable to grasp any of the lip, which is to be used in the repair, with forceps. The gloved fingers are used for most of the holding with a somewhat clumsy appearance, but with improved healing and no forceps scratches.

Angled Crile clamps which have a soft spring are used at the corners of the mouth to help control bleeding (Fig. 106F). Small mosquito forceps with rubber tubes over the jaws and a rubber band to close them gently may be substituted.

CLOSING THE LIP. A and A' are usually closed with a buried No. 000 white silk suture. If preferred, a large, firm No. 000 catgut suture is put in from the mucosal surface, picking up a good bit of tissue under both A and A' and thus in one move elevating the ala and closing the lip and nostril in the desired direction (Fig. 106G).

B and B' are closed with another fine buried silk suture and with a fine surface suture. C and C' are fitted together to test the design. An excision is then made so that a V is cut out of the cleft side's vermilion just lateral to C', opening the area and dropping a V-shaped flap of the vermilion down. This is sometimes accomplished by a single appropriate incision, simply opening the area, but this gets into the rubber idea and the "wood-working" technic usually is best (Fig. 106G).

On the sound side (after being doubly sure remnants of white skin are off of the vermilion flap below C) the largest sacrifice of tissue is made. The rather long flap of vermilion is fitted across into the open vermilion cut on the cleft side and the excess is cut off. For the incisions and trimming in this region, a fine, very sharp scissors is most useful (Fig. 106H).

C and C′ are closed with a fine surface stitch. Further surface closures are usually done between AA′, BB′ and CC′, using fine black silk. The vermilion flaps are closed with fine surface sutures, usually anchoring the points of the flaps first. Mucosal closure is continued by going right on around the vermilion clear up the inside to the buccal fornix and being sure to close the mucosa entirely even if it rests on a raw surface of the premaxilla (Figs. 106H, I).

This mucosal closure is almost as important as the skin closure. It closes the entire lip for best primary healing and thrusts the lip forward as no other part of the operation does, by being sure there is a free loose amount of tissue below even if the upper end is tighter (Fig. 106J). If this end of the wound seems too tight, it is loosened by vertical mucosal cuts on either side from the fornix downward. This is one of the few places in plastic surgery in which cutting one way and sewing another gives much help. But here the soft mucosa can actually be transposed in position from a tight purse string in the fornix to rather free flaps of mucosa that can be advanced into the lip. Complete closure of the mucosa also prevents adhesion of the lip to a raw premaxilla from occurring (Fig. 106I, J).

This point of mucosal closure is dealt with at length because it is the point most responsible for "kicking" the lip out forward. The fine mucosal sutures put the lip where it can best stay itself. Gross stay sutures may crowd the lip forward but they will not permanently hold the tissue in place. Protrusion of the lip should be accomplished before stay sutures are put in.

Stay sutures of B black silk are put in from the mucous surface if desired, going through the lip almost to the skin, usually one or two in number.

The floor of the nose is closed with surface sutures on a small full curved needle, using the flap freed on the columellar side and any part necessary of the flap left from the incision on the cleft side. Care must be taken not to include any vermilion in the floor of the nostril where it could be seen.

The nostril can be somewhat shaped by mattress sutures through it from the skin surface to pick up the mucosa, these two surfaces having been separated during the dissection. One or two are put in the alar fold, one higher up on the ala and one to try to help form an angle at the columellar-alar junction. These sutures are not very important and can be omitted (Fig. 106H).

Many operators use a mattress suture from the alar fold across the floor to tie inside the sound nostril against the septum, using small plates inside and out to prevent cutting of the sutures. If the lip is otherwise solidly closed, one can omit this suture.

The nostril is gently packed with greased gauze and a Logan bow used if desired.

At the end of the operation, the lip should be full and in front of the lower (Fig. 106J). A good flexion crease should be present. The lip should have good width and not be too long. The nostril should have a good floor, the ala should point toward the columella and the level of the ala should be the same or a little higher than the opposite one (Figs. 107, 108 and 109).

Preoperative Determinations and Care. Single clefts can be repaired at any time, but are preferably closed early in life. An early closure facilitates feeding, eliminates the necessity for constant apologies and explanations to friends by the parents, and the elastic pressure of the closed lip tends to narrow the anterior portion of any associated palate cleft during the first

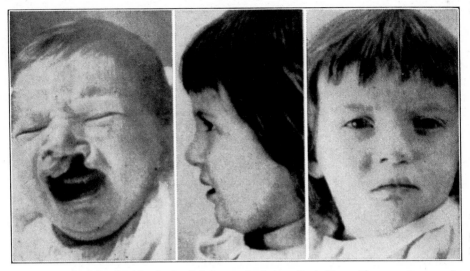

FIG. 107. Repair of wide single cleft by method described. Note the normal appearing forward thrust of the lower border of the lip and the good rotation of the cleft nostril. (From Brown and McDowell, *Surg., Gynec. & Obst.*, 80:12-26, 1945. By permission of Surgery, Gynecology and Obstetrics.)

year of life. Even very young babies, if they are well developed, tolerate the operation well, and closures have been done as early as the age of seven hours. Quite often, the father wishes to have the cleft closed before the mother sees the baby and this may be done, but one parent should see the baby beforehand. If the patient is first seen at the age of three or four days when he is losing weight, one might as well wait until he has regained his birth weight before undertaking the repair. The closure should not be done in the presence of jaundice, or in prematures or other babies weighing less than seven pounds until they have attained that weight. Upper respiratory infections are an obvious contraindication as are any pustular skin eruptions, but small areas of uninfected "miliaria" or "heat-rash" are not.

None of these children should undergo operation immediately following a trip, but they should be under observation for twenty-four to forty-eight hours for rest and to be sure that they have not contracted any upper respiratory infection.

It is still an open question as to whether these patients might not attain better general facial development if the lip and palate closures were delayed until puberty, but other factors make this choice untenable. However, this is not "emergency surgery" and should never be done under any except the most favorable conditions. A delay of one month seldom will do much harm, while a satisfactory repair may be of inestimable value to the child and conversely a faulty repair may cause irreparable damage.

Feeding is always a problem in these infants and, especially if the palate is open, they are seldom able to nurse from the breast. However, it is rarely

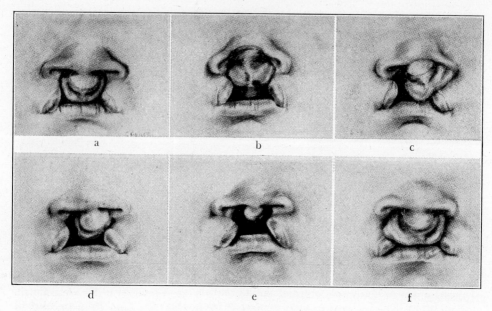

FIG. 108. Some of the common variations in size, shape and position of premaxillae in double cleft lips. (From Brown, McDowell and Byars, *Surg., Gynec. & Obst.*, 85:20-29, 1947. By permission of Surgery, Gynecology and Obstetrics.)

necessary to gavage them every three or four hours and an infant's esophagus will usually not stand this procedure long. They can be fed breast milk or a suitable formula with a medicine dropper or a syringe, best given with the baby held almost in a sitting position and taking from thirty to forty minutes for each feeding rather than the usual fifteen to twenty minutes.

Postoperative Care. No dressing is applied over the suture line when good nursing care is available. The nurses are instructed to clean the suture line with alkaline antiseptic solution on tiny gauze pledgets every few minutes for the first hour after operation and then every hour for the remainder of the day. After this, the lip is cleansed after each feeding and at other times when necessary to prevent the formation of any clots of blood or serum around the stitches. If experienced nursing care is not available, the suture line can be covered with a fine mesh grease gauze dressing which may be changed daily or oftener, cleansing the lip each time.

The grease-gauze pack in the nostril is removed in 48 hours, and the skin sutures on the lip are taken out on the fourth or fifth day. The Logan bow can be removed after one week and remaining inside sutures after ten days.

Feedings are usually given with a syringe until seven to ten days after operation, after which the baby may nurse from a bottle if the holes in the nipple are burned out and enlarged. If the baby is breast fed, the breast milk is usually given with a syringe for three or four days after operation and then the baby is allowed to nurse if the palate will permit it.

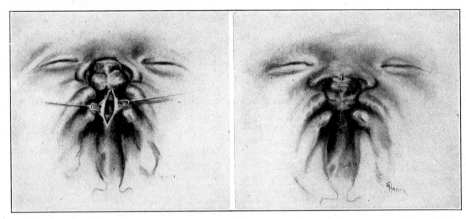

Fig. 109. Preliminary set-back of the premaxilla when absolutely necessary for closure of the lip or to prevent crumpling of the septum with subsequent blockage of the nasal airways. A small block of bone is resected submucously from the vomer just back of the premaxilla, and the latter is set back in contact with the vomer (like closing a drawer). Immobilization is obtained by nailing a straight Keith needle through the center of the premaxilla and on back longitudinally through the vomer. (From Brown, McDowell and Byars, *Surg., Gynec. & Obst.,* 85:20-29, 1947. By permission of Surgery, Gynecology and Obstetrics.)

The patient is usually discharged from the hospital on the tenth postoperative day, with the lip healed, all sutures out, no dressings, and able to nurse from a bottle or the breast, as far as the lip is concerned.

The cooperation and help of a pediatrician throughout the baby's hospitalization is solicited and gratefully received.

REPAIR OF DOUBLE CLEFT LIPS

The surgical repair of double cleft lips is about twice as difficult as in single clefts and the results are about half as good.

Normally, the frontonasal process of the embryo fuses with the two lateral maxillary processes by the ninth week. When there is total lack of fusion of these on both sides, the three processes develop independently of each other from the ninth week until term, with the result that the baby has not only a hiatus or cleft on either side, but also has severe growth distortions of the entire middle third of the face. Partial fusion on one side makes this distortion asymmetrical on the two sides and may render the interpretation and plan for repair even more difficult.

The double clefts vary a great deal in the amount and shape of the deformity, so that individual study and improvising is necessary in planning their repair. They are not considered surgically simply as two single clefts, both of which happen to occur in the same patient.

Age for Primary Operation. A fairly satisfactory rule is to close them as soon as possible after the baby weighs ten pounds, subject to variations in the extent of the deformity and the child's general physical condition. Many of these patients have an anemia and are given transfusions to bring the pre-operative hemoglobin up to 12 to 15 grams per cent. Nearly all of those with open palates will have a chronic otitis media which is not an especial contra-indication to surgery. Operations are not done, of course, during an acute exacerbation.

Until the lip is closed, feeding is done with a syringe (with a short piece of rubber tubing attached) and gavaging is usually avoided.

Treatment of the Premaxilla. The premaxilla is the separate central segment of the upper jaw and is that portion arising from the embryonic frontonasal process. Briefly, the problem of the premaxilla is that it is nearly always too far forward in the newborn baby, but only with considerable effort can it be kept from being retruded too far backward in the adult. It varies a good deal in size, shape, and position, and at times, as to the number of tooth buds it contains (Fig. 108). The large oval, or almost rectangular, premaxilla forms a better central segment of the jaw, supports the lip better, and will have the lateral incisor tooth buds inclined only slightly laterally, so that it is easier to work with for both the surgeon and the orthodontist. It overlaps the lateral processes slightly on both sides, so that if it is necessary to set it back, it will rest as a bridge on them and will not tend to tilt and cannot sink back behind them. The small, round, premaxilla may be smaller than the hiatus between the two lateral processes, so that one must try to prevent it from being forced back between and behind them, thus producing a retruded upper jaw and lip. The tooth buds are arranged in a partial circle around its periphery so that the lateral incisors may tend to grow directly into the lateral processes, or even up into the nostril floors, or forward through the lip if it becomes tilted. Some of the permanent tooth buds may be entirely missing from these tiny, round, premaxillae. Thus, the size and shape of the premaxilla greatly influences the final result.

In the newborn baby, the premaxilla is nearly always anterior to the lateral processes. It may be anywhere from just in front of them to extreme positions out on the tip of the nose where it may project forward and upward like a snout. In addition to forward displacement, it may be tilted from side to side, or rotated. If the cleft is partially fused on one side, the premaxilla may be rotated toward that side, but tilted so the open edge is farther forward.

It is not uncommon to find a bend or kink in the septum just behind the premaxilla, sometimes so marked as to occlude one or both nasal airways at birth. This may be the result of intrauterine pressure on the premaxilla.

As a rule, the premaxilla is not disturbed or set back if the lip can be closed with it in its original position unless; (a) it is badly tilted or rotated, or (b) it is so far forward that the elastic pressure of the closed lip might bend the septum and occlude one or both nasal airways.

If the premaxilla is to be set back, it is set back the least possible amount necessary to allow successful closure of the lip. This is done by splitting the mucosa over the bottom of the vomer and resecting a block (submucously) of the vomer just back of the premaxilla. The premaxilla is set back until it is in contact with the vomer again and immobilized by a wire suture through both fragments or better by nailing a straight Keith needle directly backward through the center of the premaxilla and on back through the center of the vomer (Fig. 109). In setting the premaxilla back, an attempt is made to correct any rotation or tilting so that it will be centered with respect to the lateral processes as well as possible. This is insured somewhat by having excised a block rather than a wedge of the vomer.

When the premaxilla is larger than the space between the two lateral processes, and good firm immobilization is obtained, the lip can be closed during the same operation; otherwise, the closure is done about two weeks later. Bony union between the premaxilla and vomer is rarely obtained either way, but the fibrous union helps a good deal in keeping it centered.

The Disposition of the Prolabium. The prolabium is the central segment of the lip and must be used in this position in the closure. The upper part of it is sometimes advanced secondarily into the columella at three or four years of age, but it is best not to do this primarily.

Many plans of closure have included the vermilion of the prolabium in the vermilion of the reconstructed lip, but these nearly always result in a double notch. This notching is not easy to eliminate by secondary procedures as it is due to an inherent thinning and upward direction of the vermilion on both sides of the prolabium.

Consideration of the "cupid's bow" configuration of some normal lips has somewhat confused this issue. The occurrence of the "cupid's bow" varies a good deal in normal lips and in any event it is an upward prolongation of the *upper* edge of the vermilion beneath each philtrum. The lower edge of the normal vermilion has a gradual downward curve from the center outward without any upward notches, and it is almost impossible to get this when the thin "U-shaped" vermilion of the prolabium is used as the central portion of the new lip.

It is thought best to use a plan in which an incision is made at the mucocutaneous junction all the way around the prolabium and its vermilion is turned back as a flap to be used for lining if necessary.

Design for Closure. Many of the features of the modified Mirault operation for single cleft lips are used in closing the double cleft lips. Usually a flap is turned down from the inner surface of the lateral border of the cleft on each side, and they are brought together in the midline beneath the prolabium (Fig. 110A). If the cleft is partial on one side and total on the other side a "V" excision operation may be used on the partial side and a Mirault flap on the total side (Fig. 110B). When the prolabium is unusually large and long, so that the Mirault flaps under it might result in too long a lip, 2 or 3 millimeters of skin can be excised from the bottom of the pro-

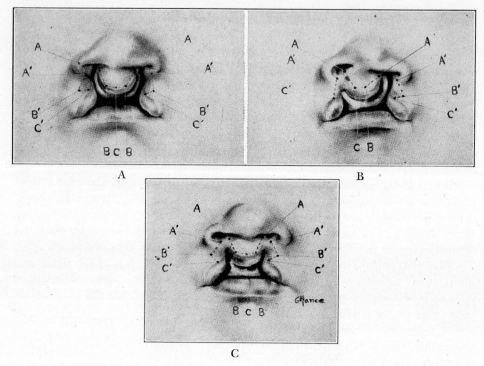

FIG. 110. (A) Closure of total double cleft with Mirault flap from each side. (B) Closure of totally cleft side with Mirault flap and partially cleft side by V-excision plan. (C) Closure of double partially cleft lip with Mirault flap from each side. See text for details. (From Brown, McDowell and Byars, *Surg., Gynec. & Obst.*, 85:20-29, 1947. By permission of Surgery, Gynecology and Obstetrics.)

labium to shorten it. If the prolabium is tiny, the lateral flaps may be designed in a rectangle (rather than a triangle) to elongate the lip (Fig. 111).

In marking out symmetrical clefts with the columella in the midline, a transverse line is imagined across the prolabium at the level of the base of the columella, and the points A are marked on either side where this line crosses the mucocutaneous junction. A′ is marked just inside the lower point of the nostril rim on each lateral side of the cleft, being careful to place it in such position that a good nostril will be formed when A′ is approximated to A, and marking it symmetrically on the two sides (Fig. 110A).

The point C is at the bottom of the skin of the prolabium in the midline and equidistant from the two A points. B is one-third of the distance from C back to A on the curved lower border of the skin of the prolabium on either side.

C' is on the mucocutaneous line of the lateral part of the lip and is opposite the most medial point where there is still full thickness of the vermilion.

To locate B', the straight line distance AB is measured with small calipers. One point of the calipers is then set on A' and the calipers rotated until the other point is BC distance from C'.

The above can be considered as a standard marking and can be altered when necessary. For instance, when the cleft is partial on one side, the line

A'–B'–C' is sometimes a straight one, so that B' can be omitted and a straight incision made from A' to C' and a "V" closure done on that side (Fig. 110B).

The Closure. The above points are punctured in and the lines scratched in with 5 per cent alcoholic methylene blue, using a fine mechanical drawing pen. The lines are then lightly incised with a knife, with care not to cut the points out. An incision is then made in the buccal fornix on each side and carried upward to separate the lip from the upper jaw (Fig. 112). This undermining is carried upward almost to the orbital border until the cheek is separated from the underlying facial bones, and the space between

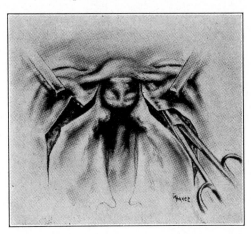

Fig. 111. Undermining to separate soft tissues of cheek from facial bones and to separate lining from covering of nostril. See text for details. (From Brown, McDowell and Byars, *Surg., Gynec. & Obst.,* 85:20-29, 1947. By permission of Surgery, Gynecology and Obstetrics.)

them is packed temporarily with gauze soaked in 1:5000 adrenalin solution.

The buccal fornix incision is then carried upward inside the lateral wall of the nostril to divide the mucosa between the upper and lower lateral cartilages of the nose until the nostril can be rotated into position and A' can be brought over to A without tension. A small fine scissors is introduced through the buccal fornix and the lower lateral cartilage of the nostril is separated from the skin covering by alternate spreading and dissecting up to the midline (Fig. 110).

The lines A'–B'–C' are then incised through the full thickness of the lip, a stab blade knife being used with a perpendicular sawing motion (Fig. 113). The small flap A'–B'–C' is rotated 180 degrees into the nostril floor. The vermilion of the prolabium is turned backward as a flap to use for lining and A–A' and B–B' are approximated on both sides, No. 000 white silk sutures being used subcutaneously and No. 000 black silk sutures in the skin. C'–C' are approximated directly under C and fine interrupted

black silk skin sutures are placed all along between A—B—C. The vermilion
closure is done by interdigitating zigzag flaps from the two sides. The inside
mucosa from the two sides is sutured to the prolabium vermilion which was

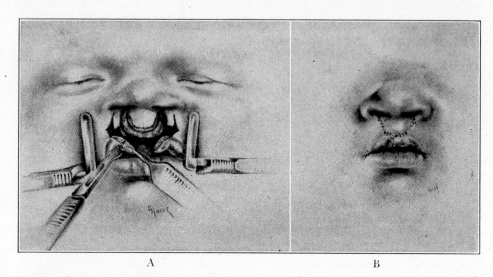

A   B

FIG. 112. (A) Perpendicular opening incisions through the lip. Knife is trimming off
tiny remnant of attached skin from vermilion flap. Note vermilion of prolabium turned
back for lining. (B) Final plan of closure with tiny ooo black silk sutures. (From Brown,
McDowell and Byars, *Surg., Gynec. & Obst.*, 85:20-29, 1947. By permission of Surgery,
Gynecology and Obstetrics.)

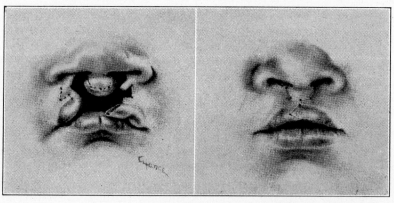

FIG. 113. Plan utilizing rectangular flaps rarely used and then only for very tiny
prolabium as this plan elongates the lip. (From Brown, McDowell and Byars, *Surg.,
Gynec. & Obst.*, 85:20-29, 1947. By permission of Surgery, Gynecology and Obstetrics.)

turned back. The nostril floor flaps are trimmed and sutured to the portion
of the prolabial skin inside the nostrils, and mattress sutures are put through
the nostril walls to aid in shaping them. Stay sutures may be put clear across
the lip from the inside, encompassing the full thickness of the lip except the

skin, to avoid any visible suture marks on the outside. (The type described by Lane is a good one.)

A Logan bow is strapped to the cheeks to protect the lip and take tension off of it while crying, and the nurses keep the suture lines free of crusts by frequent cleansing. The skin sutures are left in five days and the others a few days longer. The baby can usually be fed with a bottle after the first week, if the holes in the nipple are enlarged, and the child is discharged from the hospital after all sutures are out.

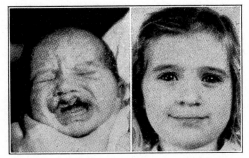

Any surgery on the palate is delayed until about eighteen months of age to permit the tooth buds to migrate out of the palate into the alveolus.

The possibility of secondary procedures on the lip is considered from the beginning with the parents, but they will be fewer in

FIG. 114. Partial double cleft shown just before operation (age 2 days) and at age of 3 years. Closed with small Mirault flap from each side. Good full vermilion obtained. (From Brown, McDowell and Byars, *Surg., Gynec. & Obst.*, 85:20-29, 1947. By permission of Surgery, Gynecology and Obstetrics.)

number and less in extent if the primary closure is a good one.

Those children who are born with a total double cleft and almost no columella will frequently require a secondary elongation of the latter so that this may be considered standard in this type of patient. Further elevation of the nose may be obtained, when desirable, by an "L-shaped" cartilage transplant.

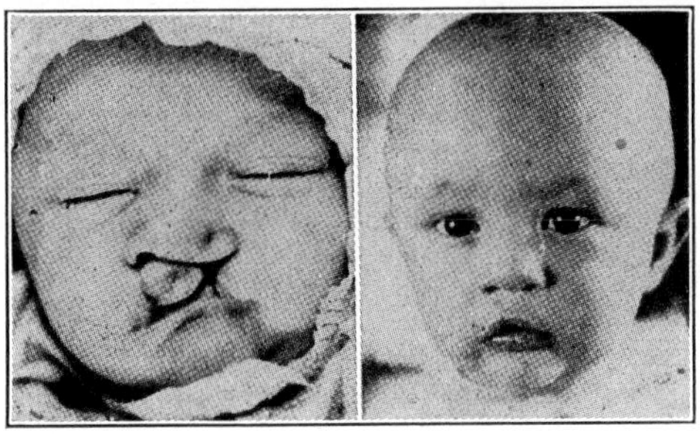

Maintenance of the size and structure of the upper dental arch is important in these patients for lip support as well as for other reasons. The child's dentist is contacted early so that proper dental hygiene may be instituted, and he may help later in providing or securing adequate orthodontic care. Limited prosthodontia may eventually be necessary in patients with total clefts.

FIG. 115. Total cleft on one side and partial on other. Closed with Mirault flap on total side and V-excision operation on partial side (all in one operation at age of a few days). The premaxilla was not moved, except by the elastic pressure of the lip. A good deal of rotation of the left nostril was necessary to get symmetry. (From Brown, McDowell and Byars, *Surg., Gynec. & Obst.*, 85:20-29, 1947. By permission of Surgery, Gynecology and Obstetrics.)

In addition to dental care, those children who have associated palate clefts may require the assistance of speech therapists and otolaryngologists. Tonsillectomies and adenoidectomies should not be done routinely, but they may be carried out if necessary for reasons of general health, or especially if the tonsils and adenoids are contributing to any loss of hearing.

The plastic surgeon can render an additional service if he will examine these patients each year throughout the growing period and advise the parents in regard to these problems as they arise. Though starting with a severe initial handicap, these children often prove to be brighter than average and succeed so well in later life that one feels well repaid for the extra time and effort required in providing the best possible care for them (Figs. 114, 115 and 116).

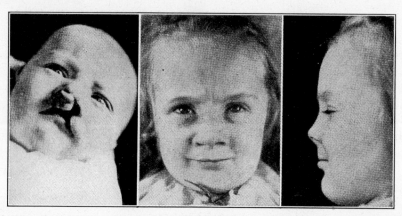

Fig. 116. Total double cleft with almost no columella and with premaxilla projecting forward from tip of nose. Premaxilla set back and lip closed early in life and columella elongated at age of 3½ years by method shown. Upper lip maintained in front of the lower one and patient has perfect speech following closure of palate at age of 18 months. (From Brown, McDowell and Byars, *Surg., Gynec. & Obst.*, 85:20-29, 1947. By permission of Surgery, Gynecology and Obstetrics.)

CLOSURE OF CLEFT PALATE

Cleft palates are preferably closed after the tooth buds have migrated out of the palate (twelve to fourteen months) and before any definite speech habits have been formed (two years). Sixteen to eighteen months of age is often a good time for the closure.

As with cleft lips, chronic otitis media is not a contraindication to operation, but acute exacerbations are. Particular attention should be paid to the preoperative hemoglobin level as these children often have nutritional anemias, and preoperative transfusions are usually given when it is low. These children should come to the operating room in a well hydrated condition.

The prevention of operative mortalities consists of preventing shock (preoperative and postoperative blood transfusions and intravenous fluids as necessary), maintenance of the airways during the operation, and maintenance of light anesthesia during the operation.

Anesthesia and Maintenance of Airways. Perhaps in no other operation is such close teamwork necessary between the surgeon and anesthetist. The anesthetist must keep the plane of anesthesia light so that the cough reflex is not lost, but so level that the child does not gag excessively and does not vomit. The surgeon must listen to each respiration throughout the operation and suction the throat or pull the tongue forward at any time if the exchange is not free and easy. These children must not be struggling for air at any time during the operation. Even slight cyanosis or enlargement of the pupils demands that the airways be cleared immediately and the anesthesia lightened. Attention to these details means the difference between an excessive mortality rate and one that is almost nil.

Induction is with drop ether and as soon as the correct light plane of anesthesia is reached, it is maintained by endopharyngeal insufflation of oxygen-ether, with a soft rubber catheter inserted through the nose on the uncleft side with the tip of it at the level of the epiglottis.

The surgeon sits at the head of the table, working upside down, with the first assistant on the right and the second assistant on the left. The child's head is extended back and is slightly dependent, placing folded sheets under the scapulae and buttocks if necessary to maintain this position. The position is important so that any blood or saliva will run up into the nasopharynx rather than down into the larynx. The second assistant steadies the head in this position with one hand and passes instruments with the other. The first assistant holds the tongue suture in one hand and uses the suction with the other to keep the airways clear at all times. The mouth is kept open with a Lane gag, but never pried so far open as to embarrass the respiratory exchange. Children over three or four years of age are most easily done under endotracheal anesthesia with the throat well packed.

The Operation. The initial incision is made with a No. 15 blade, starting over the ramus of the mandible and coming forward between the hamulus and maxillary tubercle with the blade vertically placed. The incision is then carried forward on the inside of the alveolus, turning the blade horizontally so as to cut against the alveolus, to within 1 to 2 cm. of the alveolar cleft (Fig. 117A).

A right-angled Blair-Brown palate elevator is introduced in the anterior end of the incision and the soft tissues overlying the palatine bone elevated medially to the cleft and posteriorly as far as the major (posterior) palatine artery (Fig. 117C). A Joseph nasal periosteal elevator is then introduced into the incision just back of the maxillary tubercle, pushed medially against the hamulus, or levered against it, to fracture the hamulus off medially and allow the tensor tendon to slip off of it (or the tensor tendon is cut if this is not possible). It is impossible to do one of these operations without a detailed knowledge of the anatomy of the palate, especially the triangular relationship between the maxillary tubercle, the hamulus, and the foramen for the artery.

The right-angled Blair-Brown elevator is then inserted posterior to the artery and hooked around it until the anterior edge of the blade comes up on the posterior edge of the palatine bone, getting complete mobilization of the palate all around the artery and stretching the artery out of its foramen

(Fig. 117D). The lateral wound is then temporarily packed with gauze soaked in 1:5000 adrenalin and the palate is mobilized in the same manner on the opposite side.

With a long single hook, and a No. 11 blade knife, the oral and nasal mucosa are split apart at the edge of the cleft on either side from the alveolus

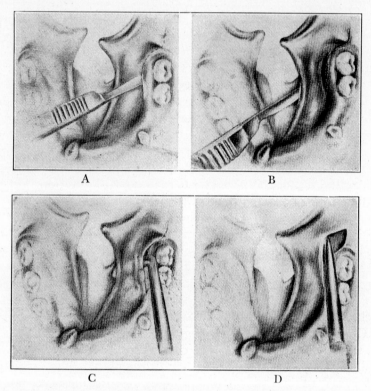

A   B

C   D

Fig. 117. Standard Dieffenbach-Warren operation for single cleft palate. (A) Initial opening incision from ramus to maxillary tubercle, around it, and forward on the inside of the alveolus. (B) Splitting the nasal from the oral mucosa at the edge of the cleft all around. (C) Right angled elevator introduced into lateral incision to elevate muco-periosteal layer from bone in front of the major palatine artery. (D) Same elevator in lateral incision behind the artery and hooking around it up on to the posterior edge of the palatine bone. (From Blair, V. P. and Brown, J. B., *Surg., Gynec. & Obst.*, 59:309-320. 1934. By permission of Surgery, Gynecology and Obstetrics.)

in front to the tip of the uvula behind (Fig. 117B). The nasal mucosa is then elevated from the septum on the uncleft side, and the palatine bone on the cleft side, until it can be rolled into a tube to line the nasal airway. It is sutured in this tubular position, using interrupted stitches of oo chromic catgut on small Lane cleft palate needles, with the knots tied on the nasal surface. This is continued on back through the soft palate, uniting the two sides of nasal mucosa flatly instead of in a tube here (Fig. 117H), and cutting the aponeurosis on one side if necessary to get enough mobilization (Fig. 117E).

One or two stay sutures are placed across the middle of the palate, being sure to get one of them opposite the hamular processes. These are of B silk on a large Lane cleft palate needle and are put in as horizontal mattress sutures, encompassing the entire thickness of the palate except the nasal mucosa. They are put in about 1 cm. from the cleft on either side, and are not tied, but have mosquito clamps hanging on them. The weight of the

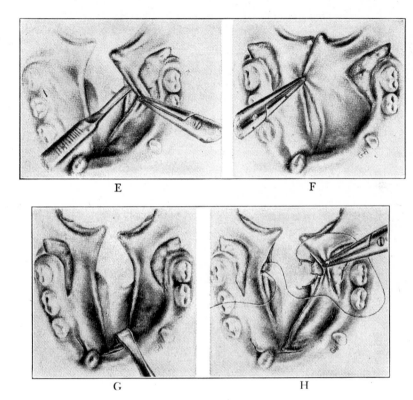

FIG. 117. (Continued). (E) Dividing the aponeurosis on one side when necessary. (F) Testing mobility of the flap. (G) Separating the nasal mucosa from the palatine bone in front. (H) Suturing the nasal mucosa of the soft palate (using fine catgut with the knots tied on the nasal surface). (From Blair, V. P. and Brown, J. B., *Surg., Gynec. & Obst.*, 59: 309-320, 1934. By permission of Surgery, Gynecology and Obstetrics.)

clamp should be sufficient to approximate the edges, a good test to see if the palate is adequately mobilized.

The oral mucosa is then closed with vertical mattress sutures (Fig. 117I, J, L) of horsehair or single strand nylon, with a few interspersed plain over sutures to get good approximation of the edges and to close the uvula, where there is not enough room for mattress sutures.

The elastic pressure of the closed lip during the first year or two of life will do a great deal to narrow the alveolar cleft anteriorly. However, it is in this area that the greatest difficulty will be encountered. Small flaps of mucosa are raised from the surface of the cleft to line the nasal airway, and

from the under surface of the lip and outer surface of the alveolus to close
the oral side. Under no circumstances should the alveolus be chiseled,
drilled, or wired, as this might damage permanent tooth buds.

At the conclusion of the operation, a small iodoform-balsam of Peru
gauze pack is placed in each lateral incision to control bleeding, the throat

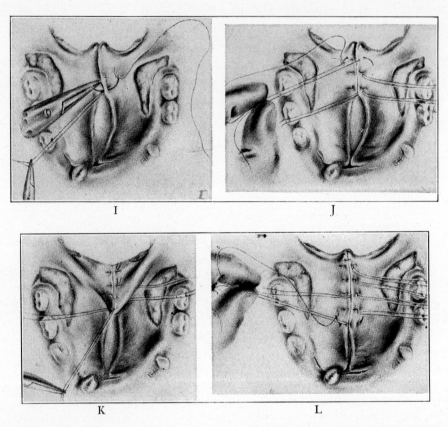

I   J

K   L

FIG. 117. (Continued). (I) Closing the oral mucosa with vertical mattress sutures of
nonabsorbable material. (J) Continuing this closure. (K) Pulling the uvula forward to
suture the nasal mucosa together at the tip end of the soft palate. (L) The vertical mattress
sutures are continued forward to the alveolus to complete the closure and small iodoform-
balsam of Peru gauze packs are inserted into the lateral incisions for 48 hours. (From
Blair, V. P. and Brown, J. B., *Surg., Gynec. & Obst.,* 59:309-320, 1934. By permission of
Surgery, Gynecology and Obstetrics.)

is cleared by suction, child turned over in the prone position, anesthetic tube
removed, and the tongue stitch taped to the cheek or chin for possible use
in the next few hours.

Postoperative Care. The child is kept in the prone position until he is
well awake and has stopped bleeding. He must be constantly watched by an
experienced nurse, anesthetist, or house officer during this period.

All postoperative feedings are given with cup or spoon and he is not
allowed to suck on a nipple at any time. The utensils are sterilized by boiling

and water can usually be started within two to three hours after operation, followed by milk in an hour or two, and thin cooked cereals and puréed foods the night of operation. These children have some difficulty in swallowing the first few hours or days, so that the intake must be closely watched and supplemented by intravenous fluids as necessary. Postoperative fever is almost always from dehydration, or a flare-up of the chronic otitis media. The otitis can be treated by chemotherapy or myringotomy as indicated.

A mild antiseptic such as 1 per cent mercurochrome can be used as nose drops and to paint the oral suture line several times daily if the child does not resist too much. Everything possible should be done to avoid excessive crying, or mechanical injury to the palate. Hard foods are avoided for one month, and the child is not allowed to put his fingers in his mouth (arm-cuffs) or have any toys that he might get into his mouth for the same period.

The hemoglobin is determined the next day and bolstered by transfusion if necessary. The child is kept in the hospital about ten days. Most of the sutures will fall out during the first month, but any remaining ones can be removed after that period.

Simple speech training exercises can be started by the mother as soon as the tenderness is out of the palate, and formal speech lessons can be undertaken usually at the age of four or five years.

ELONGATION OF THE PARTIALLY CLEFT PALATE

In the repair of cleft palates one goal should be to obtain the best possible function of the soft palate. This will require pliable tissue, sufficiently long to meet the posterior wall of the pharynx (Passavant's pad) in the sphincter-like action of this region that closes the opening between the nose and throat. Although operations may be well executed and the palates may appear normal after operation, it is extremely exceptional that perfect speech is obtained. This persistent speech defect is probably due to a leak of air into the nose which may occur if there is an opening left of only a millimeter.

Palates that are cleft only through the soft tissue or on up, part way through the bone, may have actually less tissue for repair of the soft palate than those with complete clefts; and there are also patients with uncleft palates that are so abnormally short that speech is just as bad as though the palate were cleft. Dorrance has called this "congenital insufficiency of the palate." It is in this group that the most direct attempts have been made for actually lengthening the palate, by moving the whole of the soft tissues backward and still having the bony palate in front to separate the nose and mouth.

The principle is that a direct flap of practically the entire palate is raised completely free from the bone and is immediately set back so that the anterior free edge is anchored clear back at the posterior edge of the bone. The major palatine arteries are definitely preserved and left to supply the palate flap. The palate may be allowed to heal here, the bony palate to cover com-

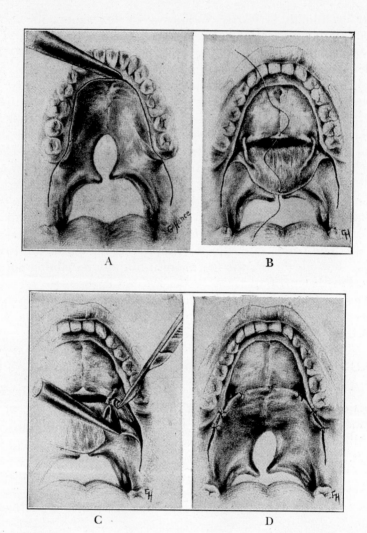

A   B

C   D

FIG. 118. Elongation of partially cleft palate, showing elongation in one operation and closure later, though both procedures are generally done in one operation now. (A) Initial incision from the ramus forward around the maxillary tubercle and all around the inside of the alveolus, around the opposite tubercle and back onto the opposite ramus. Right angle elevator introduced and entire mucoperiosteal flap raised from bones. (B) Flap turned forward, arteries stretched out of the canals and dissected free from flap for a short distance forward. The main set-back suture is inserted into the tag of nasal mucosa on the posterior edge of the bone and at the anterior edge of the flap and tied to set the entire palate back. (C) Showing cutting the tensor palatini tendon when it cannot be freed by fracturing the hamulus medialward. (D) Palate set back and held by additional sutures on either side. (From Brown, J. B., *Surg., Gynec. & Obst.*, 63:768-771, 1936. By permission of Surgery, Gynecology and Obstetrics.)

pletely with epithelium, and, at a second operation, the palate cleft itself closed, or both closure and elongation may be done at the same operation.

The Operation. An incision is made across the surface of the anterior pillar, **over the ramus and onto the maxillary tubercle; it is then carried**

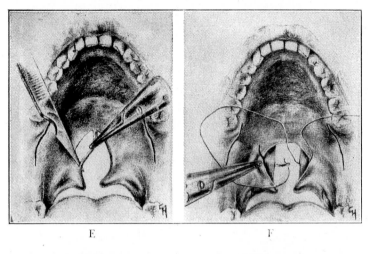

E   F

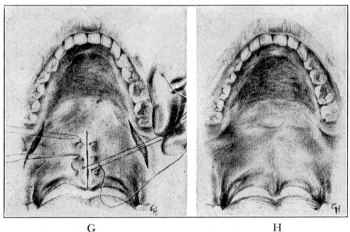

G   H

FIG. 118. (E) Paring the edges of the cleft (splitting is better). (F) Suturing the nasal mucosa (knots tied on nasal surface). (G) Vertical mattress sutures in oral mucosa. (H) Final appearance showing closure and additional length obtained without disturbance of the levator muscle-nerve mechanism. (From Brown, J. B., *Surg., Gynec. & Obst.,* 63:768-771, 1936. By permission of Surgery, Gynecology and Obstetrics.)

entirely around the palate against the alveolus and out over the opposite side (Fig. 118A).

An elevator is used to detach the mucoperiosteum completely from the bone, and the arteries are carefully preserved. When the posterior edge of the bone is reached, the nasal mucosa is carefully opened and a narrow edge is left attached to the bone to be used for the anchoring sutures that are put in later (Fig. 118B). The elevator is put behind the arteries and the space down to the hamulus and pterygoid plate is opened so that the surface and deep soft tissues throughout the entire extent of the incision may be freely mobilized. The tensor muscle may be divided at the hamulus, or the hamulus fractured over medially, and the dissection of the aponeurosis from the posterior edge of the bone is completed so that the entire mass of palate tissue is held by the remaining uncut surface over the pillars, the major arteries and the levators. At this stage, in spite of the very free dissection, it is interesting to note that the levators are still active (Fig. 118C).

The arteries are then elongated by carefully stretching them from their foramina and slightly separating them from the raw surface of the palate. We are convinced that this procedure can be successfully carried out as we do it routinely, and we do practically the same thing in repairing total clefts.

The cleft in the palate is closed by simply freshening the edges and suturing them in layers with catgut sutures on the nasal surface and vertical mattress nylon or horsehair sutures on the oral surface.

The palate is elongated by setting the anterior cut edge clear back at the posterior bony edge with a horsehair or silk suture to the little flap of nasal mucosa that is left attached here. The lateral free edge of the flap is then anchored at the maxillary tubercle on each side and one or two more sutures may be inserted (Fig. 118D).

The tissue is usually somewhat humped up, but it is definitely longer and the soft palate may be lying in contact with the posterior wall. The anterior defect is covered smoothly with a pack of balsam of Peru and iodoform gauze, and no sutures are necessary to retain it.

Recovery is usually prompt and the patient can leave the hospital in seven to ten days. The pack is removed about the sixth day, and repacking is occasionally necessary for bleeding.

Complete healing of epithelium over the bony palate occurs in twenty to thirty days, and is practically normal in appearance except that rugae are not present. At this stage the soft tissues may be somewhat humped up from side to side just behind the edge of the bone. The actual lengthening might be said to be the difference between what tissue is used in this humping up and the total distance the edge is set back. This distance may be as much as 2 centimeters, and is the space between the anterior incision to the posterior edge of the bone. Improvement in speech is usually already noted even though the palate is still a little swollen and tender.

A similar type of elongation can be done at a later operation on complete clefts that have been successfully closed, if care is taken to avoid puncturing the nasal mucosa while elevating the hard palate tissues.

REMOVAL OF SALIVARY DUCT STONES

Stones are much more common in the submaxillary gland and duct than in the parotid. They are usually radio-opaque and may be demonstrated on occlusal films in the duct (Fig. 119A) and on lateral jaw films in the gland. Symptoms are obstruction and infection in the gland with pus coming from the orifice of the duct. Stones in the duct may be demonstrated on probing, and can often be palpated.

Tiny stones can often be "milked" out of the duct by bimanually stripping it forward and expressing them out of the orifice. Larger stones are brought to the anterior end of the duct by the same maneuver, and held in this position by an assistant while an incision is made over them and through

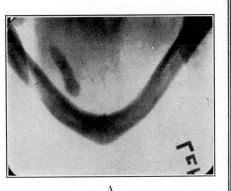

A

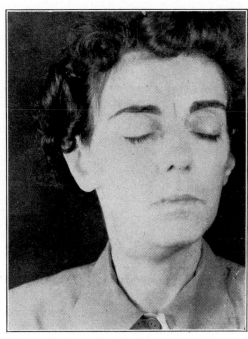

B

Fig. 119. (A) Submaxillary duct stone as seen on occlusal x-ray. (B) Typical suppurative infection of submaxillary gland secondary to stone in duct.

the orifice. As soon as the stone is extracted, the lining of the duct is sutured to the floor of the mouth to create a new and larger opening. A small blunt curet is then inserted through the duct back to the gland and any sand present removed, irrigating the duct as necessary. The patient is instructed to use natural salivary stimulants (citrus fruits, pickles, candy mints, chewing gum, etc.) for a few days to wash the gland out. If there are definite stones in the gland which cannot be expressed, removal of the gland is indicated.

Parotid duct stones can usually be seen on dental films placed between the cheek and upper gum and exposed laterally. Their removal is about the same as above, except that they are small, hard, and often stellate so that they cannot be moved in the duct. A small duct probe is usually inserted in the duct back to the stone, and dissection carried along it until the stone can be extracted. Parotid gland stones are usually small, single ones and the first symptoms may be due to a small local abscess around the stone. This is drained externally and the stone removed at the same time.

SURGICAL TREATMENT OF RANULA

These sublingual cysts are very difficult to eradicate and may tax the patience of everyone concerned (Fig. 120). They may be treated by: (1) the use of a seton; (2) marsupialization; or (3) excision. In any method, it may be advisable to insert probes into one or both submaxillary ducts beforehand to prevent injury to them during the operation.

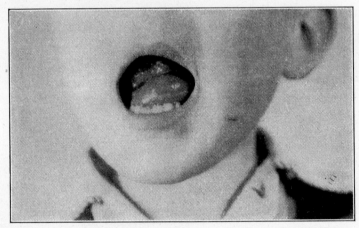

Fig. 120. Ranula. Differentiated from dermoid cyst by thin wall, bluish color and content of clear, yellow, mucilaginous fluid.

The seton is easiest for the surgeon and patient, and will cure many of them, though it may have to be repeated two or three times. After putting probes in the ducts, a piece of No. 24 silver wire on a large cutting needle is passed through the cyst and the ends cut short and twisted into a small loop. It is left in place six to twelve weeks, in order to allow epithelium to grow through the wire holes and create permanent drainage openings. Any recurrence may be treated again in the same manner, or by excision.

In marsupialization, the entire top of the cyst is cut off and the floor of it is sutured to the floor of the mouth all around. This seems like a good plan, but the circular scar created contracts down to a pin-point opening all too frequently.

Surgical excision is difficult because the sac is so thin and friable. It is done under general anesthesia (preferably with a Magill endotracheal tube) and care is taken to avoid injury to the submaxillary ducts or lingual nerve. Most of the wound can be loosely closed, but a small iodoform drain is placed to the most dependent portion. The floor of the mouth and tongue may swell a good deal afterwards, embarrassing swallowing and even breathing for a few days.

Any nodule or ulcer persisting in the vermilion of the lower lip in an adult is probably carcinoma and should be regarded as such until proven otherwise by biopsy or excision. If the lesion is small, it should be removed completely for examination.

Oval excision with the cautery, and sewing a small pack in the wound, is often the quickest and easiest method for small lesions and leaves a surprisingly small scar (Fig. 121). Sharp V-excision can be done, closing the wound in layers when small, and filling the defect with a vermilion-bordered (Abbé) flap when larger.

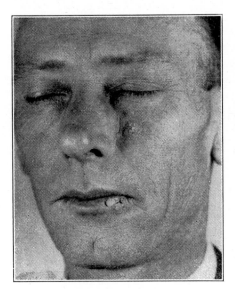 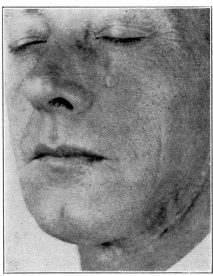

FIG. 121. Carcinoma of lip treated by wide local oval cautery excision and healed by almost invisible scar. Small carcinoma of cheek treated in same manner. Important part of treatment was the bilateral upper neck dissection.

Switching of Vermilion-bordered Lip Flaps. The blood supply through the coronary vessels makes it possible to turn a full thickness flap from one lip to the other on an extremely narrow pedicle. This is principally used for immediate repair of defects from V-excision of lip carcinomas, but may also be used for defects from cancer pastes, nomas, gummas, or other causes.

Lateral defects in the lower lip are filled by a triangle swung directly down from the adjacent upper lip, preserving the coronary vessels in a vermilion pedicle (Fig. 122). The vertical length of the lower lip defect (HF) is measured with a caliper and a flap on the upper lip of the same length is marked out with a pen and 5 per cent methylene blue. The vermilion edge of the upper lip flap should be only about two-thirds as wide as the lower lip defect, as the upper lip will be narrowed by the operation and the purpose of the operation is to restore balance between the lips.

The lines EA and E'A are lightly incised with a No. 15 blade, and then cut completely through the lip with a No. 11 blade, being very careful to avoid cutting the vermilion pedicle and coronary vessels at E. These vessels are usually at the level of the skin-vermilion junction and nearer the inside than the outside of the lip, so that it is safe to cut just through the skin down to the vermilion, but the mucosa should not be cut through down so close to the mouth opening.

The flap is then swung around down into place so that the pedicle forms the new angle of the mouth. The mucosal surface is closed first with inter-

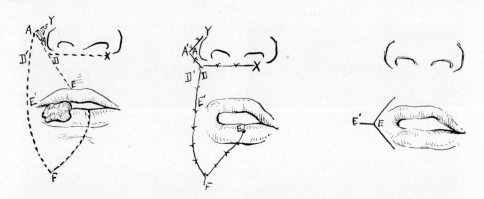

FIG. 122. V-excision of carcinoma in lateral portion of lower lip and closure with vermilion-bordered (Abbé) flap from upper lip. See text for details. (From Brown, *Surg., Gynec. & Obst.,* May 1928. By permission of Surgery, Gynecology and Obstetrics.)

rupted catgut sutures and then the skin with fine, interrupted silk sutures. The upper lip defect is closed by pulling the lip over to the cheek, excising a small triangle at A'AY if there is any tendency to a "dog-ear" at that point. DX shows a relaxation incision that is seldom necessary.

It is sometimes advisable to do a small secondary operation three or four weeks later to further open the new angle of the mouth. This may be done by making the Y opening shown and closing it as a V, or by simply opening the angle of the mouth laterally for a centimeter or so and getting a vermilion covering for the raw edges by swinging small mucosal flaps out from the inside.

Central defects in the lower lip may be closed by the procedure shown in figure 123, closing the original defect by a flap from the lateral side of the lower lip and then closing that defect with a flap from the upper lip. Both flaps can be switched in the same operation.

Curing Patients with Carcinoma of the Lip. Local lesions can be cured by radiation in any approved form, by various cancer pastes, by cautery removal, or by surgical excision. Cautery excision is often the quickest and easiest, as well as the most certain. In any event, the deaths from lip cancer are from the neck metastases, and the management of the cervical lymphatics is the important factor in saving life. Here, as elsewhere, the rule should be to do routine neck dissections (bilateral upper ones, in this instance) with occasional deviations from it when the lesion is low grade, early, and one can follow the patient closely.

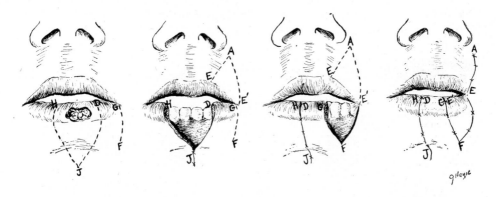

Fig. 123. V-excision of carcinoma in middle of lower lip and plan for closure, utilizing flap from upper lip. See text for details. (From Brown, *Surg., Gynec. & Obst.*, May 1928. By permission of Surgery, Gynecology and Obstetrics.)

TREATMENT OF CARCINOMA OF THE MOUTH

In an adult, an ulcer in the mouth that persists longer than three weeks, or that is indurated, should be considered as carcinoma until proven otherwise by biopsy. The commonest chronic mouth ulcer in syphilitics is carcinoma, not gumma. Vincent's organisms and yeast-like organisms can often be recovered from the surface of mouth cancers, but should not confuse the diagnosis.

Carcinoma of the mouth is usually best treated locally by radiation, unless it has invaded bone, where it becomes insensitive to radiation. Interstitial implantation of radon seed is often the most accurate method for carcinoma of the tongue (Fig. 124), floor of the mouth, buccal mucosa, tonsil, pillars, and soft palate. Seed can be obtained in $\frac{1}{2}$, 1, and $1\frac{1}{2}$ mc. sizes and implanted in a pattern to give fairly uniform radiation throughout the tumor and immediately adjacent tissues, with minimum damage to the face, neck, and other distant structures. The size of the seed used depends upon the probable sensitivity of the tumor (as shown by the gross and microscopic appearance), the thickness of the tumor, and the thickness of the structure being radiated. One millicurie seed are most often used, but they might burn a hole through a lip or soft palate of normal thickness, so that $\frac{1}{2}$ mc. seed are often used in these locations. Very thick tumors in other locations may require $1\frac{1}{2}$ mc. seed to get sufficient depth, or two layers of 1 mc. seed. The seed are so distributed as to provide the equivalent of 150 to 200 mgm. hrs. of radium to each cubic centimeter of tissue being radiated, and a margin of apparently normal tissue of at least 1 centimeter in every direction should be radiated. In computing dosage, 1 millicurie of radon is equivalent to 133 mgm. hrs. of radium. In most mouth cancers, the equivalent of 2000 to 4000 mgm. hrs. of radium is used, depending upon the size and probable sensitivity of the lesion. A lesion that is undertreated once becomes very refractory to radiation and this is important not only in providing a large enough initial total dose, but in getting an initial uniform

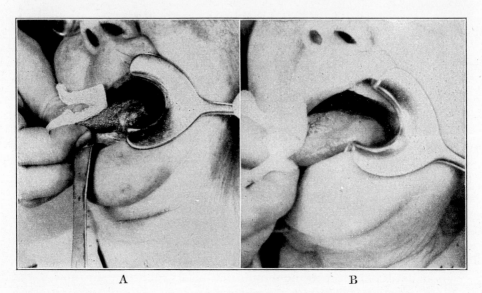

A   B

Fig. 124. (A) Squamous cell carcinoma of tongue in common location on lateral border opposite molar region. (B) Appearance 6 weeks after radon implantation. Area is healed, quite soft and mass has disappeared. The atrophy of the papillae in the area and surrounding mucositis are common early sequelae of radiation. Note extent of area radiated. Neck dissection should also be part of the treatment in nearly all patients with carcinoma of the tongue.

pattern of radiation throughout the area. Considerable experience is required in order to do this.

The small celled squamous carcinomas of the naso-pharynx, hypopharynx, and tonsil areas are often best treated by external X-radiation, or by some combination of methods. In any event, close cooperation between the radiologist and surgeon is necessary in providing the best treatment for patients with carcinoma of the mouth.

Lesions involving bone, such as alveolar carcinomas or carcinomas of the hard palate, usually require either cautery destruction of the involved bone, or wide surgical excision of it (Fig. 125). These are very resistant to radiation, and even if cured, may be followed by a very painful radio-periostitis of the adjacent bone.

The complete treatment of any mouth carcinoma always involves two phases; (1) eradication of the local lesion, and (2) the management of the cervical lymph nodes. Here, again, the rule should be to do routine neck dissections, with occasional deviations away from it, rather than to do just occasional neck dissections.

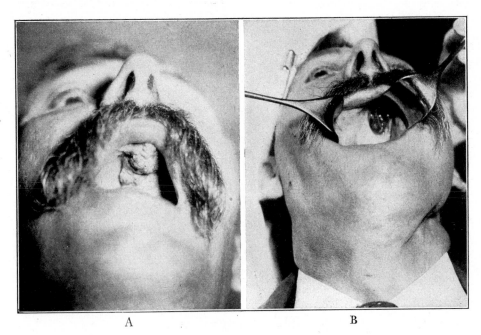

A   B

FIG. 125. (A) Large squamous cell carcinoma of hard palate. (B) Appearance 7 years later following surgical excision of lesion and cautery destruction of edges of defect. Defect left open to permit periodic inspection of the area including the interior of the antrum (these patients can wear dentures with prolongations which fit up into the defect). Note that neck dissection was also done.

TREATMENT OF OSTEOMYELITIS OF THE JAWS

Osteomyelitis of either jaw may be a part of a systemic disease involving multiple bones, but much more commonly originates by spread of a dental infection, particularly an alveolar abscess or pericoronitis.

An alveolar abscess is a pyogenic infection burrowing outward from a tooth root and as such, it is already a localized osteomyelitis. Its onset is characterized by severe, throbbing pain in the area, fever, and swelling of the surrounding soft tissues. Extraction of the tooth in this acute stage is apt to spread the osteomyelitis. The patient should be treated conservatively by chemotherapy, local heat, and analgesics until the abscess first presents on the outside of the gum. The abscess should be opened and a small gauze drain inserted just as soon as it appears, to prevent it from stripping up the surrounding periosteum. After the infection is quiescent, any extractions or necessary dental work may be done to prevent a recurrence of the trouble.

Pericoronitis is a cellulitis of a gum flap over a partially erupted tooth, usually a lower third molar. Extraction of the tooth opens up the underlying bone to the infection and may result in a serious osteomyelitis, if done in the acute stages. This cellulitis should be treated here as elsewhere, by chemotherapy, local heat, and resting the part (limiting chewing and talking). The gum flap may be excised, or the tooth extracted, after the infection has subsided.

Osteomyelitis is much more common in the mandible than in the maxilla, and the majority of cases follow local instrumentation in the presence of one of the above acute infections. The onset is accompanied by chills, high fever, prostration, and severe throbbing pain in the area. Trismus rapidly develops from spasm of the closing muscles. Initial treatment consists of chemotherapy, local heat, resting the part, and general supportive measures such as oxygen, parenteral fluids, and blood transfusions when necessary. Pain may be relieved somewhat by codeine, but morphine or other respiratory depressants should be avoided if the swelling is encroaching on the airways. A local soft tissue abscess will usually be ready for drainage on about the fourth day. The decision in regard to this is reached in reference to localization of the swelling as the area may remain hard and not become fluctuant. Drainage should always be dependent, through the upper neck (see section on drainage of jaw abscesses).

During the initial weeks, the sole surgery should consist of adequate drainage of all soft tissue abscesses. X-ray films are made at intervals, and when definite sequestrae have loosened, with enough surrounding involucrum to support the jaw, they are removed. Chisels, rongeurs, or other bone-cutting instruments should not be used on these jaws. Loose teeth are left in place, unless they are ready to fall out, as it is surprising how many of them will tighten up later and function well.

REMOVAL OF CYSTS AND TUMORS OF THE JAWS

A smooth, rounded, radiolucent area in the jaw may be either a cyst or tumor and at times, it is impossible to make a positive preoperative diagnosis. Multilocular areas in the posterior part of the body or in the ramus of the mandible are usually adamantinomas, but may be giant cell tumors. Cystic areas surrounding retained tooth root fragments are usually simple epithelial cysts, requiring only removal of the bony roof for exposure and shelling out with a small, sharp, periosteal elevator. Cysts surrounding a vestigial, unerupted tooth are usually dentigerous cysts, requiring the same treatment. Multiple cysts are apt to be on the basis of hyperparathyroidism and require removal of the parathyroid adenoma, in addition to local removal or curettage of the cysts.

The typical *adamantinoma* near the angle of the jaw can be exposed inside the mouth (Figs. 126 and 127), by splitting the overlying soft tissues and separating them to either side with an elevator, and removing the bony roof with chisels and rongeurs. If it is an adamantinoma, the tumor will be mostly cystic, filled with a clear, light yellow, thin fluid that contains cholesterin crystals that sparkle in the light. It is essential to remove all of these tumors with a small sharp periosteal elevator, preferably in one piece, and thoroughly curet the remaining cavity. If it is thought that any tumor cells may be left, the cavity may be painted with pure phenol, and then

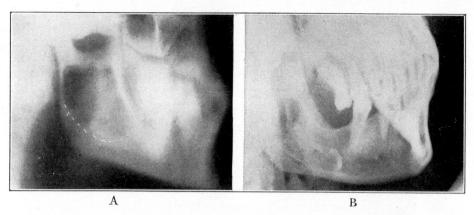

A   B

FIG. 126. (A) Initial laminagram of adamantinoma of ramus. (B) Appearance of ordinary lateral x-ray one year later following removal from the inside of the mouth. Area has healed in with new bone.

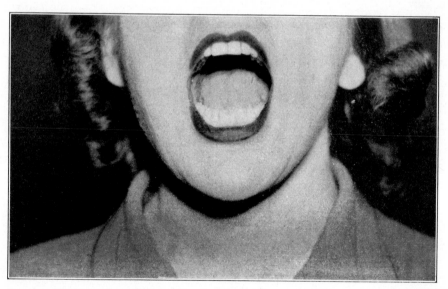

FIG. 127. Postoperative photographs of patient whose x-rays were shown in Figure 126. No external scars and continuity of jaw and occlusion maintained. Mouth opening normal.

alcohol, or may be cauterized with the surgical diathermy. It is then packed open with iodoform gauze soaked in balsam of Peru, and this packing is changed every few days until the cavity has been obliterated by granulations. If the adamantinoma has eroded through bone and extends into the adjacent soft tissues, a block resection of the involved portion of the jaw and surrounding soft tissues should be done instead.

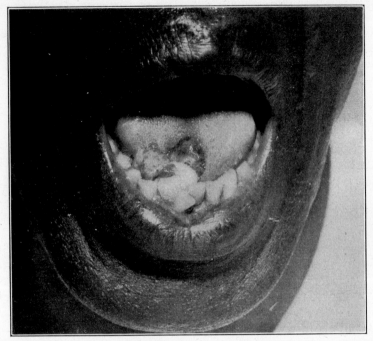

FIG. 128. Fairly typical epulis of lower jaw. This one contained a good many blood vessels and giant cells. Removal of involved teeth along with the tumor necessary.

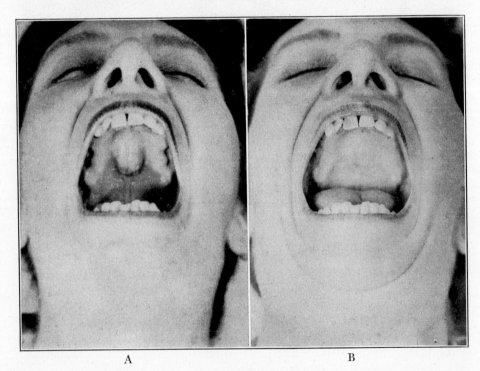

A

B

FIG. 129. Preoperative and postoperative views of a torus palatinus.

Giant cell tumors are exposed and treated in the same manner as adamantinomas, except that they are more easily cured and they may be associated with hyperparathyroidism in some instances. When first exposed, they are composed of a reddish, gelatinous material that has been described as resembling currant jelly.

One of the common tumors of the mouth is the *epulis* (Fig. 128), which is a benign fibro-hemangioma which may or may not contain giant cells.

It arises from around the neck of a tooth, or retained root fragment, and is pedunculated at that point. If composed predominantly of fibrous tissue, it will be hard and white, but if it is mostly angioma, it may be soft and spongy and either red or blue in color. Treatment consists of excision, together with removal of the offending tooth or root fragment, and cautery destruction of the peridental membrane in the socket.

Cysts of the hard palate are unilateral, occurring just behind the incisor teeth and extending from the midline, laterally over to the gum. Because they occur in the region of the incisive foramen, they are often called incisive canal cysts, but they sometimes expand upward into the floor of the nose and are then known as nasopalatine cysts. Most of them are best removed through the mouth under general (endotracheal) anesthesia.

An incision is made just inside the teeth all the way around, and the mucoperiosteal layer of the hard palate is reflected backward as

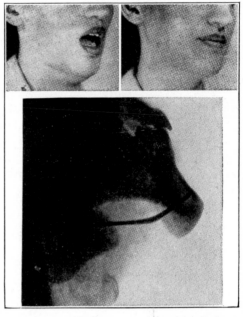

Fig. 130. Postoperative photographs and x-ray of patient who had an osteogenic sarcoma of the mandible resected 3 years ago. Continuity of jaw maintained by means of internal steel pin bridging the fragments. This can be replaced later with a bone graft, if necessary. (From Byars and McDowell, *Surg., Gynec. & Obst.*, 84:870-877, 1947. By permission of Surgery, Gynecology and Obstetrics.)

a flap, separating it with a small, sharp, periosteal elevator. The thin bone overlying the cyst is removed with a small rongeur and the cyst is then enucleated with small palate and nasal elevators, preferably in one piece and without piercing the floor of the nasal airway. The palate flap is then sutured back down in place, with a small gauze wick drain brought out between the stitches. The drain is removed in two or three days and the sutures in two to three weeks. Postoperative care is same as for cleft palate repair.

Torus palatinus is a benign exostosis occurring in the midline of the hard palate in middle aged or elderly people (Fig. 129). It usually has a groove in the middle, coinciding with the bony suture line. It is of importance only when it becomes irritated mechanically, or by hot foods, or interferes with wearing a denture. In removing it, all possible mucosa is elevated off the bone in two lateral flaps and saved. The exostosis is then chiseled off, taking care to avoid penetration into the nose, and the mucosal flaps sutured back in place.

Any bone tumor can occur in the jaws and the more unusual ones require approximately the same treatment as elsewhere in the body—simple excision for the benign tumors, and radical excision, radiation, or both for the malignant tumors (Fig. 130).

NECK OPERATIONS

General Considerations. Unless otherwise noted in the following descriptions, the operations in this area are preferably performed under general endotracheal anesthesia in adults and older children with a Magill tube brought out of the nostril and its connections over the forehead so as to be out of the way. Pharyngeal insufflation can be used in small children. In either event, it is important to have an anesthetist who knows when the patient is breathing *without effort,* and who knows what to do to secure free and easy exchange with the patient's head in an overextended position. A falling blood pressure before the operation is well started usually means that the tube is in a bronchus rather than the trachea, or that there is partial obstruction of the airway someplace between the coryna and the machine. Local anesthesia, with suitable combinations of deep third division trigeminal block, deep cervical blocks, and subcutaneous infiltration under the incision, can be used when general anesthetics are not desirable, but they are often more difficult for both the surgeon and the patient.

Pressure dressings are used after most neck operations to keep down edema, prevent serum accumulations and subsequent infections, and thus secure smoother healing. After covering any suture lines or raw areas with fine mesh grease gauze, mechanic's waste is fluffed about the neck and wrapped on with a gauze roll, making one turn around the neck, one around the forehead, and one under the chin and over the top of the head which passes in front of both ears. A final bandage may be wrapped snugly outside of this, but care must be taken to have sufficient padding over the larynx and trachea and to avoid any constricting bands of gauze in this area. The patient is checked before he leaves the operating room to see that his respirations are free and easy, and a suction machine is provided at the bedside to keep the throat clear of secretions. All participating in the postoperative care should be familiar with the signs of partial airway obstruction in this area. These are: (1) undue restlessness; (2) increasing pulse rate; (3) intercostal and suprasternal retraction; and (4) cyanosis is almost a terminal sign.

A small dose of morphine may be used as a preanesthetic drug ($1/4$ gr. doses are *not* desirable). No morphine, or other respiratory depressants, should be used in the immediate postoperative period.

Neck surgery presents many hazards because of the intimate relationship of many small, but important, structures in this area. It should be undertaken only by one who is a well trained surgeon and who, in addition, is so familiar with the minute anatomy of the neck that he can recognize all structures presenting through an incision made anyplace in the neck.

Two of the greatest safety factors in neck surgery are: (1) incisions large enough for adequate exposure, and (2) complete hemostasis at all times. This is no place for operating in a small, deep, bloody hole.

Excision of the Submaxillary Salivary Gland. INDICATIONS. Removal may be required because of tumor or stones. There are lymph nodes within the capsule of the gland so that tumors should be investigated to determine whether they might be primary lymphatic neoplasms, metastases from mouth or lip carcinomas, or primary salivary gland tumors. Of the latter, the most common are the mixed tumors and in the submaxillary gland about three-fourths of these are malignant and one-fourth benign. Malignant mixed tumors require an associated neck dissection. Malignancy can sometimes be determined preoperatively by fixation to the mandible or other contiguous structures, or by the presence of enlarged nodes in the lymphatic chain below and posteriorly. If it is thought that the lesion is a benign mixed tumor, this should be checked by frozen microscopic sections before the operative incision is closed.

Stones are usually visible on occlusal or lateral jaw x-ray films. Removal of the gland is indicated only if the stones are in the gland proper and it is thought that they cannot be extracted through the duct.

The gland can be excised through the neck, or through the floor of the mouth, but the latter may be dangerous because of difficulty in controlling bleeding from the facial artery and vein.

OPERATION. An incision is made parallel to the body of the mandible, and about two-thirds of the way down from the mandible to the hyoid bone (Fig. 131). About 3 inches is the proper length for the incision in an adult. It is carried through the skin, fat, and platysma muscle, and these three structures are raised as a flap upward to expose the gland. (The inframandibular branch of the facial nerve runs within the platysma about 1 inch below the mandible, so that it is important to raise all of this muscle in the flap to protect the nerve.) The lower end of the gland usually hangs down superficially over the digastric tendon and can be readily identified at this point. The facial vein is readily visible coming down over the gland and is divided and ligated at the lower border (Fig. 132). The areolar tissue in the fossa posterior to the gland and above the posterior border of the digastric muscle is then dissected by spreading with scissors and the tortuous facial artery is identified here, divided and ligated firmly. The lower pole of the gland is then picked up with a Jacobs or Allis forceps and rotated up out of the neck as the areolar tissue deep to the gland is divided by gauze dissection or spreading with scissors. The twelfth nerve can be identified running horizontally on the surface of the mylohyoid muscle just above the digastric tendon and it is followed anteriorly until it disappears through the hiatus in the mylohyoid. The areolar tissue and fat is cleaned out of this hiatus and it will then be seen to contain three structures. From below upward they are: (1) the twelfth nerve; (2) Wharton's duct surrounded by the sublingual gland; and (3) the lingual nerve (Fig. 133). The duct is ligated and divided as far anteriorly as possible and the lingual nerve is traced posteriorly along the superior edge of the gland. The chorda tympani branch from the lingual nerve to the gland will be found about midway along this edge and it is divided, allowing complete removal of the gland. The hemostasis is made complete, the fossa irrigated out with saline solution, a small rubber tissue drain placed from the fossa down out the middle of the incision, and the

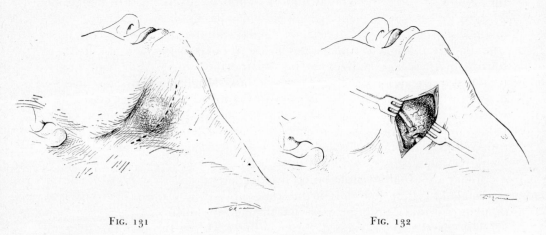

FIG. 131   FIG. 132

FIG. 131. Dotted line shows line of external incision for removal of submaxillary salivary gland.

FIG. 132. The facial vein is ligated and divided and the gland dissected out.

latter closed. Subcuticular interrupted ooo white silk sutures can be used for the main closure, with a number of tiny interrupted ooo black silk sutures for the skin, and a pressure dressing is applied. The patient is usually out of bed the next day and the first dressing is done about the fifth day, when the drain and skin sutures are removed.

Thyroglossal Duct Cysts. INDICATIONS. The presence of such a cyst or sinus is indication for its removal, though this may be postponed in young babies until they are one or two years of age. Numerous attempts have been made to obliterate these with caustics and cauteries, but complete surgical excision clear up to the foramen cecum is the method of choice. Most midline tumors in the hyoid region are thyroglossal cysts, but occasionally one sees midline dermoids (without a stalk), abscesses from lower incisor teeth (often in diabetics), or submental lymph nodes enlarged by metastatic carcinoma or tuberculosis, in this area.

OPERATION. If the cyst is acutely infected, it is drained, and removed after the infection is relatively quiescent.

When there is an opening through the skin, it may be injected with methylene blue, or a probe inserted through it on up into the mouth, or both, for purposes of identification during the excision. If the skin is freely movable over the cyst, a horizontal incision is made over the hyoid about 2 inches in length (Fig. 134). Otherwise, any area of skin attachment is surrounded by an elliptical incision, extended at either end to the desired length. If it has not been possible to insert a probe (a oo lachrymal probe is a good one) before, the cyst is carefully dissected out, opened, evacuated with

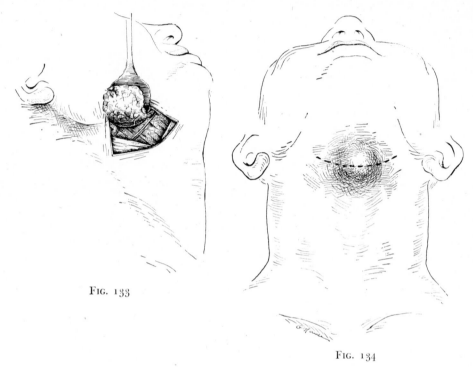

FIG. 133

FIG. 134

FIG. 133. Gland dissected out and rotated upward on to the cheek. To remove it, it is necessary to divide the facial artery (in the upper posterior angle of the wound), the duct (between the twelfth and lingual nerves in the mylohyoid hiatus), and the chorda tympani (small nerve branch to the gland from the lingual nerve).

FIG. 134. Dotted line shows external incision for removal of thyroglossal duct cyst.

a sucker, and a probe inserted through the sinus on up to the mouth. The inside of the sac is also carefully examined for the opening of any sinus track going down towards the thyroid, and a probe inserted in it, if found. A mosquito forceps is clamped on the sac and this forcep and the probe held in the left hand while the dissection is carried out with the right hand. The sinus is dissected down to the center of the hyoid bone (Fig. 135), watching carefully for any solid strand or hollow sinus of thyroid tissue extending down to the pyramidal lobe of the thyroid. Any such lower prolongation is removed, of course, and when present there may be other small cysts or aberrant bits of thyroid tissue on either side of it which should be included.

When the hyoid is reached, the periosteum is cleaned from either side of the midline with a sharp elevator and the relationship of the sinus to the hyoid determined. The sinus often passes through the upper portion of the bone in the midline, but may only be adherent to the upper surface, or may pass through the bone at a lower level. In the first instance, a small V of bone surrounding the sinus may be cut out with a sharp bone cutter, leaving a small bridge below. In the second, the sinus can be elevated out

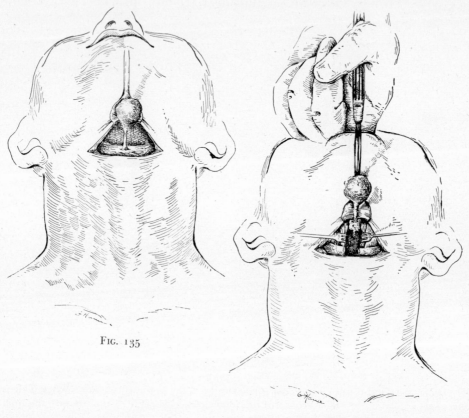

FIG. 135.

FIG. 136.

FIG. 135. The cyst, and its stalk or duct, is dissected down to the center of the hyoid bone.

FIG. 136. When the sinus passes through the center of the hyoid bone, it is necessary to resect the central block of bone surrounding it and remove it with the specimen. Dissection is then carried on up between the mylohyoid and geniohyoid muscles to the foramen cecum at the base of the tongue.

of the central groove with a small sharp periosteal elevator (the Joseph nasal elevator is useful for this). When it passes through the center of the bone, it is necessary to cut completely through the hyoid on either side and remove the central segment with the specimen (Fig. 136) (the periosteum of the two hyoid fragments can be united with a few sutures at the end of the operation).

Above the hyoid, a few mylohyoid fibers can be divided transversely for better exposure, and the geniohyoid muscles are separated with blunt retractors as the sinus is followed up between them. At this point, the surgeon hands over the specimen, mosquito clamp, and probe to an assistant, and inserts his own left index finger into the mouth on back to the foramen cecum. With his right hand, he continues the dissection on up until he can see his gloved left index finger through the oral mucosa. The sinus is removed by cutting a small buttonhole in the mucosa at this point and it is not necessary to suture it. A small rubber tissue drain is placed up to within 1

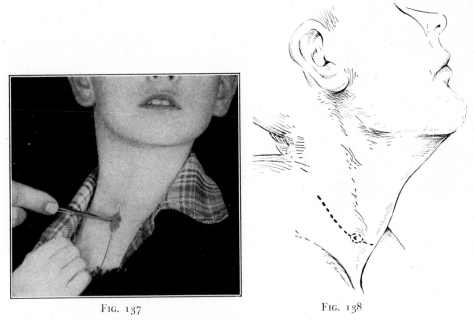

FIG. 137   FIG. 138

FIG. 137. One end of a double-ended probe is inserted into a lateral cervical fistula to show its size, location, and direction.

FIG. 138. The external incision for removal of a lateral cervical fistula surrounds a small button of skin at the orifice.

centimeter of the oral mucosa and brought out the middle of the incision. The skin and subcutaneous fat are approximated with fine, interrupted silk sutures and a pressure dressing applied. If the hyoid bone was completely divided, the patient may have trouble swallowing for two or three days postoperatively, and a stomach tube for feeding may be necessary for this period.

Lateral Cervical Fistulae. These are long epithelial tubes of tiny diameter, vertically placed, with the lower opening in the skin of the neck at the anterior border of the sternomastoid muscle about 1 inch above the clavicle (Fig. 137), and the upper opening in the oral mucosa in the general region of the palatine tonsil on the same side. They are present at birth and drain a thin, glairy fluid in small amounts unless they become infected. In each instance, it is important to remove the entire tube clear up to the oral mucosa, or there will be recurrent trouble. For this reason, it is often best to postpone the removal until three or four years of age when the work can be done under endotracheal anesthesia with greater safety and facility.

OPERATION. A small probe is introduced into the external opening and passed through the fistula up into the mouth. The external opening is surrounded by a tiny, horizontal, elliptical incision which is then prolonged forward and backward in one of the natural creases until it is about 2 inches in length (Fig. 138). The upper flap is undermined and retracted up to get

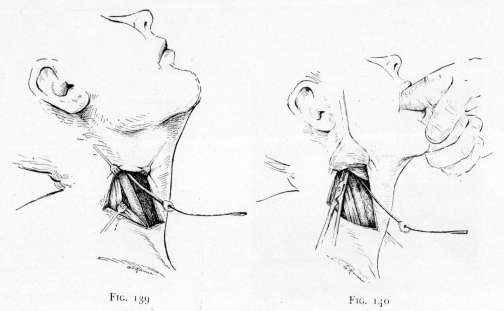

FIG. 139   FIG. 140

FIG. 139. Showing dissection of fistula up to the hyoid level. Sternomastoid muscle retracted laterally and fistula carefully separated from great vessels.

FIG. 140. Index finger inserted into mouth and placed against tip of probe as dissection is carried up underneath the digastric muscle and mandible to the oral mucosa. (In practice, a right handed surgeon would prefer to put his *left* index finger into the mouth.)

exposure and the fistula is then dissected out. It will be found to be almost subcutaneous nearly up to the hyoid level, where it goes in deep near the great vessels and up under the posterior belly of the digastric muscle (Fig. 139). This latter muscle belly is retracted upward and superficially, and the fistula is followed upward behind the submaxillary gland and inside the mandible. Occasionally, it is necessary to make a second horizontal skin incision in the upper neck for adequate exposure at this stage. Care is taken to avoid injury to the carotid, jugular, and facial vessels, as well as the important nerves in the area. At this time, the surgeon's left index finger is inserted into the mouth and placed against the tip of the probe in the tonsillar fossa (Fig. 140). The dissection is carried on upward until the gloved finger can be seen shining through the thin oral mucosa. A disc of this mucosa is then removed with the specimen. The oral mucosa is not sutured, but a small rubber dam drain is placed up to within 1 or 2 centimeters of this opening and brought down and out the middle of the skin incision in the neck. The skin incision is closed with fine ooo white silk subcutaneous sutures and ooo black silk sutures down to the drain, and a pressure dressing is applied. The drain and skin sutures are removed about the fifth day.

Branchial Cleft Cysts. There are two clinical varieties, the first branchial cleft cyst, and the lower branchial cleft cyst (Fig. 141), (the latter term is used to avoid any embryological discussion here as to its exact mode of origin). If infected, either one should be drained first and excised when

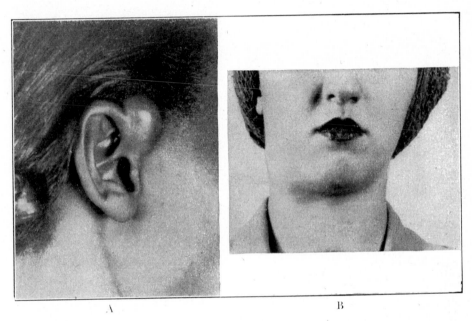

FIG. 141. (A) First branchial cleft cyst. (B) Lower branchial cleft cyst.

quiescent. The first branchial cleft cyst is a soft, subcutaneous mass, usually about 2 to 3 cc. in bulk, situated just in front of the top of the ear and just below the hair of the temple. It is associated with a skin pit or opening in the crus of the helix. Usually, a fine probe can be introduced into this opening and passed forward into the cyst. To remove it, a small elliptical incision is made around the opening and extended horizontally forward over the cyst. The cyst and its external sinus are then carefully dissected out, using the same care in separating it from the parotid as is used in removing any other small, superficial parotid tumor (see excision of parotid tumors). One must especially watch for the branches of the facial nerve to the forehead and upper eyelid. Occasionally, there are deeper sinuses extending downward and forward from the cyst into the substance of the parotid and it may be necessary to open the cyst and pass probes down into these to follow them out.

The lower branchial cleft cysts are often about 20 cc. in bulk and are in the carotid sheath (deep to the sterno-mastoid muscle) at about the level of the hyoid bone. They are usually fairly hard, spherical, and can be moved easily under the muscle and over underlying structures unless they have been infected previously. They are usually first seen between the ages of twenty and thirty years and are not associated with any masses elsewhere in the neck or mouth. A complete general examination of the patient is in order preoperatively, but even so, it may be impossible in some instances to dif-

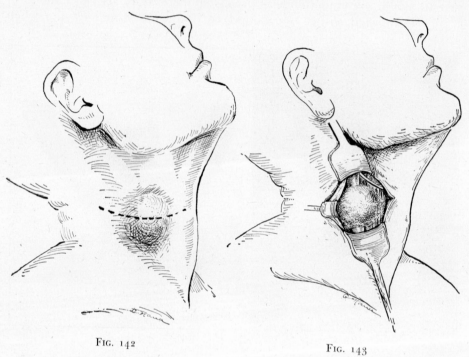

Fig. 142   Fig. 143

FIG. 142. Skin incision for removal of lower branchial cleft cyst.
FIG. 143. Sternomastoid muscle retracted posteriorly to expose the cyst. The cyst is then carefully dissected free from the great vessels and care is taken to avoid injury to the twelfth nerve which is usually just above it, or sometimes subjacent to it. The great vessels should be identified both above and below the cyst before its removal.

ferentiate them from neurofibromas or enlarged lymph nodes (primary lymphatic tumors or lymph node metastases). For this reason, the surgeon should be prepared to have frozen sections made and to do more extensive surgery if indicated after gross or microscopic examination of the mass.

OPERATION FOR REMOVAL OF LOWER BRANCHIAL CLEFT CYST. An incision about 2 inches long is made transversely over the tumor (Fig. 142), (this incision can be made part of the upper horizontal limb of a complete neck dissection incision later if necessary). This is carried down through the fat and platysma muscle to expose the sternomastoid muscle in the posterior half of the wound. The anterior edge of this muscle is lifted up and dissected free from the outer surface of the cyst until the muscle can be retracted posteriorly to expose the entire cyst. The carotid and jugular vessels and the vagus nerve are dissected out and identified below and above the cyst and one watches for possible exposure of the twelfth nerve above (Fig. 143). Following this, the cyst can often be gently enucleated with the finger, watching carefully for any possible stalk connections with the pharynx (after removal, one can squeeze on the cyst to see if there are any leaks). If the cyst has been infected, it may be necessary to split the sheath around the vessels and carefully remove it by sharp dissection to get the cyst loose. On examination, the cyst has a fairly tough, thick wall, is lined with definite epithelium which is often thrown up into wrinkles and folds, and is filled with a thick white, foul smelling, liquid or paste. Hair or other epithelial structures may be present. The skin incision is closed with deep white and surface black fine silk sutures around a small rubber tissue drain and a pressure dressing applied.

Hygromas. Hygromas are cavernous lymphangiomas of the neck and are usually first seen in infancy. They are large, soft, doughy tumors on the side of the neck which may occupy the submaxillary triangle (in which case they also present under the oral mucosa and push the tongue up) or may be in the supraclavicular fossa (where they may extend down under the clavicle into the axilla or mediastinum) or in both locations. Some consist of a few large locules; others consist of hundreds of locules, varying in size from that of tapioca to grapes. The locules have walls almost as thin as tissue paper, are lined with a single layer of endothelium, and are filled with a clear, thin, straw colored fluid. When first exposed at operation, they are bluish in color. Occasionally, they may have blood leaks into them.

The excision of a hygroma may become one of the most formidable operations in surgery and should never be lightly undertaken. Removal, or obliteration, can not be postponed indefinitely, however, because of the frequent appearance of secondary infections, or respiratory embarrassment. If the child can be observed closely, it is often wise, though, to postpone operation until six or eight months or even one year of age.

Sudden, large increases in size are usually due to a blood leak into the tumor, or to infection. In such an instance, it may be advisable to insert a large aspirating needle into the mass, and evacuate it, particularly if it is causing breathing or feeding troubles. If the fluid is bloody, about 3 cc. of 5 per cent sodium morrhuate solution can be injected (this will often seal the leak temporarily). If the fluid is pus, the needle opening can be enlarged with a knife, and a drain inserted, as well as starting general chemotherapy, etc.

OPERATION. The incision varies with the size and location of the tumor, but should be started over the largest mass. If the mass involves the entire neck, it may be necessary to extend the incision until it is exactly like one for a complete neck dissection, so this should be kept in mind. If it involves only the upper or lower half of the neck, the work can usually be done through a transverse incision.

The opening is carried down to the surface of the cysts and undermining done in all directions in this plane. The cysts are about like sacs of tissue paper full of fluid, so that great care must be taken to avoid rupturing them. After exposing a considerable area of the tumor, a decision is made as to the mode of treatment. If it consists of relatively few, but very large locules, it may be best to open one of them and then with the index finger as a dissector, convert them all into one large cavity. This cavity may be packed lightly with a long strip of 2 inch iodoform gauze (about four layers thick) wrung out of 5 per cent sodium morrhuate solution (Fig. 144). The gauze

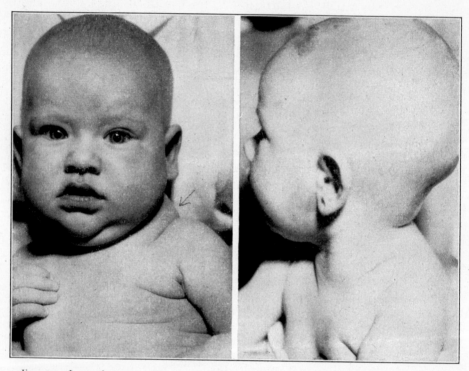

FIG. 144. Large hygroma. On surgical exposure, it was found to consist of only 3 or 4 large locules. These were converted into one cavity and the latter was packed open with 5 per cent sodium morrhuate on gauze. Result shown 2 months later.

is brought out of the center of the wound as a drain and is removed the first time on the fifth to seventh day. It is replaced with plain iodoform gauze (without sodium morrhuate) which is changed every two or three days after that until the cavity is obliterated. An external pressure dressing throughout this period of packing may help in obliterating the sacs. Recurrences happen occasionally due to the fact that all of the endothelium may not have been destroyed and are dealt with in the same manner, by opening them and repacking. It may be better to have to repeat this process two or three times than to carry out the extensive dissection necessary for complete removal.

When the mass consists of hundreds of tiny locules, the above plan is not feasible and one must proceed with complete excision of all of them. An accurate knowledge of the entire anatomy of the neck is essential, as the dissection may extend from the floor of the mouth to below the clavicle, in, around, and between the vessels and nerves in the carotid sheath and brachial plexus regions. A blood transfusion may well be necessary during the operation. The wound is closed and cared for afterward in the same manner as for a complete neck dissection. Any recurrences can be treated by surgical excision, or sodium morrhuate packing, whichever seems best when they are exposed.

It is hoped that the above is not too discouraging a picture, as these cysts can be removed or obliterated in practically all patients by the procedures outlined. Nevertheless, a good deal of work is necessary and the possibility of secondary operations should always be considered beforehand with the parents.

Biopsy of Cervical Lymph Nodes. The removal of a cervical lymph node for biopsy is not always a simple operation and should only be done by a fairly experienced surgeon in an operating room set up to deal with the contingencies that may be encountered. A careful preliminary examination is necessary, especially of the mouth, nasopharynx, hypopharynx, and larynx, to rule out the possibility

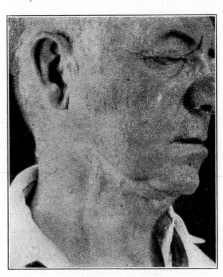

FIG. 145. Complete unilateral dissection for huge coal-black lymph nodes containing metastatic melanoma (original lesion on temple). Patient remains well after 13 years. (From Brown and McDowell, *Ann. Surg.*, 119:543-555, 1944.)

of the node containing metastatic carcinoma for which a neck dissection should be done rather than a biopsy.

A horizontal incision is made over the node, being sure that it is of adequate length to expose surrounding structures. The node is dissected out, taking time to maintain complete hemostasis and to recognize and safeguard other important structures. Never work in a small bloody hole in the neck.

Complete Neck Dissection. Neck dissection is practically the only curative measure for patients with metastatic carcinoma of the cervical lymph nodes and should be employed when the local lesion is controlled or is probably controllable (Figs. 145, 146 and 147). It is not used for tuberculosis of the cervical lymph nodes, as this lesion responds better to radiation. Localized neck lymphomas may be treated by a combination of dissection and radiation.

Complete unilateral dissection from the clavicle to the base of the skull, with removal of the sternomastoid muscle, jugular vein, and carotid fascia, is done when the nodes are limited to one side, as they are apt to be in carcinoma of the tongue, cheek, jaw, tonsil, palate, or floor of the mouth on one side. Bilateral upper dissection is done when metastases are apt to be present in both submaxillary triangles, as in carcinoma of the lip, or anterior floor of the mouth.

For complete unilateral dissection, an incision is made from the mastoid to the opposite point of the chin, passing about 3 cm. below the angle of the

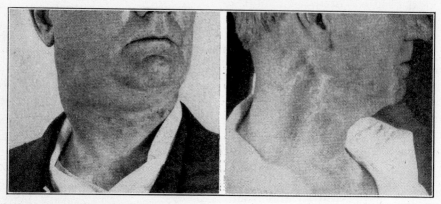

Fig. 146. Complete neck dissection for huge mass of squamous carcinoma in lymph nodes which surrounded the carotid vessels and necessitated resection of the common, external, and internal carotid arteries. Primary lesion has never been found (unless it is primary in the neck), but patient has remained well for 7 years. (From Brown and McDowell, *Ann. Surg.*, 119:543-555, 1944.)

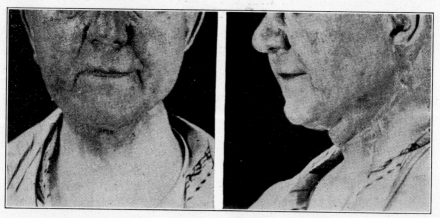

Fig. 147. Bilateral complete dissections in patient with carcinoma of tongue. Dissection done on same side when tongue was treated and crossed metastases became apparent about one year later, necessitating dissection of opposite side. Well 9 years. (From Brown and McDowell, *Ann. Surg.*, 119:543-555, 1944.)

jaw. From the middle of this incision, a vertical incision is made downward to a little below the clavicle, approximately transecting the clavicular insertion of the sternomastoid muscle (Fig. 148). The skin flaps are raised quite thin; the upper one to the upper border of the body of the mandible, the posterior one back to the trapezius muscle, and the anterior one to the ribbon muscles below the hyoid and just past the midline above the hyoid.

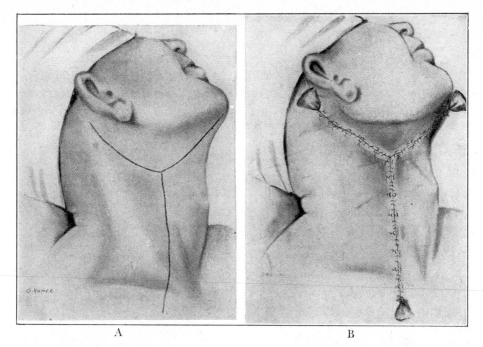

Fig. 148. (A) Original incisions for complete neck dissection. (B) Method of closing wounds and placing drains at conclusion of operation. (From Brown and McDowell, *Surg., Gynec. & Obst.*, 79:115-124, 1944. By permission of Surgery, Gynecology and Obstetrics.)

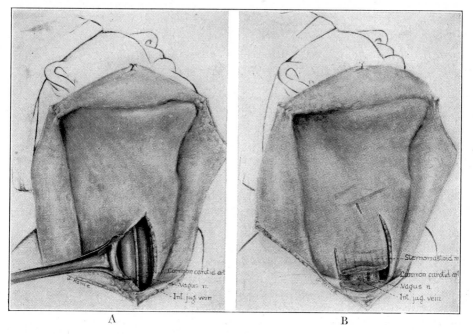

Fig. 149. (A) Skin flaps reflected back and great vessels and vagus nerve exposed through vertical incision at anterior border of sternomastoid muscle. (B) Sternomastoid muscle cut loose at lower end. (From Brown, J. B. and McDowell, F., *Surg., Gynec. & Obst.*, 79:115-124, 1944. By permission of Surgery, Gynecology and Obstetrics.)

The flaps are fastened back to expose the entire side of the neck and complete hemostasis is secured.

A vertical opening is then made at the anterior border of the sternomastoid muscle near the clavicle, and the jugular vein, carotid artery, and vagus nerve are separately identified beneath the muscle (Fig. 149A). The muscle is then cut loose from the sternum and clavicle and the end retracted

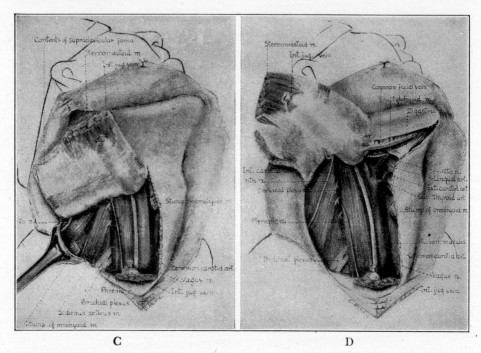

C   D

Fig. 149. (Continued) (C) Internal jugular vein divided, supraclavicular fossa dissected out, and dissection carried upward on surface of scaleni muscles. (D) Showing upward progression of the dissection to level of the hyoid and forward opening over digastric muscle. (From Brown, J. B. and McDowell, F., *Surg., Gynec. & Obst.,* 79:115-124, 1944. By permission of Surgery, Gynecology and Obstetrics.)

upward (Fig. 149B). The internal jugular vein is separated, quadruply ligated just above the clavicle, and divided between the middle ligatures. The end of the vein is retracted upward with the muscle, and the fascia surrounding the carotid artery and vagus nerve is divided and stripped upward as the dissection progresses. The supraclavicular fat is divided transversely just above the clavicle down to the scaleni muscles and back to the trapezius.

The dissection is then carried steadily upward on the surface of these muscles and the ribbon muscles, stripping the carotid artery and vagus nerve and avoiding injury to the phrenic nerve, to the level of the hyoid. (Fig. 149C and D).

A separate incision is then made horizontally just above the hyoid and just below the submaxillary gland. The tendon of the digastric muscle is identified, with the subjacent twelfth nerve (Fig. 149D). The posterior belly and stylohyoid muscle are then divided from the hyoid bone and this incision is extended laterally and down to connect with the previous one at the carotid sheath (Fig. 150A).

The subcutaneous fat is cut through down to the underlying muscles posteriorly up to the mastoid and anteriorly up to the opposite point of the chin. The submaxillary gland is rotated upward out of its fossa and freed by

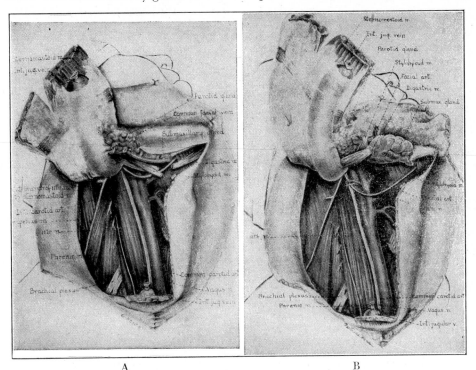

A   B

FIG. 150. (A) Posterior belly of digastric and stylohyoid muscle cut loose from hyoid bone. Eleventh nerve branch to sternomastoid cut. (B) Facial and occipital arteries and facial vein divided and submaxillary gland rotated up out of fossa. (From Brown, J. B. and McDowell, F., *Surg., Gynec. & Obst.,* 79:115-124, 1944. By permission of Surgery, Gynecology and Obstetrics.)

dividing the facial artery at its posterior border, the chorda tympani attachment to the lingual nerve at its upper border, and Wharton's duct at its anterior border (Fig. 150B and C).

The block dissection is carried on upward at the same level posteriorly as before, and on the surface of the mylohyoid muscle and mandible, anteriorly, until the upper limits of the block are reached at the upper border of the jaw and tip of the mastoid.

The jugular bulb is identified up near the base of the skull in front of the styloid process, doubly ligated, and divided below the ligatures. The upper end of the sternomastoid muscle and digastric muscle are cut loose from the mastoid, the lower third of the parotid gland is transected, and the remainder of the block is cut loose at the level of the upper border of the body of the mandible, tying the facial artery and vein on the cheek (Fig. 150D).

The entire wound is washed out with saline, the skin flaps replaced and carefully closed, bringing 1 inch drains out the anterior, posterior, and inferior incision ends (Fig. 148B). A large pressure dressing is applied. The patient's respirations are checked after the endotracheal tube is removed

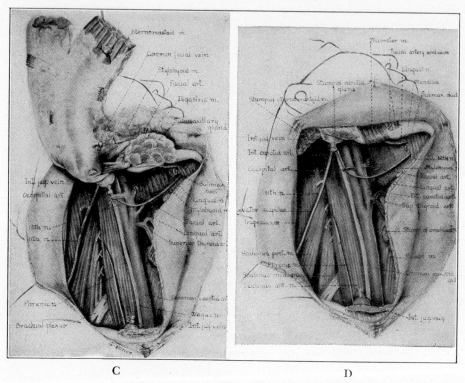

C   D

FIG. 150. (Continued) (C) submaxillary duct and chorda tympani cut. Jugular bulb ligated high and divided. (D) Sternomastoid and digastric muscles cut loose from mastoid; stylohyoid from styloid; lower pole of parotid transected; remaining tissues divided at level of upper border of mandible to remove the entire specimen in one piece. (From Brown, J. B. and McDowell, F., *Surg., Gynec. & Obst.*, 79:115-124, 1944. By permission of Surgery, Gynecology and Obstetrics.)

and he is given no morphine or other strong respiratory depressants during the early postoperative course. Patients are usually out of bed on the following day, drains removed the seventh day, sutures out and discharged from the hospital on the tenth day. It is important to maintain a good pressure dressing on the flaps, though, for the first seven to ten days, changing it as often as necessary to keep it secure.

Bilateral Upper Neck Dissections. An incision is made from one mastoid to the other, crossing the midline just above the hyoid, and the upper skin flap is raised quite thin up to the upper border of the body of the mandible and fastened up to expose the entire upper neck.

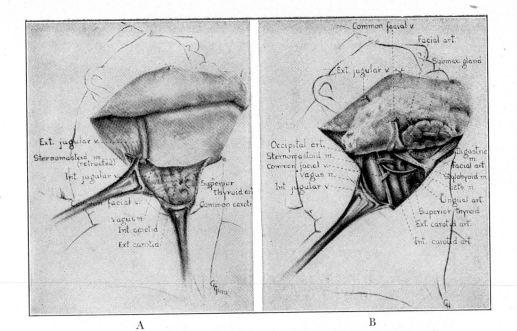

A   B

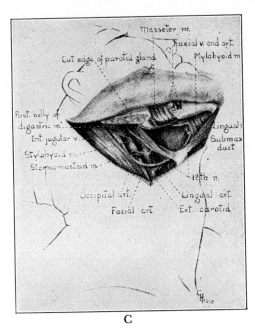

C

Fig. 151. Bilateral upper dissection. (A) Kocher incision and skin flap reflected upward. External jugular vein divided and ligated at lower end of wound. Subcutaneous fat and platysma divided all along lower edge of wound. Areolar tissue and nodes dissected out of carotid sheath down as low as possible. (B) Facial and occipital arteries and common facial vein ligated and divided. Submaxillary gland rotated up out of fossa. (C) Submaxillary duct and chorda tympani divided. Lower third of parotid transected and remainder of block removed at level of upper border of mandible. Same procedure then carried out on opposite side. (From Brown and McDowell, *Surg., Gynec. & Obst.,* 79: 115-124, 1944. By permission of Surgery, Gynecology and Obstetrics.)

One side is dissected at a time as far forward as the midline when the entire bilateral block may be removed in one piece.

The external jugular vein is divided at the edge of the lower skin flap, and the subcutaneous fat cut down to the muscle up to the mastoid and forward over the hyoid to the midline. The fat and lymph nodes in the upper carotid sheath are dissected out and reflected upward with the specimen, but the internal jugular vein is not divided (Fig. 151A). The dissection is carried upward on the surface of the sternomastoid muscle, posterior belly of the digastric muscle, internal jugular vein, and mylohyoid muscle. The submaxillary gland is rotated up with the specimen and freed by dividing the

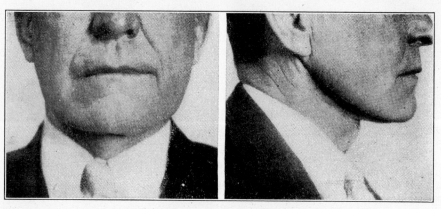

FIG. 152. Result of bilateral upper neck dissection for metastatic carcinoma from lower lip. Well 14 years. (From Brown and McDowell, *Ann. Surg.,* 119:543-555, 1944.)

facial artery at its posterior border (Fig. 151B), the chorda tympani at its upper border, and Wharton's duct at its anterior border.

The lower third of the parotid is cut loose from the remainder of the gland and the mass is taken loose from the mandible to the midline, tying the facial artery and vein on the cheek (Fig. 151C).

The wound is washed out with saline, the upper skin flap replaced and sutured. A small drainage hole is left in the midline and one at either end of the incision. A short rubber dam drain is placed in each end to the stump of the parotid, and drains are placed in the midline opening to either submaxillary fossa. A large pressure dressing is applied, taking particular care to get upward and inward pressure on the skin flaps to eliminate any dead spaces in the submaxillary fossae. Postoperative care is the same as for complete neck dissection (Fig. 152).

Drainage of Neck Abscesses of Dental Origin. These usually originate from infection of the lower molars and may occur spontaneously, or following extractions (Fig. 153). The third molar is an especially common source.

Many workers have done very meticulous dissections of the fascial planes of the neck, sometimes giving them different names which confuse the surgeon trying to find an abscess in this area. The important thing to remember is that the pus may spill over from the tooth laterally, between the ramus of the mandible and masseter muscle, or medially, between the ramus and internal pterygoid muscle and extending upward along the latter into the soft palate area.

These abscesses usually take about three to four days from the onset to "ripen" and the patient should be given chemotherapy, supportive treatment, and some relief of pain during this interval. Respiratory obstruction

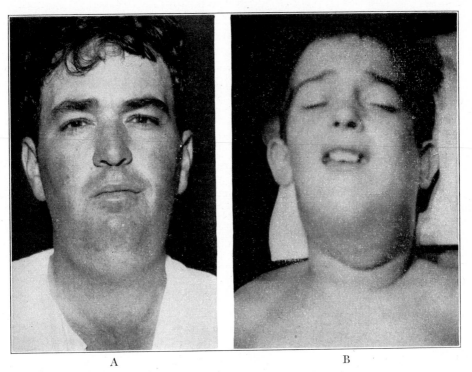

A   B

FIG. 153. Neck infections of dental origin. (A) Submental abscess originating from incisors. (B) A patient who is critically ill with masseter and internal pterygoid abscesses from a third molar. Difficulty in breathing and swallowing made emergency drainage imperative.

is one of the great dangers so that morphine or other strong respiratory depressants should not be used, and the abscess should be opened earlier than usual if the signs of early obstruction appear.

At operation, it is imperative to have a good strong suction apparatus on hand, with a catheter that will go through the nose and clear out the throat if necessary. The skin incision is about 1 inch in length, parallel to the body of the mandible, and about 1 inch below the angle of the mandible. This line may be infiltrated with novocaine, and very light pentothal anesthesia instituted. The original knife cut extends just into subcutaneous fat, and a curved hemostat is introduced and the dissection continued upward by pushing it in and forcibly spreading it until the angle of the mandible is contacted. The dissection is then continued upward first on the outer surface of the ramus, then on the inner surface of the ramus, until an abscess is encountered and drained in one or both places. When the abscess is found, an index finger is inserted into it for exploration and to insure that the drainage is adequate. A 1-inch iodoform pack is introduced and the anesthetic immediately discontinued, keeping the throat clear at all times with the suction apparatus.

Chemotherapy is continued during the postoperative period, with parenteral fluids or tube feedings as indicated. The amount of relaxation of the spasm of the closing muscles is a good indication of progress.

The patient may have a localized or generalized osteomyelitis in conjunction with the soft tissue abscess, but any sequestra are not removed until they are entirely loose. Teeth are never extracted until the whole process is quiescent.

7

THE ESOPHAGUS

W. E. Adams, M.D.

The surgical treatment of abnormalities and diseases of the esophagus has made a notable advance during the past two decades. This has been due, in part to a better understanding of the ability of the esophagus to heal following surgical incision or repair, when certain principles applied to this region are kept in mind.[1] Before describing the technic for various surgical procedures on this organ a review of the factors which make operations on the esophagus possible is in order.

Anatomy. The esophagus, a muscular organ with a mucous membrane lining, leads from the pharynx through the posterior mediastinum to the cardiac end of the stomach. It lies posterior and in close approximation to the trachea and left primary bronchus, and continues medially to the descending aorta and downward to the peritoneal cavity. Its relationship to the trachea, left primary bronchus and aorta, as well as to the pericardium, must be kept in mind in dealing with carcinoma of the esophagus since involvement of these structures by direct extension is apt to be present in long standing cases. Three constrictions of the esophagus, *i.e.,* its junction with the pharynx, as it passes beneath the left main stem bronchus, and as it passes through the diaphragm are the most frequent sites of injury due to instrumentation or to foreign bodies. The upper end of the esophagus receives its blood supply from the inferior thyroid arteries, and the lower end from the left gastric artery. The midportion receives its circulation through branches from the aorta and from intercostal vessels.

Preparation for Operations. Since many lesions of the esophagus produce some degree of dysphagia, patients frequently become undernourished and at times dehydrated. If the lesion is of long standing an anemia frequently develops. To correct these conditions adequate amounts of saline and glucose solution are administered parenterally in addition to liquids by mouth when tolerated preceding operation. Transfusion of whole blood is used to correct the anemia. Since infection is one of the hazards of these operations, attention should be given to oral hygiene and the operation is preceded by the use of chemotherapy.

Anesthesia. The development of a satisfactory method of maintaining circulation and adequate oxygenation of the tissue during a surgical pneumothorax has played a major role in the success of operations on the esophagus. The administration of anesthetic mixtures under a small amount of positive pressure with an adequate percentage of oxygen has enabled operations of several hours duration to be carried out with safety, and with a minimum of postanesthetic complications. Replacement of blood loss during operation by the transfusion of citrated whole blood will prevent the development of shock.

Postoperative Management. Following the completion of the operative procedure the residual air in the pleural cavity is aspirated and the lung fully reexpanded. This helps to avoid the development of postoperative atelectasis and pneumonitis and minimizes the danger of infection in the pleural cavity. In operative procedures where fluids by mouth are contraindicated, maintenance of water and mineral balance is obtained through the intravenous and subcutaneous routes. Nasal catheter administration of oxygen will diminish the work of the heart and help to prevent anoxia. Chemotherapy aids in preventing infection of the pleural cavity as well as postoperative pulmonary complications.

CONGENITAL MALFORMATIONS

Atresia of the Esophagus. The frequency of this congenital anomaly has been more appreciated in recent years. The malformation varies considerably as illustrated in figure 154a. Two methods of management have been successfully employed. One entails the ligation of the tracheo-esophageal fistula and exteriorization of the blind upper esophageal stump. This is later connected with a gastrostomy tube for feeding purposes. In the second procedure the tracheo-esophageal fistula is ligated and the blind upper esophageal segment is anastomosed with the mobilized lower end of the esophagus. The operation must be preceded by proper preparation of the patient and performed under local and light ether anesthesia. The approach may be from either the right or the left side, the incision paralleling the lateral border of the erector-spinae-mass between the second and sixth ribs inclusive. Portions of the third, fourth and fifth ribs are resected subperiostially and the intercostal structures are divided between ligatures. The parietal pleura is now dissected free from the parietes and retracted forward. On the right side the azygos vein is divided between ligatures and the trachea and segments of the esophagus are exposed. If too great a gap (2 cm. +) is present between the two segments, the fistula is ligated and the upper segment exteriorized and a gastrostomy performed for feeding purposes. If the two segments can be brought together following ligation of the tracheo-esophageal fistula, the lower segment is divided distal to the ligature, and the anastomosis between the two segments is carried out over a small catheter (No. 8) introduced into the two segments by way of the wound and pulled up through the pharynx by the anesthetist. This enables the anastomosis to be made more easily, an atraumatic round pointed needle with Deknatel A silk being used so as to produce minimum amount of trauma (see Fig. 154b and c). If a pneumothorax accidently occurs, the lung should be reexpanded by positive pressure oxygen administered through the face mask and the opening in the pleura closed, if possible. A soft rubber

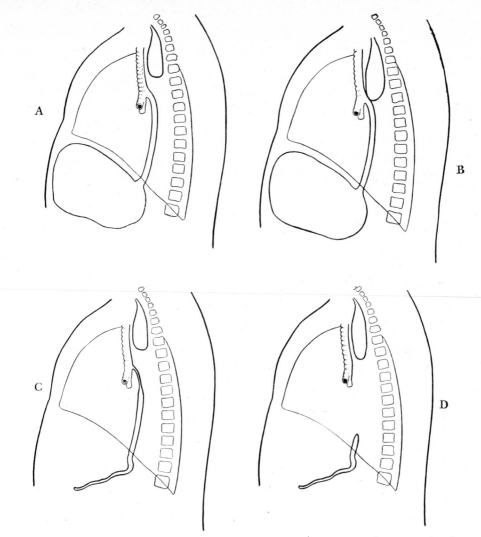

FIG. 154(1). The types of the anomaly that have been encountered at operation in 23 of the 24 cases from whom exploratory operation was performed are illustrated. (One patient died during operation before the nature of the lower segment was determined.) (From Haight, *Ann. Surg.*, 120:(Oct.), 1944.) A. The most frequent type of malformation of the esophagus. The upper esophagus ends as a blind pouch. The lower esophagus arises from the trachea at a level that is usually between 0.5 and 1 cm. above the bifurcation of the trachea. Air is present in the stomach indicating the presence of a tracheoesophageal fistula. This type of anomaly was present in 13 of the 24 patients from whom a primary exploration of the anomaly was performed. Variations in the location of the fistula were found, and in two cases the lower esophagus arose from the right stem bronchus. (From Haight and Towsley, *Surg., Gynec. & Obst.*, 76 [No. 6]: 1943. By permission of Surgery, Gynecology and Obstetrics.) B. Partial muscular continuity of the two segments. The anomaly otherwise is the same as in A (five cases). (From Haight and Towsley, *Surg., Gynec. & Obst.*, 76 [No. 6]: 1943. By permission of Surgery, Gynecology and Obstetrics.) C. The lower segment is greatly contracted for a variable distance below its origin from the trachea and air has not entered the stomach, although a tracheoesophageal fistula was present (two cases). In a third case, the lower segment was contracted, but air was present in the stomach (not illustrated). (From Haight and Towsley, *Surg., Gynec. & Obst.*, 76 [No.]: 1943. By permission of Surgery, Gynecology and Obstetrics.) D. Atresia of the upper esophagus and agenesia of the lower esophagus. The stomach does not contain air (two cases). (From Haight, *Ann. Surg.*, 120: [Oct.], 1944.)

tissue drain is placed in the wound leading to a point near the site of the anastomosis, and the wound is closed in layers with interrupted sutures.

Since these operations are performed on young infants, special care is necessary to prevent postoperative anoxia and infections. The body temperature must be kept normal by the use of an incubator and intravenous fluids and blood are given in desirable amounts.

In the early development of these operations most of the patients expired. Although the risk of the procedure is still considerable, the increasing

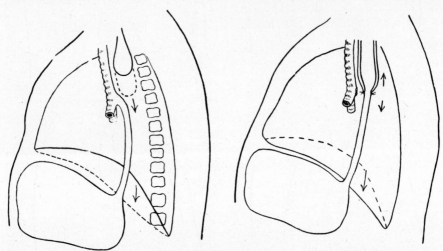

FIG. 154(2). The mobility of the upper esophagus that is seen during roentgenoscopic examination is indicated by the position of the solid and dotted lines. Solid line indicates position of the upper esophagus during the expiratory phase of respiration and during straining and crying with their attending increase in intrathoracic pressure; dotted line indicates position of upper segment during inspiratory phase of respiration. Because of the mobility of the upper esophagus, roentgenoscopic observation allows a more accurate estimation of the position and length of the upper segment than does the roentgenographic examination. Tension unavoidably occurs at the site of the anastomosis because of: (1) the gap that usually must be overcome when the two segments are united; (2) the ascent of the upper esophagus during swallowing, crying and the expiratory phase of respiration; (3) the descent of the lower esophagus during the inspiratory phase of respiration; and (4) the normal contractility of the longitudinal musculature of the esophagus. (From Haight, *Ann. Surg.*, 120:[Oct.], 1944.)

number of successful results reported justifies its use in an otherwise fatal condition.[2]

Congenital Short Esophagus. This lesion produces symptoms by the development of gastritis and ulceration of the mucosa where the stomach passes through the esophageal hiatus or in that part of the stomach above the diaphragm (see Fig. 155). Symptoms may frequently be relieved by a modified ulcer management. If this is not successful good results may be obtained by paralyzing one leaf of the diaphragm, thus relaxing the constricting influence on the stomach. The operation, phrenico-exeresis, is performed under local anesthesia through a short, oblique incision at the posterior border of the sterno-mastoid muscle, one or two fingers breadth above the clavicle. After dividing the platysmamyoides, the sterno-mastoid muscle is retracted anteriorly, thus exposing the scalenous-anticus muscle. The phrenic nerve is seen running vertically over the anterior surface of this muscle and after infiltration with novocaine it is mobilized and divided, the lower portion being slowly avulsed. The wound is closed in layers with interrupted

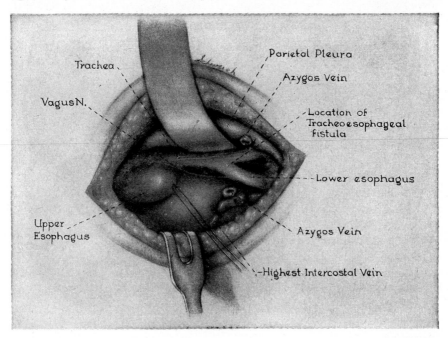

Fig. 154(3). The right extrapleural exposure of the anomaly is illustrated. The posterior portions of the third, fourth and fifth ribs have been resected and the parietal pleura has been freed from the thoracic wall. The azygos vein has been divided in order to expose the lower esophagus. The dilated blind upper segment has been partially freed from the posterior wall of the trachea. The relative size of the upper and lower esophagus, and the usual position of the tracheoesophageal fistula are shown. The right vagus nerve serves as a useful guide for locating the lower segment. (From Haight, *Ann. Surg.*, 120:[Oct.], 1944.)

sutures. By relaxing the esophageal hiatus the constricting influence on the stomach wall and the puddling of gastric secretion in the stomach above the diaphragm is lessened. Relief of symptoms is usually prompt and permanent. The risk of the operation is less than 1.0 per cent.

INJURY OF THE ESOPHAGUS

Injury of the esophagus may occur due to instrumentation, the swallowing of a foreign body, or through injuries of the chest. The wound may be a puncture or a laceration and due to contamination of the mediastinum may give rise to mediastinitis diffused or localized in character. When drainage of the site of infection is instituted as soon as toxic manifestations indi-

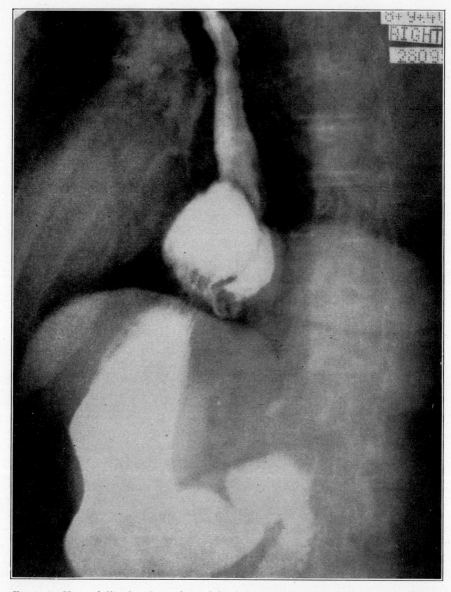

FIG. 155. X-ray following ingestion of barium by a 52-year-old housewife who complained of intermittent nausea and vomiting of 15 years' duration. She also had had some pain in the left upper quadrant and a sensation of food sticking in the chest beginning one year ago. Note position of stomach lying above the diaphragm with considerable constriction of the stomach at the esophageal hiatus.

cate the development of mediastinitis, the chances of survival (of the patient) are very good. However, if operation is long delayed a fatal outcome must be expected in a high percentage of cases.

In the case of injury from instrumentation the lesion is usually located in the cervical esophagus at its junction with the pharynx.

Anterior Approach. For injuries of the cervical esophagus and extending down to the level of the arch of the aorta the anterior surgical approach is recommended. Local anesthesia is desirable and the incision is made along the anterior border of the sterno-mastoid muscle from the episternal notch upward for a distance of 3 to 4 inches. This muscle is retracted laterally along with the vascular sheath containing the common carotid and internal jugular vein. The depressors of the hyoid bone are then split and retracted medially along with the thyroid gland, the omohyoid being drawn laterally along with the other structures. Ligation of the inferior thyroid artery is frequently necessary. Evidence of injury and infection is indicated by the presence of edema and interstitial emphysema with or without suppuration. This involvement extends to the posterior aspect of the esophagus which lies in front of the bodies of the vertebrae. Adequate dissection is necessary to expose the involved region for drainage, as well as for closure by suture of any laceration. Since most of the injuries are in the posterior wall of the esophagus, the approach for drainage of the infection and closure of a laceration may be made from either the right or the left side. After all recesses of the inflammatory process have been exposed, drainage in the form of soft rubber tissue either with or without gauze packing will allow an avenue of escape for the infection. If the inflammatory process extends to the opposite side, a counter incision is made but less dissection is necessary for the placing of drains. With the exception of partial closure of the upper angle by interrupted sutures the wound is left open.

Posterior Thoracic Approach. For injuries of the esophagus located beneath the arch of the aorta an approach through the posterior mediastinum at the desired level is indicated. This is made through an incision over the transverse processes of three or four vertebra on the right or left side. After retracting the erector-spinae-mass medially, a portion of the transverse process of the vertebrae along with the posterior ends of the corresponding ribs are resected subperiostially and the intercostal structures divided between ligatures. The parietal pleura is now dissected from the lateral aspect of the bodies of the vertebrae down to the posterior mediastinum. The wound is necessarily deep and thus care must be exercised not to open the pleural cavity during the dissection. The site of injury and inflammation is then exposed and an opening in the esophagus, if present, is sutured. The wound is packed open using soft rubber tissue drains with or without gauze enclosed. If the pleural cavity is opened and drainage of the infection is not urgent a two-stage operation is desirable. In this case the wound is packed, the lung is reexpanded and the second stage is performed at a later date. If the pleural cavity is widely opened during the operation, continuous suction drainage should be established following closure of the chest. The use of chemotherapy both before and following operation is recommended.

Prior to the use of chemotherapy and early drainage of the acute mediastinitis following injuries of the esophagus, most patients expired. When drainage is delayed for any considerable time (24 to 48 hrs.) after the appearance of toxic manifestations the chances of survival are small. The prognosis is reversed when early drainage is instituted.[3]

DIVERTICULA

This lesion is of two types; *viz.*, pulsion and traction. The former in the majority of cases is located at the esophago-pharyngeal junction, the sac extending downward posterior to the esophagus and lying in front of the

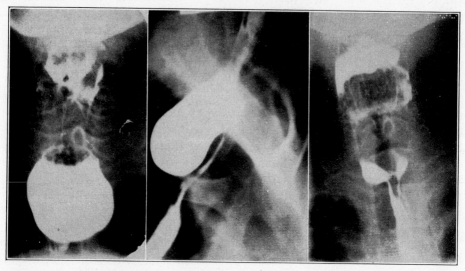

Fig. 156a. AP and lateral view before operation and AP view after operation following the ingestion of barium. This 54-year-old man complained of repeated attacks of bronchitis and pneumonitis due to spillage of contents of a diverticulum into the tracheobronchial tree during sleep. He also continued to regurgitate food several hours after eating. The pulsion diverticulum increased considerably in size during the previous three years. The patient's symptoms were entirely relieved following the excision of the diverticulum.

bodies of the vertebrae (Fig. 156a). These lesions produce symptoms by obstructing the passage of food and thus lead to malnutrition and at times dehydration. Traction diverticula seldom produce symptoms.

The approach for surgical management of pulsion diverticula is through an oblique incision in front of the left sterno-cleido-mastoid muscle extending from the episternal notch upward for 4 or 5 inches. This muscle is retracted laterally along with the vascular sheath containing the common carotid artery and internal jugular vein. The strap muscles are retracted medially along with the lateral lobe of the thyroid gland. There are no vessels to interfere with the exposure of the diverticulum except the inferior thyroid artery which may be divided between ligatures or retracted to one side. The diverticulum is then readily exposed and is carefully dissected free from the esophagus anteriorly and the prevertebral fascia overlying the bodies of the vertebrae posteriorly. The neck of the diverticulum is then identified, care being taken not to open the esophagus until the sac is to be excised. If the communication between the diverticulum and the esophagus is small, it may be closed by a single transfixion suture, the stump being buried by interrupted sutures after the diverticulum has been excised. If the communication is large as seen in figure 156b it is advisable to close the same with a row of interrupted sutures placed as the sac is being excised.

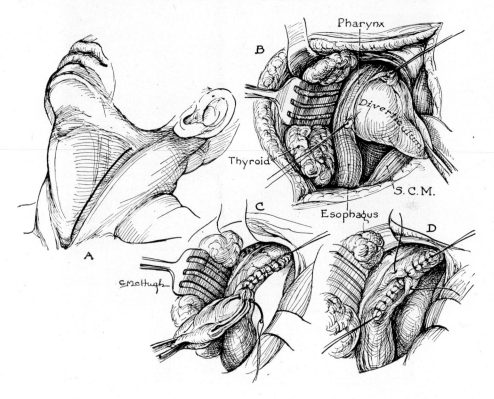

FIG. 156b. Drawing showing location of incision and exposure for mobilization of diverticulum. In this instance the neck of the sac was wide and closure following the resection was made by interrupted sutures as illustrated in (c) and (d).

This row is then inverted by a second row of silk or fine chromosized catgut sutures. If the neck of the sac is large the suture line should not run transversely in order to lessen the risk of stenosis. A rubber tissue drain is directed down to the region of closure of the neck of the diverticulum and brought out at the lower angle of the wound. The wound is then closed in layers with interrupted sutures. The use of chemotherapy following operation will aid in the prevention of serious postoperative infection.

A two-stage operation may also be employed for removing this lesion. After mobilization and elevation of the diverticulum it is sutured to the subcutaneous tissues at the first stage. The sac is then removed by a second stage operation made 3 to 6 days later, in a similar manner to that described for the one-stage operation. Good results may be expected following either

type of surgery. The obstructive symptoms are relieved and normal esophageal function is reestablished. The risk of mediastinitis following the
one-stage operation is probably no greater than in the two-stage procedure.
The incidence of esophageal fistula or other complications is also no greater

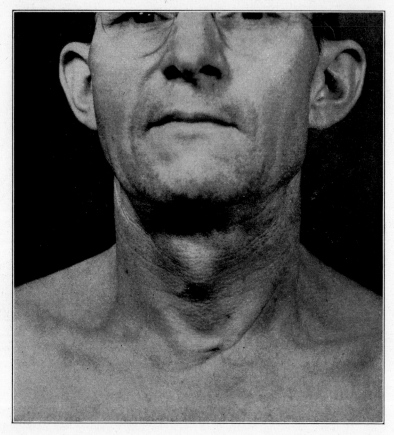

FIG. 156c. Appearance of scar following excision of pulsion diverticulum.

than in the two-stage procedure.[4] Thus the single-stage operation has continued to gain favor.

BENIGN OBSTRUCTION

Obstruction of the esophagus may be produced by a number of non-
malignant lesions. These include stenosis following the swallowing of lye
or other caustic materials, cicatricial stenosis of the lower esophagus following esophagitis from repeated regurgitation of gastric juice, and idiopathic dilatation of the esophagus commonly designated as achalasia or
cardiospasm. All of these obstructive lesions lead to some degree of under-
nourishment and at times dehydration. Strictures of the esophagus caused
by caustic materials are usually multiple and incomplete and can usually
be managed satisfactorily by repeated dilatation.

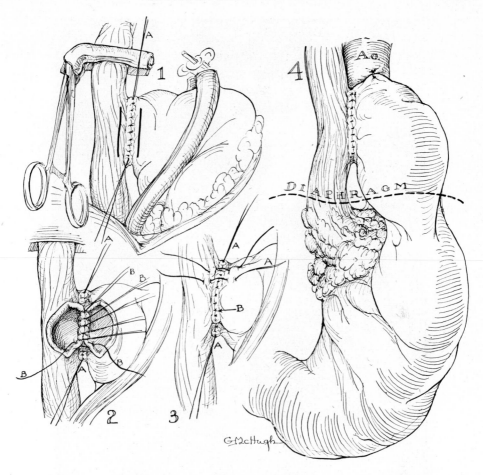

FIG. 157a. Drawing illustrating surgical technic of a lateral anastomosis between the esophagus and fundus of the stomach. The procedure may be used for cardiospasm, cicatricial stenosis of the lower esophagus or for relief of obstruction due to inoperable carcinoma in the gastro-esophageal junction.

Cicatricial Stenosis. This obstructive lesion develops in the lower portion of the thoracic esophagus and although some relief may be obtained by repeated dilatation this method of treatment is frequently inadequate and surgical management is indicated. Since the point of obstruction may extend for some distance above the cardia, the operation is best made through a transthoracic approach. The muscles of the chest wall are divided through a long incision over the left eighth rib and most of this rib is removed subperiostially. The left pleural cavity is then opened, the pulmonary ligament divided, and the lung retracted upward. The lower portion of the thoracic esophagus is then exposed by incising the mediastinal pleura and the lower 3 or 4 inches of the organ are mobilized. The obstruction usually extends up to a point just above the level of the diaphragm, thus a lateral anastomosis between the esophagus and the fundus of the stomach may be

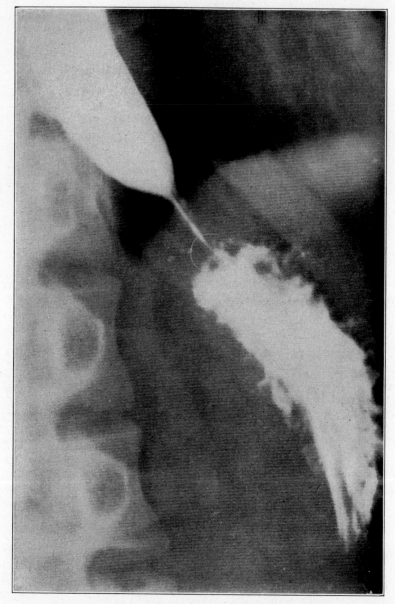

Fig. 157b. X-ray following ingestion of barium showing cicatricial stenosis of lower esophagus in a 26-year-old male. The patient had complained of difficulty in swallowing for three years and a weight loss of 45 pounds. Repeated dilatation of the esophagus failed to give satisfactory relief.

made above the site of obstruction. The fundus of the stomach is brought up through an incision in the diaphragm which extends from near its peripheral attachment to within 1 or 2 inches of the esophageal hiatus. The fundus may usually be elevated 3 or 4 inches into the lower pleural cavity without difficulty. If the spleen interferes with the technical procedure, it is removed. The surrounding structures are then protected by moist lap-pads placed about the site of the intended anastomosis. A soft right angle rubber-shod clamp is placed on the esophagus at the upper portion of the part mobilized and a specially devised curved intestinal clamp is placed across

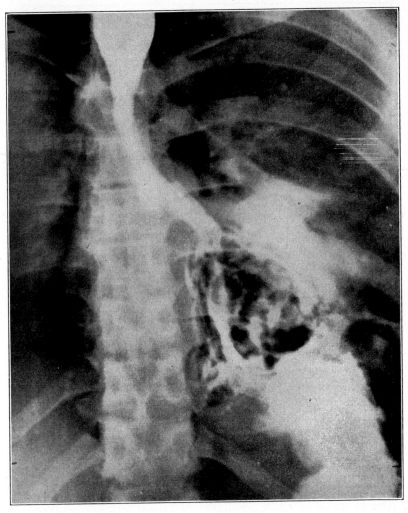

FIG. 157C. X-ray appearance following transthoracic esophagogastrostomy above the site of stricture. The patient was entirely relieved of his obstructive symptoms and promptly regained normal weight.

the fundus of the stomach to prevent contamination and to maintain hemostasis. A gastro-esophagostomy is now made using a longitudinal incision in the wall of the esophagus after first placing a row of interrupted linen sutures. The esophagus and the stomach are now opened and an inner row of interrupted sutures of the same material is used, following which two rows of sutures are placed on the anterior surface of the anastomosis (Fig. 157a). The clamps on the esophagus and stomach are now removed, and the fundus of the stomach is secured in the thorax by suturing it to the parietal pleura, thus obviating any tension on the suture line of the anastomosis. A No. 28 Pezzar catheter is now brought out through a stab

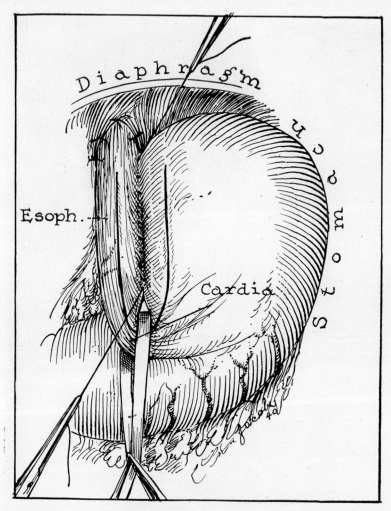

Fig. 158a. After passing a tape about the cardia the peritoneum has been divided at the esophageal hiatus. The lower end of the esophagus is mobilized by blunt dissection and at least 2 inches of it pulled down into the abdomen. The crura of the diaphragm have been reattached to the esophagus at this higher level and the outer row of the posterior layer has been completed. The line of the incision is indicated by the "U." (From Scott, *Ann. Surg.,* 122:[Oct.], 1945.)

wound in the ninth intercostal space postero-laterally for obliterating the pleural space (of fluid and air) following closure of the wound. The primary incision is then closed using pericostal sutures and a continuous running stitch for the intercostal structures. The remainder of the wound is closed in layers with chromosized catgut, and silk is used for the skin. The

Pezzar catheter is connected with a double Wangensteen suction apparatus for maintenance of complete expansion of the lung.

This operation has been found very satisfactory in relieving obstruction of the lower end of the esophagus. The procedure carries comparatively little risk, there being no deaths in 10 patients so managed.[5]

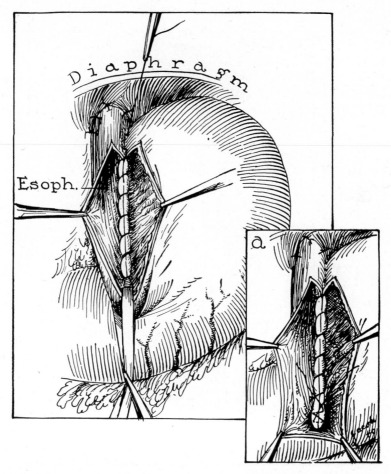

Fig. 158b. The stomach and esophagus have been opened except for the small bridge where the tape still maintains traction while the stomach and esophagus are sutured posteriorly. The tape and bridge at the cardia are now divided and one suture completes the outer posterior row. (From Scott, *Ann. Surg.*, 122:[Oct.], 1945.)

Achalasia (Cardiospasm). The majority of patients with this lesion may be relieved of obstructive symptoms by repeated dilatation of the esophagus. However, in some instances the symptoms remain rather severe and adequate nutrition is difficult to maintain under this form of treatment. Other patients become dissatisfied because of the need of repeated dilatation and prefer to have surgical management.

Two operative procedures have been devised both of which have proven satisfactory in relieving the obstruction, namely; cardioplasty, performed through an abdominal approach and esophagogastrostomy performed through a low thoracic approach.

Cardioplasty. Under spinal anesthesia, the peritoneal cavity is opened through an upper left paramedian incision. The junction of the esophagus

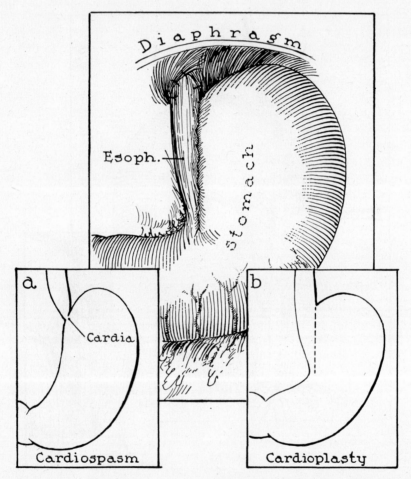

Fig. 158c. The two rows of the anterior segment have been completed making a wide opening between the esophagus and stomach. (From Scott, *Ann. Surg.,* 122:[Oct.], 1945.)

and stomach is exposed by mobilization of the left lobe of the liver. This is accomplished by dividing the triangular ligament of the liver and retraction of the left lobe of the liver to the right. A gauze tape is now passed around the cardia and is used for traction. The esophagus is mobilized from the diaphragm by incising the peritoneal fold at the esophageal hiatus as it comes from beneath the diaphragm down on the esophagus. By blunt dissection the lower 2 inches of the thoracic esophagus may be mobilized and retracted down into the abdomen. It is secured in this position by interrupted sutures to the diaphragm at the hiatus. The fundus of the stomach is now sutured to the lower 5 to 7.5 cm. of the esophagus down to the cardia and a U-shaped incision is made between the lower esophagus and the fundus of the stomach (see Fig. 158a). The posterior inner row of sutures is now placed down to the cardia at which point the traction tape is removed and the outer row posteriorly completed with a figure-of-8 stitch. The inner row is then likewise completed and the anterior two rows placed in a similar manner (Fig. 158b and c).

By adequately cleaning the esophagus prior to the operation the anastomosis may be performed with safety without the use of a clamp or a tie above the point of anastomosis. After completion of the anastomosis it is unnecessary to resuture the ligament of the liver to the diaphragm. Drainage of the site of anastomosis is unnecessary. The abdominal wound is now closed with a running stitch of silk or fine catgut for the peritoneum and posterior rectal sheath. A row of interrupted sutures is placed in the anterior rectal sheath and the remainder of the wound is closed in layers.

Transthoracic Approach. The operation for this lesion performed through a transthoracic approach is similar to that used for cicatricial obstruction of the lower thoracic esophagus (see above). Since the point of obstruction in achalasia is at the cardia, a lateral anastomosis between the lower esophagus and the fundus of the stomach may be performed lower than in the case of cicatricial stenosis.

Both supra- and infra-diaphragmatic operations have been found satisfactory in relieving esophageal obstruction. Since the operative risk is small, the choice of procedure will be determined by individual preference and familiarity with the field of approach.[6]

TUMORS

The large majority of tumors arising in the esophagus are carcinomata. They usually first produce symptoms by obstructing the lumen. Carcinoma of the cardiac end of the stomach may likewise produce obstruction by secondary involvement of the lower esophagus. Benign tumors of the esophagus, either arising from the mucosa or from the musculature are uncommon. Those arising from the mucosa are more apt to produce obstruction than those having origin in the musculature.

The surgical approach for removing benign tumors depends on the type of tumor and its location. For tumors arising from the mucosa an approach through the right side is desirable especially when the lesion is near the aorta. If the tumor arises from the musculature an approach through the left side is preferable since the stomach may be brought into the chest to re-establish the continuity of the digestive tract.

Leiomyoma of Lower Thoracic Esophagus. Through an incision over the left eighth rib the muscles of the chest wall are divided and most of this rib is removed subperiostially. The pleural cavity is opened and after dividing the pulmonary ligament the left lung is retracted upward. The

lower 10 cm. of the thoracic esophagus is exposed by a vertical incision in
the mediastinal pleura, and by a combination of blunt and sharp dissection
this portion of the esophagus and the tumor is mobilized from the surrounding structures. If the tumor arises from the mucosa and lies within the

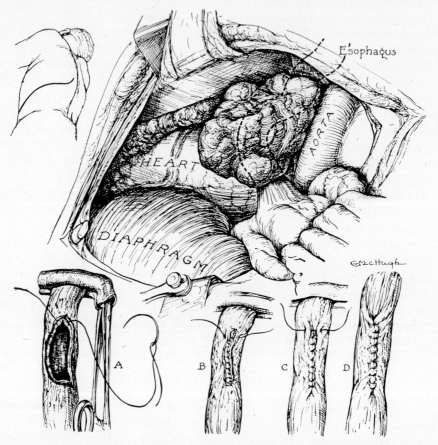

FIG. 159. Drawing showing a benign tumor (leiomyoma) of the musculature of the
lower esophagus. Exposure is obtained by resecting a segment of the eighth rib. In addi-
tion to the benign tumor the 46-year-old man had a hiatus hernia of the diaphragm.
Insert shows method of closing the defect in the esophagus after removal of the tumor.
The patient made an uneventful recovery. (From Schafer and Kittle, *J.A.M.A.*, 133:
[April 19], 1947.)

lumen of the esophagus, the esophagus is opened by a longitudinal incision,
the tumor delivered, and the pedicle divided between ligatures. When the
tumor arises from the musculature it is carefully dissected from around the
esophagus. It may involve the mucosa so intimately that opening of the esophagus is unavoidable during the dissection. The opening in the wall of the
esophagus in either case is closed with a running stitch of fine chromosized
gut placed through the edges of the mucosa. This row is then covered by
a second row of interrupted sutures of the same material, and which in turn

is inverted by a third row of sutures placed in the frayed-out musculature of the esophageal wall (Fig. 159).

The esophagus is now placed in its normal position without attempting closure of the mediastinal pleura. A Pezzar catheter is brought out through a stab wound in the ninth intercostal space postero-laterally for obliteration of the pleural cavity of fluid and air following closure of the wound. The primary incision is closed by using two pericostal sutures of a double strand of chromic 1 catgut. The intercostal structures are reapproximated by a continuous double strand of oo catgut suture. The muscles and fascia of the chest wall are then closed in layers with catgut, and silk is used for the skin. A Pezzar catheter is attached to a Wangensteen apparatus for continuous aspiration of the pleural cavity for maintenance of expansion of the lung. Although few cases of surgical removal of benign tumors of the esophagus have been reported, the results indicate that relief of symptoms may be anticipated and that the operation may be made with comparative safety.[7]

CARCINOMA OF THE ESOPHAGUS

Since 90 per cent of all carcinomas of the esophagus are located in the middle or lower third of that organ the transthoracic approach for removal of the tumor is used for the majority of cases.

Carcinoma of the Cervical Esophagus. In a small percentage arising in the cervical esophagus with or without involvement of the lower pharynx a cervical approach for removing the lesion is used. Since the larynx or upper trachea is also not infrequently involved by direct extension, removal of these structures along with the pharynx and upper esophagus *en bloc* is sometimes necessary. In spite of the fact that the operation is rather mutilating, it is a worthwhile procedure since reconstruction of the pharynx and esophagus is possible and food may again be taken in the normal manner.

Gas, oxygen and ether anesthesia are given by mask and by intratracheal catheter. A skin flap is fashioned by two horizontal incisions from the angle of the jaw on one side extending across the midline of the neck to the angle on the opposite side and connected by a vertical incision. The entire skin and subcutaneous tissue is undermined and the flap is based laterally. The sterno-mastoid muscle beneath the base of the flap is removed along with the lateral lobe of the thyroid gland on that side. The procedure from this point onward depends on whether there is involvement of the trachea and larynx by direct extension from the esophageal lesion. If this is the case the trachea is mobilized and divided below the level of the involvement and the upper cut-end is blocked by moist gauze. A tube is introduced into the trachea for the continuation of the anesthesia. After mobilization of the esophagus and pharynx a division is made just above the level of the tumor and the pharynx is packed off with moist gauze. The esophagus is then divided below the level of the tumor and the larynx divided above the level of the involvement and the tissues are removed *en bloc*. The previously prepared skin flap is placed across the area from which the tumor was removed and secured in place by two vertical lines of interrupted sutures where the esophagus is to be reconstructed. The upper edge of the skin flap is then sewed to the lower end of the pharynx with interrupted chromic catgut sutures and in a similar manner the lower edge of the skin flap is united with the upper end of the esophagus. The remainder of the flap is secured to the raw surface of the neck beyond the midline. A Levine tube is passed through the nares and down through the region of the skin flap which is to form

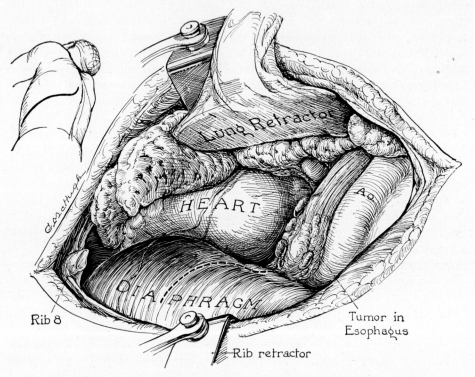

Fig. 160a. Exposure for resection of carcinoma at the lower end of the esophagus.

the artificial esophagus, and then down into the stomach for feeding purposes. The remainder of the surface from which the skin flap was removed is covered by Thiersch grafts. The upper end of the trachea is brought out to the skin surface and secured. The procedures just outlined constitute the first stage of the operation.

Sufficient time is allowed for healing before the second stage of operation is performed. This consists of incising and undercutting at the margins of the lateral sinus and suturing of the turned over edges of the skin in such a manner that the knots of catgut are within the newly formed esophagus. The first layer of sutures is inverted by a second layer of the same material. The other edges of the skin are now brought together and closed over the tube of skin forming the esophagus. Following the second stage operation a Levine tube is again passed down into the stomach for feeding purposes and maintained for approximately two weeks after which fluids and regular diet may be tolerated.

In patients where the larynx and trachea are uninvolved the procedure is essentially the same except that these structures are not sacrificed. The lateral sinus of skin is located somewhat behind these structures at the first stage. The tube of skin which is to unite the pharynx above to the esophagus below is closed at the second stage and covered by drawing the edges of the

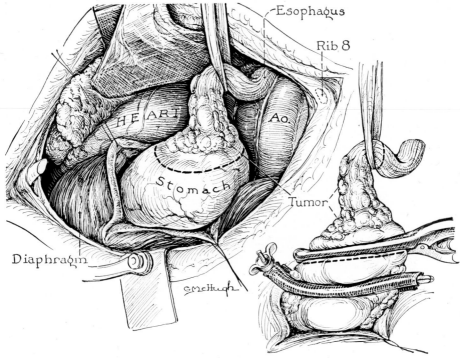

FIG. 160b. After mobilization of the stomach following incision of the diaphragm, division of the cardia is made below the tumor.

skin-flap over the same. Patients have survived this operation and enjoyed taking food in a normal manner without difficulty for a number of years.[8] This is a more desirable procedure than gastrostomy even in patients who ultimately die of recurrence of the original tumor or of metastatic lesions. The risk of the operation is comparatively little when shock is obviated by transfusion of adequate amounts of whole blood and when serious infection is prevented by careful oral hygiene and chemotherapy.

Carcinoma at the Gastro-esophageal Junction. The surgical management of carcinoma arising primarily in the lower end of the esophagus or primary in the cardia and obstructing the lower esophagus by secondary extension is essentially the same. In the latter, the line of resection through the stomach is determined by the extent of the tumor. Anesthesia is obtained by using mask ethylene-oxygen-ether administered under mild positive pres-

sure (4 to 6 mm. of mercury). Saline infusion into an ankle vein is begun
and blood loss is replaced simultaneously by blood transfusion throughout
the operation. Through a skin incision over the left eighth rib most of this
rib is removed subperiostially and the pleural cavity is opened and the left
lung explored. The pulmonary ligament is divided and the lung retracted
upward by means of a broad retractor covered by a stockinette (Fig. 160a).
The phrenic nerve is crushed. The mediastinal pleura is now incised and

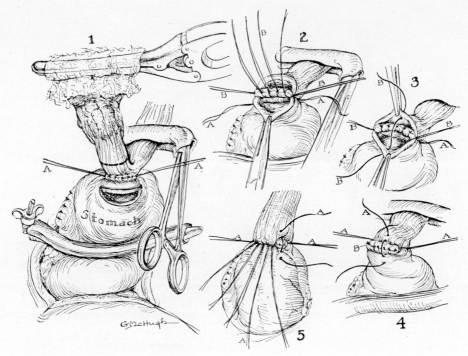

Fig. 160c. Technic for anastomosing the esophagus and fundus of the stomach by
suture.

the esophagus is mobilized by blunt and sharp dissection, the vessels between
the aorta and esophagus being divided between clamps. The peritoneal
cavity is now opened by dividing the diaphragm from the region of the
eighth costal cartilage inward to the esophageal hiatus. An exploration is
made for evidence of metastases to the liver and the extent of metastatic
involvement of the retroperitoneal lymph nodes. The spleen at times is removed to facilitate the technical procedure of anastomosis. The esophagus
and cardiac end of the stomach are mobilized from their attachment to the
peritoneum and the diaphragm. The vascular supply along the greater
curvature of the stomach is divided sufficiently to allow the fundus of the
stomach to be drawn up into the chest for anastomosis with the esophagus
following the resection of the tumor. After mobilizing the left gastric artery
and removing any adjacent suspicious lymph nodes, this vessel is divided
between clamps and ligated with linen (Fig. 160b). The cardiac end of the

stomach is now divided below the level of the tumor between a Payr clamp above and a special intestinal clamp devoid of a handle below. After closing the cardiac end of the stomach with two rows of continuous sutures, the fundus is brought up for union with the esophagus. This is accomplished by using two rows of interrupted sutures of linen, the first row is placed postero-medially before the esophagus is divided above the tumor. The remainder of the anastomosis is then carried out as illustrated in figure

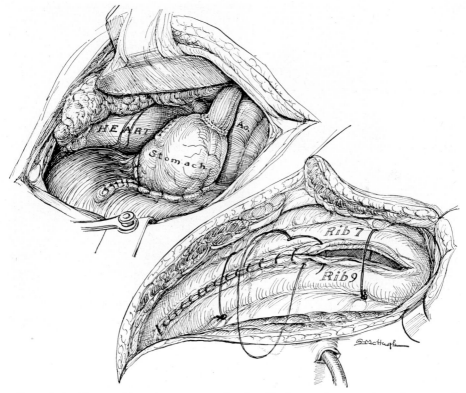

FIG. 160d. After making the anastomosis, the diaphragm is sutured to the stomach. Closure of the chest wound is illustrated.

160c. Following the anastomosis the stomach is sutured up to the pleura overlying the aorta or posterior chest wall to relax the suture line and avoid tension. The diaphragm is closed about the stomach by interrupted sutures, the remaining portion being closed anterior to the stomach with a continuous suture of chromic oo catgut. This portion of the suture line is supported by a second row of mattress sutures. A Pezzar catheter (28F) is now brought postero-laterally through the ninth interspace for maintenance of complete expansion of the lung following closure of the wound. Two pericostal sutures of a double strand of chromic 1 catgut are placed about the seventh and ninth rib, while they are held together by small toothed retractors. The intercostal structures are now brought together by a continuous suture of catgut and the muscles and fascia of the chest wall are reapproximated with the same material (Fig. 160d). The remainder of the wound is closed in layers. Following closure, all fluid and air is aspirated through the Pezzar catheter which is later connected with a Wangensteen apparatus for maintenance of constant suction of the pleural cavity.

A number of other operative procedures have been devised for removing tumors involving this portion of the gastro-intestinal tract. Most of these

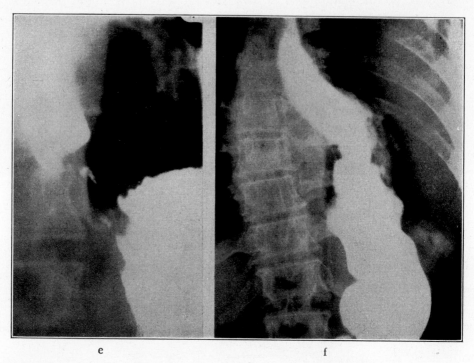

e   f

FIG. 160. (e) X-ray following ingestion of barium showing obstruction of lower esophagus due to carcinoma at the gastro-esophageal junction. The patient, a 52-year-old male, gave a characteristic history of difficulty in swallowing, weight loss and epigastric pain. (f) X-ray appearance following transthoracic resection of tumor and esophago-gastric anastomosis.

have been unsatisfactory from the stand point of risk of infection or lack of satisfactory function following the operation. The above described procedure has also been performed through an incision extending along the course of the eighth rib or eighth intercostal space and continued on to the upper left quadrant of the abdomen, both the peritoneal and pleural cavities being opened through the same incision. In this procedure the costal arch is divided and the diaphragm opened from the periphery to the esophageal hiatus. This incision allows better exposure of the contents of the upper abdomen and is of value particularly in the removal of large tumors of the stomach obstructing the lower esophagus and invading other abdominal viscera such as the pancreas and transverse colon. For lesions involving only the cardiac end of the stomach or the lower esophagus the division of the costal arch and the opening of the peritoneal cavity through the anterior abdominal wall is unnecessary.

Resection of carcinoma of the esophagus and gastro-esophagostomy is a relatively new procedure. In its early stage of development the risk of the operation was comparatively high. At the present time however, the mortality is about 10 to 15 per cent thus making the operation a very justifiable procedure.[9-11] When patients are referred for resection during the early

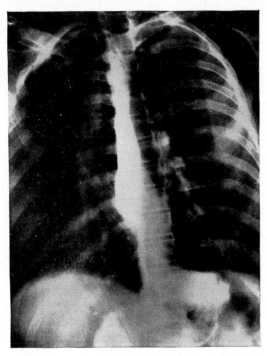

FIG. 161a. Preoperative x-ray of chest following ingestion of barium, showing an obstructing lesion of the lower one-third of the esophagus. The tumor extended approximately 1½ inches higher than the level suggested by the x-ray. (From Adams, *Surg. Clin. N. Amer.,* Chicago Number, 1946. Courtesy of W. B. Saunders Co.)

course of their symptoms, the chances of a long time cure are reasonably good. The first successful case resected by this one-stage method is living without evidence of recurrence 11 years following the operation.[12]

Carcinoma of the Middle Third of the Esophagus. The first successful case of resection of carcinoma of the esophagus (located in the middle third) was reported by Torek [13] in 1913. The operation was named after Dr. Torek and was the most successful type of procedure used for these tumors until approximately five years ago. The operation consisted of opening the pleural cavity through the lower thorax and mobilization of the entire thoracic esophagus. The lower end of the esophagus was then divided, the cardiac end of the stomach being inverted. The remainder of the esophagus was elevated from behind the arch of the aorta and through a separate incision at the base

of the neck was withdrawn from the pleural cavity. The cervical esophageal
fistula was then connected to the stomach by means of a rubber and glass
tube.

Since the development of the above described procedure for tumors
located at the gastro-esophageal junction, the application of that operation
has been extended to include tumors involving the middle third of the esophagus (Fig. 161a).[14] A long incision is made over the entire eighth left rib
and continued upward over the posterior end of the seventh, sixth and fifth
ribs. After removing the eighth rib, short segments of the posterior end of
the seventh, sixth and fifth ribs are removed and the intercostal vessels

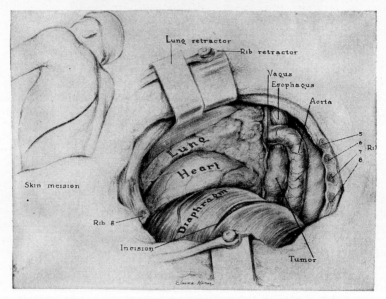

FIG. 161b. Drawing showing skin incision over the entire course of the eighth rib and
extending upward over the posterior end of the seventh, sixth, fifth and fourth ribs.
After resecting the entire eighth rib subperiosteally and a ½-inch segment of the seventh,
sixth and fifth ribs posteriorly the pleural cavity was entered along this line. With an
automatic rib spreader in place and the lung retracted, excellent exposure is obtained.
(From Adams, *Surg. Clin. N. Amer.*, Chicago Number, 1946. Courtesy of W. B. Saunders Co.)

divided and ligated. The pleura is opened along the line of this incision and
by use of a rib spreader very adequate exposure of the postero-lateral aspect
of the chest extending above the arch of the aorta is obtained (Fig. 161b).
The esophagus is mobilized from above the arch of the aorta downward to
the stomach. After opening the diaphragm from the costal arch to the esophageal hiatus, the stomach is mobilized from the surrounding structures by
division of the left gastric artery. The spleen is frequently removed to
facilitate the technical procedure. The stomach is then further mobilized by
dividing the vessels along its greater curvature just outside of the main
course of the gastro-epiploic artery, care being taken to preserve the blood

supply through this artery as much as possible. The mobilization is carried out far enough to allow the stomach to be elevated to a point above the arch of the aorta. The esophagus is then divided at its junction with the cardia, and the cardiac end of the stomach is closed by two rows of sutures. The esophagus and tumor are then elevated from behind the arch of the aorta

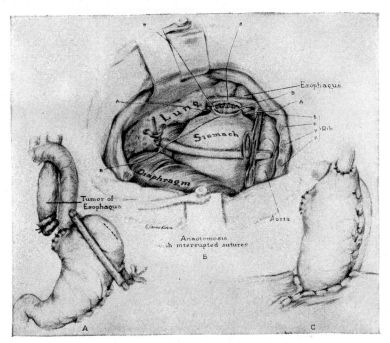

Fig. 161c. (A) The lower two-thirds of the thoracic esophagus and the upper four-fifths of the stomach have been mobilized and the esophagus divided at the cardiac end of the stomach. (B) Rubber-shod clamps have been placed across the fundus of the stomach and the upper cut end of the esophagus in preparation for the anastomosis. The posterior part of the outer row of interrupted sutures has been placed as indicated at A, and the posterior portion of the inner row of interrupted sutures has also been placed as indicated at B. (C) The anastomosis between the upper cut end of the esophagus and fundus of the stomach has been completed at a level just above the arch of the aorta. The diaphragm has been approximated about the stomach with interrupted sutures. (From Adams, *Surg. Clin. N. Amer.*, Chicago Number, 1946. Courtesy of W. B. Saunders Co.)

and the stomach is brought up for the anastomosis. The procedure from this point onward is the same as that described for the resection for carcinoma at the gastro-esophageal junction (Fig. 161c).

In view of the fact that following this operation the stomach may occupy a large part of the left pleural cavity, additional care must be exercised to maintain adequate respiratory function (Fig. 161d). At times through the swallowing of air the stomach may become dilated and may compress not only the lung of the same side but may reduce the function of the opposite lung as well. Thus during the first few days following operation the complication of atelectasis and pneumonitis must be anticipated. As experience was gained with this type of operation for carcinoma located near the arch of the aorta an increasing number of successful cases was reported. At the present time the procedure of resection and gastro-esophagostomy is preferable to the Torek operation. Complications following the operation are probably

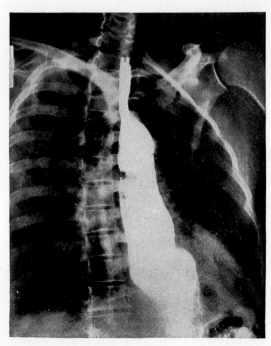

Fig. 161d. Postoperative x-ray following ingestion of barium and showing approximately four-fifths of the stomach brought up into the pleural cavity for anastomosis with the upper esophagus following resection of the carcinoma. The anastomosis is shown just below the substernal notch. (From Adams, *Surg. Clin. N. Amer.*, Chicago Number, 1946. Courtesy of W. B. Saunders Co.)

no more common than following the Torek operation and the patient has the definite advantage of being able to swallow ingested food in the normal manner. The mortality for the operation is probably very little more than for resection of tumors at the gastro-esophageal junction.

REFERENCES

1. ADAMS, W. E., ESCUDERO, L., ARONSOHN, H. G., and SHAW, M. M. Resection of the Thoracic Esophagus, *J. Thoracic Surg.*, 7:605-620, 1938.
2. HAIGHT, CAMERON. Congenital Atresia of the Esophagus with Tracheo-esophageal Fistula, *Ann. Surg.*, 120:623-655, 1944.
3. NEUHOF, HAROLD and JEMERIN, EDWARD E. *Acute Infections of the Mediastinum*, The Williams and Wilkins Company, Baltimore, Maryland.
4. HARRINGTON, STUART W. Pulsion Diverticulum of the Hypopharynx at the Pharyngo-esophageal Junction, *Surgery*, 18:66-81, 1945.

5. CLARK, DWIGHT E. and ADAMS, W. E.   Transthoracic Esophagogastrostomy for Benign Strictures of the Lower Esophagus, *Ann. Surg.*, 122:942-952, 1945.

6. SCOTT, W. J. MERLE.   Idiopathic Dilatation of the Esophagus, *Ann. Surg.*, 122:582-605, 1945.

7. HARRINGTON, STUART W. and MOERSCH, HERMAN J.   Surgical Treatment and Clinical Manifestations of Benign Tumors of the Esophagus with Report of Seven Cases, *J. Thoracic Surg.*, 13:394-415, 1944.

8. WOOKEY, HAROLD.   The Surgical Treatment of Carcinoma of the Pharynx and Upper Esophagus, *Surg., Gynec. & Obst.*, 75:499-506, 1942.

9. PHEMISTER, DALLAS B.   Transthoracic Resection for Cancer of the Cardiac End of the Stomach, *Arch. Surg.*, 46:915-929, 1943.

10. CHURCHILL, E. D. and SWEET, R. H.   Transthoracic Resection of Tumors of the Stomach and Esophagus, *Ann. Surg.*, 115:897, 1942.

11. ADAMS, W. E.   Some Recent Accomplishments of Thoracic Surgery, *Arch. Surg.*, 50:277-285, 1945.

12. ADAMS, W. E. and PHEMISTER, DALLAS B.   Carcinoma of the Lower Thoracic Esophagus. Report of a Successful Resection and Esophagogastrostomy, *J. Thoracic Surg.*, 7:621-632, 1938.

13. TOREK, F.   The First Successful case of Resection of the Thoracic Esophagus, *Surg., Gynec. & Obst.*, 16:614, 1913; *Idem. Arch. Surg.*, 10:328, 1925.

14. GARLOCK, J. H.   Re-establishment of Esophagogastric Continuity following Resection of Esophagus for Carcinoma of Middle Third, *Surg., Gynec. & Obst.*, 78:23-28, 1944.

8

ABDOMINAL INCISIONS

Frederick A. Coller, M.D. and Kenneth F. MacLean, M.D.

ANATOMY AND PHYSIOLOGY

Any discussion of abdominal incisions must, of necessity, be based upon a number of anatomical and physiological considerations. For this reason the anatomy and physiology of the abdominal wall will be reviewed. Only the practical anatomical points, which must be considered by the surgeon, who would enter the peritoneal cavity by the method which will produce the least possible damage to the abdominal wall, but still permit him to obtain optimum exposure, will be discussed.

Skin. Langer's lines of skin cleavage (Fig. 162) cross the anterior abdominal wall in a generally transverse direction. It is well recognized that skin incisions made parallel to these lines of cleavage result in much finer and firmer scars than do those which are made transverse to them. While the cosmetic end result of abdominal incisions may be of little practical importance, (except in rare instances), the fact remains that the careful surgeon desires to obtain the best possible appearance of the operative scar which he has produced. For this reason, other factors being equal, it is deemed best to make abdominal incisions parallel to, rather than across Langer's lines.

Subcutaneous Tissue. The subcutaneous fat, which is variable in amount, is contained within the areolar meshes of Camper's fascia. The deeper layer of fascia (Scarpa's fascia) is a more membranous layer and is separated from the underlying muscles and aponeuroses by areolar tissue; it contains a considerable number of elastic fibers. Both of these layers have a relatively poor blood supply, particularly when there is a heavy panniculus of fat, and for this reason are slow to heal and prone to become infected easily. Scarpa's fascia, being a definite fascial layer presents the only layer in the abdominal wall subcutaneous tissues which can readily be sutured.

Muscle and Aponeuroses. The muscles of the anterior abdominal wall may be divided into the flat or oblique muscles (external oblique, internal oblique, and transversus abdominis), and the anterior group (recti and variable pyramidalis). The fibers of the latter group run vertically while the former run in an essentially transverse direction.

The external oblique takes origin from the anterolateral aspects of the lower eight ribs. The muscle fibers from the lower two ribs pass almost vertically downward and insert into the anterior half of the iliac crest without becoming aponeurotic. The posterior border of the muscle is free. The

314

fibers from the sixth to the tenth ribs become aponeurotic along a line drawn from the ninth costal cartilage vertically downward to the level of the umbilicus, and then inclining laterally to the anterior-superior iliac spine. The uppermost aponeurotic fibers pass almost transversely but inferiorly they assume a progressively more oblique downward course. These aponeurotic fibers, together with the anterior fibers of the internal oblique aponeurosis, form the anterior sheath of the rectus muscle and insert into the linea alba throughout its length.

Contrary to the common description, however, the fibers of the external oblique aponeurosis do not fuse with the anterior fibers of internal oblique at the lateral border of the rectus muscle; on the contrary the fibers of external oblique may readily be separated from those of the internal oblique for a variable distance over the rectus, occasionally almost to the linea alba. This is particularly true below the umbilicus. Inferiorly the external oblique aponeurosis enters into the formation of the inguinal ligament and external inguinal ring which need not be discussed in this section.

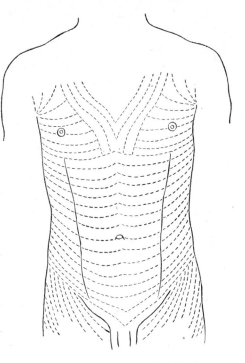

FIG. 162. Langer's lines of skin cleavage. Note the generally transverse direction in which they run.

The internal oblique arises from the lumbodorsal fascia, anterior two-thirds of the iliac crest and the lateral half of the inguinal ligament. The lowermost fibers (from the inguinal ligament) arch downward and medially to enter into the formation of the conjoined tendon. The most posterior fibers pass upward and insert into the lower three ribs without becoming aponeurotic. The remaining fibers (from inguinal ligament and iliac crest) run transversely in the lower abdomen and then, superiorly, they run upward and medially. The muscle fibers become aponeurotic at the lateral border of the rectus throughout its length. These aponeurotic fibers almost immediately split into two lamellae. The anterior lamella passes in front of the rectus muscle and inserts into the linea alba throughout its length. The posterior fibers pass behind the rectus muscle, blend with the aponeurotic fibers of transversus abdominis and insert into the linea alba. The uppermost aponeurotic fibers of the posterior lamella insert into the seventh, eighth and ninth costal cartilages. At a point 3 to 5 cms. below the umbilicus all of the internal oblique (and transversus abdominis) aponeurotic fibers pass anterior to the rectus muscle thus leaving the posterior sheath of rectus deficient below this level. The posterior sheath thus terminates at a line which is usually found 3 to 5 cms. below the umbilicus but may vary from just above the pubes to as high as the umbilicus: [9] this is named the semicircular line of Douglas (Fig. 163).

The transversus abdominis lies deep to the internal oblique and its lower origin is practically the same as that muscle. In addition it takes origin from the lumbodorsal fascia up to the level of the twelfth rib and from the inner surface of the lower six ribs, interdigitating with the diaphragmatic attachment. The lowermost fibers pass downward and medially joining with the fibers of internal oblique to form conjoined tendon. The remaining muscle fibers pass transversely and become aponeurotic as follows: at and below the umbilicus the muscle fibers become aponeurotic at the lateral border of the rectus muscle; at the xiphoid process (Fig. 163) the transition from muscle to aponeurosis does not occur until a distance 2 to 4 cms. from the linea alba is reached; from this point the transitional line gradually passes laterally until at the umbilicus the muscle fibers become aponeurotic at the lateral border of rectus. It may readily be seen then that, above the umbilicus, the lateral portion of posterior rectus sheath is formed only by the posterior lamella of the internal oblique aponeurosis; this deficiency produces an inherent weakness in closure of incisions in this region, particularly those which pass vertically through the lateral rectus sheaths. Having become aponeurotic the fibers of transversus pass behind the rectus muscle, fuse with the posterior lamella of internal oblique and insert into linea alba. Below the semicircular line of Douglas the fibers all pass anterior to the rectus muscle and insert into linea alba.

While the direction of the fibers of external and internal obliques is somewhat at an angle to the transverse plane this angle never becomes more than 30 degrees.[1] The upward and lateral pull of the external oblique is balanced by the downward and lateral pull of the internal oblique thus producing a component which, (when both muscles are contracting—as in expiration), is transverse in direction. The action of the transversus is to pull in a truly transverse direction.

The rectus sheath is commonly described (and thought of by surgeons) as a separate entity in the abdominal wall, the sole purpose of which is to enclose the rectus muscles. In reality it is formed by the aponeurotic fibers of the three flat muscles. These aponeurotic fibers are best thought of as the "little tendons" [2] of the flat muscles which insert into the linea alba and take their point of action in that structure. Thus the fibers of the rectus sheaths run transversely and a vertical incision through one or both layers of the sheath, or through the linea alba, must cut across the multiple tendons of the flat muscles. It is also worthy of note that, below the semicircular line of Douglas, the posterior rectus sheath is deficient and the rectus muscle is separated from peritoneum only by the deep epigastric vessels, transversalis fascia and preperitoneal connective tissue. McVay and Anson [9] have pointed out the wide variations in the manner in which the oblique muscle

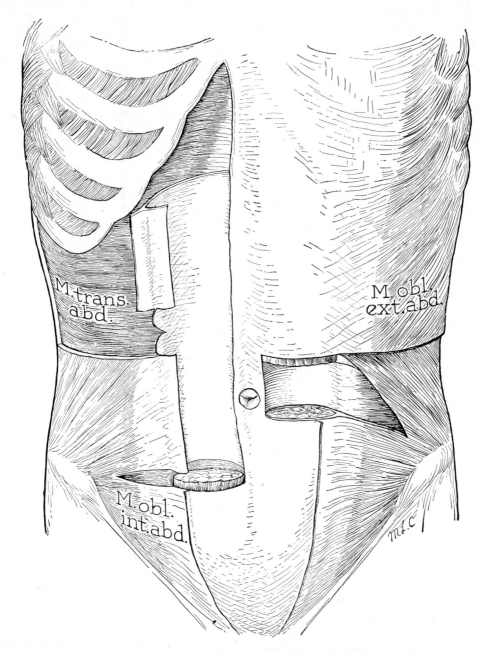

FIG. 163. The muscles and aponeuroses of the anterior abdominal wall. The semicircular line of Douglas is seldom as well visualized as is diagrammatically represented here. Note how far medially the upper transversus abdominis muscle fibers pass before becoming aponeurotic. (From Rees and Coller, *Arch. Surg.,* 47:136-146, [Aug.], 1943.)

aponeuroses split to form the rectus sheath. For all practical purposes, however, the sheath may be considered to be formed essentially as described above. They have also pointed out that the semicircular line of Douglas varies widely in its position. It may be found as high as the umbilicus; on the other hand, it is occasionally found immediately above the pubis or in any intermediate position between the two.

The linea semilunaris are two curved lines corresponding to the lateral border of the rectus muscles and marking the point at which the muscle fibers of internal oblique become aponeurotic and split (above the semicircular line of Douglas) to enclose the rectus. Above the umbilicus this line also marks the point at which the muscle fibers of external oblique become aponeurotic while below the umbilicus the same is true of transversus abdominis.

The rectus muscles attach below to the os pubis and ligaments covering the symphysis pubis. Above they insert into the xiphoid cartilage, and anterior surfaces of the fifth, sixth and seventh ribs. The muscle is thick and narrow below, thin and broad above. The superior attachment is 3 to 4 times as broad as the pubic insertion, a fact which is seldom realized until the surgeon finds that a transverse incision in the upper abdomen frequently extends laterally almost to the anterior axillary line without passing out of the rectus muscle. The medial borders of the rectus muscles are separated by the linea alba which is formed by the decussation of fibers of insertion of the flat muscles. Three (occasionally four) transverse tendinous inscriptions are found in each rectus muscle. One is commonly located at or near the umbilicus while two more are equally spaced between the umbilicus and the costal attachments of the muscles. When more than three lineae transversae are present, the additional ones are equally distributed below the umbilicus. These tendinous insertions are intimately fused with the anterior sheath of the rectus but, since they occupy only the anterior half of the muscle, they are not attached to the posterior sheath. It is apparent then that the rectus muscle is firmly adherent to the anterior rectus sheath above the umbilicus (and occasionally below). Posteriorly, however, the rectus muscle is easily separated from the posterior sheath. Because of these firm tendinous attachments of the rectus muscles to the anterior sheath there can be only minimal retraction of the rectus muscle fibers when they are cut transversely; this is particularly true above the umbilicus where tendinous inscriptions are constant.

The pyramidalis muscles attach below to the os pubis. They are of triangular shape, muscular throughout and insert by their apices into the linea alba midway between the symphysis pubis and umbilicus. They lie within the rectus sheath, anterior to the rectus muscles. They are frequently absent and play little part in abdominal incisions or their closure.

Transversalis Fascia and Peritoneum. Transversalis fascia is a thin membrane which lies between the under surface of the transversus muscle and the preperitoneal connective tissue. In the inguinal region it is relatively dense but above it gradually thins out and blends with the fascia on the under surface of the diaphragm. Beneath that portion of the transversus abdominis which is muscular this fascia presents a clear cut and readily separable layer. Beneath the rectus sheath itself, however, it blends with the aponeurotic fibers of transversus abdominis and in this region cannot be defined as a clear cut layer. It has been shown by careful dissections [9] that below the semicircular line of Douglas the transversalis fascia splits; part of it passes anterior to the rectus blending with the aponeurosis of transversus abdominis while the remainder passes behind the muscle to reach the linea alba. These posterior fibers of transversalis fascia are frequently joined by a few aponeurotic fibers of transversus abdominis. In addition it is frequently noted [9] that preperitoneal connective tissue below the semicircular line becomes a nonfatty membranous layer which may be mistaken for transversalis fascia. From the above discussion it may be seen that below the semicircular line of Douglas there is commonly a definite membranous layer which blends above with the posterior rectus sheath. For this reason the semicircular line of Douglas is seldom visualized as the clear cut crescentic lower border of posterior rectus sheath as is so often illustrated.

The peritoneum needs little description here. It is worthy of note, however, that it is closely adherent to posterior rectus sheath and linea alba; for this reason closure of the peritoneum and posterior rectus sheath as separate layers is impractical. For the same reason, closure of the peritoneum beneath the posterior rectus sheath is influenced by the same factors which pertain to the posterior sheath. Faulty closure of the posterior sheath, or separation after closure, necessarily associates itself with comparable defects in the peritoneum. Beneath the oblique muscles, on the other hand, peritoneum is readily separated from the muscles and consequently can be closed as a separate layer.

Nerve Supply (Fig. 164). The anterior abdominal muscles receive their nerve supply from the lower six intercostal and first lumbar nerves. The intercostals do not, as commonly described, run as single trunks. Davies [3,4] and Rees and Coller [1] after careful anatomical dissections have shown that, while still running in the intercostal spaces, these nerves exist as several (usually three) branches. These branches intercommunicate one with the other in the same intercostal space and from one intercostal space to the one above and below; the latter communications pass deep to the rib. These branches unite at the outer end of the intercostal space to form a single trunk. The sixth, seventh, eighth and ninth trunks then pass beneath the costal arch and enter the abdominal wall between the transversus abdominis and internal oblique. The trunks of the tenth, eleventh and twelfth intercostal nerves pass forward between the rib ends and enter the same layer of the abdominal wall. The anterior branch of the iliohypogastric nerve pierces the internal oblique 2 cms. medial to the anterior-superior spine and runs forward and downward beneath the external oblique aponeurosis. This nerve is frequently encountered in incisions of the lower abdomen; its injury, which denervates the lower fibers of internal oblique and transversus abdominis has been blamed for the occurrence of hernia following abdominal operations. While running forward between transversus abdominis and the internal oblique a further rich anastomosis [1] occurs between the intercostal nerves and between the twelfth intercostal and the iliohypogastric nerves. Upon reaching the lateral border of the rectus sheath the nerves pierce the sheath and fan out transversely beneath the rectus muscle, being distributed to its deep surface.

Because of the rich anastomosis between the intercostal nerves both in the intercostal spaces and in the abdominal wall it is possible to cut two, and sometimes even three, of the nerves without noticeable loss of function. It is apparent, however, that the nearer to the spinal cord the nerve is cut the greater is the chance of function being taken over by adjacent nerves through distal anastomoses. It is also worthy of note that once the nerves have reached the lateral border of rectus muscle little if any anastomosis occurs. For this reason any incision which passes vertically through the rectus muscle or through its lateral border, must denervate that portion of the muscle medial to the incision. On the other hand transverse incisions through the rectus muscle result in the least possible damage to its nerve supply.

The ninth intercostal nerve passes across the abdominal wall in a transverse direction at a point approximately one-third of the distance between the umbilicus and the xiphoid process. Above this point the nerves tend to run in an upward direction while below the ninth they run in a progressively downward direction. In the intercostal spaces, and as they pass beneath the costal arch the nerves are firmly fixed; in the abdominal wall, however, they are not so fixed and retraction in one direction or the other is usually feasible without injuring them. Incisions lateral to the rectus muscle which are the least likely to injure the nerves should, ideally, run down and outward in the upper abdomen, transversely at or just above the umbilicus and up and outward below the umbilicus. Such ideal incisions are not always, for other reasons, practical but the transverse types of incisions most nearly approximate this ideal. Furthermore transverse incisions encounter the nerves laterally where they are mobile and can be retracted; also if injured in the lateral abdominal wall the function of any given nerve is more apt to be taken over by anastomotic branches which lie more anterior and medially; such is not the case when they are injured near the rectus muscle.

It has been the repeated experience of surgeons [5] to note, following vertical incisions through the rectus muscle or its lateral border, weakness and bulging of the abdominal wall medial to the incision. This is undoubtedly due to denervation of that part of the muscle medial to the incision. Others [6] have noted deviation of the umbilicus to the side opposite vertical rectus incisions, undoubtedly for the same reason. Quain,[7] in experimental animals, denervated the peritoneum of one side but left the opposite side intact. Trauma and irritation were applied equally to the normal and the denervated peritoneum and he found that there was decreased resistance of the denervated peritoneum to the trauma as manifested by increased adhesions and poorer healing. It has been the experience of many surgeons to note,

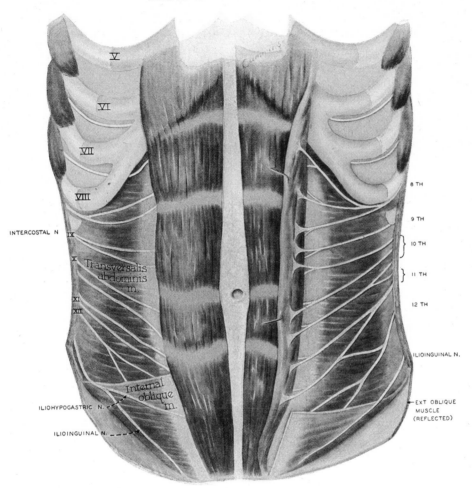

FIG. 164. Nerve supply of the abdominal wall. The anastomosis between nerves in the abdominal wall is frequently even richer than is illustrated here. The transverse tendinous inscriptions, which attach the anterior rectus sheath to the muscle are well shown here. (From Rees and Coller, *Arch Surg.*, 47:136-146, [Aug.], 1943.)

similarly, that adhesions are more frequent and extensive beneath the vertical incision than beneath the transverse. The possibility that this is due to decreased resistance of the denervated peritoneum, as well as to other factors (peritoneal separation in particular) must be considered. Bancroft [8] has pointed out that the incidence of postoperative abdominal neuromas and neuritis is more frequent than is usually believed. These cause pain and may be the seat of difficulty for years. It is apparent then, for the above reasons, that every effort should be made to avoid nerves whenever possible and to damage them as little as possible by cutting or stretching when they are encountered. The transverse incision serves best in this respect.

Blood Supply. The main blood supply to the anterior abdominal wall is derived from the superior and inferior epigastric arteries. The former is one of the terminal branches of the internal mammary artery while the latter is a branch of the external iliac. These two vessels lie posterior to the rectus muscles. There is a rich anastomosis between the two blood vessels. The remainder of the blood supply comes from the deep circumflex iliacs, intercostals and lumbar arteries, all of which enter into the anastomosis mentioned above. The inferior epigastric provides the largest single blood supply and frequently must be transected in transverse incisions in the lower abdomen; the anastomotic blood supply is so rich, however, that no danger is attendant upon this procedure. There is very little anastomosis across the midline and the linea alba is provided with the poorest blood supply of any area in the abdominal wall, a fact which undoubtedly contributes to the higher incidence of hernia and disruption through vertical midline incisions.

Function of the abdominal musculature need not be discussed in detail, however certain pertinent points, particularly as they relate to alteration of intra-abdominal pressure, deserve mention. The rectus muscles, attaching to bony points above and below as they do, play a strong role in splinting of the abdominal wall (a protective mechanism) and also in flexion of the chest and abdomen on the pelvis as in arising from the supine position. The recti also play a part in alteration of intra-abdominal pressure but this function is predominantly exerted by the oblique muscles by virtue of their origin laterally and posteriorly and insertion into the midline linea alba which is not a fixed point. The oblique muscles practically encircle the abdomen and by their contraction draw the linea alba posteriorly, decrease the circumference of the abdomen and compress the abdominal contents. During inspiration the diaphragm descends, accounting for 60 per cent of the air breathed [10] while the oblique muscles relax to compensate for this increase in intra-abdominal volume. In expiration the diaphragm relaxes while the abdominal muscles (particularly the obliques) contract, increase intra-abdominal pressure and force the diaphragm up. Strong contraction of the oblique muscles is necessary not only during expiration, but also during the acts of coughing, vomiting and defecation. In the latter instances both diaphragm and abdominal muscles contract vigorously and the intra-abdominal pressure is raised. It must also be noted that in inspiration the lower rib margins (seventh to tenth) swing up and outward (in order to increase the transverse diameter of the thoracic cavity) thus increasing the subcostal angle. This increase in the subcostal angle places tension on the rectus sheath and linea alba in a transverse direction. Vertical incisions in the linea alba or rectus sheath transect the "little tendons" of the oblique muscles which are not only under tension during expiration but which are subjected to additional tension in the upper abdomen as the rib margins flare up and outward. The predominance of the part played by the oblique muscles in respiration (and it must be great in coughing, vomiting or defecation) is well illustrated by the work of Sloan.[11] By attaching spring balances to mouth tooth forceps which in turn were attached to the abdominal aponeuroses, he was able to measure the force necessary to hold the edges of various types of incisions together with the patient under light general anesthesia. In a series of 20 cases in which an L shaped incision was employed, one side of which was vertical and the other transverse, the lateral force necessary to approximate the edges of the vertical limb was in every case 30 times greater than the vertical force necessary to bring the edges of the transverse limb together. In addition he noted that the longer the vertical incision the greater the force necessary to bring the edges together. "The force required increased in proportion to the square of the length of the incision. If the incision is lengthened to five inches it will require 45 pounds pull on each side to hold the edges of the incision together." * It becomes apparent then that the transverse incision is physiological in that it does not transect the fibers of the muscle aponeuroses which play such a predominant role in alterations of intra-abdominal pressure. The transverse incision runs parallel to these aponeurotic fibers; when these fibers are under tension the edges of the transverse wound tend to be approximated while the edges of the vertical incision are strongly separated. Any surgeon who has closed vertical incisions, with the patient straining under light anesthesia, must remember the extreme difficulty with which the peritoneum and posterior rectus sheath is closed; frequently this closure is so difficult that the peritoneum is shredded and the surgeon is forced to wonder how long the closure will stand up to the tension brought on by postoperative coughing or vomiting. Similar difficulty in closure is not encountered with the transverse incision, a fact which permits of lighter anesthesia than is possible when vertical incisions are used. Partial separation of the peritoneal closure must, in part at least, account for the high incidence of adhesions beneath vertical incisions.

HISTORY OF ABDOMINAL INCISIONS

Since the brilliant work of Pasteur and Lister made modern surgery possible it has been the custom of most surgeons to open the abdomen through various types of vertical incisions. At first only midline incisions through the linea alba were utilized and this is understandable since such an incision involves the cutting of only one almost avascular aponeurotic layer;

* Sloan, G. A., *Surg., Gynec. & Obst.*, 45:678-687, Nov., 1927. By permission of Surgery, Gynecology and Obstetrics.

opening and closure was thus made the simplest possible procedure. Subsequently other types of vertical incisions were developed and, even today, probably the majority of laparotomies are performed through one or the other of these vertical incisions. The reasons for the widespread use of the vertical incision are apparent. First, it is easier and more rapidly fashioned than any other type of incision, primarily because it does not cut across any major blood supply, nor does it transect muscle fibers. The vertical incision also allows for greater freedom of extension; an upper abdominal incision can, in the event of incorrect diagnosis, be extended from costal margin to pubes. Thus almost any portion of the peritoneal cavity is available through extension of the one incision. This consideration was of the greater importance in the earlier days of surgery, when exact diagnosis was frequently impossible, than it is in this day of modern and more exact diagnosis.

From the earliest days there has been strong prejudice against cutting across the fibers of any muscle and this is particularly true of the rectus muscle which stands out so prominently in the abdominal wall. It has long been thought that transection of any muscle violates a basic surgical principle; this feeling stems primarily from the fact that transection of most muscles (*e.g.* the biceps brachii) results in denervation of the distal portion of that muscle. As has been pointed out this is not true of the rectus for it receives its nerve supply in a segmental manner; these nerves pass across the muscle hence the transverse incision, which transects the muscle fibers, runs parallel to these nerves and is least likely to damage them. It is often stated that the rectus muscle should not be transected because it will retract thus leaving an irreparable defect which will weaken the abdominal wall. The rectus, however, is firmly attached to the anterior sheath by the lineae transversae above (and occasionally below) the umbilicus. It has been the repeated experience of surgeons that the rectus muscle does not retract beyond the edges of the sheath when it is transected; in fact the muscle remains protruding beyond the cut ends of the sheath [12] and when the latter is closed the muscle ends are approximated. Rosenblatt [13] has shown, in dogs, that the transected rectus, when approximated only by closure of the sheath, heals as a thin transverse scar comparable to an additional linea transversus. Others [2] have confirmed this finding in humans by observation of a similar thin scar in the rectus muscle when operating through old transverse incisions.

Another reason for the almost universal use of the vertical types of incisions, particularly in the upper abdomen, was the ready access it gave to the epigastric region. Approach to this region is somewhat more difficult through a transverse type of incision, particularly when a narrow subcostal angle is encountered. The transverse incision gives superior exposure for the vast majority of upper abdominal operations. On occasion, however, particularly when extensive gastric surgery is undertaken, insufficient exposure is obtained. In such instances, as described below, a vertical limb may be added to the transverse incision with resultant exposure which is superior to that afforded by any vertical incision.

For many years the vertical incision was the predominant choice of the vast majority of surgeons. With the passage of years, the accumulation of more surgical experience, better anesthesia and more exact diagnosis, more and more surgeons have been advocating the use of transverse incisions or their modifications. The day of the laparotomy which was usually emergency in nature and had to be done under poor anesthesia with the diagnosis obscure and the patient poorly prepared, (thus necessitating rapid surgery) is becoming a memory of the heroic past. A brief review of the history of abdominal incisions will contribute to an understanding of the basic types of incisions and the reasons for which they were advocated.

McBurney[14] in 1894 was the first to wander from the fold of those who used vertical incisions for operations for appendicitis. He advocated the muscle splitting incision which is universally known by his name today and which is described below. Battle[15] in 1895 countered with his incision which consisted of a vertical incision 1 cm. to 2 cms. medial to the lateral border of rectus; anterior and posterior sheaths of rectus were opened in this line and the rectus muscle retracted medially. He claimed to reduce the incidence of hernia due to the fact that intact rectus muscle was interposed between the two sheath incisions. Kammerer[16] in 1897 described an incision essentially the same as Battle's; at first he cut the branch of the iliohypogastric nerve which entered the rectus sheath but later preserved the nerve because he had noted postoperative weakness and atrophy of the rectus muscle when the nerve had been cut. In the discussion of Kammerer's presentation Weir, Meyer and others agreed that the McBurney incision did not offer enough room for the "suppurative cases" of appendicitis and furthermore they brought out the fact that any vertical incision was too far medial for any case of appendicitis in which the appendix lay lateral to the cecum. Meyer in the same discussion suggested modifying the McBurney incision by adding a vertical limb (either up or downward) in the linea semilunaris whenever additional exposure was needed. Elliot[17] in 1896 was the first to describe a true transverse incision of the skin which he carried down through the fibers of external oblique aponeurosis (thus cutting obliquely across the fibers of external oblique); he then split fibers of internal oblique and transversus as in the McBurney. He also advocated extension up or downward in the linea semilunaris for additional exposure. Harrington[18] in 1899 and Weir[19] in 1890 both pleaded for more room on occasion and to obtain it used the McBurney incision but extended it transversely across the anterior and posterior rectus sheaths, retracting the rectus muscle medially. This modification of the McBurney incision has come to be known as the Weir modification despite the fact that Harrington described it earlier. Rockey[20] in 1905 and Davis[21] in 1906 independently described a transverse skin incision similar to that previously brought out by Elliot. Rockey utilized the McBurney type of muscle splitting and extension up or downward in the linea semilunaris as necessary. Davis continued the true transverse incision through the external oblique aponeurosis as did Elliot but for additional exposure he advocated the Harrington or Weir type of extension.

Two basic types of muscle splitting incisions differing only in the skin incision have evolved for appendiceal surgery. These are the McBurney and the Rockey or Davis (which more justly should be called the Elliot) incisions. These incisions have been widely accepted although some surgeons still prefer the vertical incision of one type or the other through the rectus, particularly in females when the diagnosis is in doubt and extension inferiorly for pelvic surgery is considered as a possible necessity. On the other hand many feel that a muscle splitting incision provides adequate exposure for this purpose particularly when it is extended across the right rectus as can so readily be done. In addition the muscle splitting incision permits of ready extension laterally and upward, a step which is of great value when the appendix lies retrocecally or is lateral to the cecum. It is also now well recognized that no vertical type of incision can center over the appendix; this inadequacy of the vertical incision must lead to unnecessary contamination of the peritoneum when the suppurative appendix is drawn toward the midline. Division of limiting adhesions and the inflammatory wall about the appendix is also frequently necessary with the vertical incision.

Baudelocque[22] prior to 1847 was the first to describe a transverse incision of any type; this he advocated in the lower abdomen for use in Caesarian section. Pfannensteil,[23] however, in 1900 was the first to popularize its use in pelvic surgery. His incision, which is described below, has met favor with many gynecologists although some claim that it does not provide sufficient exposure; in such instances the rectus muscles may be transected, preferably through their tendinous lower portions as advocated by Cherney[24] in 1941. The same basic anatomical and physiological factors which apply to the rectus muscles and sheaths above the umbilicus are applicable to lower abdominal incisions despite the absence of lineae transversae and the deficiency of the posterior sheath below the semicircular line of Douglas. For additional exposure, an increasing number of surgeons have been using the true transverse incision of all layers. We have transected one or both recti in the lower abdomen in a large number of cases and have never seen harm come of this procedure despite the fact that there is a slight tendency for the muscle ends to retract beneath the ends of the sheath.

Maylard[25] in 1907 was the first to describe transverse incisions for upper abdominal surgery. In 1899 he had opened the abdomen for exploration of the stomach through an "L" shaped incision, one limb of which was transverse through all layers and the other vertical in the linea alba. He subsequently had to reopen through the same incision for gastric hemorrhage. Later he noted herniation through the vertical limb while the transverse limb healed soundly without herniation. It was this experience which stimulated his interest in transverse incisions. Subsequently other surgeons, notably Farr[12,26] and Sprengle (as quoted by Farr) have noted similar experiences with "L" shaped incisions, one limb of which was vertical and the other transverse; i.e. they have noted herniation through the vertical limb while the transverse component healed soundly. Following Maylard's description of the transverse incision of all layers, including the rectus muscles, many surgeons have written advocating some type of transverse incision for upper abdominal surgery.[32,71-76] Most of these surgeons advocated the transverse incision (essentially as described below) through all layers, including the rectus muscles, for surgery of the upper midabdomen. Most agree that it is not necessary to fix the rectus muscle to the sheath by mattress stitches (as advocated by Sprengle) and have noted perfect healing of the rectus muscle on reopening the abdomen through the same incision at a later date. All of these writers also agree that the transverse incision affords excellent exposure, involves less nerve damage, closes easier, heals more readily and is much less painful postoperatively than the vertical incision.

Sloan [11] in 1927 advocated a transverse type of incision in the upper abdomen but felt that the rectus muscles should not be transected. He described a vertical midline upper abdominal skin incision; both anterior rectus sheaths were then cut vertically near their medial borders, the rectus muscles freed from the sheath and retracted laterally. The posterior sheath and linea alba, as well as peritoneum, were then incised transversely. Singleton [27] modified this incision by using a transverse skin incision and incised the left anterior rectus sheath transversely, otherwise his incision was the same as Sloan's. Sanders [28] offered a further modification of the Sloan incision as described below. Many writers feel that this type of incision, which is designed to spare the rectus muscles, requires too lengthy a dissection and opens large fascial planes in the abdominal wall while limiting the exposure. Little harm comes from transection of the recti, by which means exposure is improved and extensive planes are not opened up for possible involvement by infection. Otherwise the Sloan incision and particularly the Sanders' modification is sound since it cuts the rectus sheath in the line of the aponeurotic fibers.

In 1917 Meyer [29] advocated a flap type of incision for upper abdominal work of all types which could be made in either of two ways. The Koenig, Kehr [30,31] incision has a vertical limb which passes through all layers at the medial border of the rectus extending down to the umbilicus from which point a transverse limb (of all layers) extended to the anterior axillary line. The other was the Perthes [32] incision in which similar vertical and transverse limbs are made as described above but extend only to the posterior rectus sheath; the flap so formed is then reflected laterally until the nerves entering the rectus sheath are visualized. An oblique incision extending downward and laterally is then made and includes posterior sheath and peritoneum; this portion of the incision is subcostal. He claimed excellent exposure, particularly for gallbladder on the right or stomach on the left. In addition no nerves were cut and the closure he felt was strong. Others have advocated flap type of incisions and, as described below, we do not hesitate to add a vertical limb to the transverse incision when necessary, although it is not used routinely.

Various other modifications of upper abdominal incisions have been described. Some [33,36] need not be described here while others have been sufficiently popular, particularly in years past, to warrant a brief description.

Kocher [34] in 1903 advocated an oblique incision 4 to 6 cms. below and parallel to the right costal margin; the anterior right rectus sheath was incised in the same line and the rectus muscle "notched." The fibers of the flat muscles were divided at the lateral border of the rectus, the nerves being retracted in so doing. Transversalis fascia and peritoneum were opened in the same line. This incision was to be 4 inches long and was intended primarily for gallbladder operations. It is necessary to point out, however, that the incision runs at right angles to the course of the intercostal nerves and is almost impossible to fashion without damaging them.

MacArthur [35] in 1915 described an incision solely for gallbladder surgery in which skin and anterior rectus sheath were incised vertically, the rectus muscle was split in its midline and retracted and the posterior sheath and peritoneum incised transversely. The same basic objection is offered here, namely that insufficient exposure can be obtained without damaging nerves.

The Mayo-Robson incision [37] described in 1903 and that of Mayo [38] which was brought out in 1938 are described below. Singleton in 1939 described a "lateral transverse" incision for operations on the gallbladder [39] and in 1940 he described a similar type of incision for splenectomy.[40] Since the two incisions are essentially the same they are described together below. From the historical review above it may be seen that every conceivable type of incision has been described for abdominal surgery. These incisions all may be divided into the two great groups of vertical or transverse although many modifications of each have been proposed.

DESCRIPTION (TECHNIC) OF INCISIONS

For all practical purposes abdominal incisions may be divided into the following groups: (1) upper midabdominal; (2) upper subcostal (right or left); (3) midabdominal (right or left); (4) lower quadrants (right or left); (5) lower midabdominal (pelvic).

The details of surgical technic, asepsis, the handling of tissues, suture materials, etc., have been discussed elsewhere in this text and will not be considered here except as they specifically pertain to abdominal incisions. In each instance that incision used and favored by us will be described first, thereafter other types of incisions will be considered.

Upper Midabdominal Incisions. TRANSVERSE OF ALL LAYERS (Fig. 165). This incision is used primarily for surgery of the stomach and pancreas. The skin incision is transverse in patients with wide subcostal angles or slightly curved upward if the subcostal angle is narrow. In either case it is designed to pass inferior to the costal margin and still reach the lateral border of both rectus sheaths. As a rule this places the incision at a point midway between the xiphoid process and the umbilicus. It may be placed slightly more to the left when extensive gastric surgery is contemplated. The anterior rectus sheaths are exposed and incised transversely from one lateral border to the other. In some cases, depending upon the surgery contemplated and the width of the recti, the incision need not extend to the lateral border of the muscles. The rectus muscles are freed at their medial borders and a finger is inserted beneath the muscle prior to cutting it. By tenting the muscles over the finger the fibers may be carefully cut across and most blood vessels clamped with hemostats before they are transected. Hemostasis of blood vessels within the muscle is obtained by means of suture ligatures. The posterior rectus sheath, linea alba, transversalis fascia and peritoneum are then incised transversely; care must be taken in this last step for peritoneum is closely adherent to posterior rectus sheath and it is possible to injure the underlying viscera if the peritoneum is inadvertently opened. The ligamentum teres is transected between hemostats and both ends ligated to control bleeding from the artery and veins located therein. Careful reconstruction of this ligament is wise, as obstruction may result from ends left free.

This incision provides excellent exposure for the average subtotal gastric resection or for work in the region of head of pancreas. When more extensive gastric surgery is undertaken the incision may be extended to the left, splitting the oblique muscles as described below. Occasionally additional exposure may be necessary. In our experience this additional exposure is required only for some very high subtotal or in total gastric resections. In such instances we have no hesitancy in extending the incision vertically upward through the linea alba. This may include skin and linea alba or, as suggested by Gurd,[41] the extension may include only the linea alba and peritoneum. Excellent exposure is then obtained for the most extensive surgery. While arguments may be put forth for the exclusive use of the transverse or the vertical incision, the fundamental necessity for adequate exposure remains. It is folly to adhere to one type of incision, no matter how basically sound that incision may be, in order to complete an operation under poor exposure and thus endanger the adequacy of the surgical procedure being performed. Although the transverse incision in the upper abdomen serves admirably for most procedures, we do not hesitate to alter it by adding a vertical limb when necessary. We feel that it is better to face the possibility of disruption or herniation through the vertical limb, as well as the increased pain and possibility of pulmonary complications which are associated with vertical incisions, rather than jeopardize the perfection of the surgical procedure being performed.

SANDERS' MODIFICATION OF THE SLOAN INCISION [28] (Fig. 166). The Sloan incision and Singleton's modification thereof have previously been described. In our opinion the Sanders' modification offers the best basic principles among those incisions which are designed to spare the rectus muscles. The Sloan incision cuts both anterior rectus sheaths vertically while Singleton cuts the right anterior sheath vertically. Sanders cuts all of both rectus sheaths transversely thereby adhering to the basic physiological principles which have previously been pointed out.

A transverse skin incision, as described above, is made. Both anterior rectus sheaths are incised transversely. The rectus muscles are freed from their sheaths and retracted laterally. The remaining layers, including linea alba, entire posterior sheath and peritoneum are incised transversely.

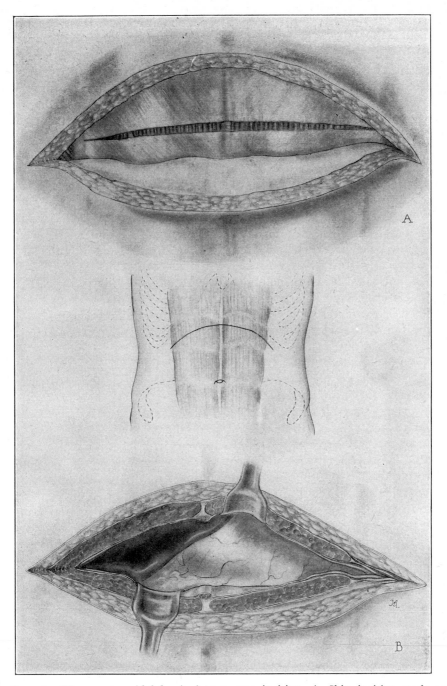

FIG. 165. The upper midabdominal transverse incision. A. Skin incision made and anterior rectus sheaths incised transversely. B. Rectus muscles transected and the incision completed. Note that the rectus muscles do not retract beneath the sheath.

This type of incision requires what, to us at least, seems to be unnecessary dissection and opens extensive planes to possible infection. Its production is time consuming. It is impossible of lateral extension, when additional exposure is necessary, without transection of the rectus muscles. There are a certain number of cases, however, in which it is necessary to explore the abdomen without being certain that the proposed surgery can be completed. This is particularly true when dealing with malignancy of the stomach or pancreas. It is suggested, particularly, for surgeons who hesitate to transect the rectus muscles, that this incision be used for exploration. If additional exposure is needed for extensive surgery the rectus muscles may be transected with impunity.

MAYO INCISION.[38] This incision is designed primarily for gallbladder operations when placed on the right or stomach when on the left. A vertical midline incision is made from xiphoid process to just above the umbilicus and is carried through linea alba and peritoneum. Midway between the two ends of the incision a transverse limb is added which includes anterior and posterior rectus sheaths as well as the peritoneum. The rectus muscle is retracted laterally. It is our feeling that the undesirable vertical limb of this incision is unnecessary if both recti are transected. The oblique incision described below serves very well for gallbladder and bile duct surgery without the use of the vertical limb which in itself offers the basic objections already pointed out.

MAYO-ROBSON INCISION.[37] This incision is designed for and used primarily in, gallbladder and biliary tract operations. It is frequently referred to as the hockey stick incision.

A vertical skin incision centering over the midrectus is started at the umbilicus (or as far below it as necessary) and extends upward to within 4 cms. of the costal margin; it then extends medially toward the xiphoid process. The anterior rectus sheath in the upper end of the wound is then incised obliquely from the midline down and laterally to its lateral border. The anterior sheath incision is then extended downward as far as the skin incision permits. The rectus muscle is freed and retracted medially. Great care must be exercised if permanent nerve damage is to be avoided for the nerves enter the lateral border of the rectus sheath. The posterior sheath and peritoneum are then opened in the same line as the superficial incision, care to prevent nerve damage again being necessary.

This incision gives reasonable exposure for gallbladder operations but, in addition to the basic objections pertaining to all vertical incisions, is almost impossible to fashion without permanently damaging two or more intercostal nerves. It has also been advocated for stomach surgery when placed in the left rectus muscle.

VERTICAL MIDLINE INCISION. This incision is quickly and easily made. A vertical incision is carried, for the desired length, through skin, linea alba and peritoneum. It has the added advantage that it can be extended from the xiphoid process to the symphysis pubis (curving around the umbilicus), with little difficulty.

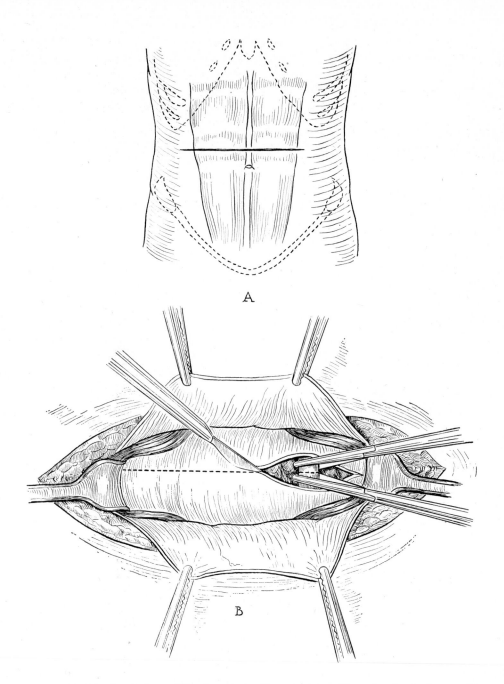

FIG. 166. The Sander's modification of the Sloan incision. Note that both the anterior and posterior rectus sheaths are incised transversely while the rectus muscles are retracted laterally without cutting. (Redrawn from Sanders, *Ann. Surg.*, 104:74-86, [July], 1936.)

Although the avascularity of the linea alba lends itself to rapid opening of the abdomen, it also makes this incision subject to retarded healing. In addition the basic objection to all vertical incisions are doubly active here since the aponeurotic fibers of both groups of oblique muscles insert at the linea alba; consequently great stress is placed on the suture line.

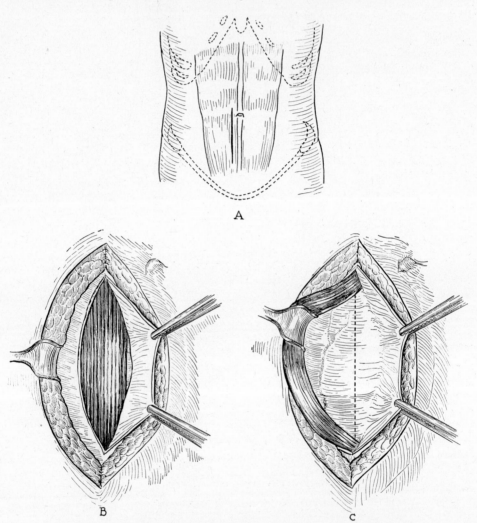

FIG. 167. Vertical paramedian incision. See text for description.

In our opinion the only excuse for the use of a vertical incision through the linea alba occurs in the need for great haste in entering the abdomen. This emergency is extremely rare.

PARAMEDIAN INCISION (Fig. 167). A vertical skin incision of the desired length, located 2 cms. either to the right or left of the midline, is made. The anterior rectus sheath is incised vertically 2 cms. from the midline. The rectus muscle is freed from its sheath and retracted laterally; the epigastric vessels usually adhere to the muscle and are retracted with it. The remaining layers are then incised vertically at the same distance from the midline.

This is a better incision than the midline (or any other vertical rectus

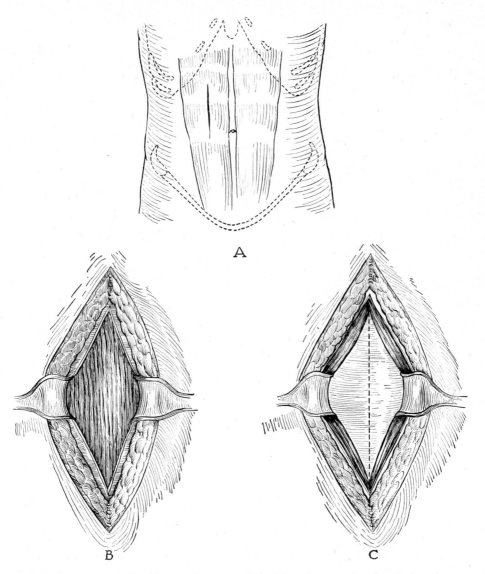

A

B   C

FIG. 168. Vertical midrectus (transrectal) incision. See text for description.

incision) but, although it sections no nerves, is subject to the same objections associated with all vertical types of incisions.

MID-RECTUS INCISION (TRANSRECTAL) (Fig. 168). A vertical incision of the desired length and in the appropriate area of the abdomen is centered over the midrectus and carried down through the anterior rectus sheath. The fibers of the rectus muscle are split and retracted and the remaining layers are incised vertically either slightly lateral or medial to the anterior rectus sheath incision.

This incision has the same disadvantages previously mentioned. In addition, in order to obtain any degree of exposure, it must extend over sufficient

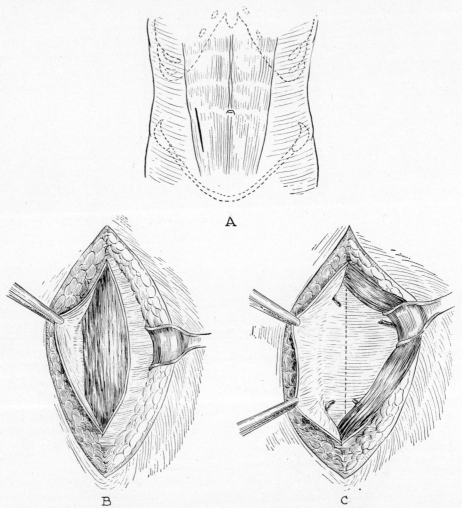

Fig. 169. Vertical pararectal incision. See text for description. Note that at least two nerves must be cut in order to provide adequate exposure.

length to result in denervation of that portion of the rectus muscle which lies medial to the incision.

PARARECTAL INCISION (Kammerer or Battle), (Fig. 169). This incision is made along the lateral border of either rectus but is usually described for use in the lower abdomen. The skin and anterior rectus sheath are incised vertically 1 cm. medial to the lateral border of rectus. The rectus muscle is freed and retracted medially. The posterior rectus sheath and peritoneum are incised vertically in the same plane as the anterior sheath.

If this incision is to be of sufficient length to be of value, two or more intercostal nerves must either be cut or remain stretching across the wound. For this reason this incision is not considered to be of real value, particularly when other types of incisions which give better exposure and have fewer inherent objectionable features, are available.

Right (Left) Subcostal Incisions. These incisions are designed primarily for surgery on the gallbladder or bile ducts when placed on the right or for spleen (occasionally stomach) when placed on the left. Similarly they may be used for hepatic flexure of colon on the right or splenic flexure on the left although the midabdominal transverse incision described below is recommended for these types of surgery.

OBLIQUE INCISION (Fig. 170). This is the incision which in our hands, has proved to be of the most value for all operations upon the gallbladder and bile ducts when used on the right or for splenectomy when placed on the left.

The skin incision begins at a point over the linea alba midway between the umbilicus and ensiform process and extends downward and laterally toward a point midway between the twelfth rib and iliac crest. For most purposes, however, the incision terminates at about the anterior axillary line. By retracting the superior skin flap slightly upwards the anterior sheath of rectus can be incised in a transverse direction (not obliquely as is the skin). The rectus muscle is freed at its lateral border and a finger inserted beneath it following which its fibers are transected and hemostasis is obtained as previously described. The posterior rectus sheath and peritoneum are then incised transversely. Occasionally it will be found that, because of the great width of the rectus muscle at this level, the incision need not be extended into the oblique muscles. The incision is usually carried transversely through the linea semilunaris. The aponeurosis of external oblique and its muscle fibers are split upward and laterally to the rib margin if necessary. A retractor pulls the lower flap of external oblique downward and the internal oblique and transversus may then be split into the flank. When the incision is extended into the oblique muscles the ninth intercostal nerve must be visualized as it runs transversely on the transversus abdominis muscle; it is readily retracted superiorly out of the wound since the incision runs almost parallel to it. Occasionally the tenth intercostal nerve will be encountered more laterally and is readily dealt with in a similar manner. When necessary (rarely) this incision may be extended to the left transversely through the linea alba, falciform ligament and left anterior and posterior rectus sheaths, either transecting the left rectus muscle or retracting it laterally as desired.

In our experience this incision gives excellent exposure for all gallbladder surgery and this is particularly the case when the common duct must be dealt with since the incision almost centers over this structure. Hyperextending the patient, by breaking the table, improves the exposure since it opens the wound and brings the abdominal contents forward. The right lobe of liver and gallbladder most commonly present in the upper margin of the wound and the liver is readily retracted and excellent exposure of the bile ducts and hepatic trinity is thus obtained. The vertical incision, in order to present adequate exposure, must extend to the umbilicus or even lower; the colon and small bowel are thus exposed and present a problem by bulging into the lower end of the wound. This is not true of the oblique incision for it limits itself to the region which is being dealt with. Heavy retraction and packing are thus not necessary.

SINGLETON'S INCISION.[39,40] As previously mentioned, the "lateral transverse" and splenectomy incisions described by Singleton are essentially the same. The lateral transverse is described primarily for biliary surgery while the name of the latter indicates the use for which it is intended.

The splenectomy incision starts at the linea alba midway between the umbilicus and xiphoid process while the splenectomy incision begins slightly lower (7 to 10 cms. above the umbilicus). Both incisions extend downward and laterally to a point just behind the anterior-superior iliac spine and just above the iliac crest. The anterior rectus sheath and external oblique aponeurosis are cut in the line of the skin incision. Thus the anterior rectus sheath is cut obliquely and the external oblique fibers are sectioned almost at right angles to the direction in which they run. The rectus muscle is freed and retracted medially. The posterior rectus sheath is incised transversely and the incision is continued downward and laterally splitting the fibers of internal oblique but cutting the fibers of transversus abdominis. Peritoneum is opened in the line of the skin incision. The intercostal nerves are isolated as they enter the rectus sheath. In the lateral transverse incision Singleton cuts or retracts the ninth and tenth intercostal nerves and states that there is numbness below the wound for several weeks. In his splenectomy incision he cuts the eleventh and retracts the tenth and twelfth intercostal nerves.

It has been the repeated observation of surgeons that interruption of the function of two or more intercostal nerves, either by cutting or excessive stretching, is associated with noticeable loss of rectus muscle function. The oblique incision described above runs more parallel to the nerves and, therefore, allows of their retraction without injury. Furthermore transection of the rectus muscle permits of less interference with the nerve supply than does freeing the muscle and retracting it medially. When the rectus muscle is cut rather than retracted medially exposure is improved to the extent that the wound need not be extended far into the flank as described by Singleton. For the same reason the oblique muscles may be split in the line of their fibers rather than transected as in the Singleton incisions.

Midabdominal Incisions. This type of incision is used for surgery of the small bowel (*e.g.* small bowel obstruction). It is also of great value for surgery upon the right, transverse and descending colon as well as upper sigmoid. By centering the various types of previously described vertical incision in the midabdomen, they may be used for these types of surgery. In our opinion, however, the vertical incision is neither as useful nor as physiological as is the transverse incision described below.

TRANSVERSE MIDABDOMINAL INCISION (Fig. 171). Depending upon the operation contemplated this incision is placed either to the right or left of the

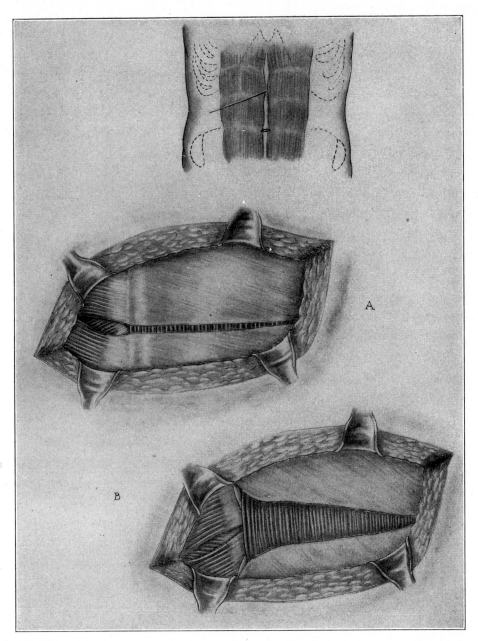

FIG. 170(1). Oblique incision. A. Anterior rectus sheath incised transversely and external oblique fibers split. B. Rectus muscle freed at lateral border and external oblique retracted. Used primarily for biliary operations on the right and splenectomy on the left.

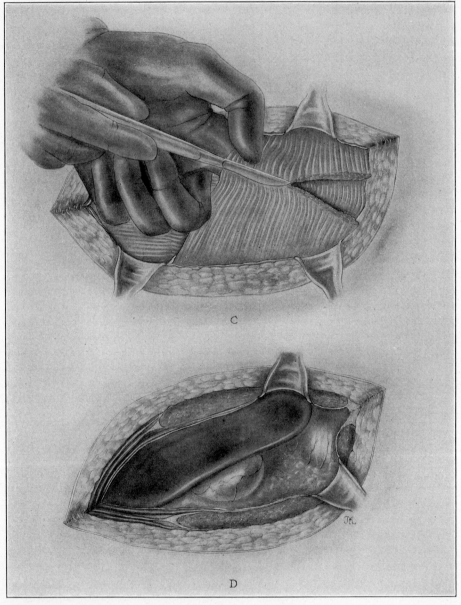

FIG. 170 (2). C. Rectus muscle transected over a finger inserted beneath it. D. Incision completed.

midline and approximately 1.5 to 2 cms. above or below the umbilicus. It is designed to be a truly transverse incision and its placement near to the umbilicus is required by the necessity of passing between the iliac crest and twelfth rib. In all four possible locations, however, the incision is identically fashioned and for that reason may be described as one incision.

The incision begins at the midline 1.5 to 2 cms. above or below the umbilicus as necessary and extends directly laterally as far as is deemed necessary for the contemplated surgery. The anterior rectus sheath is incised transversely and this incision is extended upward and laterally in the external oblique, splitting its fibers. The rectus muscle is freed at its lateral border

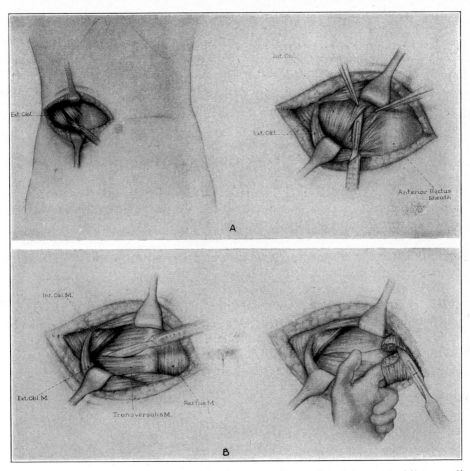

FIG. 171. Transverse midabdominal incision. A. External and internal obliques split in the line of their fibers. Note the healed left midabdominal transverse incision. B. Transversus abdominis split in the line of its fibers and the rectus muscle crosscut all or in part depending on the exposure needed. (From Coller and Vaughan, *Ann. Surg.,* 121:395-408, [April], 1945.)

and a finger inserted beneath it following which its fibers are transected and hemostasis obtained as previously described. The ninth intercostal nerve (above the umbilicus) or the eleventh intercostal nerve (below the umbilicus) is identified as it runs on the posterior rectus sheath or on the transversus muscle and is retracted upwards. The posterior rectus sheath and peritoneum are incised transversely. From the lateral border of the rectus the internal oblique and transversus abdominis are split by blunt dissection with the fingers and the remaining peritoneum opened to the lateral margin of the incision. This incision may be carried far into the flank if necessary.

This type of true transverse incision is advocated by Gurd [41] for all types of abdominal surgery; he feels that the additional exposure afforded by the lateral extension far into the flank more than compensates for the necessity of limiting the incision to the region of the umbilicus. For gallbladder surgery he retracts the right rectus muscle medially without cutting it; however, when the common or hepatic ducts must be explored he transects the right rectus muscle. For stomach surgery he uses the same incision on the left, transecting one or both recti and, when necessary he extends the incision upward in the linea alba. In our experience, however, the principles of transverse incisions can be maintained while obtaining better exposure for the upper or lower abdomen by the use of the variations described above and below.

This type of transverse midabdominal incision also lends itself readily to such retroperitoneal operations as lumbar sympathectomy or ligation of the inferior vena cava. In such instances the muscles and aponeuroses are incised as described but the peritoneum is reflected medially without opening it. For retroperitoneal work the incision is frequently carried farther into the flank and only the lateral portion of anterior and posterior rectus sheaths are transected while the muscle may either be partially transected or retracted medially as desired.

Right (Left) Lower Quadrant Incisions. For surgery in this region the muscle splitting incisions of either the McBurney or Rockey-Davis (or Elliot) type have stood the test of time and are most commonly used. As previously pointed out many surgeons still use the vertical incision of one type or another. The reasons which lead us to believe that the vertical incision is not justified for this type of surgery have been previously given. Since the McBurney and Rockey-Davis incisions are equally popular both will be described. In our hands the Rockey-Davis has served admirably for appendiceal surgery. On the left this type of gridiron incision is most useful for such operations as sigmoid colostomy. A transverse modification of the gridiron type of incision used for combined abdomino-perineal resection will also be described; this has served very well in our hands giving excellent exposure and firm wound healing.

Rockey-Davis (or Elliot) Incision (Fig. 172). A transverse skin incision is used and is designed to cross the junction of lower and middle thirds of a line extending from anterior-superior iliac spine to the umbilicus. The medial end of this incision reaches to the lateral border of the rectus muscle. When so placed the incision will usually lie approximately 1 inch above the anterior-superior iliac spine. The aponeurosis of external oblique is split in the line of its fibers (extending into the muscle fibers when necessary) and this split extends onto the rectus sheath from which external oblique fibers are usually separable. The aponeurotic junction of internal oblique and transversus abdominis is picked up at the linea semilunaris and incised transversely; this incision is then extended laterally by splitting the muscle

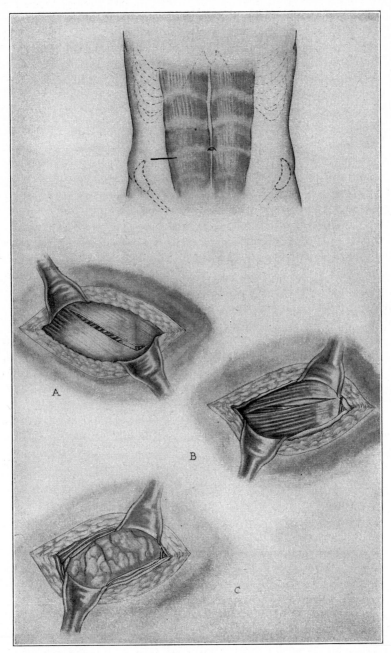

FIG. 172. Rockey-Davis (Elliot) incision. A. External oblique fibers split. B. External oblique retracted. Internal oblique and transversus abdominis split. C. Incision completed. Note the nick in lateral border of rectus sheath (Weir or Harrington modification).

fibers of the latter two muscles with blunt finger dissection thus avoiding undue handling of, and bleeding from, these muscle fibers. Peritoneum is then incised transversely. It is our practice to add the Weir or Harrington extension to this incision by nicking the lateral border of rectus sheath but the rectus muscle is not disturbed. This modification adds to the exposure without unduly complicating the wound.

McBurney Incision. The skin incision is obliquely placed and runs parallel to the fibers of the external oblique. It is 4 inches long and crosses a line from the anterior-superior spine to the umbilicus almost at right angles; it lies approximately 1 inch medial to the anterior-superior spine and its upper one-third is above the line from anterior spine to umbilicus. With the exception of the skin, this incision is identical to the Rockey-Davis and the Weir or Harrington modification may be added.

Either of the above incisions may be extended upward and laterally when necessary for additional exposure of the cecum. If more room is needed medially, one or both rectus sheaths and muscles may be transected; in such instances the inferior epigastric vessels, beneath the rectus must be ligated. In both incisions care must be exercised not to cut the iliohypogastric nerve as it pierces the internal oblique and runs downward beneath the external oblique.

Combined Abdomino Perineal Incision (Fig. 173). In recent years we have used the following incision for the abdominal portion of combined abdomino perineal resections. It is of equal value for low sigmoid resections, with or without end-to-end anastomosis.

The skin incision begins at, or just to the right of, the midline 2.5 cms. above the symphysis and extends transversely to the lateral border of the left rectus sheath; at this point it turns upward in the line of the fibers of the external oblique and terminates just above and usually about 5 cms. medial to the anterior-superior spine. If desired an alternative skin incision may be used which begins 2.5 cms. above the symphysis and extends in a straight line to the termination 5 cms. above and medial to the spine. The aponeurosis of external oblique is split in the line of its fibers and the ilio-hypogastric nerve isolated beneath it and retracted downward. The aponeurotic incision is extended transversely across the anterior rectus sheath and linea alba. The rectus muscle is then freed at its lateral border and transected over a finger as previously described. The inferior epigastric vessels are isolated running upward and medially beneath the rectus muscle; they are transected and ligated. By blunt dissection the internal oblique and transversus abdominis are then split clear to their attachment at the iliac wing. The transversalis fascia and peritoneum are then opened in the line of the aponeurotic incision. The transverse limb of this incision can be carried across the linea alba and right rectus although this is seldom necessary. If more exposure is needed the incision may be duplicated on the right.

This incision, in our experience, gives excellent exposure, closes readily, heals firmly and, as with other transverse incisions, is less painful post-operatively.

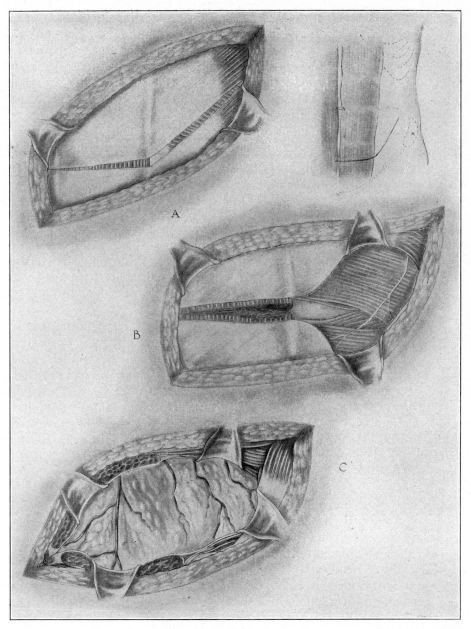

FIG. 173. Right or left lower quadrant transverse incision (combined abdomino-perineal incision). A. Anterior rectus sheath incised transversely and external oblique fibers split. B. External oblique retracted. Internal oblique and transversus abdominis split clear to the pelvic wall. C. Rectus muscle transected and the incision is completed. Note retraction of the iliohypogastric nerve.

The various types of vertical left rectus or midline incisions are frequently advocated for this type of surgery. In our opinion, however, the above described transverse type of incision gives just as good or better exposure and avoids the objections inherent to all vertical incisions. Providing the upper limb of the incision is at least three finger-breadths from the anterior-superior iliac spine the proximal limb of colon can be brought out through the upper end of the wound. If, however, the upper end of the incision lies too close to the anterior-superior iliac spine the colostomy may be made through a stab wound above and medial to the upper limb of the incision. We have used both types of colostomy construction with equal satisfaction.

Gurd [41] has advocated for this type of surgery the use of his universal incision which is located near the umbilicus and is truly transverse in all layers. He mentions the fact that it is occasionally necessary to convert this into a flap incision by extending down in the linea alba. In our experience this modification is never necessary if the incision is devised as described above. We believe that the Gurd type of incision is centered too high for adequate exposure of the deep pelvis as is necessary for sigmoid or rectal operations.

Incisions for Pelvic (Gynecologic) Surgery. The vertical incision through the linea alba or some portion of the rectus sheath is still the most popular among gynecological surgeons. The reasons for this choice have been previously mentioned. The right or left paramedian incision (as previously described) is the most popular and, if vertical incisions must be used, the most physiological since it reflects the rectus muscle without damaging its nerve supply while avoiding the relatively avascular linea alba. The vertical incisions are fashioned exactly as in the upper abdomen except for the fact that posterior rectus sheath is deficient below the semicircular line of Douglas.

PFANNENSTEIL INCISION (Fig. 174). A curved incision is fashioned which centers just above the symphysis pubis, so as to be within the hair line, and then curves upward and laterally toward the anterior-superior spines. Both rectus sheaths and linea alba are incised transversely and this incision may be extended laterally into the external oblique aponeurosis in the line of its fibers. The rectus sheaths are then reflected upward as a single aponeurotic flap as far as is necessary. Since there is no posterior rectus sheath this flap represents the entire aponeurotic strength of the abdominal wall in this region. Having reflected the flap upward the rectus muscles are separated and retracted laterally. The transversalis fascia and peritoneum are then incised vertically.

The objection has been offered by some that the Pfannensteil does not provide sufficient exposure. If such be the case the rectus muscles may be divided at their tendinous attachment to the pubes and reflected upward; [24] peritoneum and transversalis fascia may then be incised transversely.

TRUE TRANSVERSE INCISION OF ALL LAYERS. With the increasing popularity of the transverse incision for other regions of the abdomen during recent years a number of gynecological surgeons have been favoring the true transverse incision of all layers. The transverse skin incision centers at the junction of middle and lower thirds of a line extending from symphysis pubis

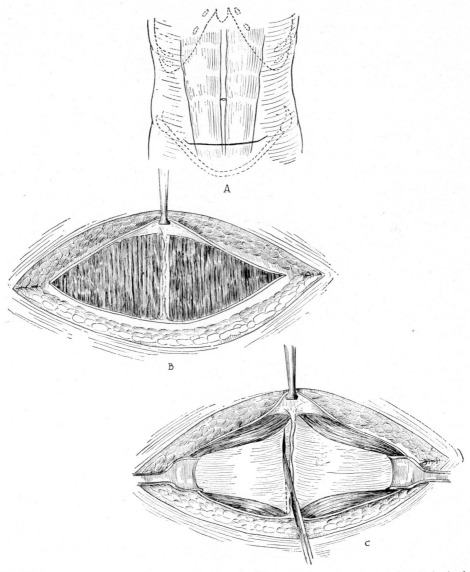

FIG. 174. Pfannensteil incision. A. Skin incision. B. Anterior rectus sheath incised transversely and reflected upward by sharp dissection. C. Rectus muscles freed and retracted laterally. Incision completed by incising remaining layers vertically.

to the umbilicus. Both rectus sheaths and linea alba are incised transversely. The rectus muscles are transected over a finger inserted beneath them. The inferior epigastric vessels are found beneath the medial third of the muscle and are transected and ligated. Transversalis fascia and peritoneum are then opened transversely. When additional exposure is necessary the incision may be extended by splitting the oblique muscles as previously described, in the line of their fibers, either to the right or left, or both, as is dictated by necessity.

CLOSURE OF ABDOMINAL WOUNDS

All abdominal wounds are closed in approximately the same manner with certain variations which are dependent upon the anatomical features of the region involved. Although wounds and wound healing have been discussed elsewhere in this text certain features of this subject, which pertain more or less specifically to abdominal incisions and their closure, will be briefly considered here.

Peritoneum. Exact approximation of the peritoneum is essential if post-operative adhesions to the abdominal wall are to be avoided. Adhesions are the commonest cause of acute intestinal obstruction, a condition in which there is a 26 per cent mortality.[1] In addition countless patients return with minor complaints of various types which are generally attributed to adhesions. Furthermore inexact peritoneal closure and healing may lay the ground-work for subsequent entrance of a wedge of omentum or bowel which may then proceed to separate the layers of the abdominal wall and result in herniation or disruption of the wound.

As previously noted, the peritoneum is closely adherent to the rectus sheath but is readily separable from the remaining portions of the abdominal wall. That peritoneum which underlies the rectus sheath is closed in the same suture layer as the posterior sheath. Elsewhere (under the obliques or below the semicircular line of Douglas) the peritoneum and transversalis fascia are closed together as a separate layer. In either case the peritoneum is carefully isolated for the entire length of the wound and its edges picked up in several fine hemostats. The peritoneum (and posterior rectus sheath where present) are then carefully closed, the cut edges being everted so that smooth serosa meets smooth serosa. It has been our custom, for a number of years, to use a continuous suture of doubled ooo chromic catgut for the peritoneum. Others prefer interrupted silk although accurate approximation makes the use of this type of closure difficult. Certainly nonabsorbable suture material should not be used as a continuous suture. Wire is not often used for closing the peritoneum because the bowel may come in contact with it and cause perforation. We have used interrupted wire closure, however, and believe it is safe providing the wire is properly tied and the ends cut closely so that sharp ends do not protrude. The difficulty encountered in closure of the peritoneum in vertical incisions has been previously mentioned. When the transverse incision is used little difficulty is encountered in the peritoneal (and posterior rectus sheath) closure. This closure is facilitated if the patient is flexed slightly in order to further approximate the edges of the wound.

Muscle Layers. Suture of the muscle layers is dependent upon the location and type of incision. Muscle is the most friable of all the tissues encountered in the abdominal wall and, when sutured, must be gently handled. In vertical incisions through the rectus, the muscle may be loosely approximated with interrupted sutures of fine silk or catgut. When the rectus muscle is transected, however, actual suture of the muscle itself is difficult, unsatisfactory and unnecessary; as previously pointed out the suture of the rectus sheath accurately reapproximates the ends of the muscle. That portion of muscle splitting incisions through the oblique muscles may best be closed by loosely tied interrupted fine catgut or silk sutures. Closure of muscle is done primarily to obliterate dead space. Little strength is added to the wound by muscle suture.

Aponeuroses. The aponeurotic layers of the abdominal wall represent the only portion of the closure in which real strength is obtained at the suture line. Muscle and fat have very little tensile strength and peritoneum has little more. The suture of the aponeuroses then is the keystone of the abdominal wall closure. Careful approximation without tension and without ischemia is obligatory.

The posterior rectus sheath, because it is adherent to the peritoneum, is closed as described above. The remaining aponeurotic layers of rectus and of the oblique muscles (external oblique in particular) are closed separately. Interrupted sutures are used because they impart the greatest strength. Furthermore it is apparent that the parting of a single interrupted suture may be tolerated without particularly deleterious results. When a continuous suture breaks the entire suture line is gone and the results may be disastrous. Catgut, as will be pointed out below, is not dependable for sufficient time to allow of firm wound healing. Nonabsorbable sutures are the most dependable and we use them exclusively for closure of the aponeuroses. Silk is a perfectly sound suture material insofar as tensile strength and nonabsorbability are concerned. The only reason to avoid its use results from the occasional difficulty encountered in infected wounds when sinuses form and small silk sutures extrude themselves over a considerable period of time. Some prefer cotton and claim that it does not offer the disadvantages of silk. For a number of years we have been using No. 30 stainless steel wire for the aponeurotic layers, particularly in the rectus sheath. It produces the least possible reaction in the tissues,[42, 43] is absolutely dependable insofar as tensile strength is concerned and does not absorb; when placed in an infected wound it does not act as a nidus of persistent low-grade infection (as silk occasionally does). Wire requires a certain amount of experience in handling for it is prone to kink and twist; when this happens the suture is likely to break. It must be tied as a perfect square knot and when so tied does not loosen or untie. Care must be exercised in tying it in order to approximate but not strangulate the tissues. This precaution is more necessary with wire than with other suture materials because the properties of the wire makes tightening of a loop require greater force than is otherwise necessary; this additional force may readily be continued and result in strangulation of tissues. The ends of the wire should be cut very close to the knot. On rare occasions, and then only in very thin people, the wire ends may cause irritation and pain if they rub on the under surface of the skin; in such cases they may readily be removed after the wound is soundly healed.

Innumerable different types of stitches and reinforcements of the aponeurotic closure have been described. These are all primarily intended to overcome the high incidence of herniation and disruption of vertical wounds. It is our opinion that, providing the basic anatomical and physiological principles of the abdominal wall are recognized and the incisions made in such manner as to interfere as little as possible with structure and function, these elaborate types of closure are not necessary. The interrupted type of suture of aponeuroses, whether mattress, figure-of-eight or simple Lembert will all serve adequately to approximate the layers and permit healing. If undue stress occurs at the wound edges (as in vertical incisions), or if tissue necrosis under the sutures results from too tight tying of the suture, the wound will give way no matter what type of stitch is used. Retention sutures that grasp large masses of tissue in a transverse direction to the wound cause pressure necrosis and diminish the blood supply to the area undergoing repair. We do not use them under any conditions.

Subcutaneous Tissues and Skin. Fat has practically no tensile strength; for this reason the finest of suture material should be used in approximating the edges of the panniculus of fat. These sutures are used only to obliterate dead space for they add nothing to the strength of the wound. In clean wounds the subcutaneous tissue should be closed. Many surgeons use the interrupted type of suture for this purpose; one or more rows of these Lembert sutures are placed in such manner as to approximate the fat and obliterate dead space. Because we feel that fine silk or cotton produce the least possible reaction in the tissues we have favored these materials for this closure.

For a number of years, in clean wounds, we have favored the use of one or more layers of subcuticular stainless steel wire sutures (Fig. 175) for the closure of the subcutaneous tissues, as well as the skin. The deeper sutures serve to effectively approximate the layers of the panniculus and interfere the least possible amount with normal wound healing since there is little tissue reaction to the wire and it is impossible to strangulate tissue with this type of suture. The most superficial wire runs just under the deep layers of the dermis and, when properly placed, accurately closes the skin. This type of closure is comfortable to the patient and affords an excellent cosmetic result, since there is no double row of suture holes to result in scarring. The smooth wire is readily removed with no more pain than is encountered in the removal of any interrupted type of suture.

Contaminated Wounds. Abdominal surgery, by its very nature is prone to result in contamination of the wound by the intestinal flora. The muscle and fascial planes, when properly closed, usually handle contamination well and infection seldom develops in these layers. The subcutaneous fat, on the other hand, has a poor blood supply and is particularly prone to be the site of development of infection. It has been our experience that the vast majority of infections develop in the subcutaneous panniculus; this is particularly true when the fat layer is thick. Experience has shown that [44] when contaminated wounds are closed primarily, the incidence of infection runs as high as 50 per cent. It is highly advantageous to close the peritoneum and aponeuroses, for reasons which are obvious. With this thought in mind, and

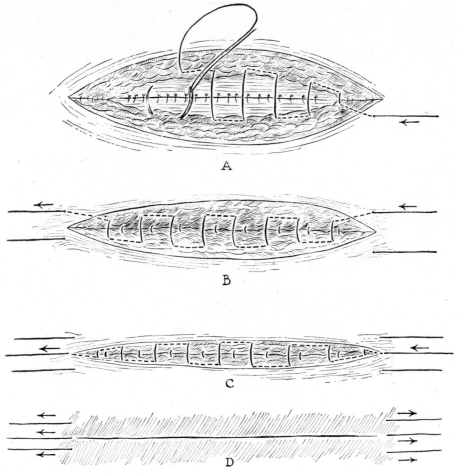

FIG. 175. Subcuticular stainless steel wire closure of subcutaneous tissues and skin (No. 28 wire used throughout). A. The first wire is used to approximate the deep fat and includes Scarpa's fascia. B. Second wire closes intermediate fat layer. C. Third wire runs immediately beneath the skin and approximates it. D. Closure completed. As is indicated by arrows the wires are run back and forth to assure that they are free and can be easily removed (knots and snares in the wire must be avoided).

believing that the majority of wound infections develop first in the fat layer, we have used a delayed type of closure in all contaminated wounds with great satisfaction.

The peritoneum, muscle and aponeurotic layers are closed as described. Near far figure-of-eight silk sutures are then placed in the skin and subcutaneous tissues (Fig. 176) but they are not tied. Gauze packs are then

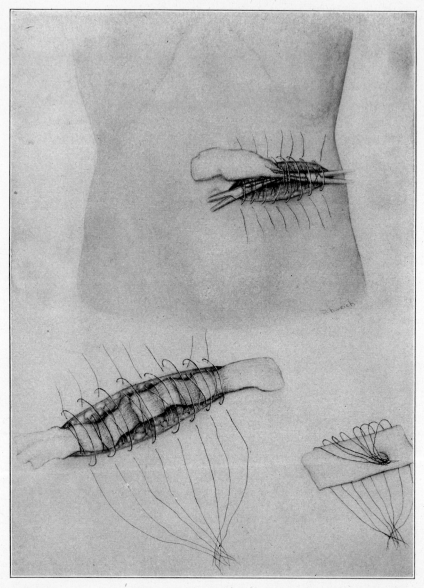

FIG. 176. Delayed closure of subcutaneous tissue and skin. Sutures and pack in place. The pack is removed in 48 hours and the sutures tied. (From Coller and Vaughan, *Ann. Surg.*, 121:395-408, [April], 1945.)

insinuated beneath the sutures from each end and meet in the midportion of the wounds; these are more easily removed than one long pack would be. The wound is then covered with a dry dressing. At the end of 24 to 48 hours the packs are removed and the sutures tied. Morphine provides sufficient narcosis for this procedure and general anesthetic is not necessary, because the removal of the pack and tying of the sutures is not particularly painful. The placing of stitches at the time of the original operation eliminates the need for a second general anesthetic and we have never seen any deleterious reaction to the sutures. As reported in 1940 [44] healing without infection was obtained in 20 of 21 contaminated abdominal wounds. Since that time we have continued to use this method with equal satisfaction.

Jones, Newell and Brubaker [45] in 1941 reported the use of a figure-of-eight alloy steel wire closure of the peritoneum and aponeurosis. A vertical left rectus incision had been used for combined abdominoperineal resection in all of these cases. The incidence of infection was reduced from 27.5 per cent to 0.85 per cent, by the use of this type of suture. From these figures

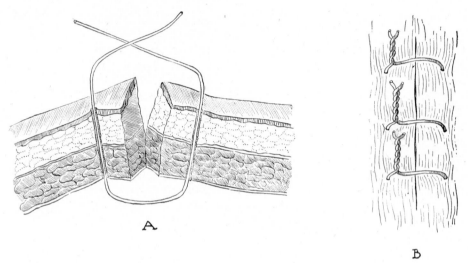

A

B

Fig. 177. Silver wire through-and-through closure of all layers of the abdominal wall. Most useful in the repair of the disrupted wound. (After Reid, *Ann. Surg.*, 98:892, 1933.)

it may be seen that a definite decrease in the incidence of infection was obtained. We feel that this suture is of definite value, particularly in the lower abdomen when contamination of a vertical incision has occurred.

Reid and his coworker [46,47] have advocated the through-and-through silver wire closure of all layers of the abdominal wall (Fig. 177) when heavy contamination has occurred, when there are chest complications with heavy coughing, when a patient's general condition demands a quick, safe closure, and for the closure of the disrupted wound. For routine use this closure does not provide accurate approximation of all layers and, for this reason, we have not used it except for the closure of the disrupted wound. The technic of this type of closure is described under disruption of wounds (page 352).

In respect to wound infections we are of the firm belief that the transverse incision, particularly in the upper abdomen, handles contamination or frank infection better than any type of vertical wound. The incidence of infection in the transverse incision is lower than in the vertical type and when it does occur it is readily handled and clears rapidly. A sound reason for this difference is apparent. With the patient lying in bed the vertical incision runs in a plane of the abdomen which is level throughout its length. Exudates or frank pus will necessarily puddle in the middle of the incision; when frank infection occurs it is difficult to clear up because, no matter how widely the wound is opened the pus will still collect in the center of the wound. The transverse (or oblique) incision, on the other hand, extends over a convex surface which is highest at its medial margin and most dependent laterally. Any exudate when it accumulates, or pus when it occurs, can readily be drained from the lateral dependent angle of the wound. Thus the principle of dependent drainage is readily established in the transverse wound but is almost impossible of accomplishment in the vertical wound.

DRAINAGE OF ABDOMINAL WOUNDS

The subject of drainage materials, indications and methods of drainage will be considered in detail under the individual sections. Certain considerations of drainage in relation to the abdominal incision are worthy of brief mention here. When vertical incisions are used the drains or drainage tubes should be brought out through separate stab wounds placed lateral to the main incision. The reasons for this are twofold. First is the consideration of infection in the abdominal wound. Drains which pass through the vertical wound may introduce infection either from within or from without; the vertical wound does not tolerate contamination well and infection is often the result. Secondly, effective drainage is difficult to obtain through the apex of the abdominal wall, *i.e.,* through the vertical incision. Laterally placed drains, on the other hand are more nearly dependent hence are more effective. In transverse or oblique incisions the drain may safely be brought out through the lateral angle of the wound for in this position it is dependent in relation to the wound and usually in relation to the area being drained; wound infection is thus less likely to develop.

DISRUPTION AND HERNIATION OF ABDOMINAL WOUNDS

Essentially the same factors must play a part in the production of both herniation and disruption of abdominal wounds. In the disruption all layers open up and various abdominal contents (usually small or large bowel and omentum) eviscerate on to the abdominal wall; this usually happens on about the ninth (fifth to eleventh) day. Herniation, on the other hand, represents the parting of one or more deep layers while the supervening layers (usually only skin) remain intact. A large percentage of hernias undoubtedly occur early and are merely an incomplete disruption in which the skin remains intact. There can be little doubt, however, that a small percentage of hernias develop late and gradually increase in size as repeated strain is placed upon the wound.

A review of the rather extensive literature on abdominal wound disruption reveals the incidence to vary between 0.22 per cent [48] and 3.05 per cent.[49] In a summary of 1526 wound disruptions and eviscerations in the literature, Bowen [50] reports an average mortality of 35.9 per cent. Some authors however, report a mortality following evisceration of as high as 75 per cent.[51] The incidence of postoperative hernia in abdominal incisions is reported at from 2 per cent to 10 per cent.[1] Mason [5] reporting a large series showed that 10.8 per cent of all herniorraphies were done to repair abdominal incisions. From these figures it may be seen that the incidence of disruption and hernia is relatively high following abdominal operations. The high mortality following disruption makes this complication a tragedy. Every effort then should be put forth in the attempt to so fashion and close abdominal wounds as to eliminate these complications or, at least, reduce them to a minimum.

Through the years a great deal has been written on the subject of disruption and herniation of abdominal wounds. Many possible causes have been listed and innumerable means of prevention have been suggested. A lengthy or even complete review of these factors is impossible in a text of this nature. However, certain factors, particularly those which we believe are important, should be considered. These may, for the sake of convenience, be divided into: (1) systemic; (2) those which are local and have to do primarily with wound healing; and (3) anatomical and physiological.

Systemic Factors. Clark [52] was the first to bring out the relation of serum protein levels to wound healing. Subsequent investigators confirmed these findings and it is now universally recognized that hypoproteinemia results in delayed wound healing; this delay occurs particularly in the fibroblastic state [53] which is so important to the tensile strength of the wound. Thompson, Ravdin and coworkers [54,55] have further pointed out that decreased proteins may result in edema at the suture line of an intestinal anastomosis (thus resulting in partial or complete intestinal obstruction) as well as decrease the general intestinal motility. These two factors may thus produce varying degrees of abdominal distention with resultant strain on the wound. They also noted that catgut absorbs more rapidly in the presence of edema, which they noted to be present in the wounds of all hypoproteinemic patients. It goes without saying then that correction of protein deficiencies by the best available method is necessary if primary wound healing is to be expected.

Lanman and Ingalls [56] established the relationship of vitamin C to wound healing although Sokolov [57] had previously suggested it and subsequent investigators [60] confirmed it in animals. That there is a very definite relationship between vitamin C and the tensile strength of human wounds was shown by Bartlett, Jones and Ryan [58,59] who found that the plasma ascorbic acid level must be below 0.2 mgm. per cent before the wound tensile strength is decreased. Several observers have noted low or absent plasma ascorbic acid in patients who have disrupted abdominal wounds. The relationship is clear. Determination of plasma ascorbic acid levels when there is any question and establishment of a normal level before operation is essential. Very large doses are frequently necessary.

In the summation of 1526 eviscerations presented by Bowen [50] 21.7 per cent occurred in cases operated on for malignancies. Similarly anemia and cachexia as well as dehydration have been blamed for disruption of wounds. The exact etiological relationship between these conditions and disruption or herniation is not clear. It seems most probable that these findings are associated with general debilitation, particularly when the gastro-intestinal tract is involved in the primary disease. Thus one would expect to find other more specific deficiencies (protein, vitamins) associated with these conditions which would account for the failure of wound healing. Carrel [62] has shown that the wound healing proceeds at a rate which is inversely proportional to the age of the patient. The average age in Bowen's compiled series was 44 years.

Local Factors. It is a well recognized surgical principle that foreign material (whether nonviable tissue or that introduced by the surgeon in the form of sutures) must be eliminated from the wound before fibroplasia can occur. The greater the amount of foreign material in the wound the longer is fibroplasia delayed. It follows then that the less suture material, blood, and tags of necrotic material left in the wound the quicker will healing progress. Foreign material may also affect wound healing by acting as a nidus in which actual infection gets a start; bacteria are able to adjust to the environment and get a start before the leukocytes can get to them. Catgut creates the greatest local reaction, silk less and stainless steel wire practically none.

Infection occurred in 25.3 per cent of the cases of disruption compiled by Bowen. Infection, whether it be subclinical or gross suppuration interferes with fibroplasia and delays wound healing. In addition, as shown by Howes,[77] catgut of any size, preparation or strength will lose all of its tensile strength in 3 to 6 days in the presence of even minimal infection. It has been definitely shown that there is a lag period in wound healing (4 to 6 days) during which the wound tensile strength is 0. The tensile strength then rapidly increases until maximum strength is reached in from 10 to 14 days. In the presence of infection then, catgut will lose its tensile strength during that phase of healing in which the tensile strength of the wound is at 0. There is increasing evidence to show that the incidence of infection in clean wounds is higher when catgut is used than when silk is used.[63] Furthermore catgut in itself produces a leukocytic reaction which must delay wound healing. Many surgeons have noted the complete absence of catgut suture material in wounds which have disrupted. The question of possible allergy to catgut has been repeatedly raised in recent years. Some [64-66] believe that it is possible to produce an allergic sensitivity to catgut which results in extremely rapid absorption of the catgut with complete loss of its tensile strength soon after it is placed in the tissues. Others, notably Pickrell and Clay [67] have been unable to produce sensitivity to catgut in animals nor have they been able to find evidence of sensitivity in humans in whom disruption has occurred. Whether or not an allergic sensitivity to catgut can occur, however, there is evidence (as outlined above) to show that catgut, of any size or preparation, cannot be sufficiently depended upon as a suture material to warrant its use in the aponeurotic layers of abdominal wall closure. Silk may lead to subsequent difficulty (as previously mentioned) hence, for reasons already put forth, we believe stainless steel to be the best suture material at present available for the closure of the aponeuroses.

In Bowen's compiled series of cases [50] 28.2 per cent of disruptions occurred through wounds which had been drained. As previously mentioned the drain may weaken the wound by the introduction of infection either from within or from outside; in addition the closure of peritoneum must be incomplete about the drain and this hiatus may offer the opening through which the entering wedge of omentum or bowel starts the process of disruption (or herniation). Drains should be used, in relation to abdominal wounds, as outlined previously.

Postoperative distention, whether it is due to adynamic ileus or actual intestinal obstruction may place great strain on the wound and result in disruption or herniation. Every effort should be made (see section on postoperative care) to combat the development of distention and to treat it in its early stages when it has developed.

Anatomical and Physiological Factors. All of the above factors undoubtedly play an important role in the production of herniation or disruption of abdominal wounds; every effort should be made to avoid or correct conditions which will lead to poor wound healing. In recent years a number of studies (previously quoted) have shown that the greatest single factor in the strength of the abdominal wall closure lies in the manner in which the incision is made. The vertical types of incision are not physiological since they cut across the major aponeurotic fibers of the abdominal wall oblique muscles; in addition they tend to denervate that portion of the abdominal wall medial to them. The transverse incision, on the other hand is, for reasons previously set down, more physiological and hence more readily closed and less apt to herniate or disrupt. Coughing and vomiting, which so frequently follow abdominal surgery are blamed for the vast majority of wound disruptions and herniations. The reason for this is apparent when it is recalled that the popular vertical incision is placed under the greatest possible strain by coughing or vomiting. These acts tend to approximate the edges of the transverse incision (which is more readily and firmly closed in the first place) hence cannot play such a major role in the disruption of the layers of this type of incision. The incidence of herniation and disruption of abdominal wounds has been previously given; these figures pertain primarily to vertical types of incisions. There is increasing evidence, however, that the incidence of herniation and disruption is very much lower in the transverse type of incision. Singleton [39] in 3147 transverse or oblique incisions found only one disruption, an incidence of 0.03 per cent. Coryloss as quoted by Farr [26] studied 2855 transverse incisions and found only seven postoperative hernias all of which occurred in infected wounds; none occurred in clean wounds. In an analysis of 1542 transverse incisions [1] only 2 hernias were reported, both in badly infected wounds; this gives an incidence of 0.13 per cent. In 225 consecutive transverse incisions in the upper abdomen studied at the University of Michigan Hospital [1] only one hernia was found; this was a small omental hernia at the site of drainage and was found only on careful examination. The only constant factor to account for the excellent statistics in these groups of cases is the type of incision. For the above reason we believe that the so-called "anatomical" or "physiological" incision (transverse, oblique, or muscle splitting) presents the best opportunity to avoid herniation or disruption of the wound.

Treatment of the Disrupted Wound. When disruption of the transverse wound does occur the bowel seldom eviscerates on to the abdominal wall as it nearly always does in the vertical wound disruption. In addition the transverse wound is much easier to close than is the vertical.

When disruption of any wound does occur it must be considered as an emergency and treatment instituted at once. Some surgeons feel that, in the poor risk patient, suture should not be attempted; under aseptic conditions they lightly pack the eviscerated bowel or omentum back in the abdominal cavity and strap the skin closed with adhesive straps. The incidence of herniation must be extremely high with this type of closure; furthermore there can be no reassurance that evisceration will not occur again nor that loops of bowel will not obstruct beneath the strapped skin wound. For these reasons we have not used the so-called conservative method of treatment. When the edges of the disrupted wound are examined it is always found that the various layers are difficult to define and that they are so friable that layer closure is almost impossible. Various types of suture have been advocated but in our hands the through-and-through silver wire [46,47] closure has proved to be the simplest, quickest and most efficient (Fig. 177). Under general anesthesia and with perfect aseptic technic the heavy silver wire is introduced, the needle passing from the peritoneum outward on both sides of the wound in order to be certain that no bowel is injured. After all of the wires have been placed they are drawn up and twisted so as to approximate the layers of the abdominal wall with the least tension which will still close the wound. The wire is heavy, malleable and nonirritating. If swelling occurs the wires may be untwisted and the tension relieved. These silver wire sutures are left in place a minimum of 14 days, or longer if adequate healing has not occurred.

POSTOPERATIVE PULMONARY COMPLICATIONS

This subject is covered elsewhere but a word as it relates to abdominal incisions is of value here. Atelectasis, (patchy or massive), pneumonia, pleuritis, and infarct or embolism account for the pulmonary morbidity. These complications are most common following operations in the upper abdomen (in from 5 to 12 per cent of cases [68]) but may follow any abdominal surgery. Vertical incision through or at the lateral border of the rectus muscle must transect some of the intercostal nerves to that area and, in many instances, other branches are traumatized by stretching and retraction; postoperative hyperirritability of the nerves must then occur and, subconsciously, the patient splints the abdominal wall to minimize the pain. Since the diaphragmatic excursion is correlated with and dependent upon free function of the abdominal musculature this splinting inevitably results in reduction of the vital capacity. Beecher [69] has reported this reduction in vital capacity to be as much as 58 per cent. Decreased ventilation then, favors the development of anoxia and atelectasis as well as pneumonia. The accumulation of secretions in the tracheobronchial tree also favors the development of atelectasis and pneumonia.[68] The best possible means of eliminating these secretions is by vigorous and frequently repeated coughing. When the vertical incision is used the pain and splinting which result markedly interfere with cough; for this reason elimination of secretions is interfered with the development of pulmonary complications is made more likely. As pointed out by Haight and Ransom [68] coughing is also one of the most efficacious means of treating pulmonary complications (atelectasis in particular) once they have developed. Pain is a much less prominent feature in the postoperative transverse wound because nerve injury is avoided and the aponeuroses are not transected. The patient is able to cough efficiently and raise the secretions in the tracheobronchial tree. Furthermore splinting of the abdominal wall is minimal or absent and a more normal respiratory excursion may be carried out. Coughing, which is so important in the prevention and treatment of most pulmonary complications places great stress on the vertical wound and at least partially accounts for the relatively high incidence of hernia and disruption of this type of incision. When the transverse incision is used, on the other hand, this stress is absent and the patient may be urged to cough without fear of producing herniation or disruption of the wound. It is also worthy of note that the use of heavy and elaborate binders for support of the abdominal wall is made unnecessary when the transverse incision is used. Thus another factor in the reduction of diaphragmatic excursions is eliminated by the use of a transverse incision. In a series of 125 transverse abdominal incisions reported by Jones and McClure [70] there were no cases of atelectasis or pneumonia although there were five cases of pulmonary emboli, two of which were fatal. In a study of comparable series of cases with vertical and transverse incisions Rees and Coller [1] show clearly the reduced incidence of pulmonary complications when the transverse incision is used.

There is a suggestion that the incidence of peripheral venous complications (phlebothrombosis and thrombophlebitis) is, in part at least, related to the venous stasis resultant upon immobility in bed. Further, there is no question as to the relationship between these venous complications and the development of pulmonary emboli. Because of the minimal amount of pain associated with transverse incisions, we have, in recent years, found it feasible to institute a program of very early ambulation following even the most major types of abdominal operations. Unless a specific contraindication exists it is now our policy to get patients with transverse incisions sitting up on the first postoperative day and in a wheelchair or walking on their second

TABLE 3. *INFLUENCE OF TRANSVERSE INCISIONS*

INCIDENCE OF PULMONARY COMPLICATIONS	TYPE OF INCISION	
	TRANSVERSE	VERTICAL
Number of cases	225	346
Patchy atelectasis	5 (2.2%)	26 (7.5%)
Massive atelectasis	0	5
Pleuritis	0	1
Infarct or embolism	1	1
Total pulmonary complications	6 (2.6%)	33 (9.5%)
Pulmonary complications chief cause of death	0	3
Pulmonary complications contributory cause of death	0	1

postoperative day. We have encountered no ill effects from this policy and feel that the incidence of pulmonary complications in general and pulmonary emboli in particular has been materially reduced. The improvement in the general welfare of the patient as well as reduction in hospital days have been gratifying to both the patient and the surgeon and represents another distinct argument in favor of the transverse incision.

REFERENCES

1. REES, V. L. and COLLER, F. A. Anatomic and Clinical Study of the Transverse Abdominal Incision, *Arch. Surg.*, 47:136-146, [Aug.], 1943.
2. MOSCHOWITZ, A. V. Transverse Incisions in the Upper Abdomen, *Ann. Surg.*, 64:268-287, [Sept.], 1916.
3. DAVIES, F. and WAKELEY, C. P. G. Abdominal Incisions in the Light of Recent Work on the Intercostal Nerves, *Australian and New Zealand J. Surg.*, 2:381-391, [April], 1933.
4. DAVIES, F., GLADSTONE, R. J. and STIBBE, E. P. The Anatomy of the Intercostal Nerves, *J. Anat.*, 66:323-333, [April], 1932.
5. MASON, J. T. A New Abdominal Incision, *Arch. Surg.*, 19:129-142, [July], 1929.
6. BARTLETT, W. and BARTLETT, W., JR. The Transverse Incision in the Upper Abdomen, *Surg., Gynec. & Obst.*, 57:93-99, [July], 1933.
7. QUAIN, E. P. Abdominal Incisions, *Arch. Surg.*, 1:585-602, [Nov.], 1920.
8. BANCROFT, F. W. Painful Postoperative Abdominal Scars, *Arch. Surg.*, 21:289-299, [Aug.], 1930.
9. McVAY, C. B. and ANSON, B. J. The Composition of the Rectus Sheath, *Anat. Rec.*, 77:213-225, [June 25], 1940.
10. BEST, C. H. and TAYLOR, N. B. *The Physiological Basis of Medical Practice*, Williams and Wilkins, Baltimore, 1945, pp. 301-302.
11. SLOAN, G. A. A New Upper Abdominal Incision, *Surg., Gynec. & Obst.*, 45:678-687, [Nov.], 1927.
12. FARR, R. E. Discussion, *J.A.M.A.*, 69:1683-1684, [Nov. 17], 1917.
13. ROSENBLATT, M. S. and COLVER, D. Transverse Upper Abdominal Incisions, *Surg., Gynec. & Obst.*, 80:641-642, [June], 1945.
14. McBURNEY, C. The Incision Made in the Abdominal Wall in Cases of Appendicitis with a Description of a New Method of Operating, *Ann. Surg.*, 20:38-44, [July], 1894.

15. BATTLE. Modified Incision for Removal of the Vermiform Appendix, *Brit. M. J.*, 2:1360, [Nov. 30], 1895.

16. KAMMERER, F. Modified Incision for Quiescent Appendicitis, *Ann. Surg.*, 26:225-228, [Aug.], 1897.

17. ELLIOT, J. W. A Modification of the McBurney Incision for Appendectomy, *Boston M. & S.J.*, 135:433-434, [Oct. 29], 1896.

18. HARRINGTON, F. B. Hernia Following Operations for Appendicitis, *Boston M. & S.J.*, 141:105-108, [Aug. 3], 1899.

19. WEIR, R. F. An Improved Operation for Acute Appendicitis or for Quiescent Cases with Complications, *M. News*, 76:241-242, [Feb. 17], 1900.

20. ROCKEY, A. E. Transverse Incision in Abdominal Operations, *Med. Record*, 68:779-780, [Nov. 11], 1905.

21. DAVIS, G. G. A Transverse Incision for the Removal of the Appendix, *Ann. Surg.*, 43:106, [June], 1906.

22. BAUDELOCQUE, C. A. NouVeau procédé pour pratiquer l'operation Cesarienne, Thesis, Paris, No. 132, 1823.

23. PFANNENSTEIL, J. Ueber die Vortheile des suprasymphysären Fascienquerschnitts für die gynakologischen Koeliotomicen zugleich ein Beitrag zu der Indikationsstellung der Operationswege, *Samml. klin. Vortr.*, No. 268, (gynäk. no. 97) :1735-1756, 1900.

24. CHERNEY, L. S. Modified Transverse Incision for Low Abdominal Operations, *Surg., Gynec. & Obst.*, 72:92-95, [Jan.], 1941.

25. MAYLARD, A. E. Direction of Abdominal Incisions, *Brit. M.J.*, 2:895-900, [Oct. 5], 1907.

26. FARR, R. E. Abdominal Incisions, *Lancet*, 32:561-569, [Nov. 1], 1912.

27. SINGLETON, A. O. Improvement in the Management of Upper Abdominal Operations, Stressing an Anatomical Incision, *Southern M.J.*, 24:200-206, [March], 1931.

28. SANDERS, R. L. Transverse Incision in the Upper Abdomen, *Ann. Surg.*, 104:74-86, [July], 1936.

29. MEYER, W. The Rectangular Flap Incision for Operations within the Upper Abdomen, *J.A.M.A.*, 69:1677-1684, [Nov. 17], 1917.

30. KOENIG, F. Über die Schnittführung bei Operationen an der Gallenwegen, *Zentralbl. f. Chir.*, 39:529-533, [Apr. 20], 1912.

31. KEHR, H. Ueber den Bauchdeckenschnitt die Bauchnaht und die Tamponade bei Gallenstein-operationen, *Arch. f. klin. Chir.*, 97:74-108, [Jan. 9], 1912.

32. PERTHES, G. Zur Schnittführung bei Operationen an der Gallenwegen, *Zentralbl. f. Chir.*, 39:1252-1256, [Sept. 14], 1912.

33. COLLINS, C. U. Some Points in the Surgery of the Bile Tracts, Describing a New Incision through Which to Reach Them and Presenting a New Instrument to Facilitate the Removal of Stones from the First Portion of the Common Duct, *Tr. West. S.A.*, 18:257-268, 1908.

34. KOCHER, E. T. *Textbook of Operative Surgery.* Authorized translation from the 4th Germ. Ed. by HAROLD J. STILES, A & C Black, London, 1903.

35. MACARTHUR, L. L. A Modified Incision for Approaching the Gall-Bladder, *Surg., Gynec. & Obst.*, 20:83-84, [Jan.], 1915.

36. DAVIS, H. H. Right Rectus Gridiron Incision in Congenital Pyloric Stenosis, *Surg., Gynec. & Obst.*, 78:213 [Feb.], 1944.

37. MAYO-ROBSON, A. W. Diseases of the Gall-bladder and Bile-ducts, Including Gall-stones, Wm. Wood & Co., New York, 1903.

38. MAYO, C. W. An Incision for Epigastric Lesions, *Proc. Staff Meet., Mayo Clin.*, 13:438-439, [July 13], 1938.

39. SINGLETON, A. O. and BLOCKER, T. G. The Problem of Disruption of Abdominal Wounds and Post-operative Hernia, *J.A.M.A.*, 112:122-127, [Jan. 14], 1939.

40. SINGLETON, A. O. Splenectomy, *Surg., Gynec. & Obst.*, 70:1051-1053, [June], 1940.

41. GURD, F. B. Abdominal Incisions. *Operative Surgery*, edited by BANCROFT, F. W., D. Appleton-Century Co., 1941, pp. 417-463.

42. BABCOCK, W. W. Catgut Allergy, with a Note on the Use of Alloy Steel Wire for Sutures and Ligatures, *Am. J. Surg.*, 27:67-70, [Jan.], 1935.

43. BABCOCK, W. W. Ligatures and Sutures of Alloy Steel Wire, *J.A.M.A.*. 102:1756, [May 26], 1934.

44. COLLER, F. A. and VALK, W. L. The Delayed Closure of Contaminated Wounds: Preliminary Report, *Ann. Surg.*, 112:256-270, [Aug.], 1940.

45. JONES, T. E., NEWELL, E. T., JR. and BRUBAKER, R. E. The Use of Alloy Steel Wire in the Closure of Abdominal Wounds, *Surg., Gynec. & Obst.*, 72:1056-1059, [June]. 1941.

46. REID, M. R., ZINNINGER, M. M., MERRELL, P. Closure of the Abdomen with Through-and-through Silver Wire Sutures in Cases of Acute Abdominal Emergencies, *Ann. Surg.*, 98:890-896, [Nov.], 1933.

47. STEVENSON, J. M. and REID, M. R. The Fundamental Principles of Surgical Technic. *Operative Surgery*, edited by BANCROFT, F. W., D. Appleton-Century Co., 1941, pp. 241-304.

48. KOSTER, H. and KASSMAN, L. P. Wound Disruption, *Am. J. Surg.*, 31:537-544, 557, [March], 1936.

49. HINTON, J. W. Allergy as an Explanation of Dehiscence of a Wound and Incisional Hernia, *Arch. Surg.*, 33:197-209, [Aug.], 1936.

50. BOWEN, A. Postoperative Wound Disruption and Evisceration, *Am. J. Surg.*, 47:3-19. [Jan.], 1940.

51. GLASSER, S. T. Evisceration and Avulsion of Abdominal Wounds, *Am. J. Surg.*. 32:63-76, [April], 1936.

52. CLARK, A. H. The Effect of Diet on the Healing of Wounds, *Bull. Johns Hopkins Hosp.*, 30:117-121, [May], 1919.

53. HARVEY, S. C. and HOWES, E. L. Effect of High Protein Diet on the Velocity of Growth of Fibroblasts in the Healing Wound, *Ann. Surg.*, 91:641-650, [May], 1930.

54. THOMPSON, W. D., RAVDIN, I. S. and FRANK, I. L. Effect of Hypoproteinemia on Wound Disruption, *Arch. Surg.*, 36:500-508, [March], 1938.

55. THOMPSON, W. D., *et al.* Use of Lyophile Plasma in Correction of Hypoproteinemia and Prevention of Wound Disruption. *Arch. Surg.*, 36:509-518, [March], 1938.

56. LANMAN, T. H. and INGALLS, T. H. Vitamin C Deficiency and Wound Healing, *Ann. Surg.*, 105:616-625, [April], 1937.

57. SOKOLOV, S. Postoperative Rupture of Abdominal Wounds with Protrusion or prolapse of the Viscera, *Vestnnk Chir.* No. 65, 66:219, 1931; *Abst. Inst. Abst. Surg.*. 55:157, [Aug.], 1932.

58. BARTLETT, M. K., JONES, C. M. and RYAN, A. E. Vitamin C and Wound Healing, Experimental Wounds in Guinea Pigs, *New England J. Med.*, 226:469-473, 1942.

59. BARTLETT, M. K., JONES, C. M. and RYAN, A. E. Vitamin C and Wound Healing, Ascorbic Acid Content and Tensile Strength of Healing Wounds in Human Beings, *New England J. Med.*, 226:474-481, [March], 1942.

60. TAFFEL, M. and HARVEY, S. C. Effect of Absolute and Partial Vitamin C Deficiency on Healing of Wounds, *Proc. Soc. Exp. Biol. and Med.*, 38:518-525, [May], 1938.

61. HOWES, E. L., SOOY, J. W. and HARVEY, S. C. The Healing of Wounds as Determined by Their Tensile Strength, *J.A.M.A.*, 92:42-45, [Jan. 5], 1929.

62. CARREL, A. Process of Wound Healing, *Proc. Inst. Med.*, *Chicago*, 8:62-66, [April], 1930.

63. ELKIN, D. C. Wound Infection. A Comparison of Silk and Catgut Sutures, *Ann. Surg.*, 112:280-282, [Aug.], 1940.

64. KRAISSL, C. J. Intrinsic Factors Altering the Absorption of Catgut, *Surg., Gynec. & Obst.*, 63:561-569, [Nov.], 1936.

65. KRAISSL, C. J., JESTEN, B. M. and CIMIOTTI, G. J. The Relation of Catgut Sensitivity to Wound Healing, *Surg., Gynec. & Obst.*, 66:628-635, [March], 1938.

66. LANGSTON, H. T. The Problem of Catgut Sensitivity and Its Relation to Wound Healing, *Ann. Surg.*, 115:141-147, [Jan.], 1942.

67. PICKRELL, K. L. and CLAY, R. C.   Wound Disruption and Catgut Allergy—Experimental and Clinical Study, with a Review of Literature, *Surgery*, 15:333-360, [Feb.], 1944.

68. HAIGHT, C. and RANSOM, H. K.   Observations on the Prevention of Atelectasis and Bronchopneumonia, *Ann. Surg.*, 114:243-262, [Aug.], 1941.

69. BEECHER, H. K.   The Measured Effect of Laparotomy on the Respiration, *J. Clin. Investigation*, 12:639-650, [July], 1933.

70. JONES, D. F. and McCLURE, W. L.   The Influence of the Transverse Upper Abdominal Incision on the Incidence of Post Operative Pulmonary Complications, *Surg., Gynec. & Obst.*, 51:208-212, [Aug.], 1930.

71. BAKES, J.   Erfahrungen mit den Sprengel'schen Bauchquerschnitten und ein neuer plastischer Querschnitt auf die Niere, *Arch. f. klin. Chir.*, 96:205-230, 1911.

72. SPRENGEL, O.   Kritische Betrachtungen über Bauchdeckennaht und Bauchschnitt, *Arch. f. klin. Chir.*, 92:536-595, 1910.

73. MEYER, W.   The Transverse Abdominal Incision, *Ann. Surg.*, 62:573-575, [Nov.], 1915.

74. SINGLETON, A. O.   The Importance of the Surgical Anatomy of the Abdominal Wall with Special Reference to Abdominal Incisions, *Proc. Interst. Postgrad. M.A. North America*, 28:101-104, 1943.

75. SINGLETON, A. O.   The Anatomic Importance of Fascia in the Abdominal Wall, *Southern Surgeon*, 3:235-243, [Sept.], 1934.

76. SOUTHAM, A. H.   A Comparative Study of Abdominal Incisions, *Brit. M.J.*, 1:513-514, [March 22], 1924.

77. HOWES, E. L.   Factors Determining the Loss of Strength of Catgut When Embedded in Tissue, *J.A.M.A.*, 90:530-532, [Feb. 18], 1928.

9

SURGERY OF STOMACH AND DUODENUM; GASTRIC VAGOTOMY IN THE TREATMENT OF PEPTIC ULCER

Waltman Walters, M.D. and Lester R. Dragstedt, M.D.

SURGERY OF STOMACH AND DUODENUM

Waltman Walters, M.D.

BENIGN LESIONS OF THE STOMACH

Benign gastric tumors may be single or multiple. They may be polypoid or they may lie within the substance of the gastric wall beneath the mucous membrane.

Polyps. Gastric polyps, like those of the colon, are potentially malignant and therefore should be removed. They produce bleeding and frequently are encountered in cases of anemia, in which the anemia is thought to be primary in type. In these cases, segmental resection of the stomach is performed and the removed tissue is examined under the microscope. If the lesion is malignant, partial gastrectomy is performed. If the polyps are multiple, partial gastrectomy is the preferable procedure provided that the polyps can be included in the portion resected. In the occasional cases in which polyps are confined to one segment of the stomach, this segment may be removed by a sleeve resection. Submucosal benign tumors such as fibroma, myoma and neurofibroma frequently cause serious although gradual bleeding; in such cases, anemia may be the only symptom. These tumors should be removed by segmental resection of the portion of stomach containing them; if evidence of malignant change is observed on microscopic examination, partial gastrectomy should be performed.

Diverticula of the Stomach. Diverticula of the stomach are rare. Cheney and Newell [1] found two gastric diverticula in 11,828 roentgenologic examinations of the stomach. Rivers, Stevens and Kirklin [2] reported that four gastric diverticula were found in 3,662 routine necropsies, and ten diverticula were removed in 11,234 exploratory operations on the stomach at the Mayo Clinic.

Most of these diverticula are false or of the acquired type. The indication is that an increase of intragastric pressure causes the diverticula.

The five patients having diverticula whom I have seen and operated on had definite, rather severe clinical symptoms which might have been attrib-

uted to distention of the diverticulum from retained food and inflammation
or bleeding from its mucosa. In the most recent case in which I operated,
the patient being a woman of fifty-seven years, a mesh of blood vessels invaded the wall of the diverticulum, and barium that had been swallowed on
roentgenographic examination seven days previously was still present in the
diverticulum at operation (Fig. 178).

Tuberculosis. Other benign surgical lesions of the stomach are tuberculosis and, in some cases, gastric syphilis. Tuberculosis of the stomach is exceedingly rare and the diagnosis has been made in less than twenty cases at the
Mayo Clinic. The diagnosis usually is not made preoperatively. Because the

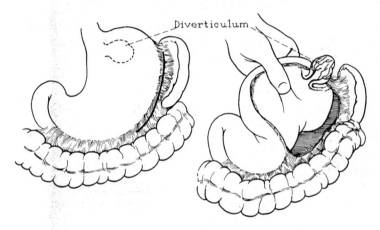

FIG. 178. Left: Portion of gastric diverticulum. Right: Exposure of diverticulum. Note
the nest of blood vessels in the diverticulum.

deformation of the stomach produced by gastric tuberculosis is similar to
that produced by carcinoma, the lesion is likely to be reported on roentgenographic examination as being malignant. However, in most cases of gastric
tuberculosis, tuberculous lesions can be found elsewhere in the patient's
body. Partial gastrectomy is the treatment for tuberculous gastric lesions. At
operation, if tuberculous lymph nodes are present in the gastrocolic or
gastrohepatic omentum, they can be removed with the portion of the
stomach containing the tuberculous lesions.

Syphilis. Gastric syphilis may produce digestive symptoms simulating
those of malignant disease. The differential diagnosis usually is made by the
roentgenologist, who is unable to palpate a tumor in spite of the fact that
the pathologic process apparently involves a large part of the stomach. In
such a case, the absence of cachexia and the presence of a normal blood
count together with serologic evidence of syphilis will usually lead to a diagnosis of gastric syphilis. Some of these patients will respond to anti-
syphilitic treatment, healing of the multiple ulcerations of the stomach
occurring without obstruction. In other cases, particularly when the ulcerations occur only in the lower third of the stomach, the healing process may
cause fibrosis and obstruction, necessitating either resection of the involved

portion of the stomach or the performance of gastro-enterostomy. I have used these methods of treatment of gastric syphilis, when indicated, with satisfactory results in each group.

Gastric Ulcer. Treatment of gastric ulcer is dependent on several factors, among which are: (1) duration and type of symptoms; (2) healing of the lesion or its failure to heal under a medical regimen carried out in a scientific fashion; (3) presence or absence of a crater, especially with respect to bleeding; and (4) presence or absence of pyloric obstruction. Age too, is an important factor.

When the symptoms have not been long present and the ulcer is small, every attempt should be made to induce healing of the lesion by nonsurgical means. Eusterman, Jordan and others have commented in detail on such methods of treatment.[3,4] A favorable clinical response to such medical treatment consists in relief of pain, disappearance of blood from the stool and disappearance of the niche seen on roentgenologic examination. In most instances, it can be assumed that these criteria are of immediate value in determining the ability of the lesion to respond to medical measures. However, a number of years ago McVicar[5] called attention to the fact that such a response may also occur in treatment of small, ulcerating, malignant lesions of the stomach. Exact information should be obtained from the patient as to whether a medical regimen has been instituted previously and the accuracy with which it was carried out and the results which have followed its use should be evaluated, for, if one or more attempts have been made to cause the lesion to heal by a carefully controlled medical regimen but the ulcerating lesion has recurred, the lesion should be removed surgically.

In the period during which our patients who have gastric ulcer are being kept under observation and medical treatment is being employed, even though the lesion appears to be healing satisfactorily, the patient is advised that he should be reexamined at intervals of three months for the first year, regardless of the presence or absence of symptoms, in order to determine with certainty that the ulcer has remained healed. If the ulcer recurs or if it does not heal, surgical exploration is thought advisable. In a few cases, unfortunately, in which response to the initial medical regimen appeared to be satisfactory, the patient failed to be impressed with the importance of repeated reexamination, either at the clinic or elsewhere, and returned later suffering from extensive carcinoma of the stomach.

PERFORATING GASTRIC ULCER WITH CRATER. A perforating gastric ulcer having a crater more than 1.5 cm. in diameter is not likely to respond to medical treatment. These ulcers, which usually are situated on the lesser curvature, will be found to have penetrated into the gastrocolic omentum, whereas some situated on the posterior wall, in most cases near the lesser curvature, may penetrate into the capsule of the pancreas. It might be inferred that malignant cells are most likely to be present in this type of lesion. Although this may be the case, especially if the lesions have large craters, fairly frequently the smaller ulcerating gastric lesions may be in a mass of highly malignant ulcerating carcinoma which already has involved the lymph nodes when the patient presents himself for examination or treatment.

GASTRIC ULCER PRODUCING PYLORIC OBSTRUCTION. If the site of ulcerating lesions of the stomach, either benign or malignant, is on the lesser curvature, they fairly frequently produce so much disturbance of motility, as disclosed both by clinical and by roentgenologic examination, that only the presence of pyloric obstruction can be determined. In some of these cases, the lesion is suspected of being a duodenal ulcer. This is particularly true if the patient has had an ulcer-like type of dyspepsia for a prolonged period. Fortunately, in cases of pyloric obstruction surgical procedures are usually advised, the presence of a gastric lesion is recognized at operation and appropriate treatment is carried out. The roentgenologist's diagnosis that an ulcerating lesion of the stomach is malignant is almost certain to be correct, particularly if the meniscus sign of Carman is seen in the course of roentgenoscopic examination. But the fact that an ulcer of the stomach is reported by the roentgenologist as being probably benign does not exclude the possibility that the lesion is carcinomatous. On many occasions at operation, with small gastric ulcerations readily visible and palpable, the fact that the lesion was carcinomatous was not recognizable until microscopic examination of the removed tissue proved the fact.

TYPES OF OPERATION FOR GASTRIC ULCER. The following types of operation are available in treatment of gastric ulcer: (1) partial gastrectomy followed by anastomosis of stomach and duodenum (Billroth I) or of stomach and jejunum (Polya-Balfour); (2) excision of a portion of the stomach containing the gastric ulcer or destruction of the gastric ulcer by cautery, in some cases combined and, in other cases, not combined with gastro-enterostomy; (3) transgastric excision of the ulcer from the posterior wall of the stomach; or (4) sleeve resection of the stomach.

The type of operation to be selected for each case depends on the type of lesion, its size, its situation, its accessibility, the amount of deformity of the stomach that would result from its removal, and the general condition of the patient. In selection of the type of operation most suited to the patient or lesion, the general statement seems justified that partial gastrectomy, particularly for large gastric ulcers, with a Billroth I, a Polya or a Polya-Balfour type of anastomosis, is the preferable procedure, provided that it can be performed with a mortality rate as low as 2 per cent. The reasons for this are: (1) the prompt relief of symptoms obtained; (2) the almost total absence of recurring ulceration; and (3) the fact that partial gastrectomy is the preferable procedure should the lesion prove to be malignant.

There is a place for destruction of the ulcer by cautery or for segmental resection of a portion of the stomach containing the ulcer, either operation being combined with gastro-enterostomy. Whereas the mortality rate associated with partial gastrectomy for large gastric ulcers, in our experience at the clinic, has been approximately 3 to 4 per cent, excision or destruction by cautery of a gastric ulcer, combined with gastro-enterostomy, usually can be performed with a mortality rate not greater than that of gastro-enterostomy. Furthermore, the risk of any operation is one of the very important factors in determining the type of operation to be chosen. One can accept the working principle that excision or destruction by cautery, combined with gastro-enterostomy, is a suitable operation of low risk for gastric ulcers located high on the lesser curvature, but that partial gastrectomy is the preferable procedure especially for large, penetrating, frequently hemorrhagic, gastric ulcers.

In some cases, similar good results can be obtained by excision of certain large, perforating gastric ulcers situated high on the posterior wall of the stomach by a transgastric approach to the lesion through an incision made in the anterior gastric wall. After the lesion has been excised the edges of the stomach are sutured together from the inside and a portion of the gastrohepatic omentum is carried posterior to the stomach, to serve as a patch over the healing anastomosis.

As has been indicated, whenever possible, I prefer the operation of partial gastrectomy for accessible, large, perforating gastric ulcers. I use the Billroth I, the Polya or the Polya-Balfour type of anastomosis; the choice of one of these procedures depends on the situation of the ulcer, the mobility of the duodenum, the amount of fat in the transverse mesocolon and the accessibility of the avascular spaces in the transverse mesocolon. Partial gastrectomy can be applied in nearly all cases of gastric ulceration. In general, the Polya or Balfour-Polya is to be preferred to the Billroth I.

Gastric ulcers situated high on the lesser curvature and those situated high on the posterior wall of the stomach frequently are reported, on the basis of roentgenologic examination, to be of questionable accessibility to surgical removal. Their high situation is likely to be considered an additional reason for continuation of medical treatment which has failed to cause healing of the ulcer previously. That all benign gastric lesions are accessible to surgical treatment is, therefore, a point which deserves emphasis. On several occasions, because of the perforating nature of the lesion and its attachment, particularly, to the capsule of the pancreas and because of contraction and fixation of the stomach in the vicinity of the lesion, the appearance has been that the lesion was higher than it really was.

For example, a man, sixty-eight years of age, had a large, recurring, perforating gastric ulcer, 3 cm. in diameter, high on the lesser curvature. No evidence of healing of the ulcer was observed on medical treatment. The reason the ulcer seemed so high was that it had perforated and had attached itself to the capsule of the pancreas and to the gastrocolic omentum. When the ulcer was freed from its attachment to the pancreas, it was found that there was a considerable amount of normal stomach above it, which enabled performance of satisfactory partial gastrectomy of the Polya-Balfour type.

Removal of that portion of the lesser curvature which contains a gastric ulcer, as in the Billroth I or the Hofmeister-Polya resection, enables the surgeon to preserve a sufficient amount of the body of the stomach and, particularly, the greater curvature, for its anastomosis with the duodenum or with the jejunum.

RESULTS OF OPERATIONS FOR GASTRIC ULCER. The results of a properly chosen, properly performed operation for gastric ulcer are among the best in surgery and recurrence of the ulcer, or disturbing symptoms without formation of ulcer, practically never are encountered. This is especially true if the operation performed is partial gastrectomy. Yet, similar good results have followed the more conservative operations of excision or destruction of the ulcer, combined with gastro-enterostomy, in most cases. Although I have not encountered a recurring ulcer after partial gastrectomy for benign gastric ulcer, I have operated on only five patients among whom gastric ulcer recurred after previous excision of a gastric ulcer, followed by gastro-enterostomy. Subsequent closure of the gastro-enteric stoma and partial gastrectomy of the Billroth I, Polya or Polya-Balfour type have been followed by excellent results and ulceration has not recurred.

In a study made of the postoperative gastric acidity of patients who previously had had gastric ulcer and on whom different types of operations had been performed, the striking thing was the high frequency with which relative achlorhydria occurred, provided adequate drainage of the stomach had been obtained following operation. This was in contrast with the effect of similar types of operation performed for duodenal ulcer.

Duodenal Ulcer. TYPES OF OPERATION FOR DUODENAL ULCER. *Pyloroplasty and Gastroduodenostomy.* Pyloroplasty and gastroduodenostomy were used more frequently in past years than at present, operation having been advised, in some cases, without an adequate attempt being made to treat the ulcer medically. In many such cases, the duodenal ulcers were small, were localized only on the anterior wall of the duodenum and lent themselves very readily to excision, division of the pyloric sphincter, or removal of a portion of it in enlarging the outlet of the stomach. In the majority of such cases, the operative results were very good, the risk was low and ulceration recurred in about the same percentage of cases as following gastro-enterostomy. In recent years, patients who have duodenal ulcer are operated on only after at least one or more attempts have been made to heal the lesion or at least control the patient's dyspepsia by a medical regimen. As a result, at operation the ulcers usually are found to be much larger, are frequently multiple and usually are associated with a considerable degree of fibrosis. As a result of this, considerable shortening of the duodenum has occurred and the patient has become fleshy; in other words, there is little motility of the duodenum, that performance of a large pyloroplasty is difficult and the stoma is not very satisfactory. Since a pyloroplasty opening which is too small may produce stasis at this point sufficient to predispose to recurring ulcer, I have felt that, in such cases, gastro-enterostomy or partial gastrectomy is preferable to pyloroplasty.

Anastomosis Anterior or Posterior to the Colon. The same indications for anastomosis posterior or anterior to the colon, whether after partial gastrectomy or in the performance of gastro-enterostomy, apply in treatment of duodenal ulcer as in treatment of gastric ulcer or gastric carcinoma. In other words, if, because of the amount of fat in the transverse mesocolon or the shortness of the transverse colon or the lack of space between the arcades of the transverse colic vessels, it would seem that the possibilities of a malfunctioning anastomosis made posterior to the colon are comparatively great, then the anastomosis is made anterior to the colon by using a longer loop of jejunum.

Exploration of the Interior of the Duodenum. On several occasions, when examination of the anterior wall of duodenum has not given evidence of ulcer, the crater of an ulcer on the posterior wall could be felt by palpating the duodenum between the thumb and forefinger. Occasionally, however, small ulcers on the posterior wall, the source of serious bleeding, are not palpable and can be recognized only by opening the duodenum and exploring its interior. This, I believe, is an essential part of gastroduodenal exploration among patients who give a history of hematemesis.

Partial Gastrectomy. Those who advocate partial gastrectomy for duodenal ulcer do so on the basis of the presence of associated gastritis and the low incidence of recurring ulceration subsequently; however, the mortality rate of partial gastrectomy for duodenal ulcer when the operation is performed by surgeons of considerable experience will vary from 2 to 5 per cent. To my way of thinking, the only object that partial gastrectomy accomplishes better than gastro-enterostomy is to produce a greater reduction of gastric acidity and gastric secretion in a greater number of cases and there are fewer recurrences of ulceration. Since it is a matter of record that but 70 per cent of the patients obtain relative achlorhydria, there is no reason why the 30 per cent who fail to do so may not be as susceptible to recurring ulceration as those who have undergone gastro-enterostomy. More interesting still is the fact that in about 12 per cent of cases achlorhydria will develop after gastro-enterostomy. After all, the crux of the matter, from the standpoint of recurrence, is whether or not the tissue resistance of the attached jejunum or duodenum has improved sufficiently so that, if free hydrochloric acid does remain in the gastric contents, recurring ulceration will not take place.

Congenital Pyloric Stenosis. For the surgical treatment of congenital pyloric stenosis the operation described by Ramstedt [6] of dividing the hypertrophied pyloric musculature with an incision extending down to the mucous membrane has been uniformly followed for many years.

Before the introduction of the Ramstedt procedure gastro-enterostomy was performed for the relief of this condition in infants. Although a small mortality rate was reported in the use of gastro-enterostomy, it undoubtedly was many times greater than that in the performance of the Ramstedt procedure. Moreover, late complications have occurred in some cases in which gastro-enterostomy had been performed for this condition. I have operated in five such cases in which the ages of the patients varied from eighteen to thirty years. In each case operation was performed for hemorrhagic gastrojejunitis or frank gastrojejunal ulcer, the symptoms of which did not appear until the patients were eighteen years of age or older. Bleeding was so severe that it was realized that radical surgical treatment was necessary to prevent the possibility of fatal hemorrhage. In one of these cases in which the patient had bled, the examination of the stomach, duodenum and jejunum by roentgenography two or three weeks later failed to reveal the lesion. Six weeks subsequently a gastrojejunal ulcer perforated. The opening was closed. Some months later, I removed the gastro-enteric stoma and resected the stomach. At this time gastrojejunitis was present. In all of these cases after the performance of partial gastrectomy I have carried out a Billroth I anastomosis (von Haberer modification) with excellent results. Two of these patients were well when they were presented three and five years respectively after their operations and letters from two of the others indicate that they have had excellent results.

Donovan and I [7] made a study of the pyloric sphincter in such cases in which resection has been performed and found that the hypertrophy of the pyloric sphincter continues to exist. Stevens and Boeck [8] and Fowler and Hanson [9] have reported similar cases in which bleeding has occurred and in which, after removal of the gastro-enteric stoma, some type of pyloroplasty was performed instead of gastric resection. In 1944 Stevens and Boeck reported their patient to have been well for one and a half years.

The technic of removal of the gastro-enteric stoma and closure of the opening in the jejunum and of partial gastrectomy with Billroth I anastomosis is described elsewhere.

MALIGNANT LESIONS OF THE STOMACH

The treatment of carcinoma as well as sarcoma of the stomach is essentially surgical. Not only does it offer the greatest possibility of relief of the troublesome symptoms of obstruction, ulceration, hemorrhage and so forth but, when the lesion is confined to the stomach or even when the adjacent lymph nodes are involved, removal of a large portion of the stomach and its adjacent node-bearing omentum will give an incidence of five year cures varying between 40 and 50 per cent if the nodes are not involved, and between 18 and 20 per cent, if the nodes are involved. Of the patients operated on, from 40 to 60 * per cent have removable lesions. At the Mayo Clinic, the incidence of resections has increased progressively, from 36 per cent in 1927 to 66 per cent in 1947.[10]

When the lesion is confined to the stomach, the surgeon must be willing to perform subtotal and, in a few cases, even total gastrectomy. The risk of subtotal gastrectomy is very little more than that of partial gastrectomy and for lesions of a comparable degree of malignancy the surgical results are comparable, for very large malignant lesions are frequently found to be of a low grade of malignancy.

As the roentgenologist is able to recognize very small lesions, similarly he is able to determine, to a considerable extent, whether or not the lesion appears within the limits of removability. This depends on whether the normal portion of the stomach above the lesion is large enough to permit of its anastomosis with the intestine. Yet, there is a possibility of error in re-

* 60 per cent in 1944.

porting some gastric lesion as being inoperable or of borderline operability when it may be removed by extensive partial gastrectomy. In other words, in such a group of cases, in 15 to 20 per cent of the cases in which the lesion is reported to be inoperable or of borderline operability there will be found to be a sufficient amount of stomach above the lesion so that the latter can be removed. For this reason it has been the custom at the Mayo Clinic for many years, to advise exploration of all malignant lesions of the stomach, regardless of their extent, provided that there was no evidence of distant metastasis. Moreover, total gastrectomy is done with increasing frequency.

Sarcoma of the Stomach. Gastric sarcoma is rare; its relative incidence is approximately 5 in 100 cases of malignant lesions. It occurs most frequently among young persons presenting the same clinical picture and roentgenologic findings as those having carcinoma. Surgical treatment and the methods used for carcinoma apply equally well to sarcoma. In cases of lymphosarcoma, however, roentgen therapy should be given after operation and also for irremovable lesions.

Operative Mortality in Cases of Resection of the Stomach for Malignant Lesions. In following out these ideas in a group of 275 cases of malignant lesions of the stomach in which patients were operated on at the clinic in 1947, the growth was removed in 148 cases with a mortality rate of 5.3 per cent. The resectability rate, therefore, was 53.8 per cent. In 125 of the 148 cases partial gastrectomy was performed with a mortality rate of 6.4 per cent and in 19, total gastrectomy was performed with a mortality rate of 5.3 per cent.

ANATOMY OF THE STOMACH

From the surgical standpoint, the arterial blood supply of the stomach and the lymphatic drainage of the stomach are very important to remember. The arterial blood supply of the stomach is so extensive that it is possible to divide both right and left gastric arteries and the right and left gastroepiploic arteries without the occurrence of necrosis of the gastric wall. As a matter of fact, that is exactly what is done in the operation of partial or total gastrectomy. The right and left gastro-epiploic arteries are ligated when the gastrocolic omentum is removed from the stomach. In the ligation and division of the gastrohepatic omentum lying along the lesser curvature of the stomach one divides the left gastric artery. Then the right gastric artery is ligated and divided when the gastrohepatic omentum of the first portion of the duodenum is divided and ligated. Branches of the left gastro-epiploic artery are ligated when the gastrocolic omentum is separated and ligated from the outer portion of the upper third of the stomach. In the ligation of the right gastro-epiploic artery in the gastrocolic omentum one must be exceedingly careful not to pick up the right transverse colic artery, a branch of the superior mesenteric artery, or else arterial circulation to the transverse colon will be interfered with (Fig. 179).

Knowledge of the lymphatic drainage of the stomach is important, and when dealing with cancer of the stomach it is advisable not only to remove that portion of the stomach involved but with it those channels of lymphatic drainage which may have become involved by extension of the malignant cells to these regions. As in surgical treatment of carcinoma of the breast one removes the efferent lymph nodes and fat, so in extirpation of the stomach or part of it, the gastrocolic and gastrohepatic omenta along the greater and lesser curvatures of the stomach containing the gastric group of

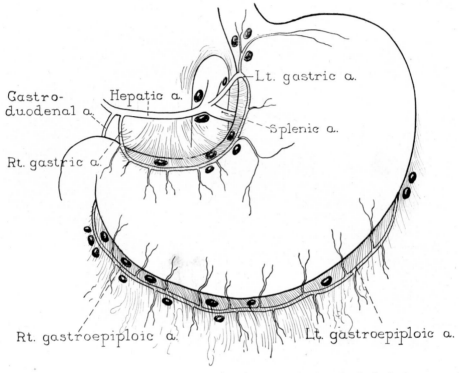

Fig. 179. Arterial blood supply and lymph nodes in the lymphatic drainage areas of the stomach.

lymph nodes, including the infrapyloric, are removed (Fig. 179). It is to be noted that efferent lymphatic vessels from all of these nodes go to the lymph nodes along the celiac aspect in front of the aorta, forming the pre-aortic nodes. It is rarely advisable to remove this latter group of nodes since in cases in which they are involved the lesion is usually inoperable.

Intramural lymphatic extension of malignant cells may occur in all directions but fortunately these usually terminate at the pylorus and at the cardia.* This makes it necessary to remove the pylorus and a small segment of the first portion of the duodenum to get beyond this region distally. Proximally one should go as far as feasible, at least 7.5 cm. beyond the upper end of the gastric malignant lesion.

* I have operated in a few cases in which intramural lymphatic involvement extended beyond the pylorus into the first portion of the duodenum.

THE BILLROTH I RESECTION: ITS MODIFICATIONS
AND RESULTS

Billroth,[11-16] in performing his first successful partial gastrectomy, sutured the end of the stomach to the duodenum, decreasing the circumference of the stomach by sutures placed in the vicinity of the lesser curvature. Péan[17-18] had performed a similar type of operation previously, but, as his

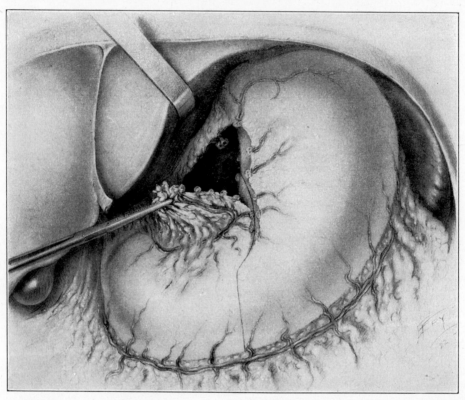

Fig. 180. Gastric vessels have been ligated high in the gastrohepatic omentum. Portion of the gastrohepatic omentum to be removed with the tumor and the pattern of stomach to be removed are shown. (From Walters, Waltman, Gray, H. K. and Priestley, J. T., *Carcinoma and Other Malignant Lesions of the Stomach*. Courtesy of W. B. Saunders Company, Philadelphia, 1942.)

patient failed to recover, his priority frequently is lost sight of. Inasmuch as Billroth, a few years after, abandoned this type of anastomosis for an indirect anastomosis of stomach to jejunum, which has been called the Billroth II,[19] it might be well to call the Billroth I the Péan-Billroth. The reason given for this change from a direct to an indirect type of anastomosis was the fact that but one patient of three on whom the Péan-Billroth procedure was performed recovered from the operation, apparently owing to leakage at the "fatal suture angle," that triangle at the upper part of the anastomosis where the three suture lines of the anastomosis approximate.

Of the various modifications of the Péan-Billroth method of direct anastomosis that of von Haberer [20] appears to be the most satisfactory, owing to the fact that the entire circumference of the stomach is sutured to the circumference of the duodenum. The larger circumference of the stomach

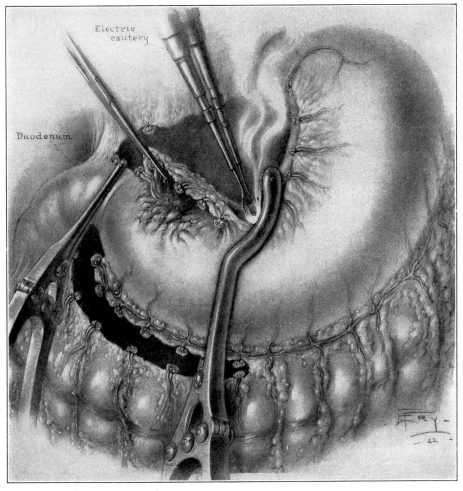

FIG. 181. Schoemaker clamp placed across stomach. Payr clamp placed across duodenum. Excision of the portion of the stomach containing the tumor with the cautery. (From Walters, Waltman, Gray, H. K. and Priestley, J. T., *Carcinoma and Other Malignant Lesions of the Stomach.* Courtesy of W. B. Saunders Company, Philadelphia, 1942.)

is decreased by interrupted sutures placed in the mucous membrane and muscularis mucosae of the gastric wall. These sutures also serve as ligatures of the larger blood vessels of the gastric submucosa.

Several methods were instituted assisting in the removal of the lesser curvature to decrease the diameter of the stomach and to prevent the formation of a diverticulum. Among these was that of Schoemaker [21,22] of The

Hague, who devised an ingenious clamp (Figs. 180 and 181) which could be placed across the stomach in such a way that when the stomach was cut along its lower margin a gastric pattern resulted in which the lesser curvature had been narrowed sufficiently so that the remaining circumference of the stomach approximated that of the duodenum. Charles H. Mayo and

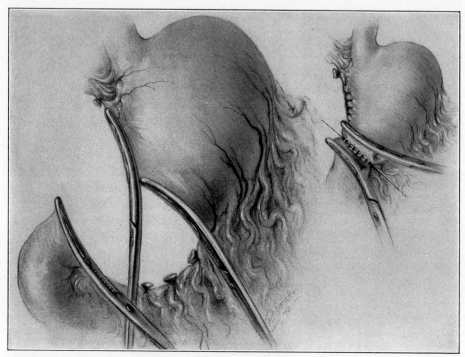

FIG. 182. Mayo method. Curved hemostats placed across the stomach and duodenum in the position to remove a larger portion of the lesser curvature. Inset shows method of making anastomosis. (From Walters, Waltman, Gray, H. K. and Priestley, J. T., *Carcinoma and Other Malignant Lesions of the Stomach.* Courtesy of W. B. Saunders Company, Philadelphia, 1942.)

William J. Mayo obtained the same result by using two curved hemostats, placing the first across the lower half of the stomach and the second almost at right angles to it so as to take out a portion of the lesser curvature (Fig. 182). In 1923, Horsley suggested that the duodenum be sutured to the lesser curvature portion of the stomach rather than to the greater curvature [23] (Fig. 183). The difference in the circumferences of the two is compensated for by a longitudinal incision down the anterior wall of the duodenum, while the greater curvature portion of the stomach is not included in the anastomosis and is closed by sutures.

The modifications of the Péan-Billroth most frequently used at the Mayo Clinic have been Schoemaker's, C. H. Mayo's and von Haberer's.*

* Finney of Baltimore and von Haberer [24] independently advised anastomosing the remaining segment of the stomach to the side rather than to the end of the duodenum.

Technic of the Billroth I Operation. The division and ligation of the branches of the gastric artery in the gastrohepatic omentum are similar in all types of partial gastrectomy, and the same applies to the ligation of the gastro-epiploic arteries. By placing the forefinger of the left hand in the

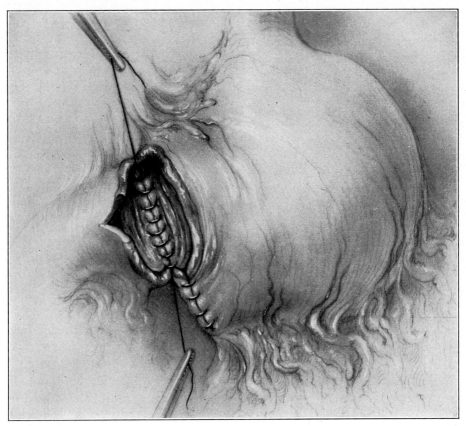

Fig. 183. Horsley's modification of the Billroth I method. (Modified from Horsley, J. S. and Bigger, I. A., *Operative Surgery,* 2:1016. Ed. 5, C. V. Mosby Company, St. Louis, 1940.)

foramen of Winslow posterior to the gastrohepatic omentum and the thumb anterior to it, wiping the upper margin of the duodenum, one is enabled to introduce a forceps accurately between the omentum and the duodenum in order to permit their separation, division and ligation. By extending the forefinger toward the midline posterior to the duodenum and the thumb

The advantage of this procedure is that it allows the entire circumference of the stomach to be sutured to the anterior portion of the duodenum after the making of an incision of equal size to that of the stomach (Fig. 184). Later, however, von Haberer[20] instituted the method previously described of narrowing the circumference of the stomach by interrupted sutures, thus permitting it to be sutured directly to the end of the duodenum. It is this latter method that I refer to when I speak of the von Haberer modification of the Billroth I.

anterior, the attachment of gastrocolic omentum to the duodenum can be well defined and forceps can be placed on the blood vessels (branches of the right gastro-epiploic artery) running through it. The gastrocolic omentum can be disconnected from the attachment to the transverse colon after the ligation of the right gastro-epiploic vessels below the pylorus, and the gastrocolic omentum can be dissected with the scalpel from the transverse colon with very little bleeding. Figure 185, showing enlarged involved

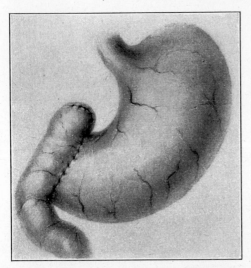

lymph nodes in the omenta, directs attention to the lymphatic drainage areas from the stomach. The inset shows the amount of gastrocolic omentum to be removed in its relation to the portion of stomach to be resected.

A curved hemostat of sufficient gripping power to hold the cut edges of the duodenum without their slipping is placed across the duodenum well below the pylorus. A second hemostat is placed above the first one (Fig. 186). The duodenum is transected between the clamps, and the stomach is reflected upward and toward the midline, where it is held by the first assistant. The surgeon wipes the gastrohepatic omentum from the lesser curvature of the stomach at the point where the gastric artery is to be divided and ligated.

FIG. 184. Diagrammatic sketch of the Finney-von Haberer terminal lateral anastomosis of stomach to side of duodenum. (From Walters, Waltman, Gray, H. K. and Priestley, J. T., *Carcinoma and Other Malignant Lesions of the Stomach*. Courtesy of W. B. Saunders Company, Philadelphia, 1942.)

Three Kocher forceps are passed through the avascular area of the gastrohepatic omentum and then applied across the omentum, which is divided between the proximal two and the distal one. The branches of the gastric artery and the blood vessels of the gastrohepatic omentum are ligated doubly, the first ligature being a suture ligature. A suction pump is introduced into the lumen of the stomach, thoroughly emptying it of any retained gastric secretion or gas (Fig. 187). This prevents fluid from the stomach being forced into the esophagus.

It is well to take out as much of the stomach above the tumor as is possible and consistent with postoperative gastro-intestinal function and motility. When the secretion and gas have been removed from the interior of the stomach, the decrease in the circumference of the stomach that will occur is surprising. This is important, since, in the Billroth-von Haberer method, the entire circumference of the stomach is to be approximated to the circumference of the duodenum. Any method enabling one to reduce the circumference of the stomach is worth while. The greater and lesser curvatures of the stomach are approximated to the inferior and superior margins of the duodenum by two interrupted sutures, and a row of continuous or interrupted sutures is placed approximating the serosal layers of the posterior wall of the stomach to the duodenum. These sutures are applied in such a

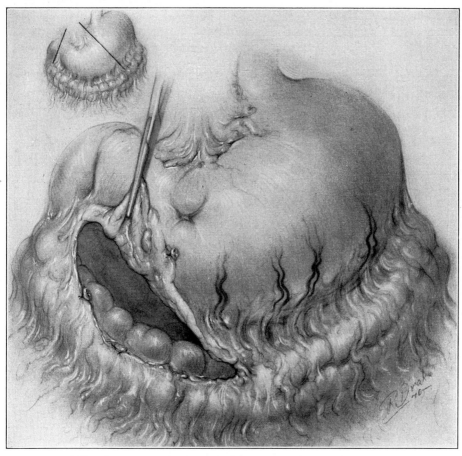

Fig. 185. Billroth I-von Haberer technic. Gastrocolic omentum containing lymph nodes separated from the colon. Inset shows the amount of stomach and of gastrocolic and gastrohepatic omentum to be removed. (From Walters, Waltman, Gray, H. K. and Priestley, J. T., *Carcinoma and Other Malignant Lesions of the Stomach*. Courtesy of W. B. Saunders Company, Philadelphia, 1942.)

way as to include larger amounts of gastric serosa than of duodenal serosa, a procedure which likewise tends to reduce the circumference of the stomach. Since the stomach has been emptied of its contents, it is unnecessary to place a clamp of any sort across it. In fact, the use of such a clamp not only reduces the amount of stomach that can be removed in some cases, but in addition, so flattens the wall of the stomach that the diameter is increased to a considerable extent. The use of a suction apparatus will keep the operative field clear of blood and duodenal secretions.

An incision, extending to the mucous membrane, is made in the posterior wall of the stomach, as shown in figure 188. Interrupted sutures are placed adjacent to each other in the mucous membrane of the posterior wall of the stomach. These sutures serve as ligatures of the branches of the gastric blood vessels, but, in addition, fulfill the purpose of reefing the mucous membrane, thus decreasing its circumference. Incision is made through the

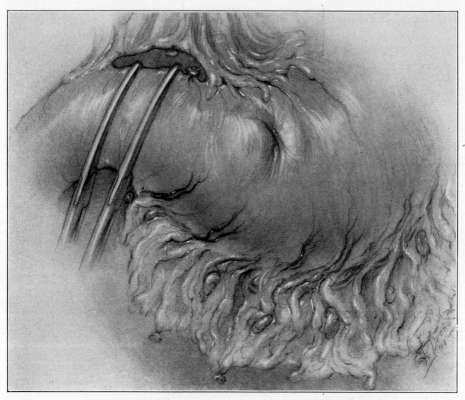

Fig. 186. Billroth I-Von Haberer method. Curved hemostats placed across the duodenum. (From Walters, Waltman, Gray, H. K. and Priestley, J. T., *Carcinoma and Other Malignant Lesions of the Stomach*. Courtesy of W. B. Saunders Company, Philadelphia, 1942.)

mucous membrane of the stomach into its lumen and the curved hemostat on the duodenum is removed. The clamped crushed tissue on the duodenum then is trimmed off. Any bleeding vessels in the submucosa of the stomach are grasped and ligated. A second row of chromic catgut sutures is used to approximate the mucosa, submucosa, and muscularis mucosae of the stomach to the duodenum. Cutting across the anterior wall of the stomach permits removal of the segment of stomach containing the tumor. If one makes an incision through the mucous membrane and the anterior wall of the stomach first, one is again able to pick up the blood vessels of the submucosa with hemostats and ligate them (Fig. 189).

After the segment of stomach containing the lesion has been removed, a point in the midportion of the mucous membrane of the anterior wall of the stomach is approximated to the midportion of the mucous membrane and submucosa of the anterior wall of the duodenum. By placing a consid-

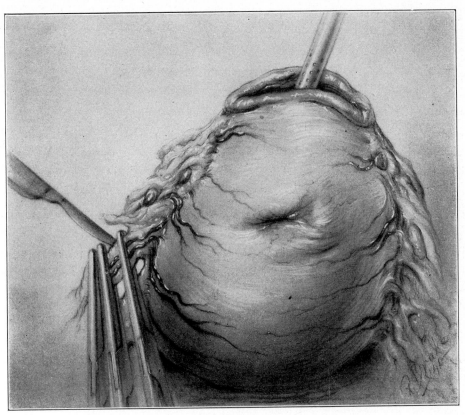

Fig. 187. Billroth I-von Haberer method. Cut end of stomach has been reflected, exposing the branches of the gastric artery and vein and the gastrohepatic omentum. Hemostats have been placed and the vessels are about to be divided. Suction pump introduced into the lumen of the stomach, emptying it of gastric secretion and gas. (From Walters, Waltman, Gray, H. K. and Priestley, J. T., *Carcinoma and Other Malignant Lesions of the Stomach.* Courtesy of W. B. Saunders Company, Philadelphia, 1942.)

erable degree of traction on the two sutures at the angles of the anastomosis one can stretch the duodenum to conform more nearly to the size of the stomach. One can enlarge the circumference of the cut end of the duodenum by making a small incision down the anterior wall of the duodenum at right angles to the circumference. Further interrupted sutures are placed in the mucous membrane of the stomach and the duodenum, each one being placed in a position so as to bisect the space between two others previously placed. A second row of sutures approximates the serosa and muscularis mucosae of the stomach to the duodenum. It is frequently advisable to start these sutures at each angle of the anastomosis, having them meet in the midline. This assists in the more accurate approximation of the structures (Figs. 190 and 191a). A third row of sutures, usually of silk and placed interruptedly, approximates the serosal layer of the stomach and the duodenum.

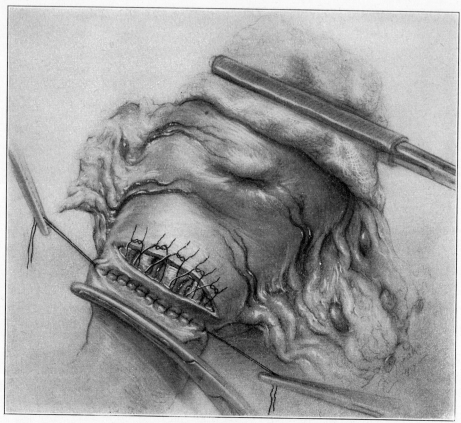

Fig. 188. Billroth I-von Haberer technic. The first continuous row of silk sutures approximating the peritoneal coat of the posterior wall of the duodenum and stomach has been applied. Incision has been made in the peritoneal and muscular coats of the stomach down to the mucous membrane and interrupted sutures of silk have been used to reef the gastric mucosa, decreasing its circumference. Sutures have been placed in the superior and inferior margins of the anastomosis, enabling one to stretch the duodenum so that its diameter nearly conforms to that of the stomach. (From Walters, Waltman, Gray, H. K. and Priestley, J. T., *Carcinoma and Other Malignant Lesions of the Stomach.* Courtesy of W. B. Saunders Company, Philadelphia, 1942.)

A portion of the gastrocolic omentum (there is usually enough lateral to the point of its removal) is brought up posterior to the anastomosis and spread out around the upper angle, where it is sutured to the stomach and the duodenum with interrupted sutures (Fig. 191a). A similar tag of omentum is placed to protect the lower angle, where it is maintained in position by sutures (Fig. 191b). The use of omentum in this fashion is a safeguard against leakage from the vulnerable points at the angles as well as the posterior wall. If possible, the gastrohepatic omentum at the points where the gastric vessels have been ligated should be brought down and

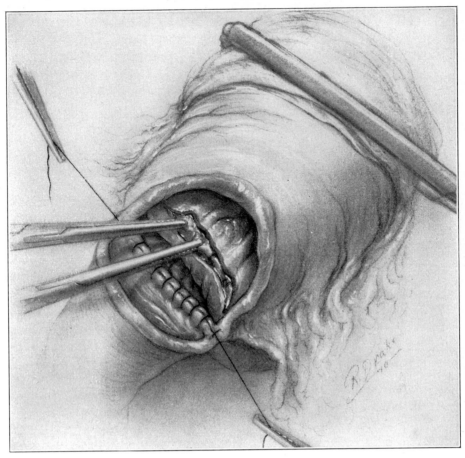

FIG. 189. Billroth I-von Haberer method. The posterior sutures have been inserted. Incision made through the mucous membrane and muscularis mucosae of the anterior wall of the stomach, enabling one to ligate the branches of the gastric vessels of the submucosa and anterior wall of the stomach and also reefing the mucous membrane, thus decreasing the size of the gastric lumen of the anastomosis. (From Walters, Waltman, Gray, H. K. and Priestley, J. T., *Carcinoma and Other Malignant Lesions of the Stomach.* Courtesy of W. B. Saunders Company, Philadelphia, 1942.)

sutured to the ligated duodenal portion of the omentum. Usually this can be done. This procedure helps to relieve tension on the anastomosis. The placing of one or two interrupted sutures between the anterior wall of the stomach and the falciform ligament holds the anastomosis to the right of the midline and assists in taking tension from the anastomosis (Fig. 192). If there has been any soiling from duodenal or gastric secretion, we frequently pour in slowly from 1 pint to 1 quart (0.5 to 1 liter) of sterile water, which is removed with the suction pump. Not only does this measure serve to dilute any gastric or duodenal secretion present, but also it is a very effective mechanical way of removing such diluted fluids. The incision in the abdominal wall is closed in the usual way.

Billroth I-Mayo Modification. This procedure differs from the Billroth-Schoemaker modification in that two long curved hemostats are placed across the stomach in the form of the pattern desired to enable approximation of the stomach to the duodenum, removing a portion of the lesser curvature.

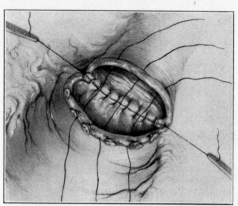

FIG. 190. Billroth I-von Haberer method. Going well beyond the tumor, the portion of the stomach containing it has been removed. Posterior anastomosis completed and blood vessels of submucosa and anterior wall of stomach ligated. Interrupted sutures shown, the first suture being placed in the center in order to approximate as nearly as possible the mucous membrane of the stomach to that of the duodenum. (From Walters, Waltman, Gray, H. K. and Priestley, J. T., *Carcinoma and Other Malignant Lesions of the Stomach.* Courtesy of W. B. Saunders Company, Philadelphia, 1942.)

The gap is closed by suture, thus decreasing the circumference of the stomach (Fig. 182). By using these curved hemostats, which are always available, one may dispense with the heavy, especially devised clamp of Schoemaker.

After division and ligation of the gastric vessels and division of the duodenum above the curved hemostat across it, as described for the Billroth I operation, a curved hemostat is placed transversely across the stomach at the greater curvature at the point where it is to be resected. A second clamp is placed across the stomach below the first clamp so that there will be no soiling, and the gastric wall between is incised. Two additional curved hemostats then are placed across the stomach almost at right angles to the first hemostat, including a segment of lesser curvature (Fig. 182), and an incision is made between them. A continuous suture of chromic catgut is placed back of this curved hemostat, not only approximating the wall of the stomach, but also serving as a hemostatic suture. The curved hemostat on the lesser curvature then is removed. A second row of sutures continuously placed, using silk, inverts the first row by approximating the serosal layer of stomach (Fig. 193). The curved hemostat on the inferior portion of the stomach then is approximated to the curved hemostat across the duodenum, enabling one accurately to insert a continuous row of silk sutures, approximating the posterior wall of the serosa of the stomach and the duodenum. When this row of sutures has been completed, an incision is made through the serosa and muscularis mucosae down to the mucous membrane of both structures and the cut edges of each are approximated. Clamps then are removed, a suction pump is introduced into the lumen of the stomach and the duodenum, and a third row of chromic catgut sutures is introduced, approximating mucous membrane of the stomach to the duodenum (Fig. 194). The anterior part of the anastomosis is completed in similar fashion, using three rows of sutures. The first row approximates the mucous mem-

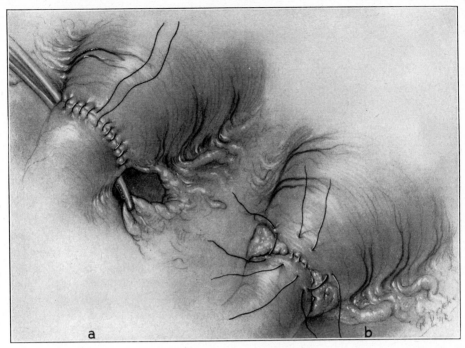

Fig. 191. a. Second row of sutures approximating the peritoneal coat of the duodenum nearly completed, separate sutures being started from the opposite sides and meeting in the center. Omentum brought posterior to the anastomosis and up over the upper angle to protect it; b. interrupted sutures approximating peritoneal coats of stomach and duodenum in the anterior part of the anastomosis. Note the omentum protecting the upper and lower parts of the anastomosis. (From Walters, Waltman, Gray, H. K. and Priestley, J. T., *Carcinoma and Other Malignant Lesions of the Stomach.* Courtesy of W. B. Saunders Company, Philadelphia, 1942.)

brane, the second row approximates the serosal and muscular coats and the third row of sutures is used to obtain an accurate serosal approximation, bringing the ends of the stomach and duodenum together without tension.

The use of omentum to protect the posterior part of the anastomosis in the upper angle is particularly valuable in this method because of the fact that the anterior and posterior lines of suture, with the sutures used to close the lesser curvature, form a triangle in which it is thought that leakage is more likely to occur than in other parts of the anastomosis because of three suture lines meeting at this angle. It is said that leakage occurred at this point in some of Billroth's cases, giving rise to the name "fatal suture angle of Billroth."

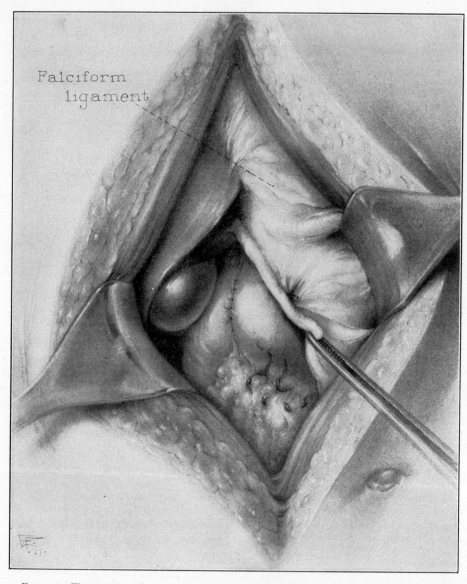

FIG. 192. Two sutures between the falciform ligament and the anterior wall of the stomach hold the anastomosis to the right of the midline and relieve tension from the anastomosis. (From Walters, Waltman, Gray, H. K. and Priestley, J. T., *Carcinoma and Other Malignant Lesions of the Stomach.* Courtesy of W. B. Saunders Company, 1942.)

Billroth I-Schoemaker Modification. Schoemaker devised a heavy crushing clamp patterned in such a way that when properly placed across the stomach it served to remove a larger portion of the lesser curvature than of the greater. The method of suturing behind this clamp and of approximating the stomach to the duodenum is not unlike that of the method used by C. H. Mayo and W. J. Mayo (Figs. 180 and 181).

Billroth I-Horsley Modification. Horsley modified the operation by suturing the duodenum to the lesser curvature of the stomach rather than to the greater, decreasing the circumference of the stomach by sutures placed at right angles to its incised portion, beginning at the greater curvature and

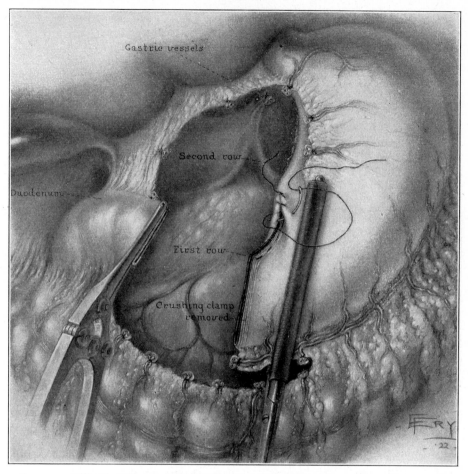

Fig. 193. Billroth I-Mayo method. Closure of the lesser curvature. (From Walters, Waltman, Gray, H. K. and Priestley, J. T., *Carcinoma and Other Malignant Lesions of the Stomach*. Courtesy of W. B. Saunders Company, Philadelphia, 1942.)

extending upward to the anastomosis. Figure 183 shows the duodenum approximated to the lesser curvature of the stomach; the posterior portion of the anastomosis, as described for the Billroth I operation, has been completed. The incision extending from the greater curvature to the anastomosis has been closed and a small incision has been made down to the anterior wall of the duodenum, enlarging the circumference of the duodenum.

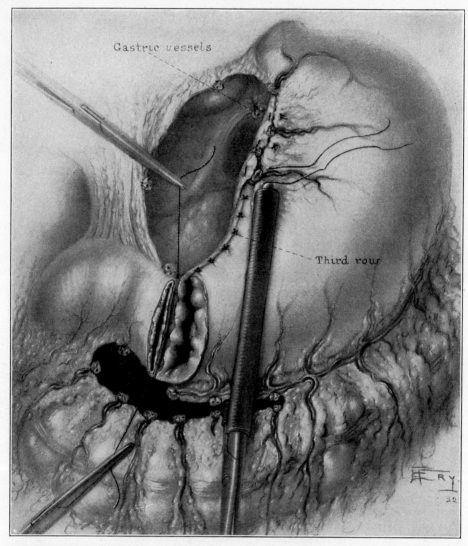

FIG. 194. Billroth I-Mayo method. Approximation of the narrowed circumference of the stomach to the duodenum. (From Walters, Waltman, Gray, H. K. and Priestley, J. T., *Carcinoma and Other Malignant Lesions of the Stomach.* Courtesy of W. B. Saunders Company, Philadelphia, 1942.)

THE BILLROTH II GASTRIC RESECTION AND MODIFICATION: POLYA OPERATION

In 1885 Billroth described his second operation of partial gastric resection. This was reported and published by von Hacker [25] in the same year. It has been known subsequently as the Billroth II operation and differs from the Billroth I operation described elsewhere in this text, in that the cut ends of the stomach and duodenum are closed and the jejunum is anastomosed to the most dependent portion of the stomach in an antecolic long loop gastrojejunal anastomosis. In 1888 von Eiselsberg[26] performed the modification now widely known as the *Hofmeister* or *Finsterer type* of Billroth II operation. He reported this modification in 1889 and advised closure of the upper portion of the cut end of the stomach, using only the lower portion in establishing continuity with the jejunum after gastric resection. Braun[27] and Jaboulay[28] in 1892 first performed and reported the establishment of an anastomosis between the afferent and efferent loops of jejunum to drain the dependent portion of the proximal loop and thus to prevent regurgitation.

Polya's[29] report in 1911 of the modification now bearing his name was more widely recognized than any previous reports of nearly the same operation. However, von Hacker[25] really first suggested the end-to-side gastrojejunostomy in 1885; Krönlein[30] apparently first actually performed this type of anastomosis on November 24, 1887, and Reichel[31] in 1908 reported several cases of terminolateral anastomosis of the now well-known Polya modification of the Billroth II operation. Polya[29] made a most interesting comment on these historical data in a footnote in a recent article:

"I was not the only one nor the first who got into difficulties and found my way out by inventing this method, but I realized at least its great practical value and saw at once that it was not only a method of necessity, but the method of choice in the majority of cases and, therefore, saw to it that it should have due publicity because this was absolutely wanting. The method was quite unknown, not only to myself, but to all my colleagues with whom I had the opportunity to discuss it, and I vainly looked for descriptions of it in the textbooks and journals which were accessible to me....*

"The great majority of surgeons, however, did not know of the method at all until I called it to the attention of the surgical world, and especially to the attention of William Mayo who saw in it the operation of the future and whose endorsement helped to make it one most widely adopted."

In the Polya modification the cut end of the duodenum is closed and a loop of jejunum is brought up through an opening in the mesocolon to form an end-to-side anastomosis with the cut end of the stomach. Balfour,[32] in 1917, emphasized, in selected cases, utilization of a longer loop of jejunum which he brought up anterior to the colon, and mentioned the advisability of establishing entero-anastomosis at the dependent part of the afferent loop with the distal loop of jejunum, if indicated. This has become known as the *Balfour-Polya modification*. Numerous other modifications of the original Billroth II procedure have been suggested, most of which have merit, but in practically every instance the fundamental principle of the Billroth II operation has been retained; namely, that the cut end of the duodenum be closed, and that gastro-intestinal continuity be reestablished by joining the remaining portion of the stomach to the jejunum.

After resection of the stomach for cancer, the most satisfactory method of restoration of gastro-intestinal continuity has been found to be the Polya or the Balfour-Polya modification of the Billroth II operation. In many

* The portion of Polya's account omitted here is given in an appendix to this chapter.

instances surgeons personally have developed slight modifications in technic that are of undoubted value. In general, the following method has been found to be satisfactory.

Two layers of peritoneum descend from the stomach and the commencement of the duodenum and enclose, near the greater curvature of the

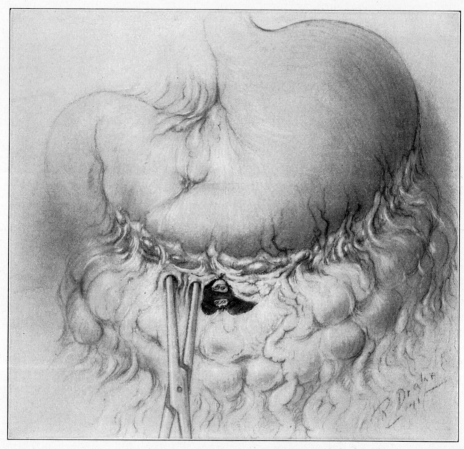

FIG. 195. An opening has been made in the gastrocolic omentum as close to the colon as possible, in order to explore the lesser peritoneal sac. Hemostat is shown in place on branch of the gastro-epiploic vessels. (From Walters, Waltham, Gray, H. K. and Priestley, J. T., *Carcinoma and Other Malignant Lesions of the Stomach.* Courtesy of W. B. Saunders Company, Philadelphia, 1942.)

stomach, the left and right gastro-epiploic vessels. After passing downward anterior to the colon, they descend for a variable distance and then turn backward and upward and ascend again as far as the transverse colon, where they separate again and enclose this structure between the anterior and posterior layers. The continuation of these peritoneal layers after they enclose the colon is referred to as the "transverse portion of the mesocolon." Usage has limited the term "gastrocolic omentum" to reference to only that portion of the greater omentum which extends between the stomach and the anterior surface of the transverse colon, to which it usually is rather densely adherent. In similar manner, the term "great omentum" usually is limited by common usage to reference to the remaining portion of these peritoneal layers that extend downward and turn back again as far as the transverse part of the colon.

To explore the lesser peritoneal sac and thus obtain added evidence as to the operability of the neoplasm, a small opening is made in the gastro-

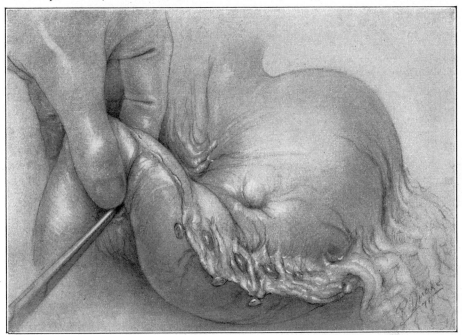

FIG. 196. A small opening has been made in the duodenohepatic omentum to facilitate mobilization of the lesser curvature of the stomach and isolation of the right gastric vessels. (From Walters, Waltman, Gray, H. K. and Priestley, J. T., *Carcinoma and Other Malignant Lesions of the Stomach*. Courtesy of W. B. Saunders Company, Philadelphia, 1942.)

colic omentum well over to the left, away from the lesion, and as close to the colon as possible (Fig. 195). This opening is then enlarged by double clamping of the branches of the gastro-epiploic vessels and by cutting of the portions of the vessels between the clamps. The mesocolon is carefully brushed away, so that the transverse colic vessels contained within it will not be injured. If, after satisfactory examination within the lesser peritoneal sac, it is decided that the lesion is operable, further mobilization of the greater curvature may be accomplished by continuance of dissection to the right as close to the transverse portion of the colon as to the region of the pylorus. By this procedure, the inferior gastric lymph nodes and the sub-pyloric lymph nodes will be included in the resection. The right gastro-epiploic vessels may then be clamped, cut and ligated. To facilitate the procedure, all the remaining hemostats may be removed at this point after the contained vessels have been ligated. It will be found, then, that there is a plexus of vessels in the region of the pylorus that has not been disturbed. To achieve satisfactory closure of the duodenal stump, these vessels must be ligated and cut close to the duodenal wall. Great care should be exercised at this point, because these vessels have relatively thin walls, and rather disturbing hemorrhage is encountered fairly frequently.

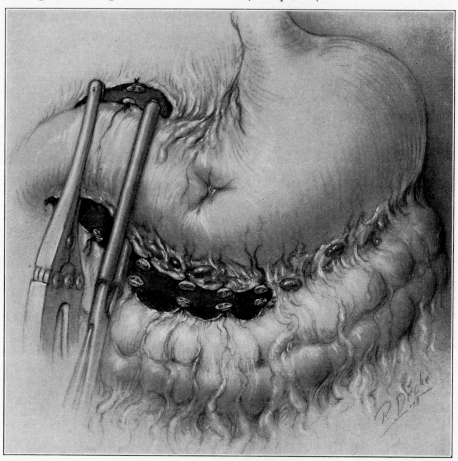

FIG. 197. The right gastric vessels have been ligated and a clamp has been placed on the duodenum distal to the pylorus and another well proximal to it so as to prevent soiling as the duodenum is divided. The gastrocolic omentum attached to the stomach contains the infragastric and subpyloric groups of lymph nodes. (From Walters, Waltman, Gray, H. K. and Priestley, J. T., *Carcinoma and Other Malignant Lesions of the Stomach*. Courtesy of W. B. Saunders Company, Philadelphia, 1942.)

To mobilize the lesser curvature of the stomach, the inferior border of the duodenum may be placed in tension and a small opening may be made through the duodenohepatic omentum close to the duodenal wall (Fig. 196). A second opening in this structure may be made easily by blunt dissection with the tips of the fingers, and an opportunity is thus afforded for placement of hemostats on the right gastric vessels. The vessels are then divided by cutting of those portions of the vessels between the hemostats. Division of the gastrocolic and duodenohepatic omentum has thus been accomplished just beyond the distal line of resection and a Payr clamp may then be placed on the duodenum well below the pylorus (Fig. 197). A second rubber-covered clamp is placed just proximal to the pylorus, but not in such a position as to crush the malignant lesion. The duodenum may be divided close to the distal clamp and the stomach is retracted upward and to the left to facilitate closure of the duodenal stump.

In closure of the duodenal stump great care must be exercised to avoid the development of a duodenal fistula. The first row of sutures may be placed as shown in figure 198a. The suture material is fine chromicized catgut. A running mattress stitch is used. By the gentle application of traction on the two ends, the clamp may be removed and the edges of the duodenal stump will be inverted. To invert the stump further, the same suture material may be utilized in the second row by a return to the starting point with a continuous mattress suture (Fig. 198b). Several interrupted mattress sutures of fine silk or cotton will give added strength to the closure (Fig. 198c). The stump of the duodenum may then be buried in the areolar tissue in the region

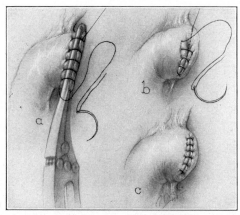

FIG. 198. Inversion and closure of the duodenal stump; a. the first line of sutures utilizes a running mattress stitch; b. the second row of sutures consists of returning to starting point with a continuous mattress suture, further inverting the stump; c. interrupted mattress sutures of fine silk or cotton form the third line of sutures to reinforce the inverted stump. (From Walters, Waltman, Gray, H. K. and Priestley, J. T., *Carcinoma and Other Malignant Lesions of the Stomach.* Courtesy of W. B. Saunders Company, Philadelphia, 1942.)

of the head of the pancreas, or any portion of available fat may be brought over in such a manner as to seal off any possible leak from the closed duodenum.

Usually, it will be noted at this point that mobilization of the greater curvature of the stomach has not been accomplished to a sufficiently great degree. Additional mobilization may be facilitated by the application of gentle traction on the gastrocolic omentum, so that an excellent view is afforded of the short vessels extending to the stomach from the left gastroepiploic vessels and of the gastro-epiploic vessels themselves (Fig. 199). The dissection may be carried as high as desired, even to the point of complete mobilization of the greater curvature if total gastrectomy should be indicated. Again, in order to facilitate final mobilization of the stomach, all hemostats may be removed after ligatures have been applied. Traction exerted straight forward on the stomach will do much to aid in the placing of a clamp on the left gastric artery. The edge of the stomach may be palpated between the thumb and index finger as shown in figure 200, and by breaking through the gastrohepatic omentum at a point beyond the line chosen for resection, the left gastric artery may be clamped and cut. It is a wise precaution to clamp this vessel doubly in case the ligature should break, and it is also advisable to apply this ligature as a double "stick-tie" of chromic catgut (Fig. 200, inset).

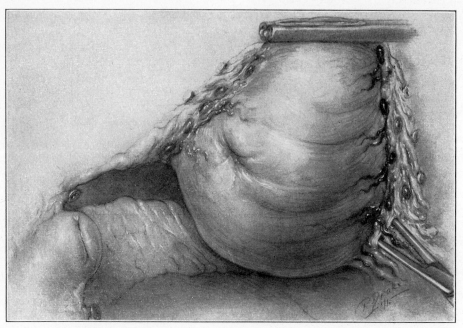

FIG. 199. Further mobilization of the greater curvature of the stomach by applying traction to the gastrocolic omentum in order to permit a clear view of the short vessels prior to clamping and ligating them. (From Walters, Waltman, Gray, H. K. and Priestley, J. T., *Carcinoma and Other Malignant Lesions of the Stomach.* Courtesy of W. B. Saunders Company, Philadelphia, 1942.)

The stomach is now thoroughly mobilized and while it is held taut in a forward position, a rubber-covered clamp may be applied just proximal to the determined line of resection. To determine the line of resection, if the stomach is distended with gas or retained contents, a trocar may be inserted through the posterior wall of the stomach and the contents of the stomach may be removed by suction. This permits collapse of the stomach and greatly facilitates approximation of the jejunum to the stomach in the construction of the anastomosis. If a retrocolic type of anastomosis has been decided on, an appropriate portion of the transverse part of the mesocolon should be selected in which to make an opening; this portion should not contain vessels and should be situated well to the left, so that the anastomosis may lie in as nearly a normal anatomic position as possible (Fig. 201). In certain instances attachment of the posterior cut edge of the transverse part of the mesocolon to the stomach will facilitate the operation but it increases the difficulty of mobilization of the stomach. Under most circumstances it is a simpler matter to attach the cut edge of the opening in the transverse por-

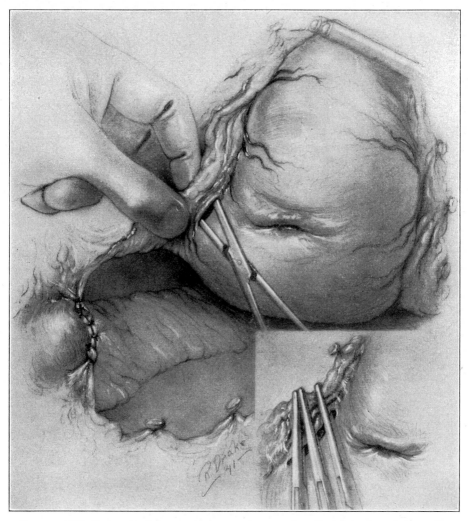

FIG. 200. To ligate the left gastric artery, the vessel and right edge of stomach are palpated between the thumb and index finger and an opening is made as close to the stomach as possible. The duodenal stump has been buried in areolar tissue and fat and has been turned into the head of the pancreas. In the inset, the vessel is shown doubly clamped. It will be ligated with double chromic catgut and a "stick-tie." (From Walters, Waltman, Gray, H. K. and Priestley, J. T., *Carcinoma and Other Malignant Lesions of the Stomach.* Courtesy of W. B. Saunders Company, Philadelphia, 1942.)

tion of mesocolon to the stomach after anastomosis has been completed. A loop of jejunum approximately 5 cm. from the ligament of Treitz is selected and is brought through the opening in the transverse mesocolon. A rubber-covered clamp is placed on the jejunum and the loop of jejunum is placed next to the retracted stomach, so that the two rubber-covered clamps are now adjacent and in such a position that the proximal limb of the jejunum lies next to the lesser curvature of the stomach and the distal limb of jejunum lies next to the greater curvature of the stomach (Fig. 202a).

To approximate the proximal limb of the jejunum to the lesser curvature of the stomach with one interrupted suture of silk and to tag this

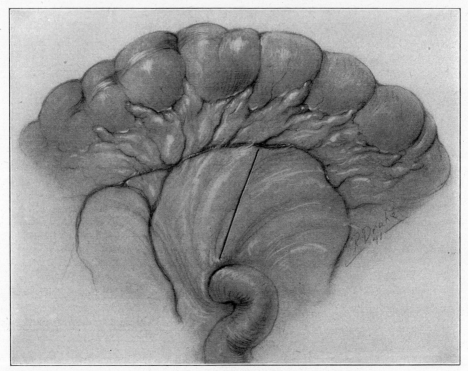

FIG. 201. Appropriate avascular region in the transverse mesocolon; the desired line of opening, the ligament of Treitz and the proximal loop of jejunum prior to being thrust through the transverse mesocolon for the retrocolic anastomosis are shown. (From Walters, Waltman, Gray, H. K. and Priestley, J. T., *Carcinoma and Other Malignant Lesions of the Stomach.* Courtesy of W. B. Saunders Company, Philadelphia, 1942.)

with a long end have been found to be convenient procedures, because the suture may be used later for retraction and also to diminish the tendency toward distortion of the anastomosis, for it marks a point toward which the first line of suture may be directed. Starting at the junction of the distal loop of jejunum and the greater curvature of the stomach, a continuous suture of silk is applied, care being taken to include if possible only the serosal and muscular layers of the wall of the stomach and jejunum; when the stay suture on the lesser curvature has been reached, this suture is tied and the ends are discarded (Fig. 202a). A third rubber-covered clamp may now be applied, in this instance to the stomach, which has been retracted upward. An incision in the posterior wall of the stomach through the extent

of the stoma should be made so that the anterior wall of the stomach is
intact. The jejunum is incised for a distance equal to that determined as
suitable for the length of the stoma, and the second row of sutures (fine
chromic catgut) may be inserted as shown in figure 202b. This suture is made

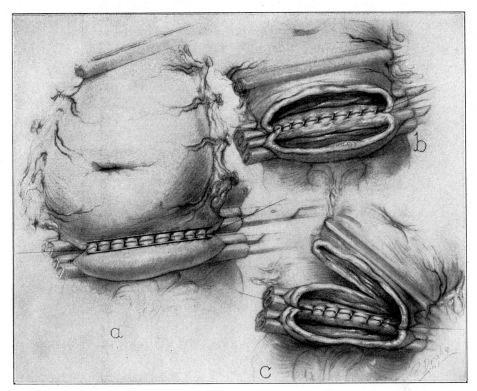

FIG. 202. The posterior line of sutures in the anastomosis; a. clamps in place on the
stomach and jejunum; the proximal loop of jejunum and the lesser curvature of the
stomach are approximated; the first row of sutures is continuous and of silk; a guide
suture has been placed between the proximal loop of jejunum and stomach for traction;
b. the second row of sutures includes all layers of stomach and jejunum and is done with
fine chromic catgut; the anterior wall of the stomach has not been sectioned; c. the clamp
on the stomach has been opened and the bleeding points on the posterior suture line
have been ligated; the clamp now has been closed and the portion of the stomach to be
resected is being cut off. (From Walters, Waltman, Gray, H. K. and Priestley, J. T.,
Carcinoma and Other Malignant Lesions of the Stomach. Courtesy of W. B. Saunders
Company, Philadelphia, 1942.)

in such a manner as to include all layers of the wall of the stomach and
jejunum, and is doubly locked when the lesser curvature of the stomach has
been reached.

   To ascertain with certainty whether or not the posterior suture line is
thoroughly dry, the clamp on the stomach adjacent to that on the jejunum
may be opened and any bleeding points may be noted and ligated individually. The advantage in having the anterior half of the stomach intact

becomes apparent at this point, for the stomach now acts as a retractor when the clamp is opened and prevents displacement of the stomach upward. When all bleeding points have been ligated, the portion of the stomach to be resected may be completely cut off (Fig. 202c).

The suture that constituted the second row posteriorly may now be continued anteriorly, the suture being locked on that side which is next to the stomach (Fig. 203a). Again the suture includes all coats,

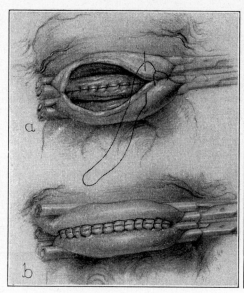

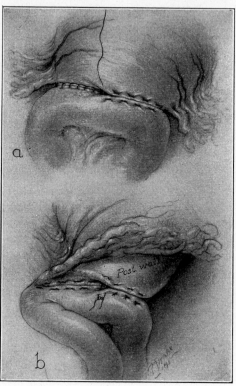

FIG. 203   FIG. 204

FIG. 203. The anterior line of sutures; a. the second row of sutures in the posterior line is continued anteriorly; the sutures are locked on the side next to the stomach and all coats are included; b. this row of sutures completed; the clamps will be removed to view bleeding points from the anterior portion of the suture line. (From Walters, Waltman, Gray, H. K. and Priestley, J. T., *Carcinoma and Other Malignant Lesions of the Stomach*. Courtesy of W. B. Saunders Company, Philadelphia, 1942.)

FIG. 204. a. The second anterior row of sutures is a continuous mattress type which serves to invert the protruding mucous membrane; b. starting posteriorly at the lesser curvature the entire suture line is reinforced with interrupted mattress sutures of silk. (From Walters, Waltman, Gray, H. K. and Priestley, J. T., *Carcinoma and Other Malignant Lesions of the Stomach*. Courtesy of W. B. Saunders Company, Philadelphia, 1942.)

but only a thin edge of mucous membrane. In this manner the mucous membrane projects slightly through the anastomosis and any bleeding point may be visualized when the clamp on the stomach has been removed (Fig. 203b).

The second anterior row of sutures (silk or fine chromic catgut) may be applied as a continuous mattress suture (Fig. 204a) and in this manner inversion of the protruding edge of mucous membrane will be accomplished. To reinforce the entire suture line, multiple interrupted mattress sutures of silk may be inserted throughout the circumference of the anastomosis (Fig. 204b).

To anchor the anastomosis below the opening in the transverse portion of the mesocolon, the colon may be retracted upward (Fig. 205) and multiple interrupted sutures of silk may be inserted so that the stomach projects

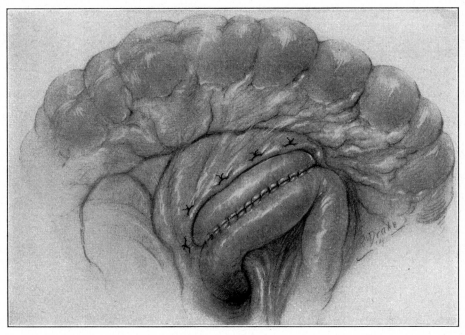

FIG. 205. The anastomosis has been brought below the colon through the opening in the transverse mesocolon and anchored there by interrupted sutures of silk, approximating the edges of the mesocolon opening to the stomach wall. (From Walters, Waltman, Gray, H. K. and Priestley, J. T., *Carcinoma and Other Malignant Lesions of the Stomach.* Courtesy of W. B. Saunders Company, Philadelphia, 1942.)

approximately 2 cm. below this opening (Fig. 205). One should be careful to insure such a position that the remaining portion of stomach will be in as nearly a normal position as possible, thus diminishing the likelihood of angulation of the jejunum at the site of anastomosis or immediately distal to it. Alternatively, if the posterior edge of the transverse mesocolon has been sutured to the stomach prior to formation of the anastomosis, the anastomosis may be pushed through the opening in the transverse mesocolon from above and the anterior edge of the transverse mesocolon may be sutured to the stomach above the anastomosis.

There are many advocates of other types of anastomosis for restoration of gastro-intestinal continuity after resection of the stomach. At the Mayo Clinic we have found the posterior Polya modification of the Billroth II in general to be the most satisfactory. In selected cases, an antecolic type of anastomosis may seem to be desirable, particularly when resection is unusually high or when a short transverse mesocolon which contains much fat is present. Rarely have we found it advisable to close a portion of the stomach according to the Hofmeister method. The same mechanical advantage as that claimed for the Hofmeister method will be obtained if the opening in the jejunum is made somewhat smaller than the diameter of the cut end of the stomach and if the anastomosis is so made that the cut end of the stomach "funnels" down to the smaller opening in the jejunum. Added advantages of this procedure lie in the saving of time in accomplishment of the completed resection and in the abolition of a very treacherous angle wherein leakage may occur (between the jejunum and the partially closed end of the stomach), such as exists when the Hofmeister technic is used.

TRANSTHORACIC RESECTION OF THE CARDIA AND ESOPHAGUS

The first successful transthoracic resection of the cardia with an anastomosis of the esophagus to the remainder of the stomach, in this country, was reported by Adams and Phemister [33] in 1938. Since that time successful operations of this type have been carried out for lesions of the cardia and the lower portion of the esophagus. At present the risk of these operations in the hands of experienced surgeons is not much greater than the risk of operation performed for carcinoma in the lower portion of the stomach by way of the abdominal route. Clagett [34] has recently reported thirty-three cases of transthoracic resection of the stomach and esophagus with but five deaths. In the last eighteen consecutive cases there were no deaths. In addition, twenty-four exploratory procedures were carried out without mortality in cases in which inoperable lesions were found.

The conciseness of Clagett's description of the technic of the operation which he has used warrants quoting in toto:

"After the patient is anesthetized and the intratracheal tube has been inserted, the patient is turned so that his right side is down and the left lower portion of the chest is readily accessible. After the operative site has been prepared and draped, a long incision is made along the ninth rib. Subperiosteal resection of the ninth rib is performed. The pleura is then opened. The lung is allowed to collapse partially and is retracted to expose the diaphragm. The left phrenic nerve is readily visualized as it passes over the pericardium. The nerve is injected with procaine to produce temporary paralysis of the diaphragm (Fig. 206). The central tendinous portion of the diaphragm is opened sufficiently so that the abdomen can be examined. The entire upper portion of the abdomen is readily accessible to examination and inspection. It is even possible to examine the pelvis.

"The extent of the lesion, its attachments and any metastatic lesions can be determined readily. If the lesion is inoperable, the diaphragm is repaired, the lung inflated and the thoracic wall is closed. If the lesion is removable.

the incision in the diaphragm is extended to the esophageal hiatus, and the upper end of the stomach and the lower end of the esophagus are mobilized (Fig. 207, left). If necessary, the spleen, the tail of the pancreas and the diaphragm adjacent to the lesion can be readily included in the resection. The stomach is severed below the lesion and the lower end of the stomach

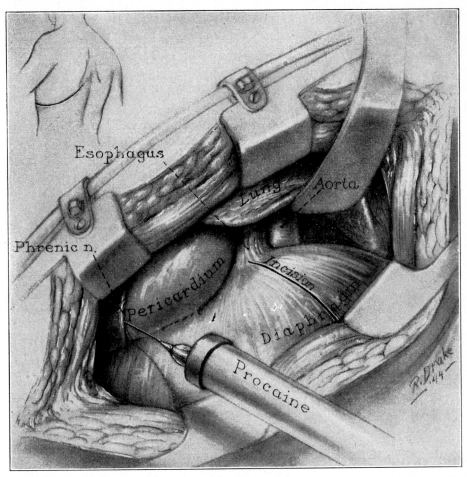

FIG. 206. Injection of the phrenic nerve with procaine. Note line of incision in the diaphragm and position of esophagus and aorta.

is closed. The esophagus is severed and the lower end of the esophagus and the cardia are removed together. An anastomosis of the end of the esophagus to the anterior wall of the remaining segment of stomach is then performed; two rows of interrupted silk sutures are used for this anastomosis. As much of the stomach as possible is brought above the diaphragm so that there will be no tension on the anastomosis. The stomach is attached to the edge of the diaphragm (Fig. 207, right).

"The operative site is washed thoroughly with saline solution. A catheter is inserted in the pleural space for temporary drainage. The phrenic nerve is crushed so that the diaphragm will remain paralyzed until healing has occurred. A catheter is inserted through the nostril and down past the anastomosis into the stomach to provide a means of early postoperative feeding. The lung then is inflated by the anesthetist. The thoracic wall is closed in layers. At the conclusion of the operation, bronchoscopy is performed in order to be sure that the tracheobronchial tree is free of secretion that may cause postoperative pulmonary complications.

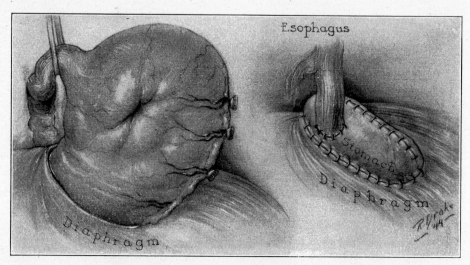

FIG. 207. Left: Delivery of the fundic end of the stomach through the incision in the diaphragm. Right: Closure of opening of diaphragm around the upper part of the stomach after the esophageal gastrostomy.

POSTOPERATIVE CARE

"The patient is placed in an oxygen tent on his return to his room. Usually not more than twenty-four hours of oxygen therapy is necessary. Five hundred to 1,000 c.c. of blood usually is administered during the course of the operation. Further transfusions are administered during the postoperative period if necessary. The catheter in the chest is connected with a water seal system so that negative pressure is maintained in the pleural space. This permits removal of the pleural effusion that results from the operation and keeps the lung completely expanded. The catheter in the pleural space usually is removed from forty-eight to seventy-two hours after operation.

"A sufficient amount of fluid is administered intravenously to maintain an output of urine of about 1,000 c.c. daily until the patient is taking adequate fluids orally. Forty-eight hours after operation water is administered through the tube inserted through the nose and esophagus into the stomach, and seventy-two hours after operation the formula devised for jejunal feeding is given. On the fourth or fifth day after operation the patient is allowed to start drinking water and is placed on a progressive type of diet. By the tenth or twelfth postoperative day, most patients tolerate without difficulty an ulcer type of diet commonly used for ambulatory patients.

"Patients are given penicillin in dosages of 100,000 units daily by intramuscular injection for one week postoperatively.

"Most patients are out of bed by the sixth or seventh postoperative day and are able to leave the hospital on the twelfth to fourteenth postoperative day." *

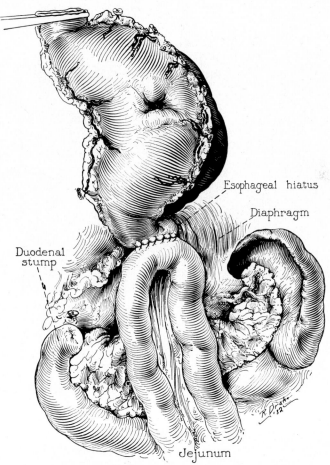

FIG. 208. Stomach used as a tractor to bring the abdominal portion of the esophagus into view. The first row of sutures is placed between the jejunum and the posterior part of the esophagus. (After Eusterman, G. B. and Balfour, D. C., *The Stomach and Duodenum*. Courtesy of W. B. Saunders Company, Philadelphia, 1935.)

TOTAL GASTRECTOMY

The following technic for total gastrectomy is one that my colleagues and I [35] have used. The operation is begun in the same way as in performance of partial gastrectomy, mobilization beginning at the pyloric end.

* Clagett, O. T., *Texas State J. Med.*, May, 1946.

The superior pyloric branch of the right gastric artery is divided by ligating the gastrohepatic omentum just below the pyloric sphincter, and the branches of the right gastro-epiploic vessels are ligated in the gastrocolic omentum below the pylorus. If the gastrocolic omentum is to be removed, it is detached from the transverse colon and any bleeding points are ligated. If only a portion of it is to be removed, the branches of the

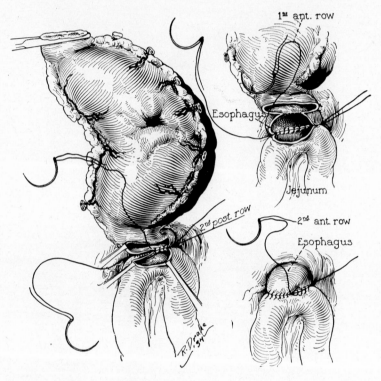

Fig. 209. Incision has been made into the lumen of the esophagus and jejunum and the second row of sutures is being applied. (After Eusterman, G. B. and Balfour, D. C., *The Stomach and Duodenum.* Courtesy of W. B. Saunders Company, Philadelphia, 1935.)

gastro-epiploic vessels in the omentum are divided between forceps and the ends are ligated. The left gastric artery is ligated adjacent to the lower end of the esophagus by separating the gastrohepatic omentum from the stomach and esophagus, dividing the artery between the forceps and ligating the proximal end with suture ligatures. Considerable care must be taken in separating the gastrocolic omentum from the spleen, and the gastrolienal ligament likewise must be divided with care so as not to tear the capsule of the spleen and start bleeding from the latter which might necessitate splenectomy for its control. The short gastric arteries should be ligated carefully.

Two curved hemostats are placed across the duodenum and an incision is made between them. The distal end of the duodenum is closed, turned in accurately, buried in the head of the pancreas and covered with omentum. Then, by use of the stomach as a tractor, the abdominal portion of the esophagus can be brought into view and the first suture line between the

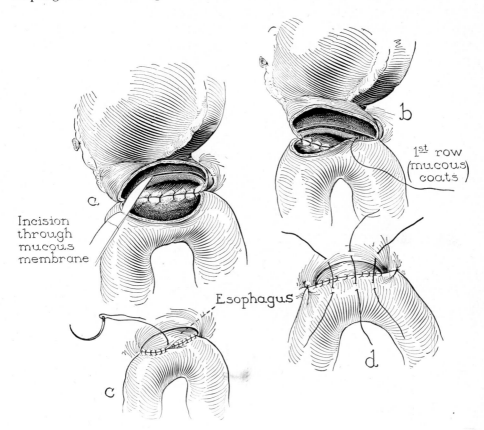

FIG. 210. a. Posterior suture line has been completed and the incision is made through the mucous membrane and submucosa of the anterior wall of the esophagus. b. The first row of anterior sutures approximating mucous membrane of esophagus and the jejunum is being inserted. Note that the esophagus is not cut through until the row of sutures has been inserted. By this method, the stomach and esophagus are used to immobilize the anastomosis. c. After removal of the stomach by cutting through serosal and muscular coats of the anterior wall of the esophagus transversely, a second row of silk sutures is inserted to approximate the peritoneal and muscular coats of esophagus and jejunum. d. Five interrupted sutures are inserted, attaching the jejunum to the peritoneum of the diaphragm adjacent to the esophagus. (From Walters, Waltman, Gray, H. K. and Priestley, J. T., *Carcinoma and Other Malignant Lesions of the Stomach*. Courtesy of W. B. Saunders Company, Philadelphia, 1942.)

jejunum and the posterior aspect of the esophagus can be placed (Fig. 208). This suture should be of silk. The jejunum and the posterior aspect of the esophagus then are opened, and a second continuous row of silk sutures is used to approximate the entire thickness of the posterior wall of the esophagus and the jejunum (Fig. 209). For further safety, additional interrupted

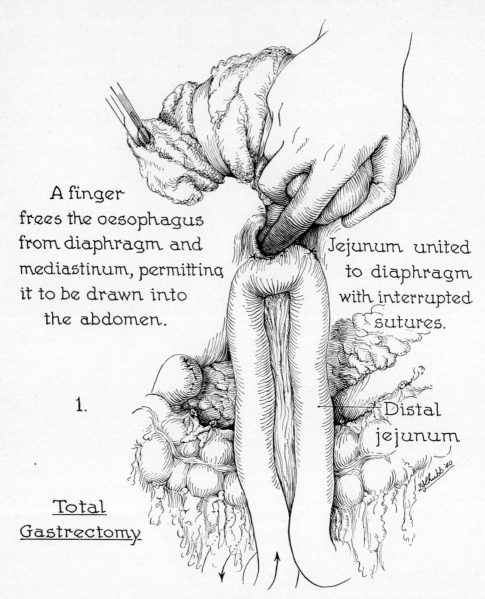

A finger
frees the oesophagus
from diaphragm and
mediastinum, permitting
it to be drawn into
the abdomen.

Jejunum united
to diaphragm
with interrupted
sutures.

1.

Distal
jejunum

Total
Gastrectomy

Fig. 211. First stage of Graham's method of anastomosing the esophagus to the jejunum in performance of total gastrectomy. (From Graham, R. R., A Technique for Total Gastrectomy, *Surgery*, 8:257-264, [Aug.], 1940.)

sutures of silk may be placed in this posterior suture line, particularly at the angles.

By making an incision through the mucous membrane and muscularis mucosae of the anterior wall of the esophagus, allowing the serosal and muscular layers to remain attached, one can insert more readily the first row of anterior sutures, uniting the mucous membrane of the jejunum to

that of the esophagus (Fig. 210a and b). With the lumen of the anastomosis
closed in this fashion the remaining two rows of anterior sutures can be
inserted with greater ease after the esophagus has been cut across. A second
row of silk sutures approximates the peritoneal and muscular coats (Fig.
210c). Interrupted sutures of silk may be placed adjacent to the anastomosis.

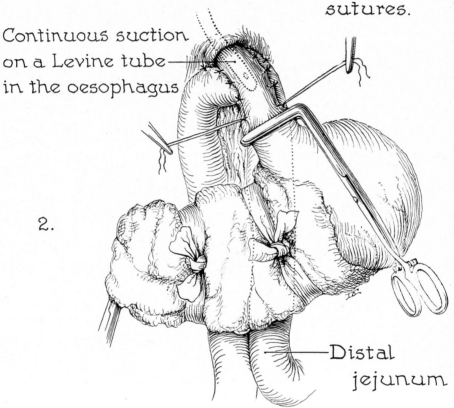

Oesophagus anchored to anterior surface of
distal jejunum by interrupted
sutures.

Continuous suction
on a Levine tube
in the oesophagus

2.

Distal
jejunum

Fig. 212. Second stage of Graham's method. (From Graham, R. R., A Technique for
Total Gastrectomy, *Surgery*, 8:257-264, [Aug.], 1940.)

These sutures attach the jejunum to the diaphragm (Fig. 210d). The safety
of the operation seems to be greater when the jejunum is carried out in
front of the colon and an antecolic anastomosis is made than when the
anastomosis is made behind the transverse colon. Although experience has
shown that it is not absolutely necessary to make an entero-anastomosis
between the loops of jejunum (jejunojejunostomy) there are many things
in its favor such as the removal of pressure of fluids accumulating in the
proximal loop and the turned-in end of duodenum and the availability of

a larger region to serve as a container of food immediately after eating. The two disadvantages are prolongation of the operation and the risk (probably small) of a supplementary anastomosis.

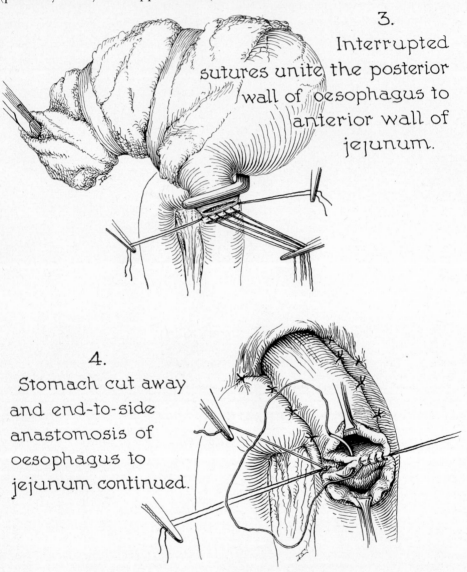

3. Interrupted sutures unite the posterior wall of oesophagus to anterior wall of jejunum.

4. Stomach cut away and end-to-side anastomosis of oesophagus to jejunum continued.

FIG. 213. Third and fourth stages of Graham's method. (From Graham, R. R., A Technique for Total Gastrectomy, *Surgery*, 8:257-264, [Aug.], 1940.)

Graham [36] has described an ingenious method of anastomosing the esophagus to the jejunum (Figs. 211, 212, 213 and 214). After the insertion of interrupted sutures approximating the posterior wall of the esophagus to the jejunum the esophagus is brought down and attached by lateral interrupted sutures to the distal loop of jejunum. After the insertion of these fixation sutures the anastomosis between the transverse opening made in the esophagus and the jejunum is made in the usual way. After its completion the proximal loop of jejunum is folded over the esophagus and the anas-

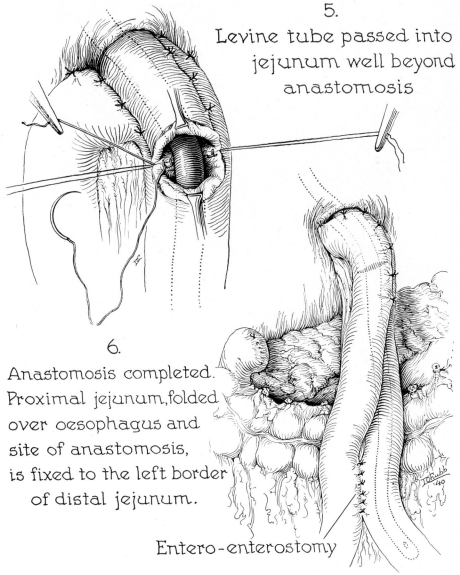

5.
Levine tube passed into jejunum well beyond anastomosis

6.
Anastomosis completed.
Proximal jejunum, folded over oesophagus and site of anastomosis, is fixed to the left border of distal jejunum.

Entero-enterostomy

FIG. 214. Fifth and sixth stages of Graham's method. (From Graham, R. R., A Technique for Total Gastrectomy, *Surgery*, 8:257-264, [Aug.], 1940.)

tomosis and is maintained in position with interrupted sutures. Thus the proximal loop of jejunum becomes a patch over the anastomosis. This procedure, however, obstructs the proximal jejunal loop in such a way that entero-enterostomy between the proximal and distal loops of jejunum is essential.

POSTERIOR GASTRO-ENTEROSTOMY

The surgeon first selects the site in the gastric wall at which he wishes to have the stoma. In order to expose the first loop of jejunum the surgeon draws the transverse portion of the colon out of the abdomen and then toward the patient's head. The assistant holds the middle portion of the transverse colon cephalad with his right hand, and by inserting the left

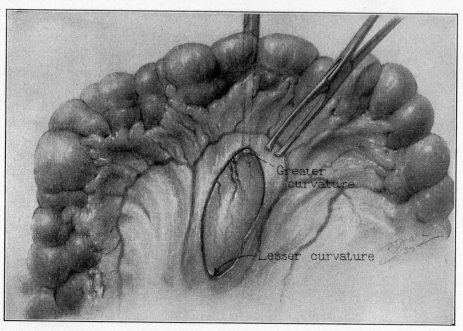

FIG. 215. Palliative posterior gastro-enterostomy for carcinoma of the stomach; a portion of the posterior wall of the stomach is brought down through an appropriate opening in the transverse mesocolon. (From Walters, Waltman, Gray, H. K. and Priestley, J. T., *Carcinoma and Other Malignant Lesions of the Stomach*. Courtesy of W. B. Saunders Company, Philadelphia, 1942.)

hand down toward the base of the mesentery of the distal portion of the transverse colon and pulling toward the left, he exposes the duodenojejunal angle. If it seems feasible to proceed, the surgeon now pulls to the right at the base of the transverse portion of the mesocolon and thus brings the proximal portion of jejunum into view. An Allis forceps is placed on the amesenteric portion of the jejunum approximately 14 to 18 cm. distal to the ligament of Treitz.

The assistant now presses the stomach down against the transverse portion of the mesocolon and an appropriate opening is made in this structure in a longitudinal line between the colon and the base of its mesentery (Fig. 215). Care is exercised to avoid the middle colic artery or any other vessel of appreciable size. By this method important vessels can be located by palpation and avoided. As the assistant pushes the stomach downward through the opening in the transverse portion of the mesocolon the posterior wall of the stomach is grasped with two Allis forceps at an appropriate distance apart (6 to 8 cm.) and the stomach is pulled well down below the transverse portion of the mesocolon. If possible, one Allis forceps is placed right on or very close to the greater curvature and the other is placed higher on the posterior wall of the stomach, toward the lesser curvature and somewhat to the right. If there are any adhesions which prevent traction

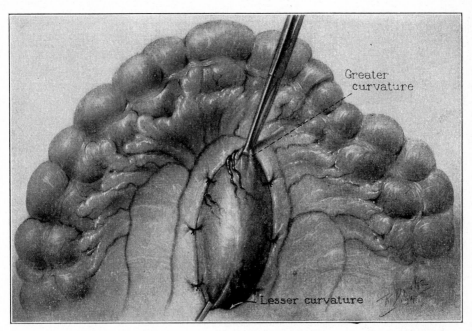

FIG. 216. Palliative posterior gastro-enterostomy: the stomach is secured below the transverse mesocolon with interrupted stitches. (From Walters, Waltman, Gray, H. K. and Priestley, J. T., *Carcinoma and Other Malignant Lesions of the Stomach.* Courtesy of W. B. Saunders Company, Philadelphia, 1942.)

of the stomach well down through the transverse part of the mesocolon such adhesions are freed at this time. After the stomach has been pulled well below the mesocolon it is sutured in this position with interrupted stitches of fine chromic catgut or silk (Fig. 216). Should it seem preferable, these sutures may be placed after completion of the anastomosis, although it is somewhat easier to insert them prior to establishment of the anastomosis. When the sutures have been inserted, the stomach is elevated out of the wound by traction on the Allis forceps previously placed on the stomach, and this portion of the posterior gastric wall is grasped with a straight rubber-covered Doyen forceps, after which the Allis forceps are removed.

The proximal portion of the jejunum now is brought into view by elevating the Allis forceps previously placed on it, and another Allis forceps is placed about 6 to 8 cm. distally on the jejunum. Both of these forceps now are held upward and another Doyen forceps is applied to the jejunum,

after which the Allis forceps are removed. Both Doyen forceps are applied
with the handles directed toward the surgeon (Fig. 217). Two small moist
gauze sponges, each with a forceps attached to the end, are placed between
the stomach and the jejunum. The stomach and the jejunum then are
approximated by bringing the Doyen forceps together in parallel position,

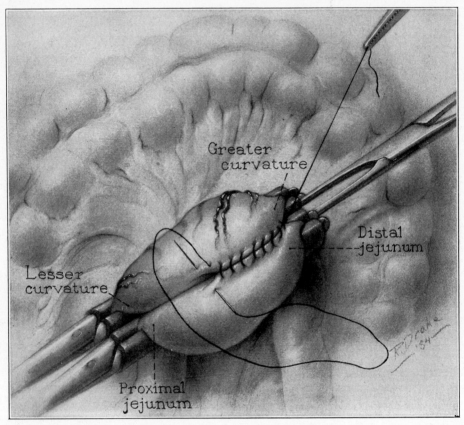

FIG. 217. Palliative posterior gastro-enterostomy: anastomosis between stomach and
jejunum. Distal loop of jejunum is in apposition with the greater curvature of the
stomach. (From Walters, Waltman, Gray, H. K. and Priestley, J. T., *Carcinoma and
Other Malignant Lesions of the Stomach.* Courtesy of W. B. Saunders Company, Philadelphia, 1942.)

so that the distal loop of jejunum lies in apposition with the greater curvature of the stomach, and the proximal limb of the jejunum is directed toward
the lesser curvature of the stomach. The stomach and the jejunum are kept
approximated in this manner by placing an Allis forceps inside of the
adjacent sides of the rubber tubes which cover the Doyen forceps. After
four large moist gauze pads have been placed around the operative site on
each side and each end of the approximated stomach and jejunum, the
surgeon is prepared to start the first row of sutures.

There are, of course, numerous different suture materials and many different types of suture which may be employed for establishing a gastro-jejunal anastomosis. The method of anastomosis which has been found to be satisfactory and which my colleagues and I usually perform is carried out as follows. Starting at the juncture of the proximal portion of the jejunum and the portion of the gastric wall closest to the lesser curvature, with fine silk or cotton (chromic catgut may be used just as well) on a straight or curved intestinal needle, the stomach and the jejunum are approximated with a running suture down to the greater curvature of the stomach and the distal portion of the jejunum. The last stitch is locked and a long end of suture is left, on which gentle traction is maintained by the hand of an assistant until it is used again; this long end of suture with needle attached is covered with a large gauze pad.

With a scalpel a straight incision now is made in the gastric wall through the serosa and the muscularis down to the mucosa. Any blood vessels of appreciable size which are visible along the base of the mucosal layer (which has not been incised) now are grasped with pointed forceps on each side of the exposed mucosa. All of these forceps then are placed to lie so that they are pointed toward the jejunum, and the jejunum now is incised to a length corresponding to the incision in the stomach. This incision is carried into the lumen of the jejunum and may be completed, if desired, with straight scissors. Any jejunal contents are carefully sponged away as the bowel is opened. The pointed forceps previously placed on the stomach now are separated and held upward. An incision is made through the gastric mucosa and this incision is enlarged appropriately with straight scissors. Any gastric contents which escape are disposed of with gauze. Vessels previously secured with the pointed forceps now are ligated with fine plain catgut.

After the exposed mucosal surfaces have been sponged with an antiseptic solution (tincture of merthiolate) the surgeon is ready to place the inner row of posterior sutures. For this purpose chromic catgut No. o on a straight intestinal needle may be employed. A running through-and-through stitch which includes mucosa and submucosa and perhaps some muscularis is utilized, beginning at the same angle at which the previous suture was begun. After this suture has been placed across the entire posterior aspect of the anastomosis the Doyen forceps are loosened temporarily to permit inspection of this portion of the anastomotic juncture for bleeding before it is hidden from view by the anterior row of sutures. Any such bleeding is controlled with interrupted sutures of fine plain catgut. The Doyen forceps then are closed again and the mucosal suture is continued anteriorly back to its starting point. An inverting type of suture for the anterior row is not necessary and is not commonly employed. When the starting point is reached, this suture is tied to the original end of silk or catgut, which previously was secured by a forceps and placed under a large moist gauze pad. The line of suture now is sponged gently with a moist gauze pad and the mucosal suture is cut. As the second assistant holds upward each end of the original silk suture of the posterior wall, the surgeon and the first assistant remove the four moist gauze sponges which originally were placed around the operative site, together with the Doyen forceps on the stomach and jejunum and the two small gauze sponges which were placed between the approximated portions of the stomach and the jejunum.

At this stage of the procedure the surgeon and the first assistant, after washing their hands, place a clean, moist gauze sponge on either side of the stomach and the jejunum while the sterile nurse places clean linen on the operating table and provides clean instruments, since those previously employed are discarded. The second assistant now relinquishes the ends of the silk suture and washes his hands. The anterior row of silk sutures is now placed, using a continuous running stitch which includes serosa and muscularis and covers the exposed mucosa of both the stomach and the jejunum. When the surgeon reaches the original starting point of this suture toward the lesser curvature of the stomach and the proximal portion of the jejunum this suture is tied to the short end which remains at this point. Additional interrupted stitches of silk which penetrate the serosa and muscularis are placed all around the anastomotic opening as a third row of sutures at a distance of 1 to 1.5 cm. from each other. Particular care is exercised at the angles of the anastomotic opening and the stitches are placed somewhat closer in these regions. A final inspection is made to be certain that everything is satisfactory, and the anastomosis is then complete. The distal portion of the jejunum is replaced so as to lie to the left, directed toward the left hip, and the transverse section of the colon is drawn downward toward the patient's feet and is replaced within the abdomen. The usual type of abdominal closure is employed and, in addition, if the surgeon desires, interrupted sutures of nonabsorbable material may be placed in the fascia.

ANTERIOR GASTRO-ENTEROSTOMY

Anterior gastro-enterostomy may be preferable when posterior gastro-enterostomy is infeasible because of a fatty, short mesocolon, or too small avascular spaces between branches of the middle colic artery and vein. Under these circumstances the same general principles are utilized in choosing the site for anterior anastomosis as when a posterior gastro-enteric stoma is created. The anterior anastomotic opening should be placed dependently in the stomach and no closer to the cardia than necessary. The opening in the stomach usually is placed transversely, close to and parallel with the greater curvature. It seems to matter little whether an isoperistaltic or an antiperistaltic type of anastomosis is made, so long as the jejunal loops hang free and unobstructed. Technical details of suture in establishing an anterior anastomosis are similar to those described for the posterior type of operation. A greater length of proximal jejunal loop than in performance of posterior gastro-enterostomy is of course necessary to provide an adequate jejunal loop to come up in front of the transverse colon without tension or angulation.

Entero-anastomosis may be performed between the two jejunal loops at an appropriate site if desired, although this joining is not essential and should be avoided if gastro-enterostomy is done for treatment of a duodenal or gastric ulcer.* If an entero-anastomotic opening is established, it usually is placed approximately 8 to 10 cm. from the ligament of Treitz on the proximal jejunal loop and in an adjacent portion of the distal loop of jejunum. In principle, anastomosis of this type is performed in a manner similar to that employed for making the gastrojejunal union. In most cases it is probably preferable to establish such anastomosis from the point of view of subsequent gastro-intestinal motor function. One need not fear subsequent jejunal ulceration if such a stoma is created, since the concentration of gastric acids almost invariably is low and the occurrence of marginal ulcer when this operation is performed for carcinoma is practically unknown.

GASTROSTOMY

In a limited group of cases gastrostomy may be employed. If such a procedure appears to be desirable, a Witzel type of operation commonly is employed. An appropriate site in the anterior wall of the stomach is selected for insertion of the gastrostomy tube. A purse-string suture of silk is placed in this region, a long loop of suture being left directly opposite the first and the last stitches. This loop then is elevated, as are both ends of the suture. Thus the anterior wall of the stomach is raised so that the tube may be inserted readily and so that spilling of gastric contents is prevented. A soft rubber catheter (size 20 to 24 F.) is prepared by cutting several extra holes near the tip and placing a hemostat a little distance from the opposite end. With the loop and the ends of the purse-string suture still elevated, a hole of appropriate size is made with a small scalpel in the middle portion of the gastric wall. This hole is encircled by the purse-string suture, the catheter is inserted quickly into the hole, and the purse-string suture is tied. The hole in the gastric wall is made somewhat smaller than the actual diameter of the catheter so that as the catheter is inserted into the stomach and the purse-string suture is tightened, the edges of the gastric wall are inverted. The catheter then is held close to and roughly parallel with the proximal portion of the stomach, and additional interrupted stitches of silk are inserted so that the tube is covered completely by the adjacent gastric wall. Perhaps six to eight such sutures in all may be employed, placed approximately 0.5 to 1 cm. apart. It is preferable to insert the tube so that it is directed distally into the stomach. The end of the gastrostomy tube may now be drawn through an avascular portion of the omentum if the surgeon desires and thence through a stab wound to the side of the incision. As this is done a forceps is inserted through the stab wound at the side of the incision. With the forceps the tube is grasped distally to the hemostat which originally was placed on the tube, and thus the tube is pulled to the outside. A strong non-absorbable suture placed through the skin at the site of the stab wound is used to secure the catheter in place.

* In 25 per cent of such cases of duodenal ulcer relative achlorhydria is obtained in contrast to 75 per cent of cases in which entero-anastomosis is not performed.

JEJUNOSTOMY

When jejunostomy is indicated it is performed in a manner similar to that described for gastrostomy. As an additional safeguard the catheter is pulled through the gastrocolic omentum. The jejunostomy tube should be inserted at a convenient site a short distance below the ligament of Treitz.

EXCLUSION OPERATION

An exclusion type of operation similar to the Devine exclusion operation may be employed in the treatment of certain fixed irremovable malignant lesions of the lower end of the stomach. This procedure is performed in a manner similar to the Polya operation, except that the distal portion of the stomach is not removed. At the second stage of the operation the growth, which lies in the gastric stump distal to the gastrojejunal anastomosis, is extirpated if removable. This operation seldom is indicated, as proper pre-operative preparation usually will enable the surgeon to perform gastric resection in one stage with as low a risk as a procedure carried out in two stages when the lesion is operable—and a gastro-enterostomy usually suffices as a palliative procedure to relieve obstruction. The operative risk, however, is high.

APPENDIX

PORTION OF POLYA'S ACCOUNT OF THE HISTORY OF HIS OPERATION

"I demonstrated my first patient operated upon with this method in October, 1910, before the surgical society of Budapest and spoke of this operation at the 1911 Congress of the German Surgical Society in Berlin (*Verhandl. d. deutsch. Gesellsch. f. Chir.*, 1911, 1:200) and when I saw that no one there knew of anything similar, I decided to publish a description of the technique, which appeared in the *Zentralblatt fuer Chirurgie*, 1911, Nr. 26. A few weeks later Wilms, then director of the surgical clinic of the University of Heidelberg, wrote an article in the *Zentralblatt fuer Chirurgie*, 1911, Nr. 32, in which he stated that a few months previously, even before reading my report, he had used a method similar to mine but with certain differences. In the *Zentralbl. fuer Chirurgie* of 1911, Nr. 42, Reichel claimed priority because he had mentioned at the 1908 Congress of the German Surgical Society in discussing a paper of Moszkovicz on aseptic intestinal operations (*Ueber aseptische Darmoperationen*) that he had performed 3 operations of the kind described by me. At the same time Bergmann, of Riga, sent to me a reprint of an article (*St. Petersburger medizinische Wochenschrift*, 1909, Nr. 52) in which he reported on 2 cases operated upon in the same manner. He did not know of Reichel's article nor did Wilms, nor did I, nor did anybody else to whom I had spoken before. The great surprise, however, came in 1916, when Narath published an article in the *Deutsche Zeitschrift fuer Chirurgie,* Vol. 136, which showed that von Hacker had advocated the idea of connecting the opening of the stump of the stomach directly with the jejunum and that it was Kroenlein, in 1888, who first performed such an operation (antecolic) . . . and that since then many surgeons including Eiselsberg . . . Mikulicz, Doyen, Graser . . . Hofmeister, Delagenière, Sasse, and others published reports of cases in which this principle was followed with various alterations in technique (antecolic, retrocolic, narrowed and unnarrowed stomach stump). These were presented usually in casuistical publications and in demonstrations before medical societies which generally do not awake public interest. Thus it happened that not one of the surgeons, who did the operation, knew of the others who had been doing it and most of those who were doing it looked upon it as a method of exceptional value, when necessity demanded, but not as a measure of great general practical value."

REFERENCES

1. CHENEY, GARNETT and NEWELL, R. R.   Large Diverticula of the Gastric Cardia, *Am. J. Digest. Dis.,* 3:920-923, [Feb.], 1937.
2. RIVERS, A. B., STEVENS, G. A. and KIRKLIN, B. R.   Diverticula of the Stomach, *Surg., Gynec. & Obst.,* 60:106-113, [Jan.], 1935.
3. EUSTERMAN, G. B. and BALFOUR, D. C.   *The Stomach and Duodenum,* W. B. Saunders Company, Philadelphia, 1936, 958 pp.
4. JORDAN, SARA M.   The Present Status of Peptic Ulcer, *New England J. Med.,* 203:917-920, [Nov. 6], 1930.
5. McVICAR, C. S.   Quoted by EUSTERMAN, G. B. and BALFOUR, D. C.   *The Stomach and Duodenum,* W. B. Saunders Company, Philadelphia, 1936, p. 768.
6. RAMSTEDT, C.   *Zur Operation der angeborenen Pylorusstenose, Zentralbl. f. Chir.,* 39:1741-1742, [Dec. 21], 1912.
7. DONOVAN, E. J. and WALTERS, WALTMAN   Unpublished data.
8. STEVENS, G. A. and BOECK, W. C.   Gastrojejunal Hemorrhage following Gastroenterostomy for Hypertrophic Pyloric Stenosis of Infancy, *J.A.M.A.,* 124:160-161, [Jan. 15], 1944.
9. FOWLER, L. H. and HANSON, W. A.   Gastrojejunal Ulcer following Gastro-enterostomy Performed Twenty-four Years Before for Pyloric Stenosis of Infancy, *Minnesota Med.,* 23:602, [Aug.], 1940.
10. COUNSELLER, V. S., WAUGH, J. M. and CLAGETT, O. T.   Report of Surgery of the Stomach and Duodenum for 1944, *Proc. Staff Meet., Mayo Clin.,* 21:17-24, [Jan. 9], 1946.
11. BILLROTH   *Offenes Schreiben an Herrn L. Wittelshöfer, Wien. med. Wchnschr.,* 31:161-165, 1881.
12. BILLROTH   *Ueber einen neuen Fall von gelungener Resektion des carcinomatösen Pylorus, Wien. med. Wchnschr.,* 31:1427, 1881.
13. BILLROTH   Excision of a Part of the Human Stomach; reported by J. A. KASSON, U. S. Minister to Austria, *Monthly Rev. Med. & Pharm.,* Philadelphia, 4:195, 1881.
14. BILLROTH   *Ein neuer Fall von geheilter Magenresektion, Wien. med. Wchnschr.,* 33:1213-1215, 1883.
15. BILLROTH   *Resection des carcinomatösen Pylorus mit glücklichem Erfolge, Anz. d. k. k. Gesellsch. d. Aerzte in Wien,* 1883-1884, pp. 121-123.
16. BILLROTH   *Ueber einen neuen Fall von gelungener Pylorusresektion, Wien. med. Wchnschr.,* 34:888-890, 1884.

17. PÉAN   *De l'ablation des tumeurs de l'estomac par la gastrectomie, Gaz. d. hôp.,* 52:473-475, 1879.

18. PÉAN   *Gastrotomie,* Cases, *Bull. Acad. de méd.,* Paris, s.2, 8:1194-1197, 1879.

19. BILLROTH   Quoted by VON HACKER. *Zur Casuistik und Statistik der Magenresektionen und Gastroenterostomieen, Arch. f. klin. Chir.,* 32:616-625, 1885.

20. V. HABERER, H.   *Meine Technik der Magenresektion, München. med. Wchnschr.,* 80:915-921, [June 16], 1933.

21. SCHOEMAKER, J.   *Ueber die Technik ausgedehnter Magenresectionen, Arch. f. klin. Chir.,* 94:541-548, 1911.

22. SCHOEMAKER.   *Zur Technik der Magenresektion nach Billroth I., Arch. f. klin. Chir.,* 121:268-271, 1922.

23. HORSLEY, J. S. and BIGGER, I. A.   *Operative Surgery,* C. V. Mosby Company, St. Louis, 1940, Ed. 5, Vol. 2, Chap. 56, pp. 1007-1024.

24. V. HABERER, H.   *Terminolaterale Gastroduodenostomie bei der Resektionsmethode nach Billroth I., Zentralbl. f. Chir.,* 49:1321-1326, [Sept. 9], 1922.

25. VON HACKER   *Zur Casuistik und Statistik der Magenresektionen und Gastroenterostomieen, Arch. f. klin. Chir.,* 32:616-625, 1885.

26. VON EISELSBERG, A. F.   *Ueber die Magenresectionen und Gastroenterostomieen in Prof. Billroth's Klinik von März 1885 bis October 1889, Arch. f. klin. Chir.,* 39:785-844, 1889.

27. BRAUN, H.   *Über die Gastroenterostomie und gleichzeitige Enteroanastomose, Centralbl. f. Chir.,* 19:102, (Beilage Nr. 32), 1892.

28. JABOULAY   *La gastro-entérostomie; la jéjunoduodénostomie; la résection du pylore. Arch. prov. d. chir.,* Paris, 1:1-22, 1892.

29. POLYA, EUGEN   *Zur Stumpfversorgung nach Magenresektion, Zentralbl. f. Chir.,* 38:892-894, 1911.

30. KRÖNLEIN   *Mittheilung über einen kürzlich beobachteten Fall von traumatischer narbiger Pylorusstenose, Cor.-Bl. f. schweiz. Aerzte.,* 18:317-318, 1888.

31. REICHEL   Discussion. *Verhandl. d. deutsch. Gesellsch. f. Chir.,* Th. 1, 137:211-212, 1908.

32. BALFOUR, D. C.   Restoration of Gastro-intestinal Continuity by Means of Anticolic Gastrojejunostomy following Partial Gastrectomy for Cancer of the Pyloric End of Stomach, *Surg., Gynec. & Obst.,* 25:473-477, [Nov.], 1917.

33. ADAMS, W. E. and PHEMISTER, D. B.   Carcinoma of the Lower Thoracic Esophagus; Report of a Successful Resection and Esophagogastrostomy, *J. Thoracic Surg.,* 7:621-632, [Aug.], 1938.

34. CLAGETT, O. T.   Transthoracic Resection of the Cardia and Esophagus, *Texas State J. Med.,* 42:7-11, [May], 1946.

35. WALTERS, WALTMAN   Total Gastrectomy for Carcinoma: Physiologic and Chemical Studies during a Period of Two Years following the Operation, *J.A.M.A.,* 100:804-806, [Mar. 18], 1933.

36. GRAHAM, R. R.   A Technique for Total Gastrectomy, *Surgery,* 8:257-264, [Aug.], 1940.

GASTRIC VAGOTOMY IN THE TREATMENT OF PEPTIC ULCER

Lester R. Dragstedt, M.D.

Complete division of the vagus nerves to the stomach as a method of treatment for peptic ulcer is a relatively new procedure. The first operations were performed in January and February of 1943, and in the intervening years, 490 patients with various types of peptic ulcer have been operated upon in this clinic by this method. A review of the surgical literature indicates that operations upon the vagus nerves to the stomach for the treatment of peptic ulcer, gastric crisis of tabes, and other diseases, were performed by several surgeons in the past. Stierlin, Bircher, Latarget, and Schiassi, as well as others have described and illustrated operative procedures on the stomach designed to sever the vagus nerve supply. Brief and incomplete reference has usually been made to the results secured. A study of these reports and an inspection of the drawings supplied suggest that the anatomy of the vagus nerves to the stomach was not very well known, and that in the operations described, a complete vagotomy was not secured. In our own experience, complete division of the vagus nerves to the stomach has provided such complete and persistent relief of ulcer distress that it seems likely, had a similar result been secured by the early workers, the operation would long since have become very widely used. The fact that the operation did not become popular is perhaps the best evidence that the earlier methods were unsuccessful in securing a complete interruption of all of the vagus nerves to the stomach. For this reason, it seems wise to present in some detail the methods that are in use at the present time in this clinic.

Gastric Vagotomy by the Transthoracic Approach. The first fifty operations on the vagus nerves to the stomach in this clinic were performed by a transthoracic approach. The anesthetic usually employed has been ethylene and ether given with a pressure mask. The patient is placed on his right side on the operating table, and a long incision made over the eighth rib on the left side (Fig. 218). The eighth rib is widely resected, and at this time, it is wise to divide the eighth intercostal nerve at the posterior margin of the incision. The left pleural cavity is then opened. The inferior pulmonary ligament to the left lung is divided between ligatures, and the left lung retracted superiorly. The pleura over the lower 3 or 4 inches of the esophagus is then divided. The esophagus is mobilized by gentle finger dissection and lifted upward into the left pleural cavity (Fig. 219). This maneuver brings the vagus nerves into view, and they can be readily palpated against the more elastic and more yielding esophageal muscle. The vagus nerves are gently separated from the lower esophagus and are divided between ligatures immediately above the diaphragm. A nonabsorbable suture such as silk or linen is used because this helps to prevent regeneration. The right or posterior vagus is usually found as a single trunk along the lower 4 inches of the esophagus. In this region, the left or anterior vagus may be represented as a single trunk or as two or more branches. It is a simple

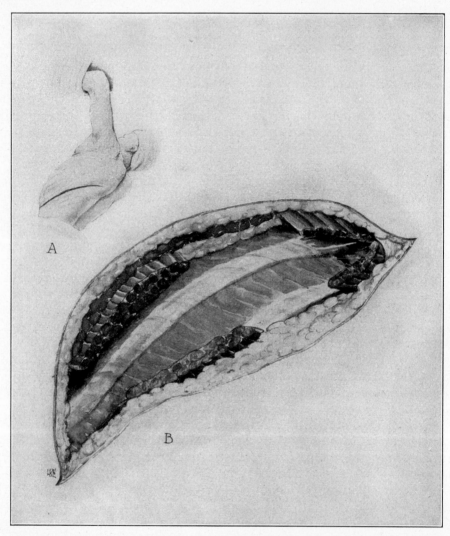

Fig. 218. Incision (A) and exposure (B) of the seventh rib for transthoracic vagotomy. (From Dragstedt, *Ann. Surg.*, 122(No. 6):975, 1945.)

matter, however, to clean off the esophagus for a distance of about 3 inches, thus making sure that all of the vagus fibers to the stomach have been divided. The esophagus is then replaced in its bed, and the overlying pleura sutured with catgut. The proximal ends of the vagus nerves are transplanted into the pleural cavity and attached to the chest wall (Fig. 220). This procedure is designed to increase the distance between the cut ends of the nerves, and thus to hinder regeneration. Moore recommends that a segment of the vagi be excised and that the diaphragm be opened to permit removal of the vagus nerves along the stomach. It seems probable, at the present time, that these precautions to avoid regeneration are unnecessary. Regeneration of the vagus fibers has not yet been observed although some of the patients have been followed for four to five years following the

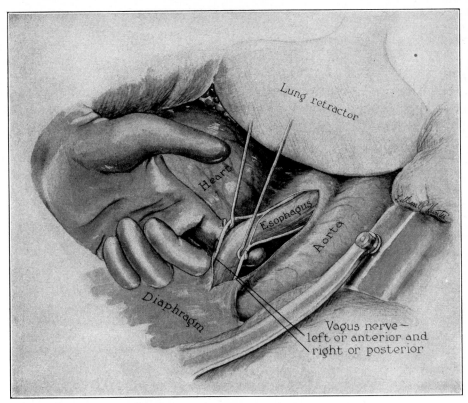

FIG. 219. Mobilization of the esophagus and isolation of vagus nerves showing the communication between the anterior and posterior trunks. (From Dragstedt, *Ann. Surg.,* 122(No. 6): 1945.)

operation. The contrast with surgery of the sympathetic nervous system is thus very striking. The lung is then inflated, the air aspirated from the pleural cavity, and the chest closed without drainage.

Transabdominal Approach. For the operation of gastric vagotomy by the transabdominal approach, it is our custom to employ a continuous spinal anesthetic. A general anesthesia with ether or with cyclopropane and curara may be equally satisfactory. It is important to secure good relaxation. A long midline or left paramedian incision is made extending from the xiphoid cartilage to 2 or 3 centimeters below the umbilicus. The stomach and duodenum are then carefully inspected and palpated, and an attempt is made to determine if there is obstruction at the pylorus. The left lobe of the liver is then secured by the surgeon and pulled downward into the operative field. This maneuver exposes the coronary ligament to the left

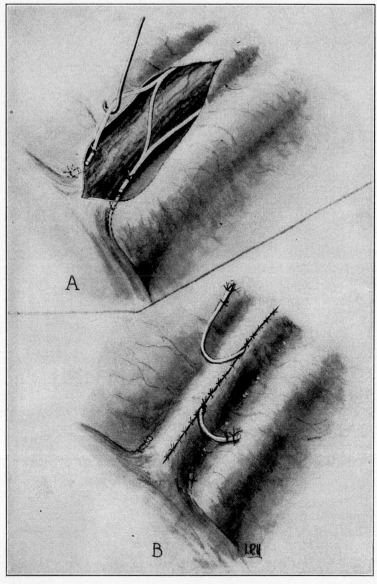

FIG. 220. (A) Ligature and division of vagus nerves just above diaphragm; and (B) transplantation of proximal ends of cut vagi into the pleural cavity. (From Dragstedt, *Ann. Surg.*, 122(No. 6): 1945.)

lobe of the liver, and this can then be most easily divided with scissors by the assistant surgeon. After division of the ligament, the left lobe of the liver is retracted to the right by a gallbladder retractor (Fig. 221). The upper part of the stomach and the lower end of the esophagus then come into view. The peritoneum overlying the lower esophagus at the margin of the diaphragm is secured by forceps and elevated. A small incision through the peritoneum is made with scissors, and the scissors are then thrust upward through the hiatus and the opening enlarged. If a Levine tube has previously

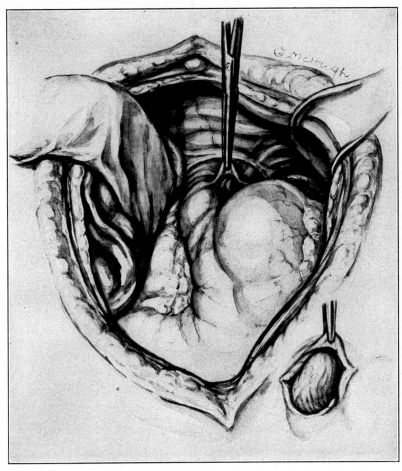

FIG. 221. The left lobe of the liver is retracted to the right and the peritoneum over the esophagus at the margin of the diaphragm is divided and the hiatus opened. (From Dragstedt, Harper, Tovee and Woodward, *Ann. Surg.*, 126(5):690, 1947.)

been introduced into the stomach, palpation of the esophagus is facilitated. The surgeon's index finger is then introduced over the esophagus into the mediastinum (Fig. 222A). By gentle finger dissection, the lower portion of the esophagus is separated from the surrounding areolar tissue. As the surgeon's fingers surround the esophagus, the vagus nerves can be felt posteriorly as they extend downward along to the lesser curvature of the stomach. The esophagus is pulled downward into the abdomen for a distance of 6 to 8 centimeters (Fig. 222B). When this is done, the left or anterior vagus nerve usually comes in view extending along the front of the esophagus toward the lesser curvature. The right or posterior vagus nerve is felt as a firm cord posterior to the esophagus and usually close to its right border. It is usually most convenient to separate the right vagus nerve from the esophageal wall by finger dissection and to pull this trunk around to the left or splenic side of the esophagus where it can be ligated and divided. In most instances, the right vagus is exposed for a distance of 6 to 8 centimeters above its

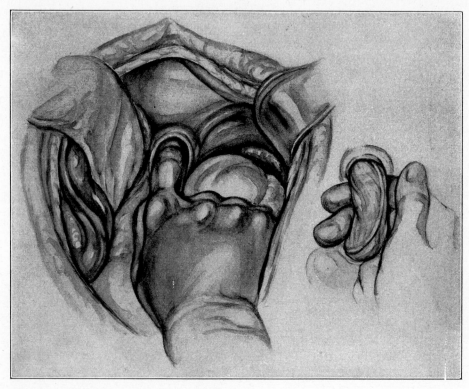

FIG. 222. The finger is introduced over the esophagus into the mediastinum, the esophagus mobilized by careful finger dissection and pulled downward into the abdomen for a distance of 2 to 3 inches. (From Dragstedt, Harper, Tovee and Woodward, *Ann. Surg.*, 126(5):690, 1947.)

entrance into the wall of the stomach along the posterior portion of the lesser curvature (Fig. 223). A clamp is placed on this nerve as far superiorly as possible, and the nerve is then divided between silk or linen ligatures. At this stage, a segment of 4 or 6 centimeters of the nerve may be resected if desired. This is unnecessary, and the distal end of the nerve may simply be pulled downward on the stomach. The left vagus nerve is similarly freed from the anterior wall of the esophagus by finger dissection and cut between ligatures. This nerve also is usually divided 6 to 8 centimeters above its entrance into the stomach. Following division of the vagus nerves, it will usually be found possible to pull the esophagus still further into the abdomen. This permits a careful review of the anterior and posterior wall to make certain that all vagus fibers have been divided. In about 50 per cent of cases, only two large trunks are seen. In the remaining 50 per cent, the anterior vagus may be represented by two or more main branches, and in a smaller number, the right or posterior vagus may be found as two or more trunks. The esophagus and proximal ends of the cut and tied vagus nerves are then allowed to retract upward into the mediastinum. The peri-

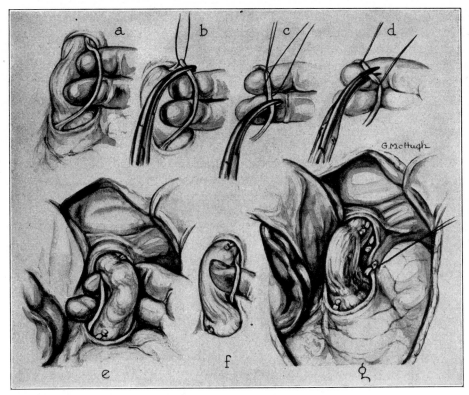

FIG. 223. The vagus nerves are separated from the esophagus by finger dissection, ligated with nonabsorbable suture material, divided and a segment 4 to 6 centimeters in length excised. (From Dragstedt, Harper, Tovee and Woodward, *Ann. Surg.*, 126(5):690, 1947.)

toneum over the esophageal hiatus is closed with several interrupted silk sutures. The left lobe of the liver is then placed in its previous position, but it is usually unnecessary to suture the coronary ligament. If cicatricial obstruction at the pylorus has been found, a gastroenterostomy or gastro-duodenostomy should now be performed.

Postoperative Treatment. Complete division of the vagus nerves to the stomach produces a profound decrease in the secretion of gastric juice, and it is upon this effect that the therapeutic value of the procedure depends for the most part. In addition to its effect on gastric secretion, the operation also causes an immediate and profound decrease in the tonus and motility of the stomach. This is most marked for the first 24 hours and recedes considerably after two or three days. Because of this decrease in tonus and motility, it is of the utmost importance to decompress the stomach for two or three days following the operation. This is best accomplished by means of an indwelling nasal tube connected with the Wangensteen suction apparatus. Parenteral administration of urecholine is sometimes useful during this period. Fluid and electrolyte balance are maintained by the daily administration of 3000 cubic centimeters of salt solution intravenously. The patient is urged to get out of bed after 24 hours. This early rising markedly decreases the incidence of pulmonary complications such as atelectasis and broncho-pneumonia.

Postoperative Complications. It is probable that all patients operated upon by the transthoracic approach develop an effusion into the pleural cavity of greater or less extent following the operation. In about 10 per cent of cases, this effusion is sufficiently great to require aspiration. In no instance, however, has it become infected or caused serious disability. Pain in the region of the intercostal incision and the costovertebral joint is the most troublesome complication of the transthoracic operation. This is present to a greater or less degree in all patients. In most cases, it subsides in a week or two, but in some patients, particularly among the older age group, pain of varying degree may persist for three or four months. In no case, however, has a patient complained that this pain has counterbalanced the beneficial effect secured by the vagotomy. The pain is decreased somewhat by previous division of the intercostal nerve and by infiltration of the intercostal nerves above and below the rib resected with procaine or eucupin. As noted above, a decrease in the tonus and motility of the stomach occurs in all patients subjected to gastric vagotomy whether by the transthoracic or the transabdominal approach. It seems probable that an increased tonus of the pylorus is also produced which lasts for a variable period. The stomach is thus very susceptible to the dilating effect of swallowed air or accumulated secretion. If gastric aspiration is not carefully maintained, an acute dilatation of the stomach may occur. I have not seen this complication in our own patients, but have been informed of its occurrence by other surgeons. An increase in the length of time required for emptying of the stomach is found in most patients following vagotomy, and in cases of cicatricial obstruction at the pylorus, retention may become very marked. Ten per cent of our patients with duodenal ulcer have required gastroenterostomy in addition to the vagus section. It is probable that a gastroenterostomy should be done in all patients with duodenal ulcer giving a previous history of vomiting or with x-ray evidence of marked pyloric obstruction. A transitory diarrhea is a troublesome complication complained of by a varying proportion of patients following vagus section to the stomach. It seems probable that this is due to a combination of retention of food for a long period of time in the stomach in the presence of a more or less complete achlorhydria. Diarrhea is very rarely seen in patients with duodenal ulcer in which a vagotomy and gastroenterostomy have been performed. It usually disappears in two or three weeks, and in no case has a patient been seriously inconvenienced by it. It is usually checked by the administration of calcium carbonate or of paregoric.

Indications for Gastric Vagotomy in the Treatment of Peptic Ulcer. At the present time, 490 patients with various types of peptic ulcer have been operated upon in this clinic by these methods. The results have been so favorable that it is possible now to conclude that a benign peptic ulcer may regularly be expected to heal following this operation. This is equally true of gastric, duodenal, and gastrojejunal ulcers. The response of bleeding ulcers has been equally favorable. Gastric vagotomy for gastric ulcer is complicated by the problem of the differential diagnosis between peptic ulcer and carcinoma. Obviously, if there is any question whatever in regard to the nature of the lesion, a gastric resection should be carried out in preference to vagotomy. In a borderline case, gastric vagotomy may be employed if repeated examinations of the stomach can be made after operation by means of the gastroscope and x-ray. If the lesion is benign, it can be expected to heal in from three to six weeks. If it does not heal within this period of time, a gastric resection had better be employed. For intractable duodenal ulcer, or for gastrojejunal ulcer, gastric vagotomy is the operative procedure of choice. The first patients have been followed for a period of almost six years, and so far, only two ulcers have recurred when the vagotomy was complete. If the present favorable outlook continues, it seems likely that the indication for the surgical treatment of peptic ulcer by this method will be markedly extended.

10

SURGERY OF THE SMALL INTESTINE *

CLARENCE DENNIS, M.D.

SMALL BOWEL OBSTRUCTION

Obstruction is not as rare as many surgeons seem inclined to think. At the University of Minnesota Hospitals, with 450 beds, a new case is seen, on the average, once every two weeks. The mortality from the disease has dropped markedly in the past few decades with more enlightened attitudes in recognition and management. The figure for the last years for which data have been collected here is about 10 per cent.

Mechanisms Causing Obstruction. (1) External hernia is responsible for slightly more than half the cases of small bowel obstruction seen at the University Hospitals. In most of these cases it represents only an incidental finding in an incarcerated hernia that is to be reduced surgically as an emergency procedure anyway. In a few, however, it is found only after careful search in patients coming with advanced obstruction without obvious cause; in such cases, careful examination for inguinal and femoral hernias *in both the prone and upright positions* has helped immensely.

(2) Adhesions of bowel to other loops or to the parietes constitute about one-sixth of the cases in our recent experience. Such situations usually follow previous operative procedures, but may be late complications of inflammatory processes such as appendicitis with extension, diverticulitis, colitis with extension, trauma, etc. The manner in which adhesion of a loop of ileum to the abdominal wall may cause obstruction is illustrated in figure 224. It has been found repeatedly that simple separation of this adhesion cures the patient.

(3) Adhesive bands account for another one-sixth of the patients in our experience. Although a few are congenital in origin, most result from a gradual stretching by intestinal activity of initially broader areas of adhesion secondary to past inflammatory processes or to former abdominal surgery or other trauma. In the series here, more than half the obstructions due to bands were an aftermath of earlier gynecological procedures. Obstructions due to congenital bands, as in Meckel's diverticulum, are included here, as well as those due to wrapping of loops around segments of bowel

* The results of certain hitherto unpublished investigations are included in this chapter. These were supported by a Research Grant from the University of Minnesota Graduate School.

and mesentery ascending to the anterior abdominal wall to form colostomies or ileostomies.

(4) Intussusception accounts for a small fraction of the University Hospital series; it is probably a larger factor in general surgical practice.

(5) Foreign body or obturation obstruction is usually due to a gallstone which has sloughed through both gallbladder and intestinal walls. About one case a year is seen here.

(6) Mesenteric venous thrombosis is probably commoner than has been considered. Obstruction results purely from loss of motility due to gangrene. Arterial occlusion must be very rare.

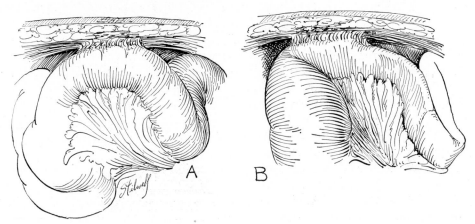

FIG. 224. The manner in which adhesion of a loop of intestine to the abdominal wall, as at the site of an old surgical wound, may cause obstruction. The bowel wall in the acute angle serves as a valve leaf, and increase in distention by increase in angulation and consequent edema renders the obstruction only more secure. Decompression of the proximal segment permits release of angulation and reduction of the secondary edema, with restoration of functional continuity. The same mechanism may apply to adhesions to other loops or viscera or to other portions of the abdominal parietes.

(7) Congenital atresias and bands are seen about once a year at University Hospitals.

(8) Volvulus is rare as a cause of small bowel obstruction in this country, although Wangensteen states it is very common in Eastern Europe. We have had two cases of volvulus of the cecum and one of the mid-ileum in ten years.

(9) Neoplasms primary in the small bowel are very rarely causes of obstruction. It is not uncommon, however, to find ileac obstruction due to adhesion to carcinomas of the stomach or colon. Encroachment on the ileocecal valve by a primary carcinoma of the cecum, and occasionally of the ascending colon, may present a typical picture of ileac obstruction.

(10) Internal hernias are very rarely the mechanism of small bowel obstruction.

Consideration of these causative agents is of paramount importance in the management of obstruction of the small intestine. Conservative therapy is based on the hypothesis that loss of bowel viability will not occur; it is therefore successful regularly only in cases due to simple adhesions and rare cases due to neoplasms. No other group can be successfully handled without surgical intervention.

The Production of Symptoms and Signs of Simple Obstruction. PAIN AND CRAMPS. Upon blockage of the lumen of the ileum to the passage of content, dilation of the gut above the area and diminution in diameter below are results to be expected. Inasmuch as intestine is sensitive to stretching, this distention causes pain; this is not localized and develops over a period of hours. Peristaltic activity in the small bowel is characterized by waves of increased muscular activity originating in the pyloric region and progressing down to the cecum (Alvarez); these waves of propulsive activity normally pass a given point at intervals of three to ten minutes. Arrival of added gas and fluid at the already distended area, with such a wave of activity, produces a sudden increase in tension, and therefore in pain. This is the cramp commonly associated with intestinal obstruction. In many instances, particularly in partial simple obstructions, this accumulation is gradual, and the inevitable stretching of the bowel wall is sufficiently slow so that pain is not appreciated by the patient except at the moments when peristaltic rushes in the gut reach the distended area.

BORBORYGMUS. With the onset of obstruction and stagnation above, gas in quantity collects above a small quantity of fluid. Each peristaltic rush forces a little more gas and fluid into this closed space, resulting at first in gurgles, audible with the stethoscope at the moment of the height of the cramp. As the volume enclosed within the bowel above the obstruction increases, the wall of the bowel is stretched increasingly more tightly, and the pitch of the audible sound coming with each cramp rises correspondingly until it becomes the familiar tinkle or borborygmus of established intestinal obstruction.

VOMITING. Retrograde peristalsis arises at intervals from the irritated bowel just above the site of obstruction, and some of the content is thus carried back to the stomach, to be evacuated by vomiting. In the first two days of the illness, this vomitus is bile-stained and may contain recognizable food. In three to five days after onset of complete obstruction, the character of the vomitus gradually changes to resemble the liquid stool seen in simple diarrhea. The fecal character is the result of the length of time the material in question has been in the intestinal tract, and is no index at all of the level of the obstruction in the gut, a fact attested to by the occasional appearance of fecal vomiting in patients with obstruction of the efferent stoma after long loop gastrojejunostomy.

DISTENTION. The degree of clinical abdominal distention depends in great measure on the level at which obstruction has occurred in the small intestine, those toward the lower end naturally resulting in distention of a greater length of bowel, and thus a greater degree of apparent distention on physical examination. By obstructing the esophagus in the dog a few days before dividing and closing the terminal ileum, Wangensteen and Rea showed that the gas found in the dilated loops is chiefly swallowed air. In the first three or four days in clinical cases, the dilated loops are filled primarily with such gas.

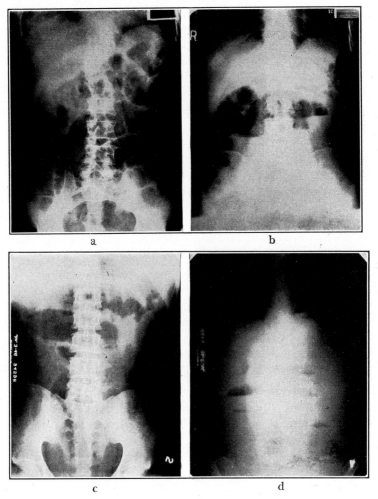

a b

c d

FIG. 225. Scout films of the abdomen in small bowel obstruction. (a) With the patient lying supine, the ladder-like arrangement of gas-filled loops is apparent. (b) With the patient in the upright position, the layering of fluid under gas is also apparent. (c) Strangulation obstruction due to an adhesive band—supine film. (d) Same patient as (c) in the upright position. The layering of fluid is again present, but without the rising of gas-filled loops in the abdomen seen in simple obstruction. Few gas-filled loops are visible, the others having filled with fluid. Presence of gas in colon after 30 hours is attributed to rapid onset of ileus due to strangulation.

ROENTGEN FINDINGS. Gas is normally present throughout the intestinal canal, but in the small intestine, where activity is great, it usually does not collect in pockets large enough for roentgen visualization (Wangensteen). With obstruction, gas collects in quantity, and because of the contrast in radio-opacity which it offers, roentgen diagnosis is accurate in the majority of cases. Scout films of the abdomen reveal a ladder-like arrangement of gas-filled coils of the small intestine. In obstructions of several days' duration, the ratio of fluid to gas increases, and upright films of the abdomen show definite fluid levels in the distended loops of bowel. In children up to four to six years of age, gas is normally present in large amounts in the ileum, and stands out in the roentgen films; the method is therefore not as valuable here as in older individuals (Fig. 225).

The degree of absence of gas visible in the colon is a good index of the completeness of obstruction, provided gas has not been injected with enemas. Although a barium meal outlines the obstructed bowel very beautifully, the barium sulfate is apt to cake and increase the completeness of obstruction. It is therefore to be condemned.

OBSTIPATION. The blockage of the ileum may occur at a time when the colon is relatively full of gas and feces. Passage of some stool and flatus for a day or even two after apparent acute onset is therefore not rare. Thereafter nothing passes in complete obstruction, even with the use of enemas.

CHEMICAL IMBALANCE. The persistent vomiting associated with ileac obstruction causes greater or less water and salt loss depending on the level involved. Lesions close to the duodenojejunal angle lie above the great water-absorbing area of the ileum and below the great water-secreting areas. The combined secretions of the salivary glands, stomach, liver, pancreas, and duodenum total 5 to 12 liters daily in the normal adult, and virtually all of this is lost through vomiting in obstructions at the level in question. But two to three days are required to produce a water, gastric acid, and salt loss sufficient to produce severe dehydration, secondary uremia due to inadequate water for renal function, hypochloremia, and occasionally alkalosis.

Observations on patients with terminal ileostomies indicate that the volume passed from that segment is usually less than 500 cc. daily. If the bowel is blocked at the ileocecal junction, therefore, the great water-absorbing area of the intestine lies above, and the degree of interference with fluid and salt balance will be so little as not to assume serious proportions before death results from other causes.

PALPABLE LOOPS. In certain cases the degree of obstruction is slight enough so that compensatory hypertrophy of the intestinal muscle above is adequate to prevent decompensation. Between these extremes are many patients with partial obstruction complete enough to give the symptoms already mentioned, but in whom sufficient hypertrophy of the intestine and sufficient wasting of the abdominal wall occur to permit visualization of the outlines of loops on the abdominal wall and palpation of them with the examining hand. This degree of change can develop in seven to ten days of chronic partial obstruction (Fig. 226).

The Production of Symptoms and Signs of Strangulating Obstruction. The term "strangulation" is here properly used to connote partial or complete blockage of the circulation to the involved intestinal segment; it is only after strangulation has been in force for one to three or four hours that loss of viability occurs. Strangulation is prone to occur in obstructions due to hernia, intussusception, adhesive bands, foreign body in the lumen, mesenteric thrombosis, and volvulus.

The symptoms and signs of strangulation in such cases are by and large simply superimposed on those of simple obstruction.

SUDDEN ONSET. In most types of strangulation obstruction, the mechanism is one of a loop passing through an aperture, into a hernial sac, or around an adhesive band, or becoming twisted on itself. These are situations in which rapid passage of the intestine into positions blocking passage of content and blood can occur. It is understandable therefore that the onset of the disease in such circumstances is frequently abrupt, with pain reaching maximal intensity within a few minutes of onset (McKittrick).

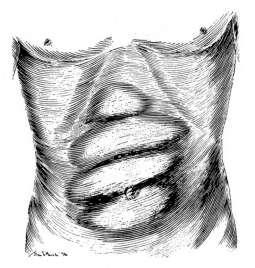

BACK PAIN. The position of the involved loop in such cases places tension on the root of the mesentery, and back pain is often associated, usually in the lumbosacral region and usually constant rather than intermittent like the crampy abdominal pain. There have also been some cases of mesenteric venous thrombosis associated with back pain for which no easy explanation has been found.

PERITONEAL IRRITATION. Interference with venous drainage of the bowel regularly precedes interference with arterial supply, the pres-

FIG. 226. Visible and palpable coils of bowel in chronic parital small bowel obstruction. These become apparent because of hypertrophy of the intestinal wall and starvation atrophy of the abdominal wall. They are usually not nearly as obvious as shown, and can best be seen by inspection with the patient supine and daylight coming from the opposite side of the patient from the observer. (From Wangensteen, *Intestinal Obstructions*. Charles C Thomas, Springfield.)

sure required to compress the veins being much the lower. Edema, engorgement, and finally hemorrhage into the lumen, into the bowel wall, and through the serosa appear before true gangrene takes place. Local tenderness is usually found in external strangulated hernias, and signs of peritoneal irritation (increased tenderness, spasm, and rebound tenderness) in internal strangulations.

FEVER AND LEUKOCYTOSIS. Impending frank gangrene, as would be expected, is accompanied by rising temperature or leukocytosis, or both.

PELVIC EXAMINATION. Experience with strangulation obstruction as a late aftermath of pelvic surgery has drawn attention to the occasional case in which the diagnosis can be made by combined pelvic and rectal examination, in which fixed or heavy, boggy loops of bowel can be palpated between the examining fingers.

SHOCK. In case more than one-fourth to one-third of the small bowel is involved, the actual blood and plasma loss from the circulating blood volume may cause the blood pressure drop and pulse rise of surgical shock.

ROENTGEN FINDINGS. L. G. Rigler has called attention to the importance of roentgen diagnosis of strangulation obstruction. In cases in which the bowel is involved in simple obstruction, the gas-filled loops are usually free to rise somewhat toward the diaphragm on assumption of the erect position. When strangulation is present, this ordinarily does not occur, and the gas-filled loops occupy identical positions on upright and recumbent films (see Fig. 225). For this reason, it is routine to take films in both positions in obstruction cases.

Further radiologic evidence of obstruction complicated by strangulation is the double coffee-bean appearance of the negative gas shadow of the strangulated loop so often seen in cases due to adhesive bands.

The Items in Diagnosis of Intestinal Obstruction. For purposes of emphasis, the cardinal findings may be grouped concisely.

Simple small bowel obstruction presents:

1. Crampy abdominal pain (3 to 10 min.) ⎤ These may be ab-
2. Borborygmi with cramps ⎦ sent very late
3. Vomiting
4. Roentgen findings—typical in most instances
5. Distention—not marked in high obstruction
6. Obstipation
7. Chemical imbalance—most marked in high obstruction.

Strangulation obstruction presents one or more of the following features in addition to the findings of simple obstruction:

1. Sudden onset
2. Back pain
3. Signs of peritoneal irritation—or local tenderness or local heat over an external hernia
4. Shock
5. Fever or leukocytosis, or both
6. Palpable soggy loops on combined pelvic and rectal examination
7. Typical roentgen findings
8. Presence of an incarcerated hernia.

Causes of Death in Intestinal Obstruction. The causes of death may be listed under three headings:

1. Strangulation
2. Chemical imbalance
3. Prolonged distention.

Strangulation in cases other than external hernia and intussusception regularly leads, in the absence of spontaneous or surgical relief, to peritonitis and death. In external hernia and intussusception, the segment which becomes gangrenous is walled off from the peritoneal cavity, in the one instance by the hernial sac and in the other by the ensheathing intussuscipiens, and drainage may spontaneously occur to the outside through the sac wall in the one or into the lumen of the bowel below the point of in-tussusception in the other.

Gross perforation occurs occasionally in experimental simple obstruction low in the ileum in dogs, commonly in colic obstructions seen in man (in whom the usually competent ileocecal valve creates a "closed loop" mecha-nism), and regularly in experimental low ileac *closed loops* in dogs. In man, however, gross perforation very rarely occurs in simple ileac obstruction, the patient dying first of other complications of prolonged distention.

An additional mechanism of death from strangulation is shock from blood loss when more than one-fourth to one-third of the small intestine is involved. This is particularly prone to occur in large hernias and in obstructions due to adhesive bands.

As has already been indicated, high small bowel obstruction leads quickly to lethal changes in water and salt metabolism. In obstructions farther down the ileum, however, these changes are overshadowed by the effects of pro-longed distention on the bowel. Studies on these effects were initiated by Whipple, Stone, and Bernheim in 1913 by means of the closed intestinal loop, and it is by the use of such blind segments that the bulk of informa-tion has been gathered. In an exhaustive study and review of the reasons for death from prolonged distention, Wangensteen concludes that venous absorp-tion of toxic materials from the lumen is diminished by increased intra-luminal pressure and that lymphatic absorption of such materials cannot be conclusively demonstrated. He notes that clinically transperitoneal absorp-tion does not occur, and the patients remain in good condition, until viability of the bowel wall has been lost in isolated areas due to stretching and com-pression of blood vessels in that wall. "The results of this experimental in-quiry are wholly in accord with those clinical observations and indicate that the chief lethal factor in simple obstruction is permeation of a gut wall whose viability has become impaired, by bacteria and other deadly agents." *

Therapy in Small Bowel Obstruction. The primary decision to be made in any case of small bowel obstruction is whether it is simple or strangu-lating. Since the development of methods of operative management of gross distention, our fear of operative intervention has lessened sharply, and ap-pearance of any one of the evidences of strangulation listed above is con-sidered adequate indication for immediate exploration.

CONSERVATIVE THERAPY. *Indications for Conservative Therapy.* The general policy at the University of Minnesota Hospitals is to treat those cases of small bowel obstruction which appear simple by nasal suction siphonage without operative intervention. In certain cases it is apparent that strangula-tion is likely to occur. Such are the external hernias, gallstone obstructions, intussusceptions, and mesenteric venous thromboses. These cases it is possible to diagnose definitively with a fair degree of accuracy upon first examination of the patient. With these cases excluded from consideration, one must have absence of any of the signs of strangulation to permit assumption that he is

* Wangensteen, O. H., *Intestinal Obstructions*, 2nd ed., 2nd printing, C. C Thomas, Springfield, Ill., 1945.

dealing with simple adhesive neoplastic obstruction rather than band obstruction, volvulus, or internal hernia. Even this early assumption often proves to be incorrect, and some signs of strangulation appear later to dictate operative intervention.

Because of this last possibility, it is not wise to embark in any case upon conservative management of small bowel obstruction unless careful reappraisal of the patient is to be performed every four to five hours; this includes abdominal and pelvic examination, temperature, blood pressure and pulse determinations, and inquiry as to the presence of back pain. Leukocyte counts twice daily and films daily are of great aid. It is by the omission of these precautions that most of the grief attributed to conservative management has been called down upon the heads of inattentive surgeons.

Hydration and Nutrition. The obstructed patient shows greater or less dehydration, depending on the level of the lesion. Reasonable evaluation of the degree is possible through hematocrit determinations. Chemical status can best be established by determinations of plasma protein level, plasma chloride level, blood urea nitrogen, and carbon dioxide combining power. In general, the patient showing clinical dehydration may be assumed to have lost 5 to 7 per cent of his body weight, and the amount of water administered intravenously in the first 24 hours should be about 7 per cent of his body weight. This infusion should be given at a rate not exceeding 400 cc. an hour and preferably is spread over the full 24 hours to minimize the danger of pulmonary edema. Hypochloremia can be corrected according to Coller's rule—namely that the number of grams of NaCl to be administered to restore the normal plasma chloride level is:

$$\frac{560 - \text{Plasma chloride (as mg.\% NaCl)}}{200} \times \text{Body wt (Kg.)}$$

A somewhat smaller amount is usually sufficient. Until the plasma chloride level has been reported, hydration can be nicely initiated by starting intravenous infusion of a mixture of equal parts of 5 per cent dextrose in distilled water and 0.9 per cent NaCl solution. In most instances hydration and chlorination can be completed with this mixture.

In cases handled in conservative fashion, the surgeon is never certain that need for surgical intervention will not arise on short notice. He therefore is well advised to try to maintain an adequate parenteral intake not only of fluid and salt, but also of vitamins, calories, and proteins. Once dehydration has been overcome by use of isotonic solutions, it has been found easily practicable to maintain a daily intake of 1800 calories by almost continuous intravenous infusion of a 15 per cent solution of dextrose in distilled water (3 liters) to which 5 grams of NaCl, thiamine, cevitamic acid, and crude liver extract have been added. The system may then be washed out with 0.9 per cent NaCl solution, and the infusion completed with 200 cc. of plasma or 500 cc. of blood, or more if the protein level has been found low. This infusion runs not faster than 4 cc. a minute. In order that long infusions may be tolerated, the needle must be placed well away from the elbow and wrist joints, preferably on the back of the forearm, permitting free use of the arm throughout.

Intubation of the Intestine. Wangensteen first showed that simple obstruction could be managed by nonoperative decompression using an indwelling duodenal tube and siphon suction apparatus. With the advent of the Miller-Abbott tube, however, we have adopted it as standard equipment for this type of case. The chief difficulty in use of the Miller-Abbott or any

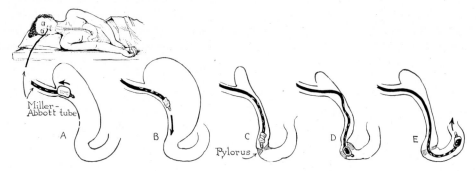

FIG. 227. Miller-Abbott intubation of the small intestine. (A) After emptying the stomach, the balloon is inflated, and the tube withdrawn until traction with deep respiration indicates it is at the cardia. The patient is placed slightly forward on his right side. (B) The balloon is emptied, and the stomach inflated with 4-500 cc. of air to hold the walls apart so the tube will slide easily to the pylorus on gradual advancement 15-18 cm. in 15 minutes. (C) The air in the stomach is removed to prevent the tube from kinking in the stomach and another 5-6 cm. is inserted. (D) Sudden, rapid injection of 2½ cc. of mercury into the balloon usually initiates pyloric contractions which carry the tube well into the duodenum. (E) The tube is advanced 6-8 cm. past the point where bile is first aspirated. Here, if a *dry* Luer syringe is held vertically, injection of 6-10 cc. of air into the balloon will indicate rhythmic contractions by motion of the syringe plunger. Ten to fifteen cc. of air may be placed in the balloon while it is advanced another 10 cm., and then the balloon may be inflated with 30-40 cc. of air. As supplied new, the balloons are too long, and the tube works more satisfactorily if a new smaller one is placed. (Method modified from Hamrick.)

other type of tube is that of passing it into the small intestine from the stomach. One method, which represents an adaptation of one described by Hamrick, is indicated in figure 227. It has the decided advantage that about two-thirds of the time it is successful in bed in these cases without need for the fluoroscope or the x-ray. When difficulty is encountered, the same procedure may be repeated under fluoroscopic control, perhaps combined with attempts to massage the tip into the pylorus.

In the great majority of cases, passage of the tube is accomplished by one method or another in the first 48 hours. It should be recalled that a portion of cases relent and recover with intragastric suction alone (Dennis and Brown).

In some cases the intestinal content is too thick and viscid to traverse the Miller-Abbott tube; here placement of the Wangensteen tube into the duodenum is worth a thorough two day trial before adopting other measures.

Dr. John Wild, a resident on the Surgery Service at the University of Minnesota Hospitals, has been experimenting with a variety of types of tube for easier intubation of the pylorus and more effective evacuation of the intestine. He has found tubes of polyvinyl chloride to be far less irritating than rubber and to offer less resistance to aspiration of bowel content. A loose bag of mercury attached by one end only to the very tip of the tube in addition to the usual balloon facilitates passage into the duodenum.

Fine and associates have demonstrated that respiration of high concentrations of oxygen aids in diminishing the gaseous distention in cases of intestinal obstruction. The method has proved of aid in some cases here, but suction is a much more direct approach to the problem of distention, and oxygen is used only occasionally as an additional measure in those cases in which suction alone has proved not quite adequate.

Relenting. Simple adhesive obstruction is the only type which may be expected to relent following conservative decompressive measures. This ordinarily occurs within two to four days after complete decompression, and delay beyond this limit is considered here an indication for operative intervention. The appearance of gas in the colon, as recognized by roentgen film, or the passage of gas by rectum, indicates that the obstructive mechanism has relented. It is customary here to allow the tube to remain in place an additional day or two and to check the tolerance of the patient to cessation of suction for one-half day before withdrawal of the tube.

Management After Withdrawal of the Tube. Mineral oil is given liberally during the next few days in conjunction with a low-residue diet, being guided in the amounts of both by the presence or absence of symptoms of partial obstruction.

In those cases in which obstruction has been an early aftermath of inflammatory processes such as ruptured appendix, it is usual that complete and permanent resolution of the obstructive process occurs. In those cases in which adhesions have caused obstruction long after subsidence of inflammatory or healing processes, it is usual that oil and dietary caution are needed for indefinite periods, and even then some cases require repeated decompression. In general, it is best to explore the abdomen in those cases suffering more than two separate obstructive attacks requiring intubation.

OPERATIVE THERAPY. *Indications.* The indications for surgical intervention in small bowel obstruction are:

(1) Strangulation—potential or suspected.
(2) Failure of decompression—either failure to intubate the intestine, or failure to decompress after intubation has been accomplished, or by gastric suction alone.
(3) Failure of the obstruction to relent on decompression.
(4) Repeated attacks of obstruction requiring intubation.

In dealing with strangulation as an indication for surgery, external hernia with obstruction, intussusception, gallstone obstruction, and mesenteric occlusion are regularly treated operatively without delay even though none of the signs or symptoms of strangulation may yet have appeared.

Appearance of any of these signs or symptoms in obstruction from other cause is a positive indication for immediate surgery.

Hydration and Nutrition. Hydration in the case admitted with definite signs of strangulation must be done expeditiously. Patients with frank dehydration do not tolerate anesthesia or surgery at all well, and, even though frank gangrene might conceivably develop in this period, it is sound practice to delay operation three hours during which a fair share of the fluid calculated as described under "Conservative therapy" may be given. The nature of the process necessitates more rapid administration here than in the simple obstructions.

Hydration may be completed during the operative procedure and postoperatively, and such transfusions may be given as are estimated adequate to replace blood and plasma loss and to maintain normal blood pressure and pulse values.

General Considerations. For repair of incarcerated or strangulating hernias in poorly prepared patients, more satisfactory and safe anesthesia may be obtained by novocaine block than by either spinal or general methods. In other instances the policy at the University Hospitals is to use a mixture of pentothal and curare intravenously, supplemented by 50 per cent nitrous oxide in oxygen, given by an intratracheal tube (Baird). The mixture used contains 25 mgm. of pentothal and 5 units of d-tubocurarine per cc. The safety of this method and the lack of unpleasant impressions on the patients have so impressed the staff that nearly all cases requiring general anesthesia are now handled in this way in both the University and the Minneapolis General Hospitals.

Placement of a No. 17 or No. 15 needle for intravenous infusion into the antecubital vein offers a large degree of security, especially if cross-matched blood is present in the operating room.

Aside from hernioplasties, most emergency operations for intestinal obstruction are exploratory, in that the site of the block in the abdomen is unknown. Longitudinal incisions are, therefore, to be preferred, as they provide wider possibilities of extension and exploration. The right midrectus is very satisfactory. Closure of the abdominal wall is most safely made with interrupted fine silk sutures of 3 or 4 pound tensile strength. Most of these patients may then safely be ambulatory the day after surgery, a measure which seems to have simplified the postoperative course immensely.

Wangensteen nasal suction tubes are placed in the stomach prior to surgery unless the case has been treated conservatively long enough already to have a Miller-Abbott tube down. Suction is maintained throughout the sojourn in the operating room and postoperatively until sounds are normal and gas is passed by rectum. This usually occurs two to three days after surgery. Nutrition by the intravenous route is continued as already indicated in these cases until oral feedings are possible.

Wangensteen Aseptic Decompression. Prior to the introduction of the conservative treatment of small bowel obstruction by Wangensteen, it was general practice to explore all cases. With the advent of nonoperative methods, most surgeons have adopted a more conservative attitude and have refrained from intervention wherever justified. This policy has been supported by three considerations: (1) Many patients have obstruction because

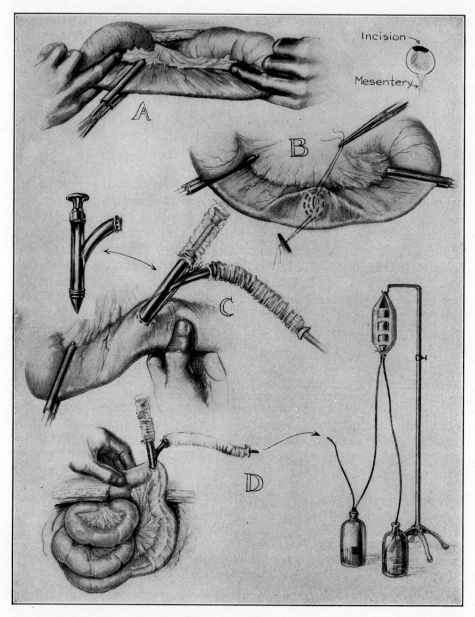

FIG. 228 A, B, C, D

they form adhesions more readily than others. Surgical intervention is then prone to be followed by reformation of many more adhesions than were there in the first place with redevelopment of obstruction, as Boys has shown experimentally. (2) The risk of manipulative perforation in the handling of hugely distended loops of bowel, and the difficulty of closure of the abdomen in the presence of that distention are dismaying considerations. (3) The knowledge that a large share of these patients would recover without operation is also discouraging to surgical intervention.

In the last few years, McKittrick has championed the policy of imme-

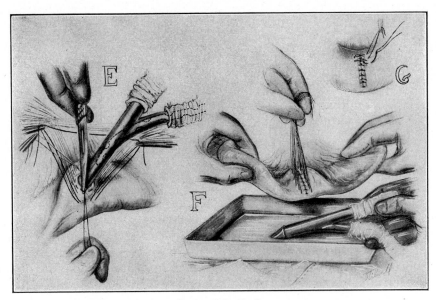

FIG. 228 E, F, G

FIG. 228. Modified Wangensteen aseptic decompressive suction enterotomy. (A) Method of emptying a distended segment of small bowel preparatory to enterotomy. The segment so emptied between the fingers should be 25-30 cm. long. Application of the rubber-shod Scudder clamps should be as light as possible, as more troubles with adhesions arise from this site than from suture lines. (B) Placement of a double purse string to secure the bowel to the trocar. Atraumatic oo catgut is used. After placement of the purse strings, a 1-cm. incision in the center exposes the intact mucosa so that easy perforation will be possible with the plunger point. (C) Securing of trocar. As an added precaution against leakage, the ends of the double purse string are tied over the side arm of the trocar. Following perforation of the mucosa, the plunger is withdrawn and the catheter is slipped into the bowel. Soiling is prevented by protection of both the plunger shaft and the catheter by soft rubber drains, lubricated with glycerine. (D) Suction decompression. Very gentle lifting of the segments of bowel will direct content to the catheter. The entire small bowel can be delivered and emptied by this means, particularly if a three-foot catheter is employed. (E) Clean removal of the trocar. A transverse row of interrupted Lembert sutures is preplaced and held up with hemostats in such manner as to support the bowel. The catheter is withdrawn into the trocar, but suction is maintained. A No. 11 Bard-Parker blade cuts the 2 purse strings, and the trocar and attachments are placed cleanly into a large basin placed for the purpose immediately beside the bowel. (F) Closure of the defect. Traction on the ends of the preplaced Lembert sutures apposes the serosa without soiling. (G) Completion of closure. Closure is reinforced by a second row of silk—Halsted mattress sutures. 30 mg. of sulfanilamide powder may be implanted between the rows. The closure process may be eliminated altogether in strangulation if a segment is employed close enough to the necrotic bowel to permit block excision of the entire area—with immediate anastomosis. (Modified from Wangensteen, *Intestinal Obstruction.* C. C. Thomas, Springfield.)

diate exploration before distention is a factor in all cases seen within 24 hours of the onset, and has a remarkable record of consecutive cases without mortality, but the fear of late adhesion formation and the likelihood of recovery of many without that surgery are valid objections to the policy.

Wangensteen has described a method of aseptic decompressive enterotomy for dealing with marked ileac distention which permits safe exploration where indicated regardless of that distention. The author has used the method with slight modifications in some 18 cases, without mortality attributable to the procedure. In many it would have been utterly impossible to deal successfully with the obstructive mechanism if preliminary decompression of the fragile, thin-walled bowel had not first been accomplished. The safety of intervention has thus been much enhanced.

Use of Wangensteen's aseptic suction enterotomy, as modified in this series of cases, may be performed with the set supplied by V. Mueller and Company or with equipment to be found in any well supplied operating room (Fig. 228). The essentials consist of an ordinary empyema trocar, a soft rubber catheter large enough just to pass through the trocar, a long piece of Penrose drain, connecting tubing, a Wangensteen suction set, and sterile glycerine. Secure ridges for provision of anchorage of the bowel to the trocar may be formed by sliding 2 or 3 millimeter segments of heavy snug-fitting rubber tubing onto the end of the trocar before autoclaving. The heat of sterilizing seals them securely. As indicated in figure 228, a piece of Penrose drain is tied on the sidearm of the trocar and covers the entire external length of the catheter, being tied securely over a glass connector in the back end of the catheter. A half-ounce of glycerine inside the soft rubber drain serves as lubricant. A second piece of Penrose drain is tied around the handle of the plunger of the trocar to avoid leakage from that source. A long segment of tubing connects the catheter to a Wangensteen suction set. About 12 holes, each 3 millimeters in diameter, are cut in the last 6 centimeters of the catheter.

In using the apparatus, the most distended free segment is delivered cautiously and milked empty between the second and third fingers of the two hands of the surgeon, and Scudder clamps are very gently applied to keep that segment empty. This maneuver allows contraction of the muscle layers and consequent thickening of the bowel wall so that a firm bite may be obtained for sutures without the danger of leakage through the paper-thin walls present before emptying. A purse string of No. oo catgut on an atraumatic needle is laid, the purse string being 15 to 20 mm. in diameter. A second purse string laid 3 millimeters wide of the first is extremely effective in eliminating leakage later. A transverse incision 1 centimeter long down to the mucosa is made in the center of the purse strings, and the end of the trocar is secured to the bowel by tight tying of the catgut strands. Greater security is afforded by tying each end over the sidearm of the trocar.

Suction is first applied, and then the plunger of the trocar is used to perforate the mucosa and then drawn back. The catheter can now be inserted into the bowel, and the Scudder clamps removed.

By very gentle threading of the catheter through the bowel in both directions and by gentle elevation of the fluid-filled loops to lead fluid to the catheter, it is now practicable to empty the entire small bowel above the site of obstruction.

Direction of attention to the obstructing mechanism is in order only after rather complete ileac evacuation. The danger of accidental tearing of the bowel wall is then minimized, and spillage in event of accident is minimal.

In some instances it will be found that strangulation has rendered a segment nonviable. In such cases it simplifies the procedure to have placed the trocar close to this area, enabling the surgeon to resect both the gangrenous bowel and the trocar site in one segment. This is usually accomplished by selection of the most distended loop, likely the lowest one, for decompression.

If simple obstruction is found and relieved without resection, closure of the decompression site must be accomplished. To do this cleanly, an effective procedure is to preplace six to eight Lembert stitches in a transverse row in such fashion that tying after removal of the trocar will invert all the bowel involved in the purse strings and one-half centimeter more on each side. After preplacement of the sutures, the catheter is withdrawn into the trocar, and the suction left in force. By traction on the catgut ties previously brought over the sidearm, each purse string can be visualized and divided with a No. 11 Bard-Parker knife blade. A discard basin held immediately adjacent to the bowel receives the trocar, etc., with minimal chance for contamination. The Lembert sutures are tied, and the closure reinforced with a layer of Halsted mattress sutures.

The rather extensive inversion of tissue which occurs does not occlude the lumen because of the marked stretching of the bowel produced by preoperative distention. In no instance has clinical obstruction in the postoperative period been recognized. On a few occasions laparotomy for other lesions at a later time has made possible reexamination of this area. Except for the presence of sutures, it is usually very difficult to differentiate this segment from others in the small intestine.

Exploration and Lysis. In cases seen very early, as McKittrick stresses, in certain cases failing to relent after partial decompression, and in the early strangulating cases, simple division of adhesive bands, or of adhesions of the involved segment to other viscera or the parietes, is sufficient to cure the patient. In case the degree of distention is moderate and the mechanism can be easily seen without fear of accident, there is no indication for any procedure in addition to the lysis needed for relief of obstruction. Obviously, results of this relatively simple operative procedure are excellent; too often, indeed, the obstruction has advanced far beyond this degree by the time the patient is first seen.

Greater degrees of distention found on laparotomy necessarily demand aseptic decompression before search for such mechanisms of obstruction.

Resection of Gangrenous Bowel. Experience at the University Hospitals has shown that resection with primary end-to-end anastomosis is a practicable and safe method of dealing with small bowel obstruction in which nonviable intestine is found. The anastomosis recommended is a modification of that of Martzloff and Burget. One of the chief difficulties which this procedure is designed to overcome is the end-to-end union of segments of

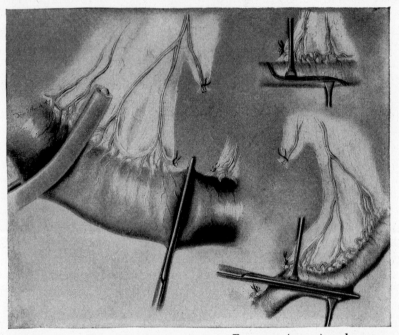

FIG. 229   FIGS. 230 (upper) and 230a

FIG. 229. Placement of the first anastomosis clamp on the distended bowel above the point of obstruction. The clamp crosses the bowel at an angle of 75 degrees and at the mesenteric border about 6 mm. from the edge of the unremoved mesentery. The bowel has been milked back and a rubber-shod clamp is applied to prevent spillage. (From Dennis, *Surg., Gynec. & Obst.*, 77:225, 1943. By permission of Surgery, Gynecology and Obstetrics.)

FIG. 230. Placement of the second anastomosis clamp on the contracted bowel below the point of obstruction. The line of crush begins 6 mm. from the unremoved mesentery, crosses obliquely 2/3 of the bowel and passes for a distance parallel with the antimesenteric border before crossing the remaining 1/3 of the bowel. (a) This length of crushed tissue, equal to that in figure 229, is obtained by distorting the bowel with Allis forceps. This clamp is placed from the mesenteric border. (From Dennis, *Surg., Gynec. & Obst.*, 77:225, 1943. By permission of Surgery, Gynecology and Obstetrics.)

widely differing diameter without the formation of blind pockets or kinks.

The mesentery is meticulously cleaned from the distended bowel proximal to the point of obstruction, a site close to the point of approach of large vessels in that mesentery being chosen (Fig. 229). A slender, crushing, anastomosis clamp is placed across the bowel, from the antimesenteric border, at an angle of about 75 degrees from the long axis of the gut. The clamp crosses the mesenteric border about 6 millimeters below the edge of the unremoved mesentery.

In order to minimize the danger of spillage of any of the content of the distended bowel during the later stages of the procedure, the contents are cautiously milked back between the fingers for 10 or 20 centimeters from the clamp, and a rubber-shod intestinal clamp is lightly applied. This clamp remains in place until the completion of the anastomosis.

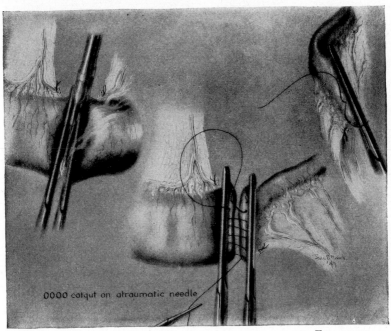

0000 catgut on atraumatic needle

| Fig. 231 | Fig. 232 | Fig. 232a |

FIG. 231. Cutting the bowel between the clamps described in figures 229 and 230 with the cautery. To prevent spillage, additional clamps are placed between those applied for anastomosis and the specimen to be removed. (From Dennis, *Surg., Gynec. & Obst.,* 77:225, 1943. By permission of Surgery, Gynecology and Obstetrics.)

FIG. 232. Placement of the posterior running fine catgut suture. The clamps are held side-by-side, so that the bowel ends are brought together with 180 degrees' rotation of one with respect to the other. The suture is laid with the clamps rolled away from each other as shown. The bites are 5 mm. long and the gaps between bites are 4 mm. (a) Placement of each end bite parallel with the long axis of the gut assures good inversion later. This suture is left loose until removal of the clamps as shown in figure 234. For very edematous bowel, oo or ooo atraumatic catgut is safer. (From Dennis,. *Surg., Gynec. & Obst.,* 77:225, 1943. By permission of Surgery, Gynecology and Obstetrics.)

Below the point of obstruction, the diameter of the bowel is usually one-third to one-half that above, and the anastomosis clamp must therefore be placed much more obliquely to attain a length of crushed tissue equal to that above. Most satisfactory stomas have been achieved by the application of the clamp from the mesenteric border with distortion of the bowel by Allis forceps lightly applied in such fashion that the line of crush, beginning at the mesenteric border, crosses obliquely two-thirds of the way to the antimesenteric border, then runs longitudinally down the bowel to gain the necessary length of crush before it crosses the remainder of the gut (Fig. 230 and 230a). The cleaning of the mesentery and the placement of the clamp with regard to the cleaned area are accomplished as on the distended intestine.*

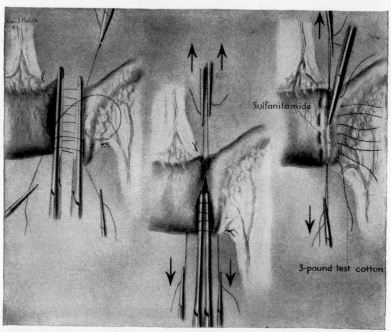

FIG. 233   FIG. 234   FIG. 235

FIG. 233. Placement of the anterior running catgut suture. The clamps have been rolled together. (From Dennis, *Surg., Gynec. & Obst.*, 77:225, 1943. By permission of Surgery, Gynecology and Obstetrics.)

FIG. 234. Removal of clamps. Tension is applied to the two ends of each of the running sutures, the clamps are carefully loosened until the tips are spread 1 or 2 mm., and the clamps are cautiously removed. (From Dennis, *Surg., Gynec. & Obst.*, 77:225, 1943. By permission of Surgery, Gynecology and Obstetrics.)

FIG. 235. Reinforcement of the suture line. The ends of the posterior running stitch have been tied to the corresponding ends of the anterior strand, and tension has been maintained during placement of Halsted mattress sutures of 2½-pound silk. With the latter placed, but not tied, sulfanilamide may be applied in small amounts between the serosal surfaces to be approximated by them. (From Dennis, *Surg., Gynec. & Obst.*, 77:225, 1943. By permission of Surgery, Gynecology and Obstetrics.)

A similar clamp is placed between the bowel to be resected and each of the clamps already described, a 3 or 4 millimeter gap usually being left

* The value of this type of placement is not limited to anastomoses performed in the presence of obstruction. In the terminal ileum under normal conditions the lumen is small enough to render anastomosis without undue reduction of the lumen difficult. This type of placement of clamps with 180 degrees' rotation has proved uniformly successful under these circumstances. In other sites where bowel ends of unequal diameter are to be joined, such as in end-to-end ileocolostomy after right hemicolectomy, this type of anastomosis has also proved uniformly successful.

between clamps. The intestine is cut in the gap between each of these pairs of clamps with the actual cautery (Fig. 231).

The anastomosis clamps are laid side-by-side, thus bringing the bowel ends together with one end rotated 180 degrees with respect to the other about the long axis of the gut (Fig. 232). Ideally the length of the area of crush in the two clamps is identical, for by this precaution the most accurate

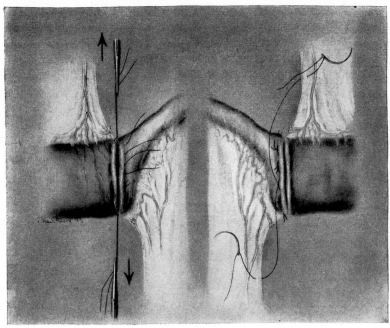

FIG. 236   FIG. 237

FIG. 236. Tying of the Halsted mattress sutures, with maintenance of tension on catgut strands. The posterior side is treated in similar fashion. (From Dennis, *Surg., Gynec. & Obst.*, 77:225, 1943. By permission of Surgery, Gynecology and Obstetrics.)

FIG. 237. Rear view of anastomosis, showing placement of stitch to close the mesenteric defect. (From Dennis, *Surg., Gynec. & Obst.*, 77:225, 1943. By permission of Surgery, Gynecology and Obstetrics.)

apposition of the two ends can be attained in making the anastomosis. The clamps are rotated away from each other, and a running basting stitch of No. oo or No. ooo plain catgut on an atraumatic needle is placed posteriorly, about 5 millimeters being taken in each bite, with a slightly smaller gap (4 mm.) being left between bites. Subsequent inversion occurs spontaneously at the time of withdrawal of the clamps only if the ends of the running sutures are properly placed; inversion of the corners with instruments, which invites contamination, may thus be avoided. Each end bite of each suture must be about 5 or 6 millimeters long and parallel with the axis of the bowel and should emerge close to the clamp (Fig. 232a).

The anastomosis clamps are now rolled together, and a similar running stitch is placed anteriorly (Fig. 233).

Tension is applied to the two ends of each of the basting sutures, the clamps are carefully loosened until the tips are spread 1 or 2 millimeters, and the clamps are cautiously and simultaneously withdrawn (Fig. 234). If the sutures have been properly placed, inversion of the cut ends of intestine will occur with no further manipulation, and clean serosal approximation will result. Tension is maintained on the basting stitches while the ends of the posterior strand are tied to the corresponding ends of the anterior strand.

With maintenance of tension on the ends of the basting stitches throughout, interrupted Halsted mattress sutures of 2½ pound test silk* are laid anteriorly, 20 or 30 milligrams of sulfanilamide (or sulfathiazole) may be implanted on the serosa between the rows of sutures if desired (Fig. 235), and the mattress sutures are tied just tightly enough for snug apposition (Fig. 236). The bowel is rolled over, and the posterior closure is similarly reinforced, tension being continued to this point on the ends of the catgut strands. Tension on the basting sutures is gradually lessened as the stoma is broken down by inverting the bowel below the anastomosis with a thumb or two fingers and thus pushing through the stoma. The catgut basting stitch, which is circular by virtue of the knots at the ends of the suture line, is held taut by this device while inversion Halsted mattress sutures are placed at the ends. The catgut ends are cut, the silk sutures are tied, and the anastomosis thus completed. The catgut sutures may be removed at this point (see below).

To close the mesenteric defect, a stitch near the center of the posterior suture line is threaded on a needle and a small bite of each mesenteric edge is taken 3 centimeters from the bowel (Fig. 237), and behind it, and thus the defect in the mesentery is tied. From this point to the root of the mesentery, interrupted silk sutures are placed. Efforts to cover the suture line with omentum have been abandoned as useless. Sulfonamides have not been generally implanted into the peritoneal cavity because it has seemed that this procedure leads to excessive adhesion formation. More recently, local implantation has been abandoned altogether.

The clamps used in making this anastomosis differ from those of Martz-loff and Burget in that they are shorter and lighter.** With the shorter clamp one may rely less on the springiness of the instrument to crush the tissue at the tip, and the clamps may therefore be more easily removed during the anastomosis. Deep, sharp, longitudinal, matching grooves are cut on the jaws of the clamp.

The advantages of this type of anastomosis over many of those described in the literature are as follows:

(1) End-to-end anastomosis avoids the formation of the blind pouches which result from closure of both ends and side-to-side anastomosis.

(2) End-to-end anastomosis necessitates but one suture line, whereas closure of the ends and side-to-side anastomosis requires three lines.

(3) Aseptic procedure permits apposition of serosal surfaces uncontam-

---

* Cotton of similar strength was used in the experimental work.

** Clamps can be obtained from V. Mueller Company, Chicago.

inated with luminal contents, a point heavily supported by experimental work.

(4) Obliquity of placement of clamps permits the best possible blood supply to the line of suture, for the vessels follow a circular course around the bowel and are not, therefore, interfered with before reaching the suture line.

(5) Rotation of one segment of bowel with respect to the other minimizes angulation and therefore minimizes possibility of obstruction at the point of anastomosis, as shown in figure 238.

(6) Rotation of the bowel avoids the dangers of closure without peritoneum at the mesenteric border; in other words, by this rotation peritoneum is provided on one surface or the other completely around the line of inversion.*

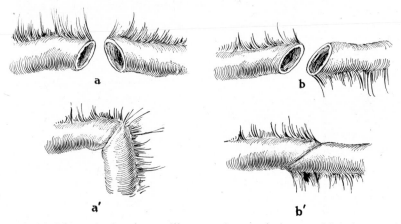

FIG. 238. (a) Schematic drawing to illustrate the angulation resulting from end-to-end anastomosis of bowel cut at 45 degrees and apposed without rotation. (b) The obviation of angulation accomplished by rotation of one segment with respect to the other is apparent. (From Dennis, *Surgery,* 5:548, 1939.)

(7) This type of anastomosis avoids the danger of stenosis at any time in the postoperative period. There has been no case of dysfunction secondary to the quarter twist imposed on each end to be anastomosed.

Use of this or the Martzloff-Burget anastomosis should not be attempted by those unfamiliar with intestinal suture until some experience has been gained in the dog. Difficulties may arise from improper placement of the catgut suture, tearing of the friable distended bowel by use of heavy instruments or too heavy sutures, and postoperative adhesion formation at the site of placement of the Scudder clamps. There is no need to resect bowel because it is distended or because it fails to contract on stimulation by snapping with the finger, or because it does not offer normal resistance to placing the needle. The greatest gentleness will be rewarded by absence of postoperative cramps or obstruction.

* In over 20 clinical cases and 60 experimental anastomoses, no instance of leakage at the ends of the suture line, *i.e.,* at the mesenteric border on one side, has occurred.

Our experience at the time of the first report comprised 16 resections with two deaths. At the present time there have been more than 40 cases, with one additional death. In only one case has a suture line leaked; here

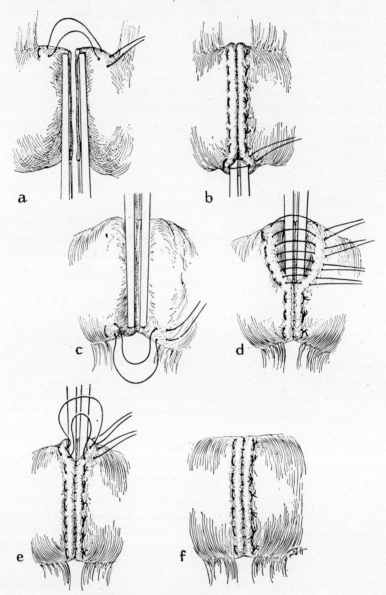

the serosa was contaminated with content on first exposure, and the silk sutures were placed too close to the catgut; a 2 or 3 millimeter space should separate them.

In the last 15 months, most anastomoses have been performed with a single layer of silk Halsted or Lembert sutures, and the method, as developed first for dealing with irreducible intussusceptions, is as follows.

Anastomosis clamps are placed somewhat obliquely and not quite completely across the prepared bowel about 1 cm. from the remaining edge of mesentery (Fig. 239). The bowel is cut across with cautery as above. Halsted or Lembert silk (2½ lb.-test) sutures are placed 7 mm. back from the cut edge of the intestine to be anastomosed (not from the clamp); they are placed first on the back side of the anastomosis and tied, closing the bowel over one blade of both anastomosis clamps. The clamps are then swung to the other side so the anterior wall of bowel can be similarly sutured and tied. Proper initial clamp placement permits closure over the tips of the clamps also. The entire suture line is now complete except at the point of exit of the clamps. Preplacement of the two sutures here permits completion of the anastomosis at once after careful removal of the clamps.

In case of wide variation in diameter of the ends to be sutured or somewhat narrow lumen, the clamps may be placed more obliquely and one end rotated, as in the oblique end-to-end anastomosis previously described. In case of difficulty in closing the bowel over both clamps, loosening or removal of the clamp from the distal or empty segment permits easy closure except at the point of exit of the remaining clamp. Because of danger of overinversion in intestine less than 2 cm. in diameter, it seems safer to use the previously described two-layer method with rotation, with withdrawal of the catgut layer after completion of the silk layer, if desired.

Adoption of the single-layer anastomosis was initially chosen because of the saving of time. It has been found, however, that omission of the catgut has shortened the period of postoperative ileus, and there is evidence that coverage of the point of apposition with mucosa is much more rapid also. Finally, this method is much less subject to accidental technical errors, with spillage, than the two-layer method.

This method has been used successfully in 19 cases, 5 with distention due to obstruction.

Catheter Enterostomy. Catheter enterostomy, of the type introduced by Wangensteen in 1933, is being employed progressively less frequently since the development of his aseptic decompression method; however, there still remain indications for the use of the method. It is employed, for example,

---

FIG. 239. Closed, one-layer, interrupted silk anastomosis. (a) Placement of first Halsted mattress sutures. Note that the clamps are placed not quite completely across the bowel. The point of exit of sutures closest to the modified Martzloff clamp is 7 mm. from the cut edge of the bowel. If the bowel is less than 2 cm. in diameter, either smaller clamps may be used, or the sutures may be placed immediately adjacent to the clamps and the clamps removed before tying the stitches, or, preferably, the two-layer, oblique, end-to-end anastomosis may be used, best with withdrawal of the inner catgut basting stitch after completion of the silk suture line. When the distance from the cut edge of the bowel to the stitches is more than one-third the length of tissue along the crushing clamps, real danger of obstruction is present. (b) Completion of back side of anastomosis, tying also over ends of clamps. (c) and (d) Front side of anastomosis. (e) Removal of clamps—delayed until all but two sutures have been tied. (f) Completion of anastomosis by tying last two sutures after removal of clamps. The total number of sutures for intestinal anastomosis has varied from 11 to 18. (From Dennis, *Ann. Surg.,* 126:788, [Nov.], 1947.)

when extensive adhesions and the fear of already present localized infection or frank pus are present. Here, in other words, is a situation in which decompression over a period of days or weeks is desired in which time it is hoped that conservative methods or subsequent surgery will result in resolu-

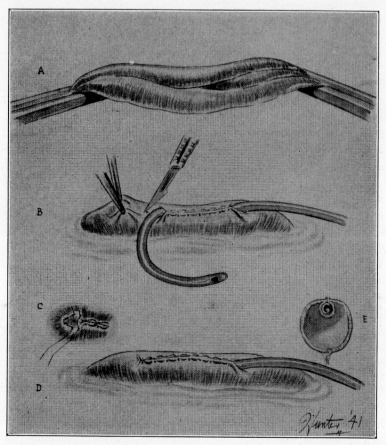

FIG. 240. Technic of catheter enterostomy. (a) Contraction of the bowel wall on relief of distention. (b) A No. 14 French catheter, preferably with several extra holes cut in the last 5 cm., is laid upon the bowel, and a few interrupted Halsted mattress sutures of 2½-pound silk are employed to make a tunnel around the catheter. The catheter is anchored to the end of this tunnel by a catgut stitch which is tied around it. The bowel is punctured in an elevated position to avoid spillage, and the tip of the catheter is inserted. (c) and (d) The inversion is completed over the catheter and puncture site. (e) The resulting peritoneal tunnel assures that fistula formation will not occur following withdrawal of the catheter. (From Wangensteen, *Intestinal Obstructions.* C. C Thomas, Springfield.)

tion of the obstructive process, or in which the conditions found dictate the simplest procedure possible.

At one time, catheter enterostomy was employed just above suture lines, as after removal of gallstones or after anastomoses. With acquisition of more confidence in suture lines, this practice has been abandoned.

In view of the limited applicability of the method, the choice of the loop to be used is narrow; the most distended available loop is employed, however. The segment is emptied as for aseptic decompressive enterotomy (Fig. 228a). A No. 14 or No. 16 soft French rubber catheter with a dozen holes in the last 5 centimeters is laid on the antimesenteric border of the collapsed bowel and buried by Halsted mattress sutures of 2½ pound-test silk (Fig. 240). A single stitch of catgut around, not through, the catheter and into the depth of the intestinal groove is placed to prevent slipping of the catheter. After 4 to 5 centimeters of closure of the gut wall around the catheter has been completed, a stab wound is made into the gut at the end of the furrow produced, and 8 to 10 centimeters of the tip of the catheter is inserted into the lumen, after which completion of the row of Halsted sutures closes the bowel over the site of passage of the catheter through the wall. The proximal end of the catheter is clamped before the Scudder clamps are removed; it is passed through a stab wound in the abdominal wall and the intestine on either side of the exit of the catheter and along the suture line is stitched with silk to the abdominal wall to seal it and prevent kinking of the catheter.

As Wangensteen points out, the advantage of this enterostomy procedure over others is that simple withdrawal of the tube, when it is no longer needed, is followed regularly by rapid spontaneous closure of the serosa-lined passage in the bowel wall.

Special Types of Obstruction. INTUSSUSCEPTION. Intussusception is not commonly found in persons over two years of age. It is more common in male than in female infants. In those cases in the older age group, there is usually some abnormality of the intestine which serves as the apex of the intussusceptum; such are lipomas of the bowel wall, polyps, Meckel's diverticulum, and hypertrophied Peyer's patches.

In the intussusceptions of infants, the process usually is initiated near the ileocecal valve. Four types may be delineated: (1) enteric, in which the intussusceptum and the ensheathing intussuscipiens are both ileum; (2) ileocolic, in which a progression of the enteric type is present, so that the apex passes for greater or less distances into the colon, but the appendix and cecum are not inverted; (3) ileocecal, in which the base of the cecum constitutes the apex of the intussusceptum; and (4) colic, entirely in the colon. By most reports, the ileocecal is commonest, ileocolic second, and enteric third (Wangensteen).

As peristaltic activity in the intussuscipiens carries the intussusceptum downward, compression of the mesentery to the latter segment causes early compression of the venous return. Engorgement, edema, hemorrhage, secretion of excessive mucus, closure of the lumen by swelling, and finally gangrene of the intussusceptum occur, the final result occurring in 24 to 48 hours.

Symptomatology in infants is almost constant. A previously healthy baby suddenly cries out as if in pain, vomits, and doubles up on the floor or bed usually into the knee-chest position. After apparent pain lasting one to three minutes, he again appears normal and resumes play. Thereafter, with regularity produced by the arrival of further peristaltic waves at the involved site, further attacks of pain occur. Vomiting initially is constant, but after 12 to 15 hours there may be a period of as long as 24 hours without more vomiting and with little pain. It is this period of decreased symptoms which is so likely to lull both parents and physician into dangerous delay. Within a few hours of onset of pain, blood and mucus are passed by rectum in the great majority of the three groups involving the colon, uncommonly in the enteric variety. In two-thirds to three-fourths of the cases involving the colon, a mass is palpable in the abdomen; in some cases it can only be felt on bimanual examination, the finger of one hand being inserted into the rectum while a nurse holds the baby upright; in the enteric type a mass is felt in a minority of cases. Fever is late, a point which aids in differentiation from enteritis.

Chronic intussusceptions are rare, and when seen are usually in the older age groups and due to some neoplasm or other anomaly of the bowel. Onset is said to be sudden and the course characterized by partial obstruction and wasting. In children it may be confused with enteritis or appendicitis.

Careful gathering of the history and evaluation with physical findings usually establish the diagnosis clearly. In those cases in which doubt remains, the diagnosis can be established with regularity in the colic, ileocolic, and ileocecal varieties by barium enema x-ray examination (Fig. 241). This method of diagnosis is exhausting to infants and should be avoided if possible in cases coming to operation. Gas in the small intestine is not a sign of obstruction, as it is normally present to the age of five to six years.

Therapy is the subject of considerable difference of opinion. Although most surgeons feel that surgical reduction is desirable, pediatricians and radiologists in the Minneapolis area have reduced many cases jointly by means of the barium enema under fluoroscopic control. The author's experience in his own family of three clinically typical intussusceptions having reduced spontaneously, before even such therapy could be instituted, attests to the ease with which early intussusceptions may be reduced. It seems perfectly feasible to reduce cases no older than 12 hours by means of cautious pressure with a barium enema under the fluoroscope, provided careful observation is maintained thereafter. Cases older than 12 hours are approaching the stage in which symptoms and signs subside even though the process persists; and in these operative reduction would seem safer.

Operative reduction is best performed under general anesthesia with intravenous fluids running, to which blood may be added if necessary. A low, 4 centimeter, right rectus incision is in order. The index and middle finger of the right hand of the surgeon may be inserted into the abdomen, and, by means of this and the left hand outside, the apex of the process can usually be gradually milked and compressed, even when found in the sigmoid region, around to the right colon. Due to the usual mobility of the right colon at this age, it can ordinarily be delivered without enlargement of the incision.

Reduction of the mass from this point may not go easily. Traction on the ileum against the ensheathing colon is to be avoided, lest the damaged bowel be torn at the point of entrance. If the whole mass is wrapped in large gauze

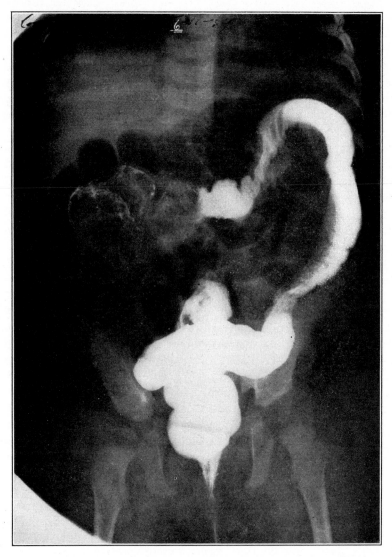

Fig. 241. Intussusception. Demonstration by barium enema roentgen examination is conclusive but exhausting to patients already sick. Coils of small intestine filling the right half of the transverse colon are beautifully outlined by the barium mixture. Gaseous small bowel distention in amount abnormal even for infants is also present.

packs wet with 0.9 per cent NaCl solution at body temperature, pressure may be exerted by the whole hand on the mass so as to reduce the edema present. This is best maintained four to five minutes. In our experience at Minnesota, the process can then usually be reduced, at least entirely past the ileocecal junction, by further gentle compression and milking from the hepatic flexure toward the junction.

Usually reduction is simple and complete as soon as the process has been driven out of the colon. In five cases, however, in our experience here in the last five and one-half years, the remaining enteric intussusception has been demonstrated at this stage to be frankly gangrenous. Exteriorization and secondary closure were employed in one, and resection and primary end-to-end closed anastomosis were employed in the others. All babies have recovered. Anastomosis is simpler at this site than might be imagined because the bowel above and below the gangrenous area has been dilated enough by the pathologic process to render the procedure much less minute than it would be in the normal bowel at this age.[8]

GALLSTONE OBSTRUCTION. Gallstone obstruction, as we have seen it at the University Hospitals, occurs from passage of a sufficiently large stone to block the intestine, through an abnormal communication between the biliary tract, usually the gallbladder, and the intestine, usually the duodenum. Exceptions have been reported, in which stones small enough to traverse the choledochus and ampulla have caused areas of spasm and therefore obstruction.

As Rigler and associates have shown, acute flare-ups of disease in the gallbladder or choledochus associated with presence of a large stone result, in some cases, in sealing of the involved viscus against the intestine, usually the duodenum; in a period of one to two days erosion of the walls permits passage of the stone into the intestine. In view of the progressive decrease in diameter of the ileum as the cecum is approached, large stones sooner or later become impacted. Gallstone obstructions of the sigmoid colon have been reported, but are very rare.

The history alone should establish the diagnosis in most cases. There is usually antecedent history of bouts of biliary colic, and the present bout ordinarily has been initiated in a manner identical to the previous ones, although it is likely more severe. After a day or two the right subcostal and back pain merge into intermittent generalized cramps, the previous pain persisting between peaks, and vomiting, often of much bile, becomes more persistent.

The obstruction caused by a gallstone usually is transient or intermittent. It relents for a few hours or a day or two, only to recur again as the stone becomes impacted at a lower level. Finally it becomes firmly impacted with continuing symptoms, this time usually of obstruction alone. There is danger of pressure erosion and gangrene of the wall against which the stone is impacted, and this is most safely considered therefore a potentially strangulating obstruction from the start.

Intestinal obstruction is recognized as due to a gallstone on the basis of two findings: (1) There is more abdominal tenderness than would be expected, especially in the right upper quadrant, and (2) Rigler's roentgen sign is regularly present. Rigler, Borman, and Noble pointed out that distention due to obstruction of the bowel leads regularly to filling of the biliary tract with air which can be visualized on plates taken in the upright position (Fig. 242). Presence of this finding with roentgen signs of bowel obstruction

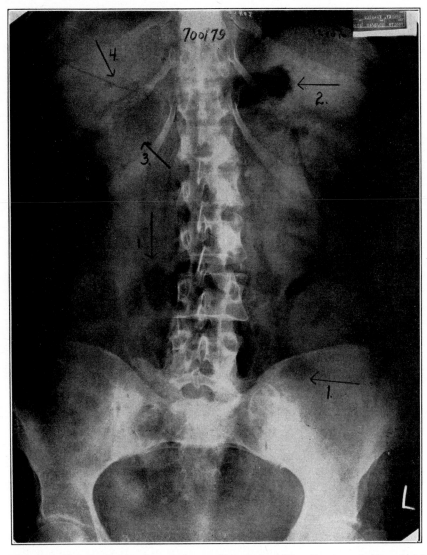

Fig. 242. Gallstone obstruction of the small intestine. Visualization of distended loops of small intestine (1) duodenum (3) and stomach (2) indicates small bowel obstruction; the presence of gas in the biliary ducts (4) indicates presence of an enteric biliary fistula. This combination of findings (Rigler's sign) is almost diagnostic of gallstone obstruction. The stone is only occasionally discernible in the small intestine by roentgen study. (From Rigler *et al., J.A.M.A.,* 117:1753, 1941.)

is almost pathognomonic of gallstone obstruction. Roentgen visualization of the stone is not ordinarily possible, but search for it by oblique films, etc., should be made if there is doubt. Barium ingestion makes beautiful pictures, but is not necessary; it incurs the added dangers of caking in the lumen and spillage of barium sulfate in subsequent surgery, which is poorly tolerated.

Surgical removal of the stone without delay is indicated. Delivery of the involved loop is made through a short rectus or a short transverse incision. The loop is milked empty and Scudder clamps are applied. If possible, the stone is dislodged upward 6 or 8 centimeters to permit employment of less traumatized tissues than are found over the stone; it is usually impossible to move it downward.

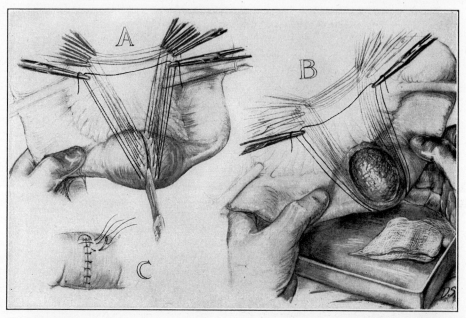

Fig. 243. Technic of removal of an obstructing gallstone. The segment containing the gallstone is delivered and emptied as in figure 228A. (A) After the stone has been dislodged upward a few centimeters, a transverse row of Lembert presection silk sutures is laid and a transverse incision made in the bowel now overlying the stone and between the two portions of each suture. (B) The sutures are held out of the way, and the stone is popped out by a finger behind the bowel, directly and cleanly into a basin. (C) Traction on the ends of the sutures closes the defect, and closure is reinforced with a row of Halsted mattress sutures, preferably with implantation of 20 to 30 milligrams of sulfanilamide between rows. (Modified from Wangensteen, *Intestinal Obstructions*. Charles C Thomas, Springfield.)

Even in cases in which the bowel wall has been apparently badly damaged, healing has been uniform. Presection Lembert sutures are laid as in removal of the decompression trocar, and a transverse incision over the stone permits evacuation of the stone from the otherwise empty gut directly into a basin (Fig. 243). Presence of facets on the stone should encourage search for more stones. A row of Halsted mattress sutures reinforces the presection layer, 30 to 40 mg. of sulfanilamide being placed on the serosa between layers, if desired. It is not necessary to invert all the tissue originally found stretched over the stone, nor is protective proximal catheter enterostomy needed or desirable. Recovery is the rule.

Subsequent care should include cholecystectomy and closure of the chole-cystenteric fistula.

EXTERNAL HERNIA WITH STRANGULATION. In hernias in which incarceration and obstruction are of less than five or six hours' duration and in which no signs of strangulation have yet appeared, the sac may be boldly opened and repair accomplished as in elective hernioplasty. In cases of longer duration, or in cases presenting signs of strangulation, particularly in femoral hernias, special precautions are in order to prevent contamination of the

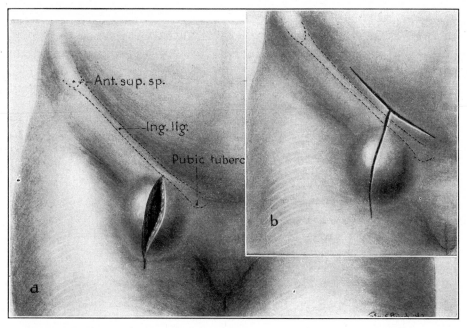

FIG. 244. Repair of femoral hernia with gangrenous bowel. Skin incision: (a) For recognition of gangrene, without opening sac. (b) Completion of incision after recognition of gangrene. (From Dennis and Varco, *Surgery*, 122:312, [Aug.], 1947.)

operative field. Here, in the femoral canal, a narrow, rigid, sharp margin surrounding the defect results in a high incidence of strangulation.

The stomach is emptied with a Wangensteen suction apparatus, and the patient is supplied with water and salt as needed. A catheter is placed in the bladder. Under local block anesthesia a vertical incision is made over the bulge in the groin and carried cautiously down to the peritoneum. The contents of the sac can be visualized through the wall, and bloody fluid, pus, feces or black bowel can usually be readily recognized.

If any of these indicates the presence of gangrenous bowel, dissection in this area is discontinued, and an incision is made 2 cm. above the inguinal ligament and parallel to it, and the vertical incision is continued upward to it to make a T-shaped incision (Fig. 244). The aponeurosis of the external oblique muscle is split parallel to the ligament and about 1 cm. above it, and extended into the external inguinal ring. The margins of the internal oblique and transversus muscles (and the cord if the patient is a male) are elevated, the deep epigastric vessels are divided and ligated, and the peritoneum is incised parallel to the oblique skin incision.

From this vantage point, the viscera entering the hernia may be easily seen. Omentum, if involved, is divided and ligated close to the neck. The small bowel entering the sac is prepared by division of the mesenteric attachment from the proximal to the distal side of the incarcerated loop of bowel. Because of the tension, it is best to ligate the vessels before division. Two Ochsner clamps are placed across each of these limbs of bowel, and the ileum is severed between each pair with the cautery.

The gangrenous sac contents having been freed from intra-abdominal attachments, the inguinal ligament is divided close to the pubic attachment and split laterally, leaving enough heavy aponeurotic tissue applied to the front of the neck of the sac to prevent relaxation of the neck and release of the soiled content. The sac is encased in a rather firm layer of fascia derived from the femoral canal. Dissection outside it frees the entire sac except for the residual fibrous portions of the ring, which can then be cut under direct vision from the surrounding tissues and left on the neck of the sac (Fig. 245). Palpation for an anomalous obturator artery adds safety. The entire contaminated area may be then removed intact, without soiling the remaining field.

The bowel ends remaining are anastomosed as already indicated. Closure of the peritoneal defect is easily accomplished because of the mobility of the peritoneum in this area. Closure is usually made by interrupted mattress sutures of 2-pound-test silk, thus approximating the margins of the defect resulting from excision of the sac in a vertical line and closing the original oblique peritoneal incision in a line parallel to the original opening. Repair of the hernial and surgical defect is simplified by application of the principles of the McVay-Harkins modification of the Lotheisen hernioplasty. The margins of the internal oblique and transverse muscles are sutured to Cooper's ligament as far laterally as the femoral vein and to the inguinal ligament lateral to that point. A McVay-Harkins relaxing incision may be made in the posterior layer of the anterior rectus sheath if the incision is needed to gain approximation without tension. The inguinal ligament is restored by interrupted sutures of 3-pound-test silk, approximating it as far medially as it will go, without undue tension, to the lacunar ligament and to Cooper's ligament. The aponeurosis of the external oblique muscle is finally approximated with interrupted silk sutures (over the cord in the male), thereby completing the hernial repair proper. Silk closure of the skin is used without drainage.

If no evidence of necrosis is apparent on first exposure of the sac, it is well to dissect the sac rather widely and to place moist packs about it before incision of the sac wall. In one case clean omentum overlay gangrenous bowel and dirty fluid in the sac. Use of this preliminary dissection permitted closure of the opening in the sac so that the operation could be completed essentially as described.

If no nonviable bowel is encountered, the sac may be widely opened, the hernia reduced by enlarging the neck medially, and repair done entirely from below.

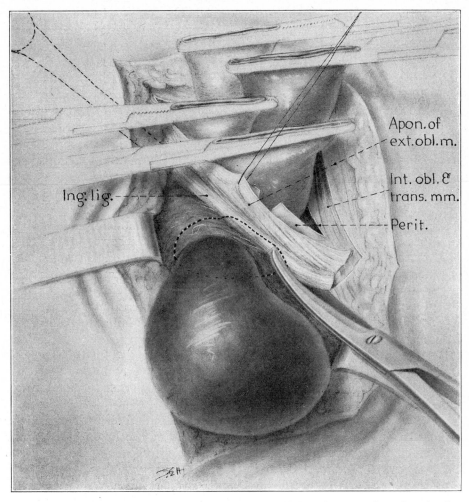

FIG. 245. Repair of femoral hernia with gangrenous bowel. Separation of neck of sac with retention of intact fibrous ring. (From Dennis and Varco, *Surgery*, 122:312, [Aug.], 1947.)

Fourteen femoral repairs have been done in the University of Minnesota Hospitals and in the Minneapolis General Hospital. There have been one superficial wound infection, and one recurrence of herniation. One patient in the latter group has died (ruptured aortic aneurysm 29 days after surgery). The safest procedures which have been reported to date (Gatch) involve external drainage of the sac and secondary repair of intestinal continuity, without repair of the hernial defect. The present method seems more direct, simpler, and safer.

MESENTERIC VASCULAR OCCLUSION. In the experience at the University Hospitals, mesenteric venous thrombosis without evident inciting cause is by far the commonest form of mesenteric vascular occlusion. Onset may be insidious or acute, but it is found in half the cases that a relatively mild course of several days of moderate pain and occasional cramps, with diarrhea and vomiting, precede recourse to the physician. Distention is not constantly marked, and, when present, is due rather to peritoneal irritation than to the obstruction caused by paralysis of the congested nonviable segment of bowel. Blood is commonly aspirated through the Miller-Abbott tube or passed by rectum. Involvement of the superior mesenteric vein is many times more frequent than of the inferior.

The diagnosis of venous thrombosis is commonly missed preoperatively because it is not considered. It is more common than gallstone obstruction, for instance, and should be borne in mind. One differential diagnosis, that from twisted ovarian cyst, is particularly difficult to make. A finding of considerable help is the palpation of heavy, soggy loops of bowel between the fingers on combined rectal and pelvic examination.

Therapy consists in resection and primary anastomosis of the involved intestine with 25 to 30 centimeters of margin along the bowel and wide excision of the mesentery. In the past several years only one case has been encountered at the University Hospitals in which further thrombosis after resection has been shown to occur.

CARCINOMA OF THE CECUM. Three cases have been encountered in which apparently typical simple small bowel obstruction has failed to relent after Miller-Abbott decompression. In two cases exploration revealed carcinoma of the cecum with encroachment on the ileocecal valve, and the third showed carcinoma of the ascending colon with incompetent ileocecal valve. All three recovered after primary right hemicolectomy and ileo-transverse colon anastomosis.

MISCELLANEOUS TYPES OF OBSTRUCTIONS. Congenital obstructions of the newborn are not discussed because of the rarity of the lesion and lack of space; an excellent account is found in Ladd and Gross's *Abdominal Surgery of Infancy and Childhood*.

Obstruction due to diaphragmatic and retroperitoneal hernias and due to congenital malrotation of the intestine are omitted because of the rarity of the conditions and the author's paucity of experience with them. They are amply discussed by Wangensteen.

ILEOSTOMY

The situations in which ileostomy is demanded are not common, but the grief to be encountered if the procedure is performed with neglect of certain fundamental principles warrants a discussion of the methods to be employed.

Ileostomy is used in the following circumstances:

(1) Chronic, nonspecific, ulcerative colitis

(2) Pan-colectomy for polyposis of the colon or other conditions

(3) Acute, complete obstruction due to cancer in the right colon; a procedure more commonly to be recommended is end-to-end ileo-transverse colostomy with exteriorization of the ends of the colon and ileum communicating with the right colon.

Since it is by far the commonest of these conditions, chronic ulcerative colitis here will serve as the basis for discussion.

Review of the statistics on cases of nonspecific ulcerative colitis at the University of Minnesota Hospitals for the ten years ending January 1, 1944, showed an 8 per cent mortality in twenty-five patients treated surgically, and a 28 per cent mortality in fifty-seven cases treated by conservative types of management. This present emphasis on the surgical management is, of course, a temporary one to be employed only until the true nature of the disease shall have been discovered, when it is presumed that less radical measures may suffice.

Experience in the past 15 months with 22 patients with ulcerative colitis indicates that those cases having not yet lost much flexibility in the intestine through fibrosis benefit greatly from the performance of division of the vagus nerves. Observations thus far available indicate that most cases of less than 2 years duration need no other therapy than vagotomy, and that some of longer duration also react favorably. Those cases with advanced fibrosis have no longer sufficient storage capacity for stool, and do not benefit from vagotomy; these are the patients in whom the risks of carcinoma of the colon and cirrhosis of the liver rise steeply with the passage of time.

As the previous study pointed out, until 1946 the safest procedure in those cases requiring any surgery at all was to perform ileostomy and to allow at least three months to pass before undertaking colectomy. The very mild cases can usually be handled medically. All others were candidates for ileostomy. Emergency indications were: uncontrollable hemorrhage; fulminating disease; impending perforation; and obstruction. Elective indications were: chronic ulcerative colitis resisting all forms of medical treatment; segmental ulcerative colitis; very early ulcerative colitis; and polyposis including those cases with possible malignancy.

The type of ileostomy now employed has developed gradually in the past few years. At first, all ileostomies were of the double-barreled type, the loop being brought out through the main incision. Most of these wounds healed nicely, but about one-third of them broke down under the influence of the unspent digestive ferments poured forth from the ileostomy. This has, in the past, been one of the great objections to ileostomy posed by internists and surgeons alike. Excoriation of the skin, which results from constant bathing in the unspent secretions coming from the bowel, has been a second factor. Finally, the progressive emaciation born of loss of appetite and seepage of plasma from painful raw surfaces has caused many clinicians to throw up their hands in horror at the suggestion of ileostomy in any but the most extreme cases.

These problems seem to have been largely overcome by the employment of the ultimate regimen indicated below. It has become the impression of most members of the surgical and medical staffs at the University of Minnesota Hospitals that ileostomy is less a burden than any but the most mild cases of colitis.

It has been learned by painful experience that the most extreme care and precision must be exercised with every detail of the preoperative, operative, and postoperative care of these cases, and with this finding in mind, the procedures employed are described.

Preoperative Preparation. The bulk of the candidates for ileostomy have been troubled with profuse liquid stools many times a day, the frequency and debilitating effect of which have been only increased by administration of the high-protein, high-caloric diets ordinarily employed at Minnesota on poor-risk patients. It has, therefore, been the practice to fortify these individuals for ileostomy by continuous intravenous infusion of from 2 to 3 liters of 15 per cent dextrose solution in distilled water during the 24 to 36 hours before surgery. This is usually supplemented with plasma, as the plasma protein is ordinarily depleted. Crude liver extract (Campalon *) and the available purified vitamins are added to the dextrose solution. Use of the veins of the legs is scrupulously avoided because of the danger of thrombophlebitis in these cases.

Preoperative preparation includes 100 mg. of pentobarbital the night before surgery, repeated in the morning if the patient is not drowsy, also morphine and hyoscine as in routine preparation for other procedures. Wangensteen nasal suction is instituted before the patient leaves the ward, and is maintained usually the next two days. Enemas are scrupulously avoided.

Operation. ANESTHESIA. The patient is made as comfortable as possible on the operating table and an 8 centimeter left lower rectus incision is made under 0.50 per cent metycaine local infiltration (Fig. 246). The rectus sheaths are not infiltrated with 1 per cent solution until exposed, as a precaution against puncturing the bowel. The rectus muscle is retracted laterally, and the abdomen entered.

CHOICE OF LEVEL. No manipulation of the colon is performed. The desired segment of bowel can almost regularly be easily identified by the presence on the antimesenteric border of the terminal 10 cm. of ileum of the ileocecal fold. It is delivered into the field; the diameter of the bowel is measured and it is carefully inspected with a view to making the ileostomy definitely above the level of involvement.** The mesentery is infiltrated with metycaine as far posteriorly as possible, and is divided at the chosen point for from 8 to 10 centimeters toward the root, tying the well-isolated vessels encountered with No. 0 chromic catgut or 0000 silk (Fig. 247).

DIVISION OF ILEUM. After careful evaluation of the circulation of the bowel following this division of the mesentery, a segment is removed between clamps and both remaining ends are closed with Parker-Kerr catgut sutures, each suture being reinforced by three or four Halsted mattress sutures of

---

* Winthrop Chemical Company, New York, N. Y.
** The terminal ileum has been involved in one-third of our reported cases.

No. 4-0 Deknatel silk. The distal stump is sutured to the mesentery (Fig. 247) to prevent intussusception, the ties are left long on the upper end to ease re-identification, and both are dropped back into the abdomen.

The resected segment is opened at once by the pathologist and examined for evidences of disease at this level. Presence of diseased bowel at the site of ileostomy favors fecal fistula formation and postoperative diarrhea, and dictates ileac resection upward until good bowel is reached.

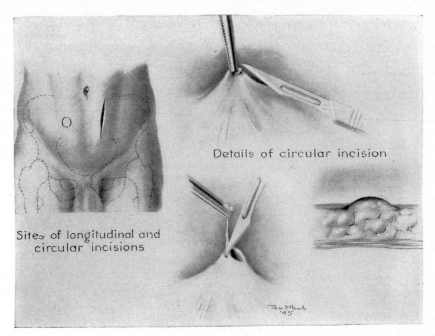

Details of circular incision

Sites of longitudinal and
circular incisions

FIG. 246. Ileostomy. Details of the incisions employed for single-barreled terminal ileostomy. An 8-cm. left lower rectus incision is made. A circular skin incision equal to the diameter of the ileum to pass through it is made 6 cm. below the umbilicus and from 2 to 3 cm. to the right of the midline. The cuticular surface of the skin projects farther toward the center of the circular defect than the deeper layers; local anesthesia. (From Dennis, *Surgery,* 18:435, 1945.)

PREPARATION OF CIRCULAR ILEOSTOMY INCISION. The optimal site for ileostomy on the abdominal wall is dictated in a large measure by the characteristics of the Koenig-Rutzen ileostomy bag. It should be from 6 to 7 centimeters below the belt line, and well away from the anterior-superior spine of the ilium and the inguinal fold. In practice the usual position is 6 centimeters below the umbilicus and 3 centimeters to the right. The skin is infiltrated at this point, picked up, and buttonholed with a scalpel (Fig. 246). A circular defect, equal to the original diameter of the ileum to be passed through it, is made in such fashion that the cuticular layer projects farther toward the center of the circle than the deeper layers of the dermis, and may thus later be spread upward along the ileum somewhat (Fig. 246).

The rectus sheath is bluntly exposed and longitudinally incised just

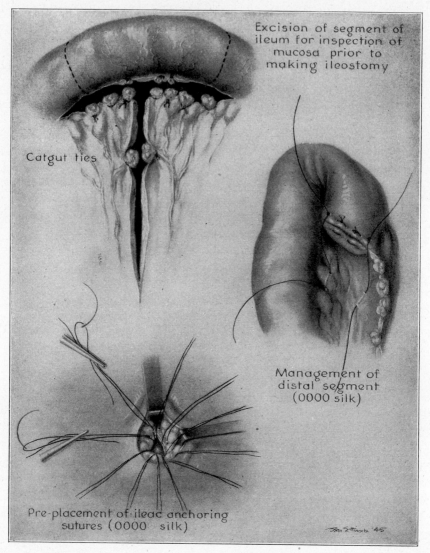

Excision of segment of
ileum for inspection of
mucosa prior to
making ileostomy

Catgut ties

Management of
distal segment
(0000 silk)

Pre-placement of ileac anchoring
sutures (0000 silk)

Fig. 247. Single-barreled ileostomy. At the site chosen for ileostomy the mesentery is divided 8 to 10 cm. toward the root, using catgut ties. A segment of intestine is removed for immediate gross pathologic examination to rule out ulcerative ileitis at this level. Both remaining ends are closed by Parker-Kerr catgut and Halsted mattress No. 4-0 silk sutures. The distal end is sewed to the mesentery to prevent intussusception. Lower figure shows placement of fine (No. 4-0, two-pound test strength) silk anchoring sutures in the rectus sheaths and peritoneum. (From Dennis, *Surgery*, 18:435, 1945.)

sufficiently to permit easy passage through it of a finger of the surgeon equal in diameter to the ileum as first exposed.

ILEAC ANCHORING SUTURES. Fixation of the ileum to the abdominal wall by fine silk (No. 4-0 Deknatel rather than 5-0) sutures is best accomplished by preplacement of these sutures, usually from ten to twelve in number, in

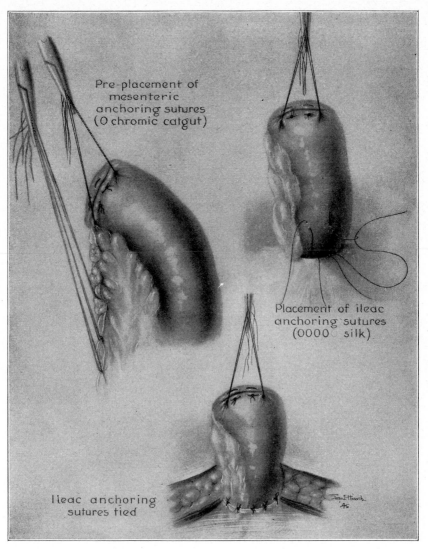

Pre-placement of
mesenteric
anchoring sutures
(O chromic catgut)

Placement of ileac
anchoring sutures
(0000 silk)

Ileac anchoring
sutures tied

FIG. 248. Single-barreled ileostomy. Sutures for anchoring the mesenteric cut edge to the anterior abdominal wall are placed before the closed orad stump of ileum is brought through the circular incision, to avoid inaccessible hemorrhage. No. 4-o silk is just as satisfactory as o chromic catgut for this purpose. After passage of the bowel through this incision, the sutures already anchored to the rectus sheath and peritoneum are all completely placed by submucosal bites (*avoiding mucosa*) in the ileum and sub-serosal bites in the mesentery. The bowel is then slipped back into place, and all sutures are tied and cut. (From Dennis, *Surgery*, 18:435, 1945.)

the rectus sheaths and peritoneum before passage of the bowel through the defect (Fig. 247). Completion of these sutures is accomplished after delivery of the closed ileum by small submucosal bites in the bowel and serosal bites in the mesentery; the bowel is then slipped back into position for tying of the sutures (Fig. 248).

MESENTERIC-ANCHORING SUTURES. Prior to passage of the ileum through the ileostomy defect, two or three sutures are placed on the mesenteric border and left temporarily without tying (Fig. 249). After securing the ileac-anchoring sutures already described, these mesenteric-anchoring sutures are employed to fix the mesenteric border to the peritoneum and posterior rectus sheath for from 4 to 5 centimeters caudad to the ileostomy opening through the abdominal wall in an effort to minimize both prolapse and torsion of bowel about the loop coming to the ileostomy (Fig. 249).

The ileum should now project about 3 cm. beyond the skin surface, and there should be good color to the bowel and an obvious pulsation of the arteries of the mesentery outside the skin, measures which have been found to militate against later stenosis of the stoma.

SKIN SUTURES. Fixation of the skin edge to the bowel is essential to the subsequent comfort of the patient, as will be indicated. It is best accomplished with No. ooo chromic catgut sutures or 4-o silk sutures catching just the cuticular margin. The bowel is worked down into the subcutaneous tissue and the skin edge elevated in the process, so that the attachment ultimately lies one and one-half centimeters out from the point where the skin at first lies naturally against the ileum (Fig. 249). This is best done at once after tying the deep anchoring sutures, before the edema from manipulation is marked.

The left rectus incision is closed with interrupted silk, No. ooo and oooo Deknatel, and a dry gauze dressing is applied. Petrolatum gauze is placed around the ileostomy and a No. 14 French, soft rubber catheter with from 10 to 12 holes is inserted from 6 to 7 centimeters, and secured with a catgut purse-string suture (Fig. 249). This intubation may be delayed as long as 48 hours.

Postoperative Care. INTUBATION. The patient returns to the ward awake and comfortable. Full Wangensteen suction is applied to the nasal gastric tube and about one-half suction to the ileostomy catheter. After the first 24 hours, appreciable amounts of fluid are usually removed through the catheter. Usually the nasal tube can be removed in 48 hours without subsequent discomfort. The ileac catheter must be removed in four days to avoid leakage, and at this time healing is adequate to discontinue aseptic management of both incisions.

SKIN CARE. In removal of the catheter, the following procedure has proved most satisfactory. All dressings are removed, and the skin for from 12 to 14 centimeters around the bowel, including the rectus incision, is covered with a one-half centimeter layer of the paste described by Ladd and Gross (as used here: aristol 100, castor oil 600, zinc oxide 320, and petrolatum 1280). By the actual cautery the catheter is loosened and the end of the bowel widely opened, care being taken to remove completely the valve-like inverted lips of ileac wall and to amputate the ileum 8 to 10 mm. from the skin. Drainage is thereafter rather profuse and liquid. The patient now assumes much of the care of the ileostomy, and keeps the skin carefully protected from the ileac secretions by free application of paste and hourly changes of dressings. Nursing help is needed chiefly during the night for the next three days.

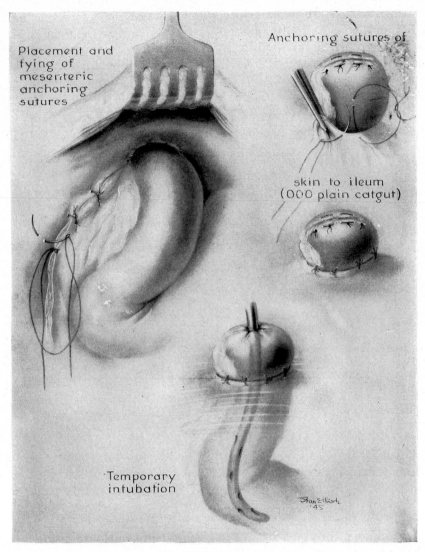

Placement and tying of mesenteric anchoring sutures

Anchoring sutures of

skin to ileum (000 plain catgut)

Temporary intubation

FIG. 249. Single-barreled ileostomy. The mesenteric-anchoring sutures are completed and tied. The skin is sutured to the ileum at a point 1.5 cm. distal on the bowel to the point where it lies naturally. The serocutaneous juncture is covered with petrolatum gauze and the ileum intubated. (From Dennis, *Surgery*, 18:435, 1945.)

About seven days after surgery the patient is fitted with a temporary Koenig-Rutzen bag, and may be up and about the ward (Fig. 250). As soon as the patient masters the management of the bag, usually in another two to three days, he goes home.

Twenty-five days after surgery, shrinkage of the exposed ileum is complete. At this time the patient returns for measurement of the exact outline and position of the mucocutaneous junction, data required for preparation of the patient's Koenig-Rutzen bags.*

Double-barreled Ileostomy. In certain instances stricture or actual obstruction of the colon may be present, or the patient may be too desperately ill to withstand such a procedure as that outlined, even under local anesthesia. In these patients it is safer to perform a double-barreled ileostomy, making the initial 5 to 6 centimeter incision under local anesthesia at the

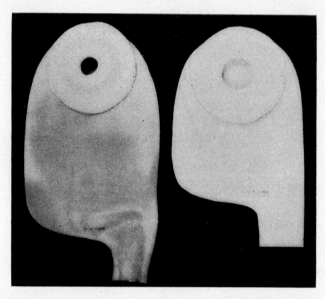

Fig. 250A. The Koenig-Rutzen bag is a rubber-covered brass facing with an opening made individually to fit the bowel, and a bag to hold discharges. (From Dennis, *Surgery,* 18:435, 1945.)

site chosen for ileostomy, and filling this incision with the loop of bowel instead of attempting any skin-to-skin approximation at all. A glass rod is passed through the mesentery to support the ileum, but the No. 4-0 silk peritoneal anchoring sutures and skin sutures are used nevertheless (Fig. 251). Spillage into the distal loop can be prevented for about six weeks by a tie of umbilical cord tape around the distal ileum just outside the skin.

Postoperative care is essentially the same as in the single-barreled ileostomies. The bowel is cut longitudinally down to the glass rod one week after operation before the application of a bag.

* Obtained from H. W. Rutzen, 3952 N. Lowell Avenue, Chicago 41, Illinois. The patient is supplied with two bags, one for day and one for night use. The bag is made of soft rubber and has a flat brass, rubber-covered facing made to order to fit the patient to hold it against the skin around the stoma. Bland rubber cement is used to fix this facing to the skin for 3 cm. around the mucocutaneous junction. Bags are removed for change each morning and night by application of petroleum naphtha with an eyedropper. They may be emptied between changes through a vent in the lower corner of the bag, otherwise secured by a rubber band.

Rationale of Procedures. ANESTHESIA. Early in the surgical management of the disease in this clinic, the anesthetic of choice was ethylene supplemented with ether. Under this anesthesia one of these debilitated patients died before the skin incision was completed. Another died upon exposure of the peritoneum. More recently we have had one apparently good-risk patient go into shock during ileostomy under spinal anesthesia. Another patient went into deep shock following administration of a low spinal anesthetic by a physician-anesthetist, requiring over 2 liters of plasma and blood

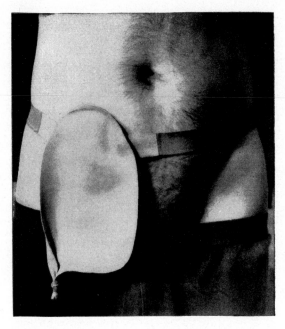

FIG. 250B. The Koenig-Rutzen bag is cemented to the skin, and may be emptied from the lower end when necessary. (From Dennis, *Surgery*, 18:435, 1945.)

to restore the pulse and blood pressure without surgery at all. Two days later, after intravenous infusion of 20 per cent glucose solution, he underwent ileostomy uneventfully under local anesthesia.

Following the adoption of McKittrick's suggestion that ileostomy be done under local anesthesia, no patients have developed shock during this operation. This includes about two dozen cases.

THE CIRCULAR INCISION. The policy among most surgeons is to perform ileostomy by exteriorization of a loop or end of the bowel through the incision, with closure of the abdominal wall around the ileum. This was the policy at the University of Minnesota Hospitals also, until one unfortunate case of marked wound breakdown led to a review of the cases. The policy since has been to avoid skin-to-skin approximation in the neighborhood of the stoma. Since the adoption of this policy, primary union of both the main and the ileostomy incisions has occurred in every case.

Double-barreled ileostomy is more commonly used elsewhere than single-barreled ileostomy, but the latter has been preferred here because of greater ease of later colectomy, absolute prevention of passage of ileac contents into the colon, and lower frequency of hernia formation beside the bowel.

REPLACEMENT OF DISTAL STUMP INSIDE THE ABDOMEN. Secure closure methods have been described. Martzloff and Burget found that properly closed loops of ileum, dropped back into the abdomen of dogs, perforated

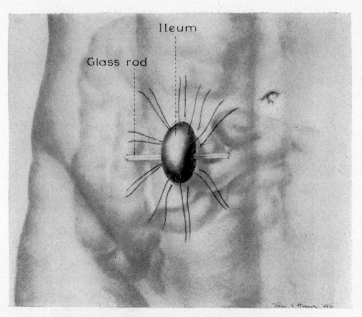

FIG. 251. Double-barreled ileostomy. This is reserved for patients with obstruction or too severe a disease to stand the longer procedure. It is performed through a 5-cm. incision which is completely filled by the bowel. Peritoneal and skin sutures are placed as in the single-barreled ileostomy. (From Dennis, *Surgery*, 18:435, 1945.)

elsewhere than at the suture lines. It has been found in the experimental laboratory here that simple obstruction in the dog's ileum by division and proper closure culminates ordinarily in perforation of the bowel well apart from the suture line.

With these facts in mind, we have had no fear of the procedure described, and have had no reason to regret dropping the closed end back into the abdomen in over 60 cases.

CLOSURE OF ORAD STUMP IN PREPARATION OF ILEOSTOMY. Closure of the orad ileac stump prior to bringing it through the abdominal wall was adopted because it decreased contamination, both from the cut end otherwise held in a clamp of some sort and from tearing of the ileum which was found frequently to occur, in trying to pass it through the necessarily narrow ileostomy opening in the abdominal wall. It also facilitates clean temporary catheter intubation at the end of the procedure.

FIXATION SUTURES IN PREVENTION OF PROLAPSE. Certain factors have proved particularly important in eliminating prolapse and herniation around ileostomies. The most important of these is the accurate suturing of the wall and mesentery of the ileum to the parietal peritoneum and rectus sheaths just as securely with fine silk sutures as if the bowel were being anastomosed.*

Prolapse in two cases seen at this clinic has been completely relieved by approaching the ileostomy from within the abdomen, narrowing the fascial orifice, and placing fine silk anchoring sutures of the type described.

MESENTERIC ANCHORAGE IN PREVENTION OF PROLAPSE. Garlock has recommended inclusion of the mesenteric cut edge in the peritoneal closure caudad to the single-barreled stoma as a means of reducing prolapse development. Cattell follows the same procedure. The procedure of suturing this edge to the anterior abdominal wall was adopted in line with this suggestion, and seems to have been partially effective. There has been one case of prolapse for almost 15 centimeters in this group, however, and the only factor which seemed likely to play a role in this failure was that the rectus sheath incision had been made large enough to admit two fingers. Since adoption of a rectus sheath opening only large enough to admit one finger equal in diameter to the ileum as first exposed, no prolapse has occurred.

SIZE AND TYPE OF SUTURE MATERIAL. Ileostomies were early done with heavy silk sutures. Many of these wounds drained for weeks or months beside the bowel, with discharge of sutures from time-to-time and great disability, long hospitalization, and psychic disturbance to already unstable patients. Catgut was, therefore, adopted for all sutures and ligatures except the ileac-anchoring sutures, where silk was known to be more reliable. Fine silk sutures of No. 4-0 Deknatel, two-pound-test, at this point, are at least as strong as the ileum in which they are placed, and in no instance has use of this size stitch for ileac anchorage been followed by discharge of serum, pus, or suture material from the wound.

PLACEMENT OF ILEAC ANCHORING SUTURES. Two ileostomies recently performed by other methods at the clinic have been followed by development of fecal fistulas, one through the main incision and both through the skin close to the bowel. In one of these the segment employed was involved with extension of the disease from the colon. In both of them the ileac-anchoring sutures were of heavier grade and were placed from within the abdomen, making precise submucosal placement without entering the lumen virtually impossible.

In a third case of placement from within the abdomen, the lateral side could not be reached or visualized, and sutures were not placed there. Herniation developed on the lateral side only.

* This policy was adopted after careful dissection of a series of colostomies during the procedure of closure. Certain other observations were made at autopsy and clinically. With but one exception, no colostomy (or ileostomy) was found to be free from herniation beside the bowel unless a colostomy had been performed which included placement of sutures as described. Almost every case of stenosis of colostomies was found to be associated with such herniation and apparently secondary to it. Of those made as described, only one colostomy hernia has developed.

The adequacy of the suture method just described is testified by the finding at autopsy of clean healing of the ileum to the abdominal wall in the case of involvement of the entire stomach, ileum, and colon, even though the mucosa was largely ulcerated away and the entire ileac wall heavily involved at the site of ileostomy.

DURATION OF ILEOSTOMY PROCEDURE. The rather meticulous procedure outlined cannot be done hurriedly. Under local anesthesia there is little premium on time except for the convenience of the surgeon. The average time including anesthesia in the twenty cases reported was two hours and thirty minutes. Recollection of prolonged suffering from painful open wounds, extensive excoriations, and repeated operations, as well as of the weeks and months I have spent trying to salvage the situation for patients in whom the operative procedures have been done hurriedly and improperly, is adequate incentive to continue to spend this amount of time with them in the proper performance of the ileostomy in the first place.

SKIN CARE. It is true, as much in the postoperative care as in the operative procedure, that a little time spent with the patient is an ounce of prevention.

Various methods of management after ileostomy are feasible. Tincture of benzoin, tannic acid, petrolatum, and vinylite resin have proved entirely inadequate to prevent excoriations. The use of rubber dam cemented to the skin with Koenig-Rutzen cement is satisfactory, but requires close watching and changes at least twice a day. The most useful preparation found so far at this clinic is the paste of Ladd and Gross, which coats the skin with a good protective layer.

It is at this stage that the failure of many ileostomies is caused. Excoriation and breakdown of the skin are relatively easy to prevent but extremely difficult to heal in the constant bath of irritating ileac discharge. Early excoriation at this stage or later often may be aided by use of rubber dam precisely fitted around the bowel and cemented to the skin. This may be removed two to three times daily for one-half hour warm baths, with the water level well above the stoma. Dusting the area lightly with zinc stearate powder before application of the skin cement is also helpful. Very occasionally patients have been placed face down on a mattress with a hole in it so secretions fall away without touching the skin.

Application of special hooks to the ileostomy bag so a tight elastic belt fastens 5 to 6 centimeters from the skin has been shown by Rutzen to apply sufficient pressure of the bag against the skin to heal most skin erosions.

Avoidance of difficulty is facilitated by cutting the bowel no more than 1 centimeter from the skin on the fourth day. Longer segments mushroom so that a bag with stoma the size of the mucocutaneous junction cannot be passed over the end of the bowel. It is also important that no mesentery project outside the skin, as this also tends to mushroom.

Once the patient has progressed to use of the Koenig-Rutzen bag, other measures are usually unnecessary. The management is quickly learned by the patient, who is the one person most interested in care of his skin, but in the experience of this clinic is not to be turned over to most internes or to nurses not specially tutored, for trouble and even disaster have almost invariably followed such delegation of care.

Proper choice of time of day, usually three or more hours after eating, so that constant discharge is not occurring, greatly facilitates clean changes of bags.

THROMBOPHLEBITIS. Pulmonary embolus has killed two patients here in the last eighteen months, one nine days postoperatively and one preoperatively.* This is such a common complication of the disease that patients are now regularly kept up and active, when possible, up to the time of surgery, and are routinely given 200 mg. dicumarol the night before surgery and postoperatively sufficient to keep the prothrombin time 2 to 3 seconds above the control level.

POSTOPERATIVE WEIGHT GAIN AND PLACEMENT OF SKIN SUTURES. When management and care are performed as has been described, most patients have returned to the active life followed before onset of the disease. The weight gain following ileostomy is prompt and marked. Of thirteen patients in whom proper procedures were employed and data are available, the average weight gain in the three months after surgery was 22.7 per cent of the body weight at surgery. The extremes were no gain and 71 per cent gain. No dietary restrictions are employed.

This weight gain is largely due to deposit of fat between the skin and the deep fascia. The result is likely to lead to bulging of the skin except close to the ileostomy, where the surface will necessarily funnel down to the bowel, which, of course, has not increased in length (Fig. 252). In order to permit a flat skin ultimately, to which an ileostomy bag can be well fitted, it is best at the time of ileostomy to lift the skin out immediately adjacent to the bowel and to suture the two thus (Fig. 252).

Meckel's Diverticulum. According to Bell, Meckel's diverticulum is found in 1 to 2 per cent of autopsies. It may be situated anywhere from the ileocecal junction to the ligament of Treitz, but is most commonly found 25 to 100 centimeters from the cecum. It may be represented by a simple patch of gastric mucosa without outpouching; by a simple blind diverticulum without distal attachment; by a diverticulum with a heavy or light cord extending from the tip to umbilicus, other loop of intestine, or base of mesentery; or, finally, by a complete fistula to the umbilicus, occasionally with atresia of the fistula at one or more points with cyst formation.

The difficulties attributable to the anomaly are usually seen in children or young adults and are:

(1) Ulcer formation due to local gastric secretion, causing:
   a. Perforation

---

* Embolism also killed the only patient who had been subjected to ileostomy (double-barreled) elsewhere by this method. The patient had had a perforation and had a large mass in the sigmoid region. He died following embolism occurring less than 72 hours after operation. Dicumarol had been started at 60 hours. The drug should be given preoperatively.

    b. Latent or gross bleeding
    c. Diverticulitis.
(2) Intestinal obstruction due to:
    a. Intussusception
    b. Strangulation of intestine around or beneath the terminal band
       attachment—most common when that band attaches to the base
       of the mesentery.

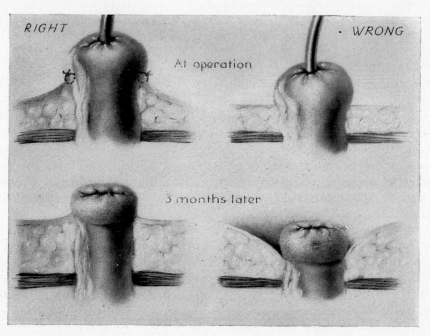

FIG. 252. Skin fixation. At ileostomy the skin is elevated before suture to the bowel. Increase in subcutaneous fat with the usual weight gain then ultimately leaves the patient with the skin flat, so that the bag will fit nicely and excoriation next to the ileum can be avoided. Without this protection, a funnel-shaped depression can defeat efforts to preserve the skin. (From Dennis, *Surgery*, 18:435, 1945.)

Perforation, probably due to penetrating acid ulcer, has occurred twice at the University Hospitals in the recent past. In one of these cases, the anomaly lay in the jejunum and was proved to be gastric mucosa by resection of the segment. Bleeding has been encountered very rarely in the experience here, and diverticulitis has not been seen. In the cases suffering perforation, the onset is sudden, with maximal pain, boardlike abdomen, and other evidences of peritoneal irritation appearing abruptly. Such a story and findings should warn the surgeon against the usual diagnosis of appendicitis. Roentgen evidence of free gas also helps.

In those cases producing obstruction, the diagnosis may be suggested by absence of abdominal scars or history of inflammatory processes in a young individual, but can hardly be established without exploration.

A question frequently debated is whether a Meckel's diverticulum found incidentally at operation should be removed just as most surgeons favor removal of the appendix. In view of the absence of any symptoms prior to potential catastrophe in most cases, and in view of the virtual absence of risk of excision in experienced hands, it is wiser to remove the diverticulum and band if present, particularly in young people, unless some strong contra-indication, such as peritonitis, is present.

The manner of removal is important. In case of a very narrow stalk, ligation and inversion with a purse string stitch is in order. Usually the stalk is broad, and such inversion causes stenosis of the ileum. Here a small hemostat should be placed across the base *perpendicular to the axis of the ileum,* and clean closure accomplished over it, after cautery removal of the pouch, using interrupted Halsted silk sutures placed far enough back from the hemostat to permit tying all but the end one next to the joint of the instrument before removal of the clamp. The area may be emptied and protected during this process by Scudder clamps as in aseptic decompression. Resection of a segment of intestine is rarely necessary.

Regional Ileitis. Regional ileitis was first described by Crohn, Ginzburg, and Oppenheimer in 1932. Although the literature on the subject is large, the etiology is still unknown. Usually the involvement is limited to the terminal ileum, but may be more extensive or may solely involve segments such as upper ileum or jejunum. The occasional case which develops classical chronic nonspecific ulcerative colitis after resection of the involved small bowel would suggest the identity of these two processes.

In early stages the disease is characterized by inflammatory and fibrotic thickening of the ileac wall with round cell infiltration and mucosal ulceration. The course is chronic and the clinical findings are those of abdominal cramps without obstruction, malaise, and, on exacerbations, fever and peritoneal irritation. In later cases the process becomes sufficiently massive to cause partial or functionally complete intestinal obstruction. In still more advanced stages, fistulas also are found, and communicate, in our experience, with other loops of small intestine, with colon, or with stomach; spontaneous external fistulas also have been reported.

Diagnosis usually rests on evaluation of the findings listed and on roentgen study, in which marked narrowing of the stream in this region and radiolucence of the immediately surrounding area due to thickening of the bowel wall are superimposed on stasis due to partial obstruction; the barium may be introduced by rectum—or by mouth if obstruction is partial. In many cases the patient comes as an acute emergency, the severity of the symptoms having led to overlooking of the chronic nature of the disease. Faced with a patient with signs of small bowel obstruction and peritoneal irritation, the surgeon usually will explore with a working diagnosis of strangulating obstruction. Such physical findings may arise in any one of three relatively common conditions:

    (1) Strangulating small intestinal obstruction
    (2) Acute appendicitis with extension and consequent obstruction
    (3) Acute exacerbation of regional ileitis.

It is only by delving into the history with all possibilities in mind that a correct diagnosis can be consistently reached.

Therapy is debated, and the policy at the University Hospitals is not entirely settled, but resection of the involved area is favored by most, regardless of the stage of the disease. In the acute exacerbations, fear of neglecting a strangulating obstruction has usually led to immediate exploration, and the confidence gained in closed anastomosis has led to immediate resection and anastomosis, the resection being radical enough to remove all involved bowel and mesentery and 15 to 30 centimeters of normal-looking, non-edematous intestine as well, including the right colon if so indicated. Results have been very gratifying in this group.

In three of the 22 cases of ulcerative colitis subjected to vagotomy, mentioned in discussion of ileostomy, regional enteritis was not only also present, but the cause of the bulk of the findings. In two of the three patients, complete prompt clinical remission has occurred, and the patients are entirely asymptomatic today. In the third case, the colon had been removed and an ileoproctostomy had previously been performed, permitting proctoscopic examination of the ileum; it was seen to revert from an angry inflamed segment immediately after vagotomy to a segment with normal-appearing mucosa 4 weeks later. All three of these patients are well, one to two years after vagotomy. It is of course too early to consider the role of vagotomy in this disease settled.

Management of cases with fistulas is usually facilitated by ability to establish the diagnosis by roentgen study, the diagnosis less often being confused with strangulating obstruction. Preparation of the patient by a good oral and parenteral high caloric regimen with use of succinyl sulfathiazole is in order, following which resection of the entire involved area *en bloc* has been regularly successful. Patients seem much improved, even after removal of more than half the small bowel. More is to be feared from fistulization through anastomoses in involved bowel than from loss of normal intestine.

Tumors. Tumors of the jejunum and ileum are rare; in the order of frequency they are:

    (1) Adenocarcinoma

    (2) Argentaffine tumors

    (3) Myomas, polyps, lymphoblastoma, etc.

Both adenocarcinoma and argentaffine tumors may metastasize to the lymph nodes or liver. Myomas and simple polyps are benign lesions. Any of these growths except the myoma is most likely to be announced by partial or complete obstruction. Occasionally myomas and polyps may produce obstruction by serving as the apex of an intussusception. Bleeding and perforation occur, but are much more rare.

Diagnosis has been indicated in the section on obstruction; and is not likely to be established until exploration.

Therapy depends on wide excision of the lesion and mesenteric involvement, if present, with primary anastomosis. Even in the presence of hepatic

metastases the patient rarely will do as well with a short circuiting procedure as he will with resection.

REFERENCES

1. ALVAREZ, W. C. *The Mechanics of the Digestive Tract*, 2nd Ed., Paul B. Hoeber, New York, 1919.
2. BAIRD, J. W. Pentothal-curare Mixture, *Anesthesiology*, 8:75-79, [Jan.], 1947.
3. BELL, E. T. *A Text-book of Pathology*, 3rd ed., Lea and Febiger, Phila., 1938.
4. COLLER, F. A. and MADDOCK, W. G. Water and Electrolyte Balance, *Surg., Gynec. & Obst.*, 70:340, 1940.
5. CROHN, B. B., GINZBURG, L. and OPPENHEIMER, G. D. Regional Ileitis: a Pathologic and Clinical Entity, *J.A.M.A.*, 99:1323, 1932.
6. DENNIS, C. Oblique, Aseptic, End-to-end Ileac Anastomosis, Procedure of Choice in Strangulating Small Bowel Obstruction, *Surg., Gynec. & Obst.*, 77:225, 1943.
7. DENNIS, C. Ileostomy and Colectomy in Chronic Ulcerative Colitis, *Surgery*, 18:435, 1945.
8. DENNIS, C. Resection and Primary Anastomosis in the Treatment of Gangrenous or Non-reducible Intussusceptions in Children, *Ann. Surg.*, 126:788, [Nov.], 1947.
9. DENNIS, C. and BROWN, S. P. Treatment of Small Bowel Obstruction, *Surgery*, 13:94, 1943.
10. DENNIS, C., EDDY, F. D. and WESTOVER, D. Vagotomy in the Treatment of Idiopathic Ulcerative Colitis and Regional Enteritis, *Minnesota Med.*, 31:253, 1948.
10A. DENNIS, C., EDDY, F. D., McCARTHY, A. M., WESTOVER, D. and FRYKMAN, H. M. The Response of Vagotomy in Idiopathic Ulcerative Colitis and Regional Enteritis, *Ann. Surg.*, (In Press).
11. DENNIS, C. and EDDY, F. D. Evaluation of Vagotomy in Chronic Non-specific Ulcerative Colitis, *Proc. Soc. Exp. Biol. & Med.*, 65:306, 1947.
12. DENNIS, C. and VARCO, R. L. Femoral Hernia with Gangrenous Bowel, *Surgery*, 22:312, [Aug.], 1947.
13. FINE, J., BANKS, B. M. and HERMANSON, L. The Treatment of Gaseous Distension of the Intestine by Inhalation of 95% Oxygen, *Ann. Surg.*, 103:375, 1936.
14. GATCH, W. D. External Hernias Containing Gangrenous Bowel, *J.A.M.A.*, 129:736, 1945.
15. HAMRICK, W. H. A Technic for Introducing the Miller-Abbott Tube, *U. S. Nav. M. Bull.*, 41:1737, [Nov.], 1943.
16. LADD, W. E. and GROSS, R. E. *Abdominal Surgery of Infancy and Childhood*, W. B. Saunders, Phila., 1941.
17. McKITTRICK, L. S. The Diagnosis and Management of Acute Obstruction of the Small Intestine, *N. Eng. J. Med.*, 225:647, 1941.
18. MARTZLOFF, K. H. and BURGET, G. E. Closed Intestinal Loop: Aseptic End-to-end Intestinal Anastomosis and Method for Making Closed Intestinal Loops Suitable for Physiologic Studies, *Arch. Surg.*, 23:26, 1931.
19. MILLER, T. G. and ABBOTT, W. O. Intestinal Intubation: Practical Technique, *Am. J. Med. Sc.*, 187:595, 1934.
20. RIGLER, L. G. *Outline of Roentgen Diagnosis*, J. B. Lippincott, Phila., 1938.
21. RIGLER, L. G., BORMAN, C. N. and NOBLE, J. F. Gallstone Obstruction: Pathogenesis and Roentgen Manifestations, *J.A.M.A.*, 117:1753, 1941.
22. WANGENSTEEN, O. H. New Operative Techniques in Management of Bowel Obstruction: Aseptic Decompressive Suction Enterotomy, Aseptic Enterotomy for Removal of Obstructing Gallstone, and Operative Correction of Non-rotation, *Surg., Gynec. & Obst.*, 75:675, 1942.
23. WANGENSTEEN, O. H. *Intestinal Obstructions*, 2nd ed., 2nd printing, C. C Thomas, Springfield, Ill., 1945.

24. WANGENSTEEN, O. H. and REA, C. E.   The Distension Factor in Simple Intestinal Obstruction: Experimental Study with Exclusion of Swallowed Air by Esophagostomy, *Surgery*, 5:237, 1939.

25. WHIPPLE, G. H., STONE, H. B. and BERNHEIM, B. M.   Intestinal Obstruction: a Study of a Toxic Substance Produced by the Mucosa of Closed Duodenal Loop, *J. Exp. Med.*, 17:307, 1913.

26. DENNIS, C.   Oblique, Aseptic, End-to-end Intestinal Anastomosis, *Surgery*, 5:548, 1939.

11

THE PANCREAS AND ADRENAL

Alexander Brunschwig, M.D.

THE PANCREAS

Exposure of the pancreas is obtained through a variety of upper abdominal incisions (see Fig. 253). When the gastrohepatic omentum is redundant, the stomach is pulled downward and the gastrohepatic omentum is incised; this exposes the body and tail of the pancreas. The conventional exposure of the body of the pancreas is by transection of the gastrocolic omentum, retraction downward of the transverse colon and elevation of the stomach (see Fig. 254). The head of the pancreas is exposed by incision of the base of the transverse mesocolon as it courses over it, and retraction downward of the transverse colon to pull the freed mesentery with it. Care is exercised to avoid injuries to the middle colic vessels which emerge from beneath the neck of the pancreas. Mobilization of the head of the pancreas is obtained by incision of the peritoneum along the convex borders of the duodenum. The thumb is inserted behind the head of the pancreas and with the index finger on its anterior surface, palpation of the head is easily carried out (see Fig. 255).

Wounds of the Pancreas. These result from stab or bullet wounds usually in the abdomen. Incised wounds are closed by interrupted suture with a soft rubber drain placed to the site of repair.

Comminuted pancreatic tissue is excised with a ligature placed about the proximal stump. Intact pancreatic tissue distal to a comminuted segment is also removed (see below, section on partial pancreatectomy).

Incision and Drainage of the Pancreas. This procedure was followed in the past for acute pancreatitis. The body was exposed, as described above (see Fig. 254). Single or multiple incisions of the parenchyma were made, soft rubber drains inserted to these incisions and the abdominal wound closed about the drains. When vigorous oozing of blood was encountered hemostasis by apposition of gauze packs was secured. The packs, if employed, should be removed in 24 hours; the drains may remain *in situ* for longer periods. In the presence of evidence of cholecystitis or cholelithiasis, cholecystostomy or cholecystectomy is also performed; in the former, the tube is preferably brought out through a separate stab wound in the right upper quadrant.

More recently, experience would suggest that the conservative treatment for acute pancreatitis offers greater opportunity for survival. In the absence of operative interference supportive measures for the treatment of concomitant shock are instituted. Subsequent signs and symptoms of upper abdominal abscess require surgical intervention for drainage. In this event incision of the pancreas itself would not be necessary, simple evacuation of purulent exudate will suffice together with removal of any necrotic fragments of tissue (pancreas or omentum) that may be encountered.

Operations for Pancreatic Duct Lithiasis and Calcification in the Pancreas. Calcification in the pancreas may or may not be associated with symptoms severe enough to warrant surgical intervention. The fact that in roentgenograms of the abdomen, varying degrees of calcification may be observed unaccompanied by symptoms referable to the pancreas, renders a true evaluation of such findings very difficult when such symptoms are present. The outstanding symptom associated with calcification of the pancreas is severe epigastric pain. The excision of calcified areas, when indicated, is carried out by exposure of the pancreas and resection of the visible or palpable calcified foci. The defects in the parenchyma are closed by interrupted silk sutures and the peritoneum closed over the wounds when possible. Soft rubber drains are placed to the sites of operation.

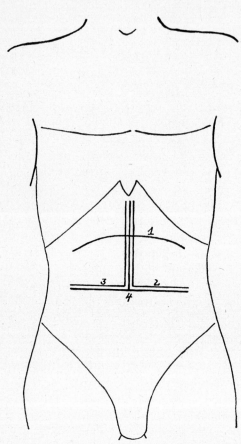

Fig. 253. Diagrams of various incisions for operations upon the pancreas. (1) High transverse. (2) L-shape. (3) Reverse-L. (4) Inverted-T.

Recently it has been shown that sympathectomy, including particularly splanchnicectomy, relieves the pain in calcification of the pancreas. Preliminary to operation a high dorsal sympathetic block is performed to determine whether or not pain is relieved. For obvious reasons, splanchnicectomy is preferable to total resection of the pancreas for relief of pain.

Pancreatic duct lithiasis may be visible upon roentgenographic examination of the abdomen but cannot be definitely differentiated from calcification in the parenchyma. In fact, the two conditions may be coexistent. To probe the pancreatic ducts, the lower portion of the second segment of duodenum is isolated and a linear incision about 3 to 4 cm. in length is made on the anterior aspect of the bowel to exposure of the papilla of Vater. A fine probe is passed backward into the main pancreatic duct. The presence of calculi may be readily appreciated as the tip of the probe strikes them; also, a grating sensation may be felt as the probe may pass beyond calculi. A grooved director may be passed into the main pancreatic duct and the parenchyma incised over it. Calculi are picked out of the duct with

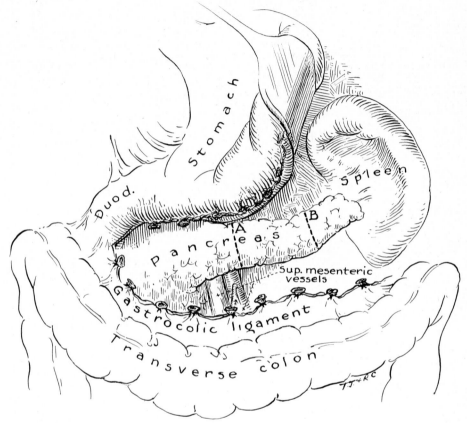

FIG. 254. Diagrammatic representation of exposure of body of pancreas. The gastrocolic omentum has been divided, the stomach retracted upward and transverse colon retracted downward. A and B, levels of elective transection for removal of various segments of the body and tail of the gland. As related in the text, the spleen may be elevated and used as a handle to elevate various portions of the body of the pancreas; in such instances the spleen is also removed.

forceps or washed out by means of saline squirted out of a syringe. Accurate apposition of the parenchyma over the opened duct by means of interrupted silk sutures, serves to close the duct. Soft rubber drains are placed to the site of incision into the pancreas. The incision in the duodenum is closed by two layers of interrupted silk sutures.

The Management of Pancreatic Cysts. True cysts of the pancreas are blastomas with definite fibrous connective tissue walls lined with epithelium. Pseudocysts about the pancreas are collections of fluid that have become

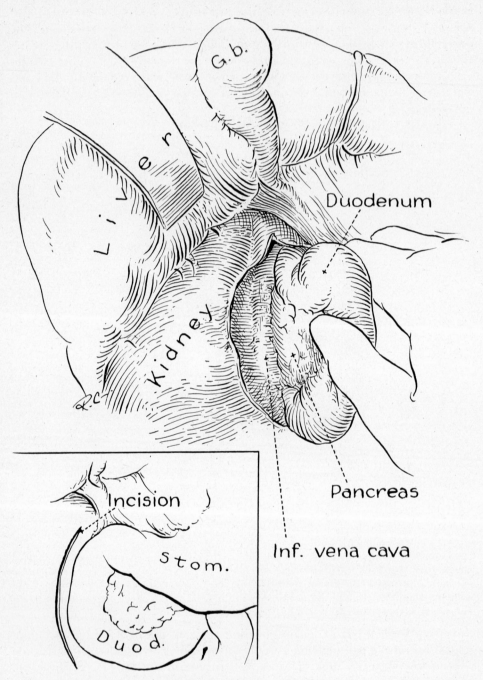

Fig. 255. Diagrammatic representation (inset) of mobilization of head of pancreas and duodenum. An incision is made along the greater curvature of the duodenum. The head of the pancreas and duodenum are grasped between thumb and index finger.

walled off by fibrinous exudate that has become organized by connective tissue proliferation; the omentum and surfaces of the stomach, transverse mesocolon, colon and small intestines may contribute to the walls of a pseudocyst.

The incision of choice is a high midline incision that may be extended downward or to the right or left (L, or reverse-L).

A small cyst (usually a true blastoma) may be enucleated.

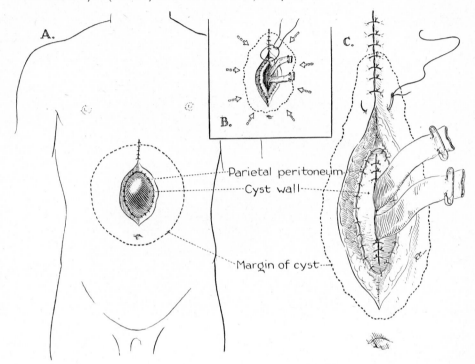

Fig. 256. Marsupialization of pancreatic cyst. (A) Suture of cyst wall into lower angle of midline incision. (B) The cyst wall has been opened and contents evacuated with insertion of rubber drains. (C) The wound is closed loosely around the drains.

Moderate size cysts may also be excised rather easily when the proper cleavage plane is entered at the site of attachment to the pancreas. Preliminary aspiration of its contents to collapse the walls may facilitate excision. The collapsed cyst is grasped by several hemostats and traction upon them reveals the extent of attachment to the pancreas.

Large pseudocysts are marsupialized. This may be done in one or two stages (see Fig. 256). If it is done in two stages, the first step consists of attaching an elliptical area of the most protuberant portion of the cyst wall, by interrupted sutures, to the anterior parietal peritoneum of a segment of the abdominal wound and closing the latter tightly above or below this area. Gauze is packed into the wound to favor adhesive exudation at the junction of the cyst wall with the parietal peritoneum. Two or three days later a linear stab wound is made in the exposed wall of the cyst, the contents evacuated by suction and the interior of the cavity packed with gauze. The latter is changed daily for several days and then soft rubber drains are inserted until the cyst cavity becomes spontaneously obliterated—a matter of a few weeks.

When the operation is performed in one stage a stab wound is made in the most protuberant portion of the cyst wall and its contents evacuated completely. The collapsed cyst is then opened more widely and the edges of the opening attached by interrupted sutures to the margins of a segment

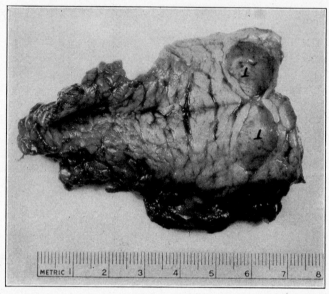

FIG. 257. Photograph of surgical specimen consisting of the distal half of the body and tail of the pancreas resected without the spleen to include T, an islet cell adenoma that produced hyperinsulinism.

of the midline abdominal incision, the latter being closed tightly above and below. The subsequent treatment is the same as for the second stage of the two-stage procedure described above. The one-stage procedure is safe and most surgeons prefer it.

True cysts of moderate size are best resected. Cysts with purulent contents are best marsupialized and evacuated in two stages. Hydatid cysts should be excised in toto at one stage, if possible, great care being exercised not to rupture them. If they are very large, a two stage evacuation will be necessary.

Multilocular cysts should be excised, but if marsupialized, the various locules must be opened into a common cavity.

CYST-GASTRO-OR-ENTERO-ANASTOMOSES (internal drainage). Some operators have been successful in treating pancreatic cysts by evacuation and then anastomosing them with the stomach or a loop of small bowel, the rationale being that the contents are continuously evacuated internally. The writer's limited experience with these methods has not been fortunate and he cannot recommend them. In one patient subjected to a second laprotomy (the first having been done elsewhere) there was a multiloculated cyst, only one locule of which had been anastomosed to the jejunum and the remainder of the cyst was still intact and producing symptoms.

Resection of Small Solid Tumors (Islet Cell Adenomas). Benign islet cell adenomas of the pancreas usually measure 1 to 2 cm. in diameter, and are purplish or greyish in color with texture quite different from that of normal pancreatic parenchyma. Macroscopically, they are sharply demarcated. They may be removed by cuneiform resection of a segment of pancreatic tissue bearing the tumor with closure of the defect by interrupted silk sutures. When the firm nodule is palpated deeply within the body or tail of the gland, resection of that segment, together with all pancreatic tissue distally is carried out (Fig. 257). Because of the likelihood of multiple

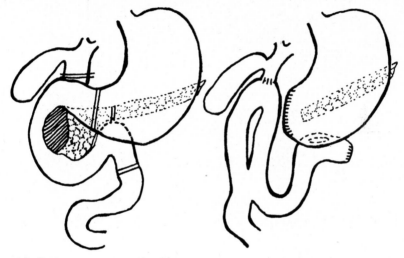

FIG. 258. One-stage pancreatoduodenectomy with occlusion of the neck of the pancreas (author's technic). The lower stomach, dilated common bile duct, neck of pancreas, and jejunum have been transected for removal of the head of the pancreas and duodenum. The upper alimentary tract has been reconstituted by posterior gastro-enterostomy, choledochojejunostomy, and jejunojejunostomy.

islet cell adenomas, the surgeon should not be assured, when one is found and excised, that the procedure may be terminated. The entire body and tail must be thoroughly inspected and palpated, and the head of the gland mobilized and also palpated and inspected for additional adenomas.

Partial Pancreatectomy (Body and Tail). Resection of segments of the body or tail of the pancreas with apposition of the distal remaining segment to the proximal one should not be envisaged since the distal segment will continue to secrete and give rise to a pancreatic fistula. Varying portions of the body and tail may be removed beginning at any level, but all of the gland distal to the elected level is excised.

Exposure of the gland is secured by division of the gastrocolic omentum, retraction upward of the stomach and downward of the transverse colon. The peritoneum over the anterior surface of the body is quite mobile and may be lifted with a toothed forcep and incised along the long axis of the organ (when not invaded by carcinoma). The blood supply of the body and tail is derived from several branches of the splenic artery which courses either behind or superior to the gland. When only the body and tail are to

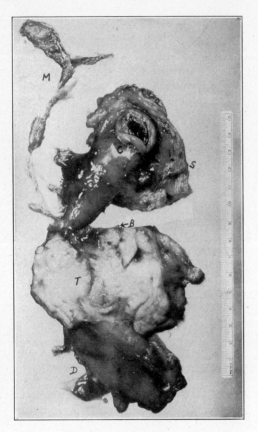

FIG. 258A. Photograph of surgical specimen obtained from pancreatoduodenectomy. M, metastatic nodes from porta hepatis; S, lower stomach, and C, site of cholecystgastrostomy performed previously to relieve intense jaundice; D, lower duodenum; T, bisected head of pancreas largely replaced by tumor; B, opened common bile duct.

be resected a curved hemostat is inserted beneath the organ at the prospective level of transection and the parenchyma divided. The proximal stump is closed by a mass ligature of linen tied tightly, but not so tightly that it cuts into the parenchyma. The segment of gland to be removed is then elevated and the vessels on its deep surface or along its upper border are secured, ligated and transected. Excision may commence with the tip of the tail and proceed proximally to the desired level, when the gland is then transected after that portion to be removed has been completely mobilized.

A maneuver that has been employed by the writer with success is the following: after elevation of the stomach and depression of the transverse colon, the spleen is mobilized by division of the splenocolic and splenodiaphragmatic ligaments, and splenogastric vessels. It is then attached only to the tail of the pancreas by means of the splenic vessels. It is grasped by the right hand and brought forward into the field. In this manner, it brings upward the tail and body of the pancreas and the latter may be mobilized to the neck. With transection of the latter the spleen, body and tail of the pancreas are removed.

RESECTION OF THE HEAD OF THE PANCREAS: PANCREATODUODENECTOMY. Malignant tumors of the head of the pancreas are resected by pancreatoduodenectomy. The head of the pancreas may not be resected alone without concomitant removal of the duodenum because the blood supply of the head of the pancreas and duodenum are so closely related. (Obviously, well circumscribed small benign tumors may be enucleated from the head, and the bed in the parenchyma closed by interrupted sutures.)

Pancreatoduodenectomy was performed first as a two-stage procedure with a 4 week interval between each stage. In patients with marked debility and severe icterus, a first stage operation consisting of choledochostomy or choledochojejunostomy alone may be performed (see Fig. 258). When feasible, it is better to perform the whole operation in one stage. The procedure employed by the writer is as follows:

1. A high midline, transverse, or inverted-T incision.

2. The head of the pancreas and duodenum are mobilized by in-cision of the peritoneum along the greater curvature of the duodenum. This step aids in ascertaining if the neoplasm has invaded the first por-tions of the portal vein.

3. The lower stomach is tran-sected and the upper segment is closed. The superior pancreatodu-odenal artery is divided near the duodenal wall.

4. The common bile duct is transected at or slightly below the level of the upper margin of the first portion of the duodenum.

5. The neck or proximal por-tion of the body of the pancreas is transected at the level of, or slightly to the right of, the superior mesen-teric vessels. In the stump of the pancreas, the main pancreatic duct is secured by a hemostat, twisted through a 90 degree arc, and ligated with silk. The pancreatic parenchyma is sewed by interrupted interlocking mattress sutures that are not tied too tightly (see Fig. 259).

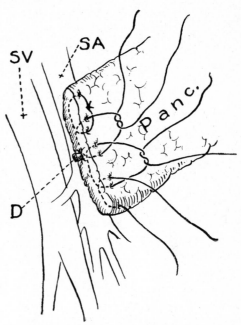

FIG. 259. Showing method of occlusion of the stump of the pancreas after pancreatoduo-denectomy without implantation of the pan-creas into the bowel. SV and SA, superior mesenteric vein and artery respectively. The pancreatic duct, D, has been ligated. Inter-locking mattress sutures are placed in the transected parenchyma and tied firmly. (Silk technic.)

6. The superior mesenteric vessels are elevated from the uncinate process of the pancreas and third portion of the duodenum.

7. The ligament of Treitz is incised, thus freeing the duodenojejunal junction and facilitating transection of the jejunum distally.

8. The jejunum 3 to 6 centimeters distal to the ligament of Treitz is transected, and the lower segment is closed by three concentric purse-string sutures (linen). Duodenum, head of pancreas, and lower segment of common bile duct are removed.

9. A posterior gastrojejunostomy is performed.

10. The transverse mesocolon is incised to permit the first long loop of

the jejunum to be brought upward for the choledochojejunostomy. The latter may be done "anteriorly."

11. A jejo-jejunostomy is made below the opening in the transverse

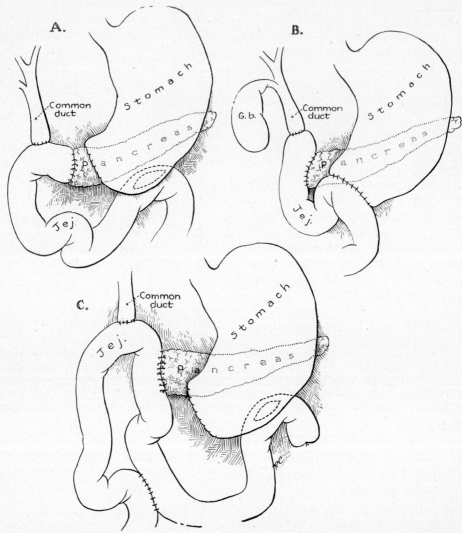

FIG. 260. Showing various methods of reconstituting the upper alimentary tract after pancreatoduodenectomy with implantation of the pancreatic stump into a loop of jejunum. (A) The transected end of jejunum is brought up for implantation of the common bile duct and stump of pancreas, followed by anastomosis of the jejunum to stomach; (B) Essentially similar procedure to the above with higher gastro-jejunostomy; (C) Implantation of common bile duct and pancreas into long loop of jejunum.

mesocolon between efferent and afferent loops of jejunum going to chole-dochojejunostomy.

12. A soft rubber drain is applied to the site of the head of the pancreas and the abdominal wound is closed.

Variations of the above procedure have been described (see Fig. 260), the principal difference being that the transected neck of the pancreas is implanted into the jejunum with the hope that pancreatic juice may be returned to the bowel (see Fig. 261). Up to this writing, no necropsy observations have been reported to indicate that such implantations function in this respect; it is the author's impression that cicatricial obliteration occurs in such pancreatic stumps and that the external secretion of the pancreas in the end is occluded. However, burying the stump of pancreas into jejunum is a method for obviating pancreatic fistulae. The latter step does prolong the operation.

Total Pancreatectomy. Total pancreatectomy is compatible with life but the patient is rendered diabetic. The severity of the diabetes is not as marked as might have been anticipated; 20 to 40 units of insulin daily usually suffices to control carbohydrate metabolism. Following total pancreatectomy patients may exhibit an insulin hypersensitivity and therefore might develop hypoglycemia after the injection of small doses. The postoperative care must be carried out with the close cooperation of the internist, who is well aware of this.

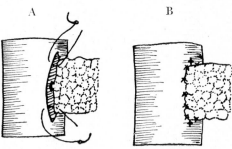

FIG. 261. Method of implanting transected neck of pancreas into loop of jejunum. (A) Linear incision through serosa and muscularis to exposure of submucosa. A small opening is made in the mucosa of the bowel and the pancreatic duct is sutured to it. The pancreatic parenchyma is sutured to the margin of the wound in the bowel musculature by interrupted silk sutures. An alternative method (B) is simply to suture the pancreatic duct into the mucosa by a transfixion suture without actually incising the bowel mucosa, in anticipation of the transfixion suture sloughing away with creation of a pancreatic fistula into the bowel. The remainder of the procedure is carried out as described above.

Total pancreatectomy (see Fig. 262) is a combination of the procedures described above for pancreatoduodenectomy and for resection of the body and tail of the pancreas. Splenectomy at the same time may facilitate the procedure as outlined above since the spleen may serve as a handle to elevate the body of the pancreas. The operation may begin with mobilization of the head of the pancreas and duodenum, then the body and tail; or first, the tail and body (with or without the spleen) are elevated and dissection proceeds from the patient's left toward the superior mesenteric vein, in which region the final dissection is performed to remove the entire pancreas, as described for pancreatoduodenectomy.

Occlusion of External Pancreatic Secretion. This is not incompatible with more or less adequate assimilation of fat and proteins. In some instances the stools are nearly normal; in others, they may be numerous, fatty and bulky. Where the latter situation exists pancreatin is indicated and alleviates the steatorrhea. Otherwise, a liberal general diet is recommended without special additions. It would appear that sufficient nutritional requirements are met when there is absorption of 30 to 40 per cent of fat ingested.

Pancreatic Fistulae. Pancreatic fistulae develop after excision of the head of the pancreas and duodenum and where the transected pancreas has not been reimplanted into the jejunum. Such fistulae are to be expected and accepted and after several months close spontaneously.

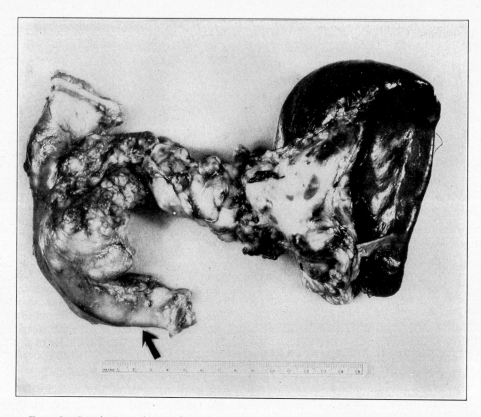

Fig. 262. Surgical specimen of total pancreatectomy (performed for diffuse carcinoma of the pancreas) showing in addition to the pancreas, the lower pylorus, small segments of jejunum (beyond white arrow) and spleen. This specimen is from first total pancreatectomy performed in man, 1943. The patient died on the ninth postoperative day of lobar pneumonia. During the first three days he had profound hypoglycemic attacks resulting from injections of 10 units of insulin, because of insulin hypersensitivity.

Fistulae may persist at the site of a marsupialized pancreatic cyst. They have also been observed following drainage of the pancreas for acute pancreatitis or drainage following injury to the pancreas where the latter has been comminuted and the area drained.

A serious situation obtains when there are concomitant pancreatic and biliary fistulae. Continuous suction through catheters inserted well into the fistula should be instituted as soon as the condition becomes apparent.

The presence of infection favors digestion of the abdominal wall. In the absence of infection there is little digestion but the skin becomes markedly irritated, erythematous and excoriated.

In the absence of infection, protection of the skin by aluminum paste may be carried out for prolonged periods in anticipation that the fistula will close spontaneously. The patient should be encouraged to indulge in normal physical activity. Specific dietary and drug therapy (atropine) have

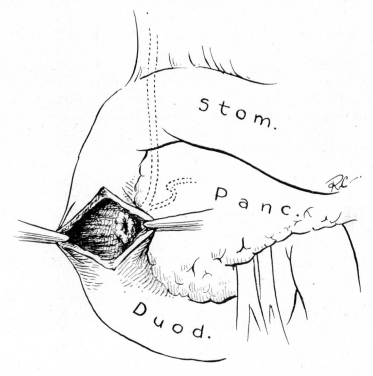

FIG. 263. Transduodenal exposure of small neoplasm of papilla of Vater. A linear incision on anterior aspect of lower portion of second segment of duodenum is spread by Allis hemostats applied to the margins of the wound with retraction.

not been successful in the author's experience, in reducing the discharge from pancreatic fistulae.

The injection of sclerosing solutions into the sinus tract, *i.e.* sodium morrhuate, Zenker's solution, etc., may prove to be of benefit. For some unknown reason, a silver nitrate stick applied into the sinus has been regularly observed to be followed by severe pain but did not bring about appreciable healing and the writer strongly advises against such measures.

X-ray therapy in moderate doses has sometimes been reported to decrease the discharge of pancreatic juice and favor healing of the fistulae.

Operative treatment consists of dissection of the sinus tract to the pancreas and excision of the deeply situated "blind end" together with a small portion of pancreatic tissue from which the fistula appears to arise. If the fistula derives from an isolated portion of the tail, the latter is completely excised. Another, but more complicated procedure, is to dissect out the superficial opening with 2 or 3 mm. of skin about it and after suitable mobilization of the tract, implantation of the stoma into a loop of small bowel or even into the stomach.

Fistulae are sometimes caused to persist because the attending physician inserts tubes or drains under the assumption that they must be kept open to "heal from the depths"; this is erroneous, as healing is facilitated by the absence of such drains.

Operations Upon the Papilla of Vater. It is difficult to palpate the normal papilla of Vater through the intact duodenum. Small neoplasms or impacted calculi are readily felt after incision of the parietal peritoneum along the greater curvature of the duodenum, elevation of the latter and palpation of the ampullar region between thumb (behind) and index finger.

To test for patency of the ampulla, the common bile duct is opened by linear incision below the entrance of the cystic duct, and a probe or rubber urethral catheter pushed downward in the common duct; its entrance into the duodenum is readily appreciated.

Transduodenal exposure of the papillary region is made by incision through the anterior wall of the duodenum in the lower half of the second segment. The wound margins are held widely apart by Allis forceps (see Fig. 263).

Impacted calculi in the ampulla of Vater are liberated by incision of the stretched-out mucosa over the calculus which permits lifting the calculus out with forceps or with a small spoon (see also Chapter 12). Usually this incision in the mucosa is not repaired since it contracts after the stone is removed.

Growths of limited size are resected by elliptical incision through the duodenal wall to include the lesion. The transected common bile and main pancreatic ducts are reimplanted into the duodenum by suturing them to the wound margins with interrupted fine silk. If the wound is large, the rest of it is closed by a single layer of similar sutures. If the common duct is small and there appears to be some likelihood of subsequent stenosis, a cholecyst-duodenostomy or -jejunostomy may be performed after closure of the incision in the anterior duodenal wall by two rows of interrupted sutures.

Large carcinomas of the papilla of Vater with invasion of the subjacent head of the pancreas present a surgical problem identical with that afforded by carcinoma of the head of the pancreas. They are excised by pancreatoduodenectomy.

THE ADRENAL GLANDS

The adrenal gland may be excised for a neoplasm developing in it. Usually the entire gland is removed, even though the tumor is of such size that it might be enucleated or removed by partial resection of the gland. The neoplasms peculiar to the adrenal are: cortical adenomas, benign or malignant, with or without endocrine activities, pheochromocytomas (arising from the medulla), neuroblastomas, and very rarely, cysts.

There are numerous small arteries and veins supplying the adrenals: the most important branches arise from the corresponding renal vessels. Other important vessels are derived directly from the aorta and inferior vena cava and from the subdiaphragmatic branches of the aorta and inferior vena cava. The sympathetic nerve plexuses for the most part accompany the principal vessels especially those from the renals, and enter the hila of the glands. In operations upon the adrenals it is important that the location of the principal vessels be borne in mind in order that they may be properly secured and ligated to avoid hemorrhage which renders the operation much more diffi- cult, especially when performed via the abdominal approach.

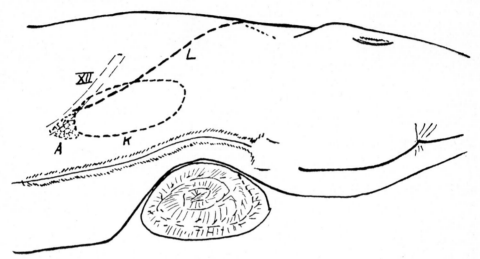

Fig. 264. Showing L, loin incision in relation to twelfth rib. A, right adrenal gland and K, right kidney. Patient lying on left side with sand bag under left flank.

The diagnosis of endocrinologically active adrenal tumors is made from clinical findings, and for details the reader is referred to appropriate works in this field. Palpable masses caused by such tumors (except hypernephromas) are rarely observed. Retroperitoneal insufflation of air prior to radiography is sometimes successful in affording visualization of the outlines of tumors too small to palpate, but negative findings are of limited significance. Such in- sufflation, however, is not without danger.

Lumbar Incision. The conventional approach to the adrenal gland is via the lumbar or loin incision (see Fig. 264).

This incision extends from a point over the outer edge of the erector spinae at the level of the twelfth rib and courses downward and outward in oblique direction toward the junction of the lateral third of Poupart's liga- ment with the mesial two thirds. The length of the incision depends upon the size of the mass to be excised, etc. The lower portion of the latissimus dorsi is divided and the oblique and transversalis muscles are separated or divided for exposure of the transversalis fascia. This is incised the length

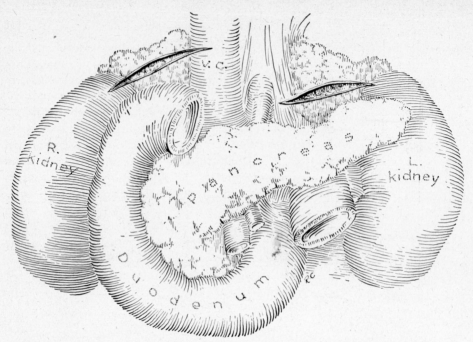

FIG. 265. Diagram illustrating incisions through posterior parietal peritoneum for exposure of right and left adrenal glands respectively (abdominal approach).

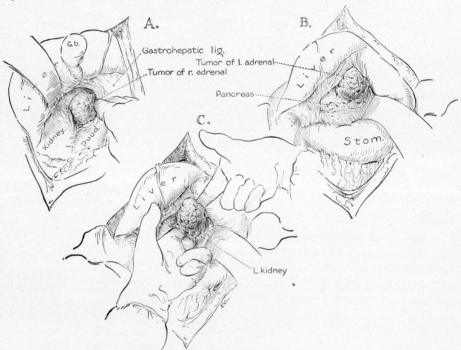

FIG. 266. Abdominal approach to excision of adrenal tumors. (A) Tumor of right adrenal gland being enucleated (with the adrenal) through posterior parietal incision above upper curvature of duodenum. (B) Exposure of tumor of left adrenal gland through gastrohepatic omentum after retraction of the stomach downward. (C) Excision of tumor and left adrenal gland through incisions in gastrohepatic omentum and posterior parietal peritoneum.

of the wound. The quadratus lumborum is also divided to facilitate a widening of the exposure. Incision of the transversalis fascia exposes the perirenal fat which is separated to direct visualization of the kidney. The twelfth rib is retracted upward, the kidney depressed, the posterior aspect of the suprarenal gland is exposed.

Sizable tumors of the adrenal gland are, of course, immediately apparent and it is readily determined whether or not there is infiltration of the underlying kidney. In the latter event a nephrectomy with excision of the suprarenal en masse is performed.

Following simple adrenalectomy drainage is not necessary but when the kidney is also removed, it is well to leave a large soft rubber drain to the excision site.

Closure of the loin incision is carried out in layers, preferably by interrupted sutures. The transversalis fascia is approximated with care, the incised wounds in the muscle are likewise repaired.

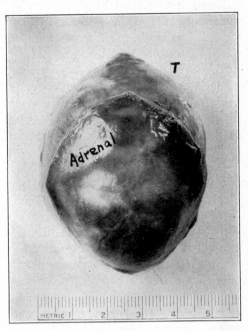

FIG. 267. Photograph of pheochromocytoma and right adrenal gland removed from patient with proxysmal hypertension. The tumor, T, and flattened adrenal were excised en masse (abdominal approach) after manual exploration revealed a normal adrenal on the left side. Patient is well, 5 years postoperatively.

Abdominal Approach. There is considerable difference of opinion as to the choice of incisions for operations upon the adrenal gland; some prefer the loin incisions routinely, others the abdominal route unless the diagnosis of a bulky tumor is apparent, under which circumstances a nephro-adrenalectomy is envisaged and the lumbar route is unquestionably indicated.

The abdominal approach is indicated when there is doubt concerning the presence of a small adrenal tumor (cortical adenoma or pheochromocytoma) and as to which side may be involved. This approach affords the advantage for exploration of both adrenals, the retroperitoneal regions and in the female, the ovaries, through one incision and on one occasion.

The supra-umbilical midline incision is made, and manual exploration of both adrenal regions is carried out (see Figs. 265 and 266). The glands are palpated throughout their entire extent and special care is exercised to ascertain their thickness as well as their general size and outlines. Congenital absence of one adrenal is not extremely rare; in a relatively limited number of cases, removal of one of the glands has resulted in death of the patient from adrenal insufficiency, because of the absence of the adrenal on the other side. The importance of ascertaining the thickness of the remaining gland is illustrated by an experience of the writer, who was satisfied that the right gland was normal because its outlines were palpated, but following removal of a large left adrenal cortical carcinoma, death ensued from acute adrenal insufficiency. Necropsy revealed that while the remaining adrenal was normal in length and breadth, it was extremely thin and obviously atrophied and incapable of proper function.

The right adrenal is approached as illustrated in figure 266A. The stomach is retracted to the patient's left, the liver and gallbladder are retracted upward. The posterior parietal peritoneum is incised, along the upper curvature of the duodenum where first and second segments join. This opening exposes the right adrenal gland which lies in an upward and backward direction.

The left adrenal is approached as illustrated in figure 266B. If the stomach is redundant and the gastrohepatic ligament is long, the former is retracted downward and the ligament incised for exposure of the body of the pancreas. The posterior parietal peritoneum along the upper border of the gland is incised and behind the middle third of the gland lies the left adrenal. When the stomach is not redundant and the gastrohepatic omentum is short, the body of the pancreas is exposed by transection of the gastrocolic omentum with retraction of the stomach upward and the colon downward. The left adrenal is located as described above. In figure 267, the entire adrenal gland, together with a neoplasm arising from it, has been removed.

Partial adrenalectomy and denervations of these glands are procedures of historic interest only and, on the basis of present knowledge, cannot be classified as operations that have general surgical approval.

12

THE GALLBLADDER AND BILE DUCTS

Warren H. Cole, M.D.

NORMAL ANATOMY

Gallbladder. The gallbladder is a pear shaped organ situated in a fossa on the inferior surface of the liver between the right and quadrate lobes. It measures 7 to 10 cm. in length and when filled contains 30 to 40 cc. of bile. The dome or broadest portion is designated as the fundus and the narrowest part as the neck; the intervening portion is the body. The neck of the gallbladder projects inferiorly, forming a sacculation known as Hartmann's pouch, which at times may project so far downward as to lie against the common duct or duodenum. The exposed surface of the gallbladder is covered with peritoneum which is derived from the surface of the liver. In people with average build, the gallbladder may be located approximately beneath a point where the tip of the ninth right costal cartilage crosses the midclavicular line.

Bile Ducts. The neck of the gallbladder terminates in the *cystic duct* which is 3 to 4 cm. in length and 2 to 4 mm. in diameter. The duct curves with an invariable course, and empties into the hepatic duct at an acute angle. The inner wall of the cystic duct contains folds designated as valves of Heister, which traditionally are supposed to have a spiral pattern. This pattern is rarely seen in the specimen removed at the operating room, suggesting that variations in the valves of Heister may be associated with gallbladder disease.

The *hepatic* or *common hepatic duct* is formed by the junction of the right and left hepatic ducts just within the liver at the hilus. In slightly less than 10 per cent of cases, the duct bifurcates into the right and left branches just outside the liver. The duct varies in length, but averages about 4 cm. in length and 7 mm. in diameter (see Fig. 268).

The *common bile duct* is formed by the junction of the cystic and hepatic ducts. It is 8 to 10 cm. long and about 1 cm. wide. On the average, less than 2 cm. of the duct lie above the duodenum. At this point the duct lies in the hepatoduodenal ligament to the right of the hepatic artery and anterior to the portal vein. The foramen of Winslow is an opening posterior to these structures, connecting the greater peritoneal cavity with the lesser. The remainder of the duct extends down posterior to the duodenum, traversing the periphery of the head of the pancreas or lying in a sulcus adjacent to the pancreas. In slightly over half the cases it unites with the pancreatic duct

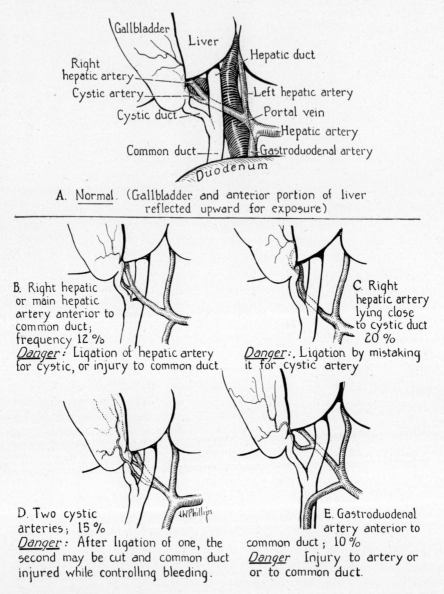

A. Normal. (Gallbladder and anterior portion of liver reflected upward for exposure)

B. Right hepatic or main hepatic artery anterior to common duct; frequency 12%
Danger: Ligation of hepatic artery for cystic, or injury to common duct.

C. Right hepatic artery lying close to cystic duct 20%
Danger: Ligation by mistaking it for cystic artery

D. Two cystic arteries; 15%
Danger: After ligation of one, the second may be cut and common duct injured while controlling bleeding.

E. Gastroduodenal artery anterior to common duct; 10%
Danger Injury to artery or to common duct.

FIG. 268. Anatomy of the biliary system. There are so many anomalies in this region that the "normal" as depicted in A, is in reality a composite of the most common variations encountered. The remainder of the types shown (B to K) represent the anomalies most apt to lead to difficulty or complications of operation on the biliary tract. (Prepared for movie on Anomalies and Strictures of the Common Duct, for the *American College of Surgeons*, 1947. Courtesy of American College of Surgeons.)

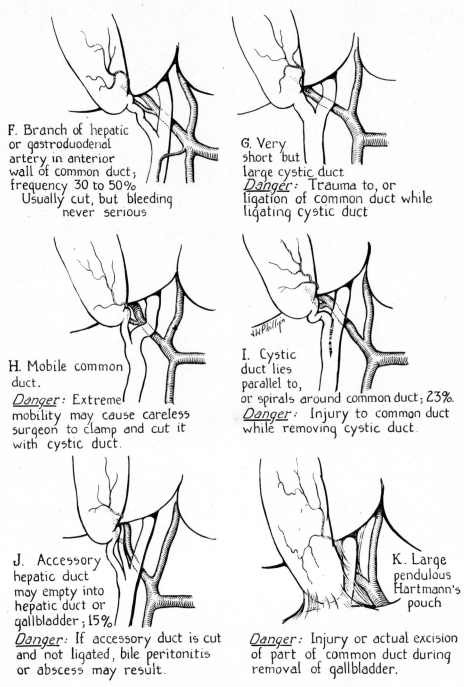

F. Branch of hepatic
or gastroduodenal
artery in anterior
wall of common duct;
frequency 30 to 50%
Usually cut, but bleeding
never serious

G. Very
short but
large cystic duct
Danger: Trauma to, or
ligation of common duct while
ligating cystic duct

H. Mobile common
duct.
Danger: Extreme
mobility may cause careless
surgeon to clamp and cut it
with cystic duct.

I. Cystic
duct lies
parallel to,
or spirals around common duct; 23%.
Danger: Injury to common duct
while removing cystic duct.

J. Accessory
hepatic duct
may empty into
hepatic duct or
gallbladder; 15%
Danger: If accessory duct is cut
and not ligated, bile peritonitis
or abscess may result.

K. Large
pendulous
Hartmann's
pouch

Danger: Injury or actual excision
of part of common duct during
removal of gallbladder.

FIG. 268. Anatomy of the biliary system continued.

to form an ampulla 2 to 4 mm. from its entry into the duodenum. Frequently the two ducts pierce the duodenal wall separately. The ampulla is surrounded by circular as well as longitudinal muscle fibers, constituting the sphincter of Oddi.

Hepatic and Cystic Arteries. The hepatic artery divides into the right and left hepatic artery at about the level of the junction of the cystic duct with the hepatic. The cystic artery usually is a branch of the right hepatic (see Fig. 268A). The right hepatic artery normally lies posterior to the common duct, but is extremely variable in location, as discussed later.

The right hepatic artery supplies the right lobe of the liver, and the left branch the left lobe. With very few exceptions, each artery enters the liver adjacent (and slightly superior) to the respective branch of the portal vein (see Fig. 268A). In about 10 per cent of cases the *portal vein* enters the liver before bifurcation. When this anomaly exists, there is more tendency toward anomalies of the hepatic arteries, particularly relative to their point of entry into the liver.

ANOMALIES

Nowhere in the human body are anomalies more common than in the biliary tract, particularly the ducts and arteries. Furthermore. these anomalies probably have greater surgical significance than anywhere else in the body, as will be discussed under Dangers and Precautions. Variations in this region are so common that it is difficult to determine just what is normal. For example, in a study of 200 consecutive autopsies studied by Flint,[1] only 34 per cent could be classified as normal.

Gallbladder. Anomalies of the gallbladder are more spectacular than anomalies of the ducts or arteries, but of much less surgical significance because they are much less common and rarely the cause of technical accidents. Complete absence is extremely rare and perhaps most commonly observed in infancy, with atresia of the hepatic or cystic duct, particularly the former. Occasionally, at operation the surgeon finds a small nubbin of tissue at the proximal end of the cystic duct; this may be of congenital origin but more commonly represents atrophy of the gallbladder following gangrene of the wall or other similar pathologic process. Likewise, on rare occasions, the gallbladder is found buried in the liver. A double gallbladder is 4 to 5 times more common than complete absence. Incomplete duplication is more common than complete duplication with two cystic ducts. When the duplication is incomplete, the anomaly may be trabecular (dependent on outgrowth of hepatic tissue), or diverticular, or created by a septum. Floating gallbladders having little or no attachment to the liver, are very rare, but have been observed. All of these gallbladder anomalies are commonly associated with cholecystitis or gallstones.

Hepatic, Cystic and Gastroduodenal Arteries. Anomalies of the arteries are of more surgical significance than other anomalies. In 79 per cent of cadavers Flint noted that the right hepatic artery arises from the main hepatic trunk (normal), and in 21 per cent from the superior mesenteric. In 4.5 per cent of cadavers Flint found an accessory right hepatic artery, which usually arose from the superior mesenteric. In 12 per cent of autopsy specimens the right hepatic artery crosses to the right, anterior to the common hepatic duct instead of posterior (Eisendrath [2]) as shown in figure 268B. In fully 95 per cent of the cases the cystic artery arises from the right hepatic artery. In at least 20 per cent of patients coming to the operating room for operation on the biliary tract, the right hepatic artery projects far to the right and is parallel to the cystic duct. In about 15 per cent of autopsy specimens there are 2 cystic arteries (Flint [1]); the second artery usually arises from the

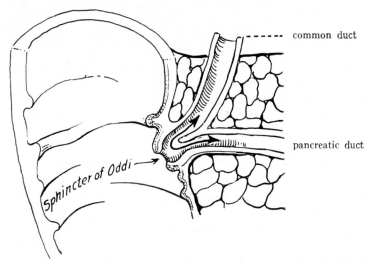

FIG. 269. Although there are numerous variations in the relationship of the terminal end of the common bile duct and the pancreatic duct, the communication illustrated above is found in about one-half of adult humans. (Cole and Elman, *Textbook of General Surgery*, 5th ed., D. Appleton-Century Co., New York, 1948.)

right hepatic artery, but commonly is derived from the gastroduodenal. In 20 per cent of cases, the gastroduodenal artery lies anterior to the retroduodenal portion of the common duct (Eisendrath [2]). Perhaps the most common arterial anomaly is a small artery lying in the anterior wall of the common duct; it may arise from the hepatic or gastroduodenal artery and is present in fully half of patients operated on for biliary tract disease (see Fig. 268F).

The Bile Ducts. Anomalies of the cystic duct are of important significance to the surgeon because they complicate cholecystectomy. A short wide cystic duct is observed in about 5 per cent of patients and may allow passage of small stones into the common duct; when short, the surgeon may mistake the common duct for a continuation of the cystic duct and ligate it during cholecystectomy. On the other hand, the cystic duct is very long and closely adherent to the common duct (see Fig. 268I) in 20 to 25 per cent of patients (Eisendrath). In 15 per cent of autopsy specimens an accessory right hepatic duct is encountered (Flint) arising from the right lobe of the liver and joining the common hepatic duct at almost any level (see Fig. 268J). Less commonly, an accessory duct extends from the right lobe of the liver and empties into the gallbladder on the hepatic side. Unusual mobility of the common duct or projection to the right at the junction with the cystic is fairly common and of importance because of possibility of injury during ligation of the cystic duct, as will be discussed later.

Atresia of the common duct is quite rare and is usually encountered only during infancy because such an anomaly is usually fatal within a few months unless corrected by operation. The normal anatomy at the terminal end of the common duct is illustrated in figure 269.

SURGICAL PHYSIOLOGY

The function of the gallbladder is to store bile, particularly during periods between meals; in the normal gallbladder, the bile is concentrated 8 to 10 times by removal of water through the mucosa (Rous and McMaster [3]). The gallbladder mucosa secretes mucus which accumulates in the gallbladder after obstruction of the cystic or common duct. If the obstruction should extend over a period longer than a few days, the bile pigment may be absorbed and oxidized to such a degree that the contents of the organ are colorless and transparent (white bile). By means of its musculature, the organ is able to contract and empty; fatty food is particularly effective in causing contracture. This contraction usually takes place only at meal time aided by the stimulus of a hormone, cholecystokinin (Ivy and Oldberg [4]) derived from the duodenum and jejunum. Removal of the gallbladder is followed by dilatation of the extrahepatic bile ducts and to a lesser extent the intrahepatic ducts. The function of the gallbladder is by no means vital, since people get along very well following cholecystectomy without any digestive disturbances.

Bile is important in the digestion of fats, and metabolism of vitamin K, but the absence of bile from the intestinal tract can be tolerated for months with very little damage to the nutritional status of the patient unless infection develops. The secretion of bile by the liver may be maintained up to a pressure of 300 mm. of water or more. The gallbladder musculature is able to exert a pressure of about the same degree. Under the influence of severe spasm, the sphincter of Oddi can withstand a pressure equal to or actually greater than this figure, thus accounting for the syndrome of *biliary dyskinesia*. However, under ordinary circumstances the sphincter will open with much less pressure, particularly when the stimulus of food is present.

The sphincter of Oddi is a very valuable structure, protecting the biliary tract from reflux of food and consequent infection. This fact is very important in consideration of the type of operation to be considered; obviously the sphincter should be preserved if at all possible, since the human hand is unable to construct a sphincter with the same degree of protection from reflux and infection.

DANGERS AND PRECAUTIONS IN OPERATIONS
ON THE BILIARY TRACT

As will be discussed later, operative trauma accounts for the majority of strictures of the common duct; erroneous ligation of the right hepatic artery will frequently result in death. Since these technical errors are so serious, it is obvious that all possible effort must be extended to prevent their occurrence.

Not the least important of the pitfalls in gallbladder surgery is hurry on the part of the surgeon. If he fails to take the time to identify the cystic and the common ducts at their junction, the common duct may easily be ligated or constricted by the cystic duct ligature. When in doubt about the identity of the common duct, it should be aspirated with a syringe and hypodermic needle. If the structure in question happens to be the portal vein, no harm is done by the needle puncture.

The anatomy of the biliary tract and its anomalies have been discussed in moderate detail because of their tremendous importance to the safety of operative procedures. Although a complete knowledge of anatomy is essential to the surgeon, anomalies in the region of the biliary tract are so common that the surgeon must see and identify every structure in that area before cutting it. One of the most serious errors made because of anomalies is the mistaken identity of an anomalous right hepatic artery curving toward the cystic duct, and its ligation for the cystic artery. If that vessel is ligated, death will ensue in at least half the cases (R. Graham and Connell [5]). Dissection along the anterior surface of the hepatic duct must be carried out carefully since the right hepatic artery crosses the duct anteriorly in 10 to 15 per cent of cases instead of posteriorly. After identification and ligation of a cystic artery, the surgeon must bear in mind that an accessory cystic artery exists in about 15 per cent of cases. If the accessory cystic artery is cut before grasping with a forceps, it tends to slip back toward the right hepatic artery lying normally under the hepatic duct. Careless grasping of tissue in the region of the spurting vessel is apt to result in clamping of the common duct along with the stump of the cystic artery. When exposure is poor following such accidents, as it usually is because of difficulty in obtaining a dry field, it is usually helpful to insert the left index finger into the foramen of Winslow (if open) and compress the hepatic artery against the thumb or adjacent structures. This will control the hemorrhage and permit exact location of the bleeding point. A much more common source of bleeding is the incision of a small artery (branch of the right hepatic or gastroduodenal artery) in the anterior wall of the common duct when the duct is opened. This artery is present in about 50 per cent of cases, but is so small that its control is rarely difficult.

Anomalies of the cystic duct also requires identification. If the cystic duct is short and the common duct unusually mobile, the common duct may be mistaken for the cystic and ligated, because traction on the gallbladder will make the cystic and common ducts appear as one continuous structure erroneously identified as the cystic alone. Some surgeons emphasize the necessity of dissecting the cystic duct thoroughly from the common duct because in 20 to 25 per cent of cases it is long and adherent to the common duct. They contend that if the cystic duct is ligated too far proximally, the stump may enlarge and form a "pseudo gallbladder," perhaps with recurrence of symptoms. Although the author admits this may occur, he has never seen such a case and is of the opinion that thorough dissection may result in more damage (through injury to the common duct) than good (by elimination of the "pseudo gallbladder"). A remnant of the cystic duct left *in situ* may contain a stone but it will probably produce no symptoms unless it drops into the common duct, which rarely happens. After completion of cholecystectomy the raw area should be inspected closely for the cut surface of accessory hepatic ducts. Looking for escape of bile is not sufficient precaution because a depression of the blood pressure incident to the operation or anesthesia may temporarily cause cessation of bile secretion. If these aberrant ducts are cut and not ligated, a collection of bile followed by peritonitis or abscess formation may develop unless the area is drained and drainage is effective. The greatest danger or complication of collection of bile (with or without abscess formation) in the region of the common duct, is formation of a stricture of the common duct at a later date.

CHOLECYSTOSTOMY

When gallbladder surgery was initiated several decades ago, cholecystostomy was the operation usually performed. However, it was soon discovered that recurrence of symptoms was common following this operation. It is now estimated that 40 to 50 per cent of patients having cholecystostomy for gallbladder disease will have return of symptoms within 5 years. Cholecystectomy has, therefore, become the procedure of choice, but there are occasions when cholecystostomy is definitely indicated instead of cholecystectomy.

Indications. Not infrequently the decision to do a cholecystostomy instead of cholecystectomy may be life saving. Indications are as follows:

1. Since gallbladder disease, including cholelithiasis, is a disease of adult life, it naturally will be common in elderly people who are very *poor operative* risks. If life expectancy is short in these patients and they are such poor risks that cholecystectomy is dangerous, cholecystostomy will be the operation of choice, particularly since it may give complete relief for the few remaining years of life.

2. In the presence of *severe inflammation,* cholecystectomy itself may be extremely difficult and dangerous, particularly if infection has become superimposed on the acute inflammation. Aspiration of the contents of the gallbladder and a stained smear of the material will reveal the presence or absence of bacteria. If infection is present, and the local signs are indicative of a fulminating infection, cholecystectomy may be contraindicated. Chole-

cystostomy is not indicated in all cases of empyema because in many instances infection is of trivial importance or even absent.

3. Patients having severe symptoms due to gallbladder disease, but likewise having some other serious *complicating disease,* may not be able to withstand cholecystectomy.

Technic. The type of incision will vary with different surgeons. Either a paramedian, transrectus or transverse incision may be utilized. For the routine cholecystectomy the author prefers a right paramedian incision because it allows better opportunity for exploration of the rest of the abdomen, although many surgeons feel that patients have less discomfort following a transverse incision (see also Chapter 8).

If the operation is being performed for acute cholecystitis, the adhesions surrounding the area should not be broken up except at the dome of the gallbladder. If there are no adhesions, wet laparotomy pads should be inserted around the gallbladder, protecting the intestines from contamination which may result during the operation. To minimize contamination, a small trochar is inserted into the fundus of the gallbladder and the contents evacuated. To evacuate the gallbladder more completely, the fundus of the gallbladder is then grasped with two Allis forceps and an incision made through the wall with a sharp pointed knife, having a suction tube ready to insert and remove the remainder of the contents. After the fluid is evacuated, the stones are removed with scoops. After all stones have been removed, it is usually wise to insert the finger down toward the cystic duct to see if additional stones can be palpated. Previous to this maneuver the area of the neck of the gallbladder and the cystic duct itself should be palpated, if the field is not obliterated by adhesions, to detect stones in the cystic duct or neck of the gallbladder which might not be detectable from within the gallbladder. A rubber tube with a diameter of about ½ inch is then placed in the gallbladder and a purse-string suture of continuous No. o chromic catgut taken around the tube (see Fig. 270). The inversion of the serosa is made more complete by applying a second purse-string suture around the rubber tube. The tube is anchored to the gallbladder wall by passing the needle through the wall of the tube before tying the suture. If the gallbladder is located very far to the right of the incision, it is usually preferable to make a stab wound at the appropriate place and bring the rubber tube out through this stab wound. The gallbladder should be anchored to the anterior peritoneum, and omentum sutured in place around the area to wall it off as much as possible from the rest of the peritoneal cavity. If the cholecystostomy tube is brought out through the main incision, two or three interrupted sutures can be taken, anchoring the gallbladder wall to the parietal peritoneum, at the same time securing the omentum with the sutures. The wound is then closed around the tube after it is brought out through the original incision. If inflammatory signs are very pronounced, a small Penrose drain should be inserted down to Morrison's pouch (unless obliterated by adhesions), and brought out to the exterior along with the cholecystostomy tube.

The cholecystostomy tube must be anchored thoroughly lest movements of the patient pull it out of the gallbladder. A suture is taken through the skin and wall of the tube and tied. The skin is so sensitive that the patient is not apt to pull the tube out when so anchored. It should be left in 2 or

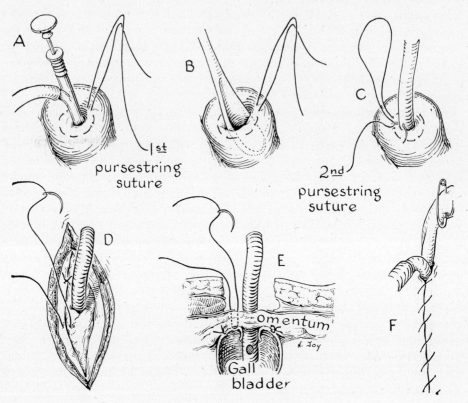

FIG. 270. Technic of cholecystostomy. (A) The gallbladder is evacuated by insertion of a trocar into the fundus; (B) stones are removed with gallbladder scope; (C) a rubber tube is anchored in the gallbladder with a double purse string; (D and E) the gallbladder is anchored to the anterior abdominal wall and the area sealed off with omentum; (F) insertion of a Penrose drain leading down alongside the gallbladder to Morrison's pouch is desirable.

3 weeks, depending upon the progress of the patient. The Penrose drain is removed in 48 to 96 hours depending upon the course of the patient.

Results. When cholecystostomy is performed for removal of stones, the immediate symptomatic results are excellent, but stones as well as symptoms are very apt to recur. For example, in a follow up study made by Black,[7] he noted that 24 per cent of patients upon whom cholecystostomy had been performed had required an additional operation, compared to only 1.8 per cent of patients needing an additional operation following cholecystectomy. Actually the figure of 24 per cent is lower than the experience of many surgeons. It is conservative to estimate that at least 50 per cent of patients having cholecystostomy will have serious symptoms within 4 or 5 years after operation. The mortality rate of cholecystostomy will be 6 to 8 per cent, which is actually higher than that of cholecystectomy. This relatively high mortality is not indicative of the seriousness or magnitude of the operation, but reflects the condition of the patient; cholecystostomy is rarely performed now unless the patient is a very poor operative risk.

CHOLECYSTECTOMY

Since it has been shown that cholecystostomy is so frequently followed by recurrence of symptoms within one to three years, cholecystectomy is now the procedure of choice except under circumstances just described under cholecystostomy.

Indications. 1. *Abdominal pain* of gallbladder origin is an indication for cholecystectomy, but considerable difficulty may be encountered in determining just how much pain the patient must have before operation is justified. The surgeon may obtain considerable assistance from the patient in making such decisions by questioning him closely as to the severity of pain. In other words, is he, the patient, having so much pain that he is willing to undergo the expense and discomfort of an operation to eradicate the pain? However, as described below, cholecystectomy may be indicated, even though pain is minimal or absent.

2. *Cholelithiasis* is considered by many surgeons to be adequate indication for cholecystectomy regardless of the presence or absence of pain. The author agrees that all people under the age of forty-five or fifty should have cholecystectomy for stones even though no pain is present. Justification for cholecystectomy as just indicated for asymptomatic gallstones is based on the fact that if the patient must carry gallstones for 20 to 30 years, the chance of development of a serious or fatal outcome from a complication such as acute cholecystitis with perforation, cancer of the gallbladder, obstruction of the cystic or common duct, or perforation of a stone into a loop of intestine is far greater than the danger of cholecystectomy itself. However, there would appear to be little indication for removal of gallstones if life expectancy is short (*e.g.* 2 to 4 years) since the possibility of development of complications just mentioned would be greatly diminished.

3. *Tumors* represent an indication for cholecystectomy but they are extremely difficult to diagnose.

4. *Secondary disease of other organs* may be a strong indication for cholecystectomy. The common secondary lesions produced by cholecystitis are hepatitis, pancreatitis and intestinal obstruction caused by duodenal adhesions.

5. *Obstruction of the cystic or common duct* usually demands operative interference. When the cystic duct is blocked, hydrops follows and in many occasions empyema develops. When a stone is present in the common duct, cholecystectomy as well as choledochostomy is usually advisable along with removal of the stone because many stones in the common duct no doubt

originate as small stones in the gallbladder and are passed into the common duct by way of the cystic duct.

6. *Trauma* may be an indication for removing the gallbladder but if the perforation occurs at the dome, cholecystostomy may be adequate.

Technic. A paramedian, transrectus or transverse incision will give adequate exposure for a cholecystectomy. The surgeon should use the one which he is accustomed to and prefers. The author prefers a right paramedian. Thorough exploration is made to confirm the diagnosis and exclude other important lesions. The common duct is palpated, particularly with the index finger in the foramen of Winslow. It may be desirable to incise the peritoneum over the common duct so it can be exposed for more thorough examination. If exposure is unsatisfactory or the operation appears difficult, the falciform ligament is grasped with a forceps, cut, and the liver rotated upward to facilitate exposure. The fundus of the gallbladder is grasped with forceps and another applied to the neck of the gallbladder; traction upward will improve exposure of the junction of the cystic and common duct (see Figs. 271 and 272).

In the average case, the author prefers to start dissection in removal of the gallbladder at the cystic duct, and dissect upward toward the fundus. The incision of the peritoneum over the common duct is extended toward the junction of the cystic duct with a scissors or by blunt dissection. The cystic duct is isolated first and two clamps applied to the lower end and the duct cut between the clamps. This allows exposure of the cystic artery which lies superior and slightly posterior to the duct. Again with blunt dissection the artery is isolated and clamped and cut as was the duct. Before dissecting the gallbladder from its bed, it is helpful to inject some saline with a hypodermic needle and syringe into the margin of the gallbladder bed on either side to facilitate incision. The attachments of the gallbladder to the gallbladder fossa are then cut by sharp dissection from below upward, watching for an accessory hepatic duct or cystic artery. If an accessory duct is cut during excision of the gallbladder, it should be ligated carefully lest bile accumulate later and produce a bile peritonitis or abscess. On most occasions there will be a moderate amount of hemorrhage from the gallbladder fossa. These vessels cannot be tied if the bleeding is from the liver itself, but is controlled by a gauze pack until the surgeon is ready to suture the gallbladder bed. The cystic artery and duct are tied separately, using strong silk or cotton. The gauze pack is then removed from the gallbladder fossa and the raw area approximated with a running suture of No. 000 chromic catgut. This will control bleeding from all points except spurting vessels which should be controlled by an individual suture. The wound is then closed around a Penrose drain inserted down to the stump of the cystic duct to allow exit of bile in case an accessory duct is cut and not tied, or in case the suture slips off the stump of the cystic duct. It is well known that a single drain does not drain the peritoneal cavity. However, when the abdominal cavity has been drained following cholecystectomy the author has never seen bile peritonitis, or a local abscess secondary to accumulation of bile, fol-

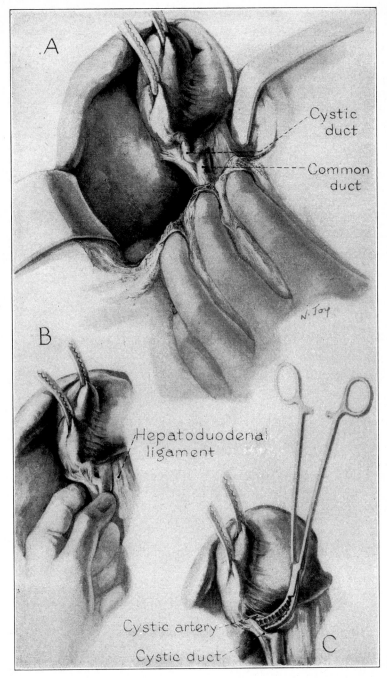

FIG. 271. Technic of cholecystectomy. (A) The junction of the cystic and common duct is isolated; (B) the common duct is palpated for stones by inserting the index finger into the foramen of Winslow; (C) the cystic duct is dissected from the cystic artery.

lowing leakage of bile into the peritoneal cavity, although he has seen large amounts of bile escape through the drainage site on innumerable occasions. The answer to this seemingly contradictory situation probably lies in the fact that it takes a large quantity of bile to give rise to an abscess, and the major portion of bile escaping from a duct will drain to the exterior alongside a properly placed drain. The omentum is brought up and placed over the duodenum and other organs to protect them from adhesions to the suture line in the liver.

The wound is closed in layers around the drain, unless more direct drainage is achieved by bringing the drain out through a stab wound. The author closes the peritoneum with No. o chromic catgut and the fascia with interrupted cotton. The drain is removed in 48 hours.

When cholecystectomy is being performed for *carcinoma of the gall-bladder* a variation in technic will be necessary, with removal of that portion of the liver adjacent to the gallbladder. Unfortunately, carcinoma of the gallbladder is a rapidly invading tumor and very difficult to diagnose in its early stages. For the two reasons just noted, the 5 year cure rate is very low, being much less than 10 per cent. Obviously, if metastases are present in the liver or elsewhere, cholecystectomy will not be indicated.

Resection of liver tissue adjacent to the gallbladder can be accomplished readily along with removal of the gallbladder by application of several through-and-through sutures (preferably catgut) on each side of the gall-bladder for the control of hemorrhage. These sutures are inserted from the dorsal side of the liver to the ventral surface and back again; each one is tied before resection of the gallbladder and adjacent liver tissue is begun. In spite of numerous sutures taken through the liver for control of bleeding, considerable hemorrhage will usually take place during resection. Therefore, once incision is begun it is preferable to proceed rapidly with excision of the mass since bleeding points cannot be controlled until the entire mass is removed, except that digital pressure between the hilus and dome of the liver often minimizes bleeding. Rarely will a large pack fail to control hemorrhage; by removing the pack gradually, additional sutures may be taken to control bleeding points. If the hemorrhage arises from numerous points and under low pressure, application of a large piece of gelfoam or similar absorbable hemostatic agent will be efficient in controlling the bleeding.

Results. The symptomatic results following cholecystectomy are comparatively good, but are directly related to the correctness of diagnosis and type of symptoms. All surgeons have observed better results following cholecystectomy when "typical" gallbladder pain is present than when dyspepsia or mild indefinite pain is the important symptom. At least 90 per cent of patients with gallbladder pain of severe degree will have good results following cholecystectomy. Results are likewise better if stones are present. For example, in a study of 610 cholecystectomies, Lehman and associates [8] noted satisfactory results in 79 per cent of patients with stones contrasted to only 64 per cent good results in patients without stones.

The results of cholecystectomy on duration of life is well illustrated by the study conducted by Dublin and associates,[9] who noted that the death

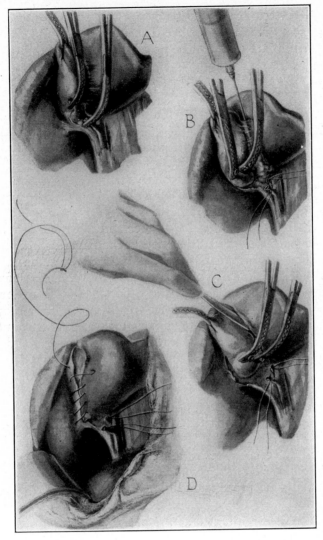

FIG. 272. Technic of cholecystectomy, continued. (A) The cystic duct and cystic artery are ligated separately; (B) injection of saline alongside the gallbladder will facilitate its dissection from the liver bed, but is by no means necessary; (C) the peritoneum at the edge of the gallbladder is incised, and the gallbladder removed from below upward; (D) the raw area in the liver bed is obliterated with a continuous suture of fine catgut. When the area around the common duct is covered with dense adhesions, it is safer to start dissection from above downward.

rate in patients having had cholecystostomy was 155.7 per cent of the expected rate, compared to 115.1 per cent in patients treated medically, and only 95.9 per cent of the expected rate in patients who had had cholecystectomy. The above figures prove rather conclusively that the gallbladder is not necessary to life, and that removal of a diseased gallbladder is often a life saving procedure.

Previous to the advent of sulfonamides and penicillin, the mortality rate following cholecystectomy alone was 6 to 7 per cent. Although insufficient time has elapsed to obtain data since that period, it can be estimated fairly accurately that the rate now will be no higher than 2 or 3 per cent.

CHOLEDOCHOTOMY AND CHOLEDOCHOSTOMY

When stones are present in the common duct, it should be opened, the stones removed, and the gallbladder likewise taken out unless there are contraindications such as might exist when emergency operation is performed for suppurative cholangitis.

Since malignant tumors (particularly carcinoma of the head of the pancreas or ampulla of Vater) as well as stones, may result in dilatation of the common duct, the surgeon must at all times be mindful of the significance of Courvoisier's law. For example, jaundice and obstruction of the common duct induced by a carcinoma of the head of the pancreas is accompanied by a dilated gallbladder, whereas jaundice produced by stone in the duct is accompanied by a small, shrunken and usually fibrotic gallbladder.

Indications. On most occasions, the common duct is opened to search for and remove stones. However, they are by no means always palpable. Certain pathologic features, as discussed below, may be encountered which suggest the presence of stones and serve as indication for opening the duct:

1. When a *stone is palpable* in the common duct it is obvious that incision into the duct and removal of the stone is indicated.
2. *Dilatation of the duct* is a strong indication of obstruction distal to the dilated area. Such obstruction, particularly when caused by stones, is usually located in the pancreatic portion of the duct or at the ampulla of Vater, although stones may shift about and be found at variable positions in the duct.
3. *A thickened wall of the common duct* is usually indicative of a chronic inflammatory process and likewise is usually caused by stones within the duct.
4. The *presence of jaundice with pain* is a fairly accurate indication of common duct obstruction. A history of jaundice may or may not be an indication for opening a duct because one of the most common causes of jaundice of several days' or a few weeks' duration is a medical disease, namely virus hepatitis (acute catarrhal icterus).
5. There are several *miscellaneous* indications, including suppurative cholangitis, strictures, tumors and obstructions due to lesions in the pancreas.

Technic. Exposure may be obtained satisfactorily by one of three types of incision, namely: paramedian, transrectus and transverse, as described in Chapter 8. One important precaution is that good exposure be obtained so that good vision of the operative field is possible. The incision is lengthened until satisfactory exposure is achieved. Exposure is facilitated very much indeed by the assistant's skillful use of his hands and gauze packs. The stomach and duodenum can be held away from the common duct by his hand probably better than by retractors although mild retraction on the sides will be advantageous.

Opinions may differ as to whether a cholecystectomy should precede or follow choledochostomy, assuming that cholecystectomy is also indicated. In general, surgeons are apt to explore the common duct first, leaving the gall-bladder in for use as traction to elevate the liver and bile ducts. The main disadvantage of leaving the gallbladder in while the common duct is being explored is that small stones might drop down through a large cystic duct into the common duct during the procedure of the cholecystectomy. This can be obviated by putting a clamp on the cystic duct before the common duct is explored. Palpation of the common duct for stones must always be done from above downward because of the danger of forcing stones upward into the liver. It is much more difficult to get a stone out of the intrahepatic ducts than out of the pancreatic portion of the common duct.

The peritoneum over the common duct is incised and fatty tissue dissected bluntly from the anterior surface of the duct to allow identification and exposure of the duct. During this dissection it is essential that the surgeon watch constantly for an anomalous hepatic artery which may cross anterior to the duct or protrude over it. With very few exceptions positive identification of the common duct by aspiration with a syringe and hypodermic needle is indicated before opening it. Before incising the duct, it is advisable to attain fixation by placing a stay suture of silk, cotton or catgut on each side of the proposed incision. By elevating the duct there is less danger of cutting through both walls and perhaps injuring the portal vein below. When an incision 1 to 2 cm. long is made in the common duct, suction is applied to minimize contamination because very frequently the bile is infected with *E. coli, streptococci,* etc. (see Fig. 273).

A scoop which can be bent at an angle is chosen to explore the ducts. A long thin scoop is preferable to a large circular one because a large scoop is apt to push the stone ahead of it. This problem of the choice of a scoop and its manipulations is much more important than assumed by most surgeons. It is very easy by careless manipulation to push the stone ahead either into one of the hepatic ducts or into the pancreatic portion of the common duct. If the scoop is pushed posteriorly against the wall of the duct, as it is inserted upward or downward in the duct, it is less apt to push the stone ahead of it. Likewise the angle of insertion into the duct is important, since if the neck of the scoop is bent too much the end of the scoop will encroach on the anterior wall and thus tend to push stones forward ahead of it.

In general, faceted stones indicate the presence of more than one stone. A small catheter may be inserted upward and downward into the duct and the duct flushed out with saline, hoping to wash out stones. Occasionally suction applied with a syringe and catheter will dislodge stones. It is always advisable to palpate the duct more than once because the manipu-

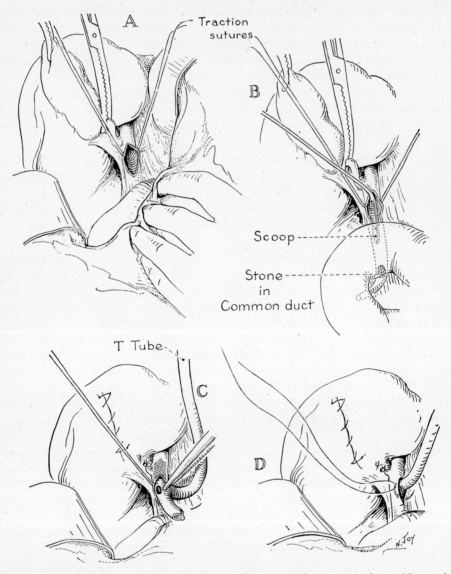

FIG. 273. Choledochostomy. (A) After identification of the common duct with a syringe and hypodermic needle, two stay sutures are taken in the wall and the duct opened; (B) stones are removed with proper gallbladder scoops; (C) after removal of all stones, a T tube is inserted; (D) the opening in the duct is closed around the tube. The gallbladder may be removed before or after exploration of the common duct; if afterward, the cystic duct should be clamped with a forceps as in A, to prevent stones from slipping through a dilated cystic duct into the common.

lation of exploration may dislodge stones and make them palpable, whereas upon first examination they were not. Nodules in the pancreas may confuse a surgeon a great deal. When there is doubt about the identity of the nodule, it is helpful to insert a large probe into the duct and then palpate the area for relationship of the nodule to the probe. This problem becomes more important when we realize that many stones are rather firmly lodged in the lower end of the common duct, and may actually ulcerate through the duct to become "encysted" and therefore difficult to remove; "encysted" stones are usually located at the ampulla of Vater.

Opinions differ as to the use of dilators for the sphincter of Oddi. Some surgeons prefer to pass a sound up to 20 to 22F hoping that this may encourage passage of small stones and other debris in the common duct and will discourage any tendency toward spasm of the sphincter. However, the author does not believe in dilatation of the sphincter of Oddi, although he is convinced of the necessity of insertion of an appropriate sound or thick probe through the sphincter to be sure that no stricture or stone is present at the ampulla. As a matter of fact, the operation cannot be considered to be complete until the surgeon is convinced that he is able to pass a sound or probe through the sphincter of Oddi into the lumen of the duodenum. It is very easy to misinterpret the position of the probe in the terminal end of the common duct. Ordinarily, after it is in the lumen of the duodenum, pressure of the probe against the anterior duodenal wall will make it obvious that only the anterior wall intervenes.

When the stone cannot be dislodged after a moderate amount of manipulation a transduodenal approach should be made to remove it. The duodenum is mobilized by cutting the peritoneum on its lateral border and a longitudinal incision made in it over the ampulla of Vater, which is located at the lower end of the second portion of the duodenum (see Fig. 274). After opening the duodenum, search is made for the sphincter of Oddi. If it cannot be seen, as is frequently the case, the stone is pushed forward with the finger against the wall of the duodenum and search is then made for the sphincter. The sphincter is dilated with blunt forceps and an incision made at an appropriate place to allow evacuation of the stone. If any incision is required in addition to dilatation of the sphincter, it is made directly over the stone so as to obviate danger of penetrating into the open tissues posteriorly. After extraction of the stone, it may be necessary to suture the mucosal surface of the common duct to the mucosa of the duodenum to prevent stricture formation or invasion of infection posteriorly. After additional palpation and insertion of probes has convinced the surgeon that no more stones remain in the common duct, the incision in the anterior wall of the duodenum is closed in a transverse direction, utilizing continuous catgut for the first layer and interrupted silk or cotton for the second layer. It is usually desirable to take a few sutures to act as a third layer because of the seriousness of leakage at this point if it should occur. However, too much inversion of tissue at the site of incision may actually produce an obstruction.

After the stones are removed from the common duct a T tube should be inserted to allow drainage of bile. The tube should be smaller than the common duct to facilitate its easy removal, and likewise to allow passage of bile around it in case it does become plugged. However, it must be emphasized that small tubes of the 14 to 16F size are apt to supply inadequate drainage on occasions when drainage is important. The two ends of the T tube are cut so that each arm is no longer than 1.5 cm. It is highly desirable to cut a small piece out of the posterior part of the T tube just opposite the junction of the two tubes to facilitate removal (see Fig. 273). The opening in

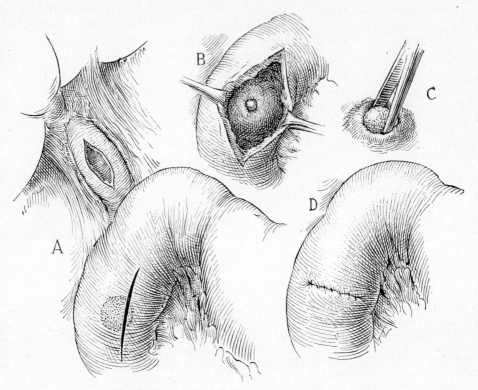

FIG. 274. Transduodenal removal of stones impacted in the distal end of the common duct. (A and B) When the stone cannot be removed through an opening in the common duct, a longitudinal opening is made in the duodenum over the ampulla of Vater; (C) the stone is extracted, frequently only after a slit is made in the sphincter; (D) after removal of the stone the opening in the duodenum is closed in a transverse direction. (From Cole, W. H., *Illinois State M. J.,* 1939.)

the common duct is then closed around the tube with interrupted sutures of catgut. Nonabsorbable sutures must not be used for this purpose because they would prevent removal of the tube, and likewise might encourage deposition of bile precipitates at the point where they pierce the internal wall of the duct.

After the surgeon has achieved a water tight closure around the T tube, the gallbladder is removed as indicated and as described previously. A Penrose drain is left in the wound leading down to Morrison's pouch and is brought out of the wound alongside the T tube through the upper portion of the wound or through a stab wound to the right of the wound, depending upon which may allow better drainage.

Results. Removal of stones from the common duct is associated with a high incidence of fairly complete relief (60 to 70 per cent) but numerous complications prevent much better results. Overlooking a stone is one of the most important causes of failure. Pancreatitis, hepatitis, severe inflammation of the common duct, and biliary dyskinesia represent complications which may prevent good results. Rarely indeed does a stricture form at the site of choledochostomy. Previous to the use of sulfonamides and penicillin the mortality rate following choledochostomy for stone was about 10 per cent. During recent years the rate is probably no greater than 4 or 5 per cent.

STRICTURES OF THE COMMON DUCT

Etiology. All surgeons have been impressed with the fact that most strictures of the common duct are secondary to operations on the biliary system, and in fact are produced by trauma, itself. In a series of 49 cases encountered at the Illinois Research and Educational Hospital we [10] found that in 65 per cent the cause could be designated without question as being traumatic in origin. In our series [10] there was an additional 23 per cent which we designated as being inflammatory in origin. In this group, symptoms of the stricture did not develop for several months (4 months to 5 years) following operation. However, it is safe to assume that probably in half of these the stricture was secondary to the operation. In a study of 188 cases, Flickinger and Masson [11] concluded that 73 per cent of the strictures resulted from surgical trauma. Figures presented by other authors are usually higher, *e.g.* Cattell [12] 80 per cent and Walters [13] 90 per cent. See figure 275 for types.

There are three major factors giving rise to surgical accidents leading to stricture; (1) carelessness and haste, (2) insufficient knowledge of anatomy and appreciation of anomalies, and (3) injury to the common duct while controlling the hemorrhage. Perhaps the most common error is excision of part of the duct when traction on the gallbladder distorts it and pulls it into the position normally occupied by the cystic duct. When Hartmann's pouch is unusually large and densely adherent to the common duct there is great danger of injury to the duct during cholecystectomy, as has been emphasized by R. Graham.[6] Short, thick cystic ducts likewise may be responsible for injury to the common duct because of close proximity. When accessory hepatic ducts are cut and not ligated the resultant accumulation of bile may give rise to fibrosis and obliterative cholangitis unless effective drainage is established to the exterior. Many injuries to the common duct are sustained while the surgeon is attempting to control hemorrhage. If the surgeon loses his presence of mind and commences to stab blindly in the bloody field, he may include a portion of the common duct in the clamp or ligature controlling the bleeding point.

Of the remaining causes of stricture of the common duct, diffuse sclerosing pancreatitis is probably the most important, although it has not been emphasized in the medical literature. In our series of 49 patients, the stricture was caused by chronic sclerosing pancreatitis in 10 per cent of cases.

Abscess about the duct, ulceration through the wall of the common duct by stone, and suppurative cholangitis are other etiologic factors producing stricture. Numerous etiologic factors and mechanisms are illustrated in figure 276.

Prevention of Strictures. Since trauma is the most common cause of stricture of the common duct, it is obvious that the surgical profession must take all precautions to prevent stricture. Listed below are numerous precautions, which if heeded will minimize possibility of stricture formation.

(1) Obtain good exposure during operations on the biliary tract.

(2) Do not be in a hurry when dissecting structures in the neighborhood of the common duct.

(3) Keep constantly in mind possibilities of anomalies.

(4) Isolate the junction of the cystic and common ducts before ligating the former.

(5) Cut no structure until identified.

(6) Ligate no artery in the region of the ducts until it is proven that the vessel enters the gallbladder.

(7) Ligate the cystic duct and artery separately.

(8) When hemorrhage is encountered control it by insertion of the index finger in the foramen of Winslow and compression of the hepatic artery between the finger and thumb (Fig. 277). This procedure will allow accurate ligation of the vessel without inclusion of other structures.

(9) Start dissection of the gallbladder at the fundus when adhesions around the common duct are dense.

(10) During cholecystectomy observe the field closely for severed accessory hepatic ducts and ligate them if present.

(11) Maintain good aseptic care and technic, which will minimize abscess formation.

(12) Avoid delay in the surgical treatment of cholecystitis, particularly if symptoms of disease of the common duct exist.

Operative Repair of Strictures. As in many other surgical lesions, no one type of operation will be applicable to all types of strictures. The need for several types of operation is dependent largely upon the amount of duct involved. The authors have had very poor results with the conventional operation of anastomosis of the hilar duct to the duodenum (see Fig. 278).

If the injury to the duct is detected soon after operation, repair should be effected immediately, since early repair, up to within 10 days of the operation is possible without encountering significant adhesions. Between the third and tenth week following the accident, operation is very difficult because adhesions during this period are very dense and vascular. However, any delay to avoid the complication of adhesions is undesirable because of the danger of development of hepatitis and suppurative cholangitis.

The author prefers a right paramedian incision. Care must be exercised in making this incision since the intestines are usually densely adherent to the peritoneum. Dissection is started along the margin of the liver approaching the hilus from the anterolateral direction. With this approach there is less danger of injury to vital structures such as the portal vein and hepatic artery, since the common duct would be encountered first. However, if the common duct is absent near the hilus, the portal vein will be encountered

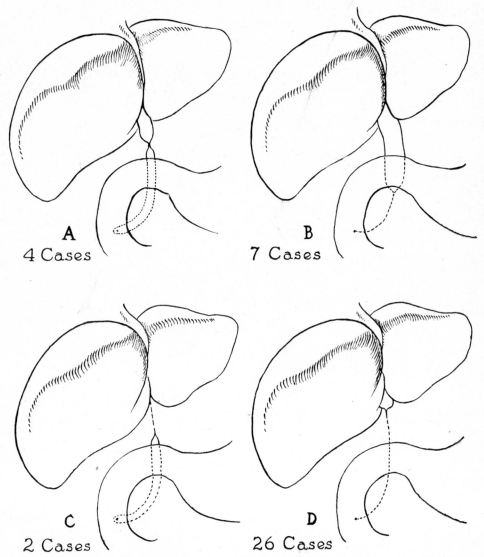

A
4 Cases

B
7 Cases

C
2 Cases

D
26 Cases

FIG. 275. Types of strictures of the common duct. (A) Local stricture; (B) stricture of distal end; (C) stricture of upper portion of duct; (D) absence or stricture of entire duct. (Modified from Cole, Ireneus and Reynolds, *Ann. Surg.*, 122:494, 1945.)

first and may be injured unless the surgeon is extremely careful. Aspiration of the structures in this region with a syringe and hypodermic needle will aid greatly in identifying the stump of the common duct and portal vein. Exposure of the hilar area is achieved as shown in figure 279.

The duodenum and head of the pancreas should be thoroughly mobilized in the search for the distal end of the common duct, because the sphincter of Oddi is such an important structure and cannot be duplicated by the

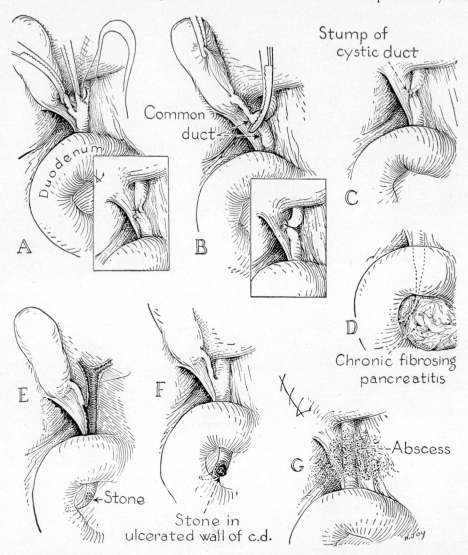

FIG. 276. Mechanisms in production of stricture of common duct; (A) transfixion with a needle; (B) ligation with the cystic; (C) ligation of the cystic duct too close to the common; (D) chronic diffuse sclerosing pancreatitis; (E) cholangitis; (F) ulceration of the wall by stone; and (G) abscess or local collection of bile. (From Cole, *Can. Med. Assn.*, 1948.)

surgeon. Cattell [12] advises splitting the head of the pancreas in the effort to find the distal end of the common duct. If the distal end can be found it can usually be brought up to meet the proximal end, and an end-to-end anastomosis performed as described below.

REPAIR OF LOCAL STRICTURES. If the stricture is confined to a small area in the duct there will be no difficulty in excising the stenosed area and approximating the two ends. When this repair is possible, insertion of one row of interrupted sutures is usually all that need be done, except that

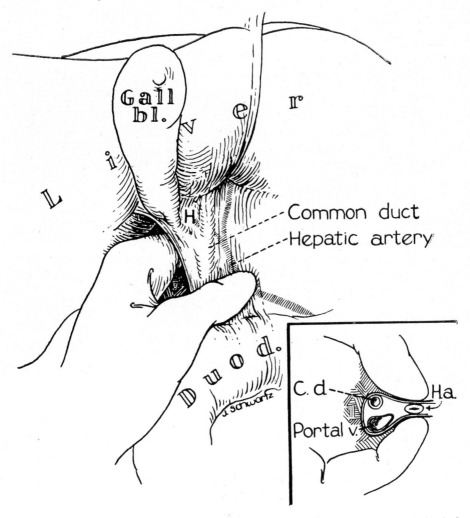

FIG. 277. Control of hemorrhage in region of common duct by insertion of the index finger in the foramen of Winslow and compression of the hepatic artery between the index finger and the thumb.

support of some type for the suture line must be supplied. In repair of this type, the author is of the opinion that a rubber T tube offers the best support, providing it is inserted through an opening separate from the suture line, with one of the longitudinal arms of the T tube extended past the suture line (see Fig. 280). Vitallium tubes have been used by some surgeons in the repair of local strictures, but the author emphatically recommends a T tube, and does not favor use of a vitallium tube in such a repair because these tubes occasionally become plugged with bile precipitates. A rubber tube consisting of part of a catheter, extending from the hilus of the liver downward into the duodenum, may be used for support and held in position by a silk suture anchored to the tube and extending out through the wound, as recommended years ago by McArthur.[14] The suture is anchored to a button or similar object on the skin, and cut three or four months after operation to allow the tube to progress downward into the intestinal tract.

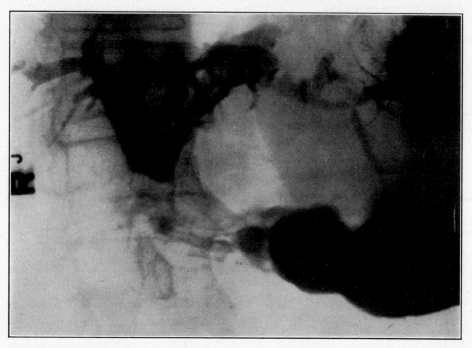

FIG. 278. Reflux of barium (after a barium meal) through the stoma after the old conventional operation of anastomosis of the duodenum to the hilar duct. The patient is having numerous attacks of chills and fever and should have another operation, preferably another type. (From Cole, Ireneus and Reynolds, *Ann. Surg.*, 122:503, 1945.)

ANASTOMOSIS OF THE SIDE OF THE COMMON DUCT TO THE DUODENUM. When more than 2 or 3 cms. of common duct are found, and particularly when there is possibility that the stricture may not be permanent, anastomosis of the common duct to the duodenum is justifiable. There are two or three methods of performing this operation, but the one emphasized by Sanders,[15] in which a longitudinal opening is made in the common duct as well as in the duodenum, is the one preferred by the author. In this operation it will be necessary to mobilize the duodenum and head of the pancreas so that the duodenum can lie adjacent to the common duct (see Fig. 281). An outside layer of silk or cotton is placed between the duct and duodenum. Longitudinal incision is then made in the common duct and in the duodenum adjacent; a second or inside row of interrupted fine catgut sutures is then placed. Both rows of sutures are completed throughout the entire circumference. Use of a longitudinal incision in the common duct, as described, should minimize the danger of stricture formation.

In another operation anastomosing the common duct to the duodenum, incision in the common duct is made transversely and the duct sutured to the duodenum, which is brought up to meet the duct. Two rows of interrupted sutures are taken around the stoma, as described above. In either

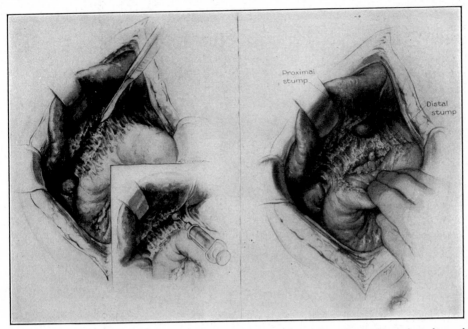

FIG. 279. Exposure of the hilar region is achieved only after sharp dissection through very dense adhesions. (A) The approach is safer from the anterolateral side; the stump of the duct is identified with a syringe and needle; (B) search is made for the distal end of the duct by incision of the peritoneum alongside the duodenum and rolling that structure medially and inferiorly. The distal end of the common duct with the sphincter of Oddi are so important in repair that the head of the pancreas should be split (Cattell) before giving up search for the duct. (From Cole, Ireneus and Reynolds, *Ann. Surg.,* 122:495, 1945.)

operation the surgeon must be careful in obtaining mucosa-to-mucosa approximation.

TRANSPLANTATION OF THE COMMON DUCT INTO THE DUODENUM. On numerous occasions when the stump of the common duct is long and very well mobilized it may be preferable to transplant the duct into the duodenum, particularly when the stricture is complete and there is no chance of restoration of patency. The end of the duct should be excised so that fairly healthy duct wall is obtained for the suture line. A longitudinal incision is made in the duodenum and mucosa-to-mucosa approximation obtained by interrupted sutures of fine catgut. An outside layer of interrupted sutures of silk or cotton should be placed to minimize development of a duodenal fistula (see Fig. 282).

ANASTOMOSIS OF HILAR DUCT TO ROUX Y ARM OF JEJUNUM. The author is convinced that use of the Roux Y arm of jejunum in repair of complete absence of the common duct is preferable to other types of operations.

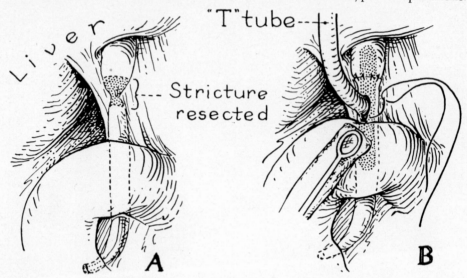

FIG. 280. Repair of local stricture. (A) The stenosed area is resected; (B) A T tube is inserted into the duct through an opening above or below the suture line.

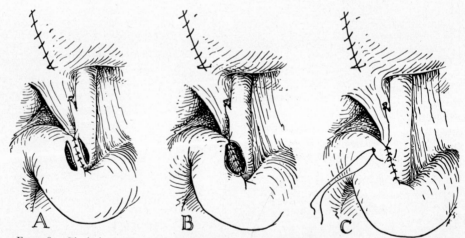

FIG. 281. Choledochoduodenostomy utilizing a longitudinal incision in the common duct (Sanders). (A) A posterior row of interrupted silk or cotton is placed before making the incision; (B) an inside row of interrupted catgut is taken around the stoma; (C) the outside row of silk or cotton is completed.

Obviously this procedure should be utilized only when it is impossible to find the distal end of the duct with preservation of the sphincter of Oddi. The jejunum is severed about 2 feet from the ligament of Treitz. The proximal end is then sutured to the distal end about 18 inches from the point of section. This arm of jejunum is brought up to meet the hilar duct anterior to the colon if the mesentery is long. If the mesentery is short it will be necessary to make an opening in the mesocolon and bring the arm up posterior to the colon as illustrated in figure 283. Some type of support is necessary at the suture line. A vitallium or rubber tube may be used, but recently the author has been using a T tube, inserted through an opening in the terminal end of the jejunum about 3 cm. from the anastomotic line, with one arm extending past the stoma. It is removed in 4 or 5 months.

Use of Vitallium Tube. When utilizing the Roux Y arm of jejunum, use of the vitallium tube (as introduced by Pearse) is a fairly satisfactory method of maintaining patency of the stoma. The bell end of the tube is inserted up

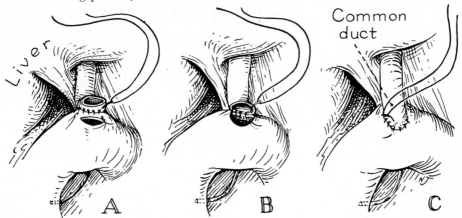

Fig. 282. Transplantation of the common duct into the duodenum. (A) An outside row of interrupted silk or cotton is taken; (B) the inside row consists of interrupted sutures of fine catgut; (C) the outside row is completed.

into the hilar duct and anchored with a purse string (see Fig. 283). The end of the Roux Y arm of jejunum is closed by inverting sutures leaving a small opening in the center through which the vitallium tube is to be threaded. Interrupted sutures are taken between the hilus of the liver and the end of the jejunum, but none are tied until all are placed. The distal end of the tube is then threaded into the arm of jejunum and held in position while interrupted sutures are tied, holding the end of the jejunum against the hilus of the liver. Maintenance of position of the tube in the arm of jejunum is best accomplished by insertion of a long clamp through a hole in the wall of the jejunum about 2 inches from its end. After the approximation is completed this opening is closed. The wound is closed in the usual fashion and a drain is left down to the anastomotic site and left in place for five or six days in case a fistula should develop. Omentum is pulled upward and placed in position over the intestines to minimize reformation of adhesions.

Use of Rubber Catheter. In 1945, Allen [16] suggested use of a rubber catheter in supporting the suture line between the Roux Y arm of jejunum and hilar duct. The bell end of the catheter is inserted upward into the hilar duct and anchored with interrupted sutures. The end of the jejunum

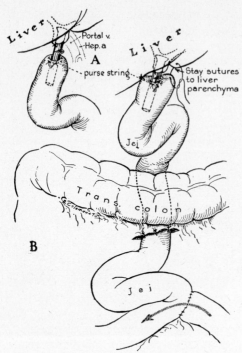

FIG. 283. Two methods of anchoring vitallium tube and end of jejunum are available. In method illustrated the purse string taken in the duct stump and end of jejunum will make a water-tight anastomosis. However, a second method recently utilized by the author consisting of fixation of flange of tube to liver anteriorly with a silk suture, and fixation to liver posteriorly with a silk suture around the tube may slightly minimize tendency toward recurrence of stricture. In this second method there will usually be leakage of bile for a few days alongside drain placed at completion of operation. Although end of jejunum is attached firmly with interrupted sutures to liver around the stump of the bile duct; the tube anchored by this method will remain in place 3 to 6 months. The author has also used the McArthur principle of attaching a silk suture to vitallium (or rubber) tube and bringing it to outside with fixation over a button; 3 or 4 months later the suture is cut allowing tube to pass on down intestine. (Modified from Cole, Ireneus and Reynolds, *Ann. Surg.*, 122:499, 1945.)

is turned in with formation of a cuff (see Figs. 284 and 285). The distal end of the catheter is threaded into the arm of jejunum and brought out through an opening in the wall of the jejunum so that the catheter can be extended anteriorly to the exterior. A hole is made in the rubber catheter 2 or 3 inches from the end so that bile may flow through the catheter into the lumen of the intestines as well as to the exterior through the catheter itself. The opening in the jejunum is surrounded with omentum to prevent diffuse contamination. The catheter is left in place for three months.

Allen [17] has recently modified this method by inserting a Blakemore vascular vitallium tube over the catheter so that the metal tube will act as support to the suture line.

Use of Mucosal Flap of Jejunum (Modified Hoag Operation). In 1937 Hoag [18] suggested the use of a mucosal flap of stomach supported by a short piece of rubber catheter for establishing continuity with the hilar duct. The author believes this method has definite merit, but has modified the procedure by constructing a tube of mucosa at the end of the Roux Y arm of jejunum (see Fig. 286). After the mucosal flap has been anchored to a short rubber tube, obtained by cutting off the bell end of a catheter, the end of jejunum is inserted upward into the opening at the hilus of the liver and anchored in place with interrupted sutures. This operation would appear to have its greatest usefulness when the stump of the common duct does not protrude beyond the liver, but is actually found within the liver. On numerous occasions it is necessary to cut through scar tissue at the hilus of the liver before normal duct mucosa can be found. As much scar tissue should be excised as possible without jeopardizing the portal vein and the raw areas at the hilus of the liver can then be covered with the mucosal flap. As stated previously, it is probably preferable to use a T tube for this purpose, utilizing one arm of the tube for support at the stoma.

ANASTOMOSIS OF LEFT INTRA-HEPATIC DUCT TO ROUX Y ARM OF JEJUNUM. Recently Longmire and Sanford [19] have reported a method consisting of cutting across the left lobe of the liver to obtain exposure of the cut end of a major intra-hepatic duct, particularly when the common hepatic duct cannot be found at the hilus. The cut is made across the lobe slightly to the left of the round ligament, controlling vessels with mattress sutures. When a satisfactory duct is found the remainder of the lobe is resected so that a loop of jejunum can be brought up against the cut surface of the liver and the end of the duct sutured to a small opening in the intestine obtaining mucosa-to-mucosa contact. The jejunum is anchored to the cut surface of the liver with numerous interrupted silk or cotton sutures. An entero-enterostomy is performed between the two arms of jejunum going to the liver. If desirable, a Roux Y arm of jejunum can be constructed, anastomosing the cut end of bile duct to a small opening near the closed end of jejunum. This method will be very useful when the bile duct cannot be found at the hilus.

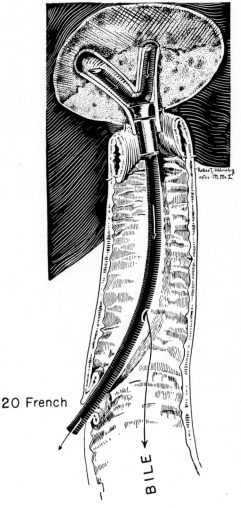

20 French

BILE

FIG. 284. Allen has modified his original operation and now inserts a Y rubber tube into the two arms of the hepatic duct; a vitallium tube is threaded over the tube which is brought to the exterior through a hole in the wall of the jejunum. (Courtesy of Arthur Allen.)

CHOLECYSTENTEROSTOMY. When the gallbladder is present and not seriously diseased, it may be used in performance of the anastomosis between the biliary tract and the intestinal tract. Under ordinary circumstances this is a poor operation if the patient is expected to live very long because the stoma tends to constrict down and stenose. However, when there is possibility that the patency of the common duct will be restored and when it is very difficult to obtain exposure of the common duct, such an operation

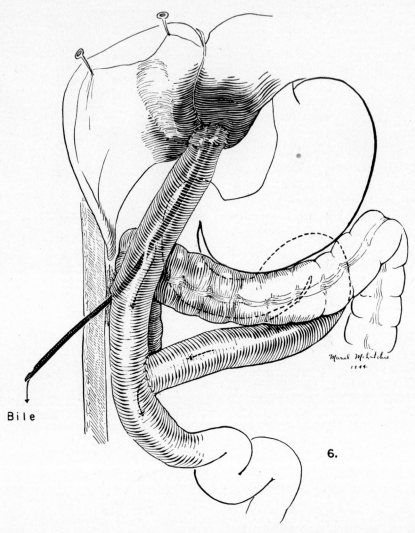

Bile

6.

FIG. 285. Schematic representation of Allen's operation after completion. The proximal end of the jejunum has been reimplanted into the side of the distal end at a low level; and the tube in the hepatic duct brought out through an omental tab; and a stab wound in the abdominal wall lateral to the incision. (From Arthur Allen, *Ann. Surg.*, 121:420, 1945.)

is entirely justifiable. Obviously, the surgeon must prove, by aspiration of the gallbladder or otherwise, that bile is passing through the common and cystic ducts into the gallbladder. The author is strongly of the opinion that when the gallbladder is used in anastomosis of the intestinal tract a loop of jejunum should be utilized for the anastomosis so that an enteroenterostomy can be performed and the food stream shunted away from the gallbladder (see Fig. 287). The performance of an enteroenterostomy between the two arms of jejunum will not effectively shunt the food stream

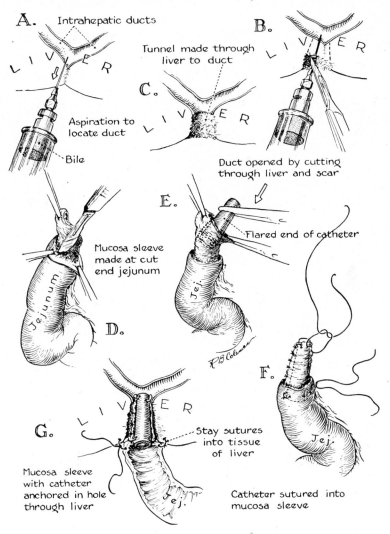

FIG. 286. Method (modified Hoag operation) utilized by the author when no duct remains at the hilus, and scar prevents the conventional mucosa-to-mucosa approximation, the fibrous tissue is excised and the mucosa at the end of the Roux Y portion of jejunum used as a graft to bridge across the scarred area thereby hoping to minimize contracture at the hilus which is the location of most recurrent strictures. (From Cole, *Can. Med. Assoc.*, 1948.)

away from the gallbladder. To obtain effective shunting it is necessary to make two or three folds in the proximal arm of jejunum.[20] This operation is very applicable to cystic dilatation of the common duct. If the gallbladder is absent or so badly diseased that it cannot be used for an anastomosis, the loop of jejunum may be anastomosed directly to the cystic area in the common duct to relieve the obstruction which usually exists in the duct

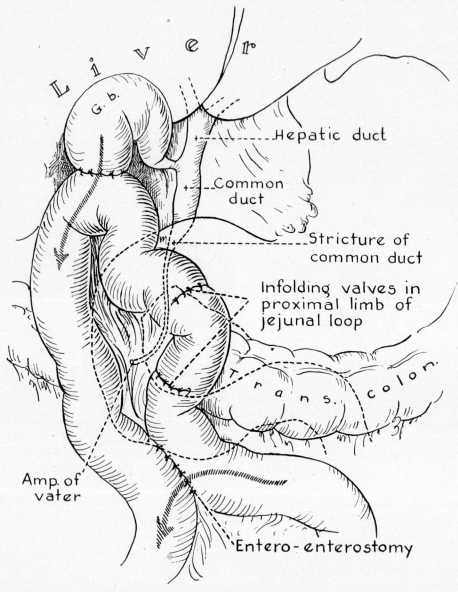

FIG. 287. Cholecystenterostomy utilizing a loop of jejunum. This operation is recommended only in inoperable carcinoma of the head of the pancreas or in strictures of the common duct which may be only temporary, as in pancreatitis localized to the head of the pancreas. (From Cole and Peterson, *Arch. Surg.*, 51:18, 1945.)

distal to the cystic dilatation. In either event, folds should be placed in the proximal arm to prevent regurgitation of food into the dilated common duct or gallbladder.

ANASTOMOSIS OF THE HILAR DUCT TO THE DUODENUM. Years ago the most popular operation for stricture of the common duct was anastomosis of the hilar duct directly to the duodenum when the distal end could not be found. However, the author has had such poor results with this operation that he has abandoned it. If performed, it is essential that mucosa-to-mucosa approximation be obtained. It is only fair to state, however, that some surgeons still utilize this procedure and feel that they have good results with it.

ANASTOMOSIS OF THE HILAR DUCT TO A LOOP OF JEJUNUM. Some surgeons anastomose the hilar duct to a loop of jejunum, performing an

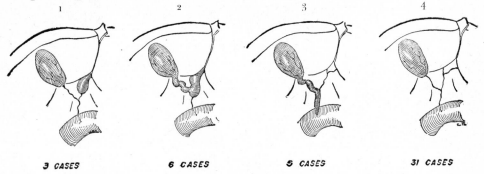

FIG. 288. Sketch of types of atresia of the extrahepatic bile ducts as found in exploration of 45 cases. (1) Hepatic duct patent and connecting with liver. (2) Hepatic and part of common duct patent (gallbladder may be atresic or patent). (3) Hepatic duct atresic, gallbladder, cystic and common duct normal. (4) Hepatic and common ducts atretic. (From Ladd and Gross, *Abdominal Surgery in Infancy and Childhood*, W. B. Saunders Co., Philadelphia, 1941.)

enteroenterostomy between the two arms of jejunum to shunt food away from the anastomosis between the hilar duct and intestine. However, our experience at Illinois Research and Educational Hospital has been very unhappy with this method. Early in our experience with repair of common duct strictures we [21] anastomosed a loop of jejunum to the hilar duct as described above in 5 patients with stricture. One of the patients died postoperatively. All of the 4 remaining patients developed chills and fever indicative of suppurative cholangitis. In 2 of these we severed the proximal arm of jejunum but did nothing to the stoma which appeared adequate; the chills and fever ceased abruptly and the patients have remained well ever since. For 2 years we lost track of the third patient, but she returned shortly thereafter with severe chills and fever which proved fatal within a few days after admission to the hospital. We advised operation in the fourth patient who was having frequent chills with fever, but she did not consent; shortly thereafter the chills became less frequent and are now so mild and infrequent that operation is no longer indicated. X-ray examination with barium in all 4 cases revealed regurgitation into the intrahepatic bile ducts. However, we wish to emphasize that x-ray examination in such instances must be more than momentary. In our experience observation

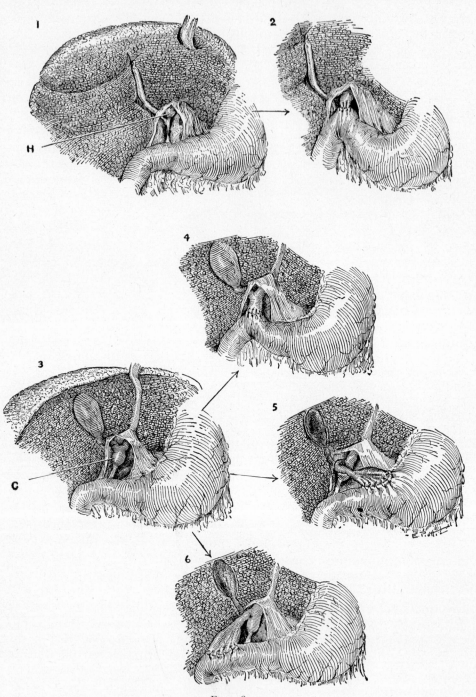

Fig. 289

at intervals of 60 minutes or longer with manipulation of the abdomen, has revealed regurgitation in all cases even though an enteroenterostomy between the two arms of jejunum was performed. Accordingly, we are convinced that regurgitation of food into the intrahepatic ducts can result in suppurative cholangitis, although we emphasize that *obstruction is a much more common cause of the infection.*

Operation for Congenital Obstruction or Atresia of the Common Bile Duct. Unfortunately, not over 25 per cent of infants with congenital atresia of the bile duct are amenable to surgical therapy because important structures are so often absent when anomalies of the biliary tract are present. In general, two types of operation are available for repair of atresia of the common duct in infancy. If the gallbladder is absent, but the proximal stump of the common duct found, it may be anastomosed to the duodenum. Although this operation is a poor one for adults, it is tolerated well by infants and suppurative cholangitis rarely appears to develop.[22] If the gallbladder is present and is receiving bile through the hepatic and cystic ducts, it may be anastomosed to the duodenum. It may be necessary to mobilize the gallbladder somewhat from the bed of the liver to achieve anastomosis (see Figs. 288 and 289).

Results of Operations for Stricture. In a large series good results can be expected following repair of strictures in 70 to 80 per cent of patients, although the experience of the operator is a very important factor in results. In general, results are jeopardized by numerous previous operations since scar tissue around the hilar duct will be increased by successive operations. When enough proximal and distal duct can be found to do an end-to-end anastomosis, the results should be perhaps slightly better than in the other types of lesions.

In our series of 63 operations in 49 patients we had 4 postoperative deaths or a mortality rate of 6.0 per cent. Eighty per cent of the series had results classified as good to excellent. On a few occasions chills and fever were present for a year or two after operation, but later disappeared.

CARCINOMA OF THE BILE DUCTS

Malignant lesions of the bile ducts are not as common as those encountered in the gallbladder, although of recent years their incidence appears to be increasing. In carcinoma of the gallbladder, stones are present in 75 to 80 per cent of cases, but in carcinoma of the bile ducts only in 30 to 35 per cent. Contrary to the greater incidence of carcinoma of the gall-

Fig. 289. Types of operative relief which have been effective for atresia of bile ducts. 1. Atresia of hepatic duct treated by hepaticoduodenostomy, as shown in 2. 3. Atresia of the common duct treated by choledochoduodenostomy, cholecystogastromy and cholecystoduodenostomy, as shown in 4, 5 and 6, respectively. Choledochoduodenostomy is believed to be a better procedure than cholecystogastrostomy or cholecystoduodenostomy. H. Blind end of hepatic duct. C. Blind end of common duct. (From Ladd and Gross, *Abdominal Surgery in Infancy and Childhood,* W. B. Saunders Co., Philadelphia, 1941.)

bladder in women than in men, the ratio is reversed in malignancy of the bile ducts, this lesion being about twice as common in men as in women.

In a study of 92 cases of carcinoma of the bile ducts Rolleston and McNee [23] noted that the lesion was distal to the cystic duct in 37 per cent, at the junction in 30 per cent and above the junction in 20 per cent. In only 6.5 per cent did the growth involve the cystic duct primarily.

Grossly, the tumor is not very hyperplastic, although moderate thickening of the wall at the point of obstruction is usually present. When the tumor is located in the pancreatic portion of the common duct it frequently resembles a stone upon palpation. Exploration of the mass with a hypodermic needle will differentiate tumor from stone. When the lesion is located proximal to the junction of the cystic duct with the common, the gallbladder will be collapsed. On the other hand, when the tumor is located distal to the junction with the cystic duct, the gallbladder will be dilated, unless previous inflammation has scarred and shrunken the gallbladder.

The *diagnosis* is very difficult to make with accuracy. The onset is usually insidious with painless jaundice being the most prominent symptom although occasionally pain is very severe. The stools are acholic and remain so once obstruction becomes complete. Occult blood is usually present, but gross bleeding is rare. Itching is common.

Resection of Carcinoma of the Bile Ducts. The location of the tumor is a very important factor in the ease with which resection can be carried out. When located at the hilus near the junction of the right and left hepatic ducts resection will be difficult and in fact useless because tumors in this location tend to metastasize rapidly into the liver. When located at the midportion of the duct, near the junction of the cystic duct with the common duct, resection with primary anastomosis will usually be possible. Wide excision is necessary. In such instances cholecystectomy will be indicated. In order to bring the two ends of the ducts together, it will be necessary to mobilize the stump of the duct, the duodenum and head of the pancreas so that the distal stump can be brought up to meet the proximal. Anastomosis is carried out as described for benign local stricture. Usually one layer of sutures is adequate. Drainage of the duct is carried out by insertion of a T tube into an opening proximal or distal to the suture line, but not through the suture line.

When the tumor is located in the distal portion of the common duct near or in the head of the pancreas, resection of the duodenum and head of the pancreas, as described in Chapter 11, for carcinoma of the ampulla of Vater and carcinoma of the head of the pancreas will be necessary.

REFERENCES

1. FLINT, E. R. Abnormalities of the Right Hepatic, Cystic and Gastro-duodenal Arteries, and of the Bile-ducts, *Brit. J. Surg.*, 10:509-519, [Apr.], 1923.
2. EISENDRATH, D. N. Anomalies of the Bile Ducts and Blood Vessels as the Cause of Accidents in Biliary Surgery, *J.A.M.A.*, 71:864-867, [Sept. 14], 1918.

3. Rous, P. and McMaster, P. D.   The Concentrating Activity of the Gallbladder, *J. Exper. Med.*, 34:47-73, [July], 1921.

4. Ivy, A. C. and Oldburg, E.   Hormone Mechanism for Gallbladder Contraction and Evacuation, *Am. J. Physiol.*, 86:599, 1928.

5. Graham, R. R. and Connell, D.   Accidental Ligation of the Hepatic Artery, *Brit. J. Surg.*, 20:566, 1933.

6. Graham, R.   Personal communication.

7. Black, J. M.   Review of 100 Consecutive Gallbladder Operations, *Brit. M. J.*, 1:11, 1935.

8. Wilson, W. D., Lehman, E. P. and Goodwin, W. H.   Prognosis in Gallbladder Surgery, *J.A.M.A.*, 106:2209, 1936.

9. Dublin, L. I., Jimenus, A. D. and Marks, H. H.   Factors in the Selection of Risks with a History of Gallbladder Disease, *Proc. Ass. Life Insur. M. Dir. Amer.*, 21:34, 1934.

10. Cole, W. H., Reynolds, J. T. and Ireneus, Carl, Jr.   The Surgical Treatment of Strictures of the Common Duct in Advances in Surgery, *Interscience Pub. Co.*, N. Y., 1948; Strictures of the Common Duct, *Ann. Surg.*, 128:332, 1948.

11. Flickinger, F. M. and Masson, J. C.   Reconstructive Operations for Benign Stricture of the Bile Ducts, *Surg., Gynec. & Obst.*, 83:24, 1946.

12. Cattell, R. B.   Benign Strictures of the Biliary Ducts, *J. Am. Med. Assn.*, 134:235, 1947; personal communication.

13. Walters, Waltman.   Study of Results of Operations in Eighty Cases, *J.A.M.A.*, 113:209-213, [July 15], 1939; Walters, W. and Lewis, E. B.   Strictures of the Common and Hepatic Bile Ducts with a Report of Ninety-eight Cases, *Frank H. Lahey Birthday Volume*, Charles C Thomas Publisher, Springfield, Ill., 1940.

14. McArthur, Lewis L.   Repair of the Common Bile Duct, *Ann. Surg.*, 78:129-138, 1923; Repair of the Common Bile Duct, *Surgery*, 78:129, 1923.

15. Sanders, R. L.   Indications for and Value of Choledochoduodenostomy, *Ann. Surg.*, 123:847, 1946.

16. Allen, A. W.   A Method of Re-establishing Continuity Between the Bile Ducts and the Gastro-intestinal Tract, *Ann. Surg.*, 121:412, 1945; personal communication.

17. Allen, A. W.   Personal communication.

18. Hoag, C. L.   Reconstruction of the Bile Ducts; New Method of Anastomosis, *Surg., Gynec. & Obst.*, 64:1051, 1937.

19. Longmire, W. P., Jr. and Sanford, M. C.   Intrahepatic Cholangiojejunostomy with Partial Hepatectomy for Biliary Obstruction, *Surgery*, 24:264, 1948.

20. Peterson, L. W. and Cole, W. H.   Use of the Defunctionalized Loop of Jejunum in Bile Duct Obstruction and Other Intra-abdominal Lesions, *Arch. Surg.*, 1948.

21. Cole, W. H., Ireneus, C. and Reynolds, J. T.   The Use of Vitallium Tubes in the Treatment of Strictures of the Common Duct, *Ann. Surg.*, 122:490, 1945.

22. Ladd, W. E. and Gross, R. E.   *Abdominal Surgery in Infancy and Childhood*, W. B. Saunders Co., 1941.

23. Rolleston, Sir Humphrey and McNee, J. W.   *Diseases of the Liver, Gallbladder and Bile Ducts*, Macmillan and Co., London, 1929.

13

THE LIVER AND SUBPHRENIC SPACE

ALTON OCHSNER, M.D. AND MICHAEL E. DEBAKEY, M.D.

SUBPHRENIC INFECTIONS

The treatment of subphrenic infections is primarily conservative because the majority will resolve spontaneously and relatively few will progress to suppuration. Many nonsuppurative lesions are not diagnosed, the infection subsiding without the condition's being suspected. If, however, patients with intraperitoneal infection, regardless of cause, are carefully examined for a possible subphrenic infection, the diagnosis can be made readily. Repeated examinations of the upper abdomen are particularly indicated in patients with such continuing signs of infection as pyrexia and leukocytosis. As already mentioned, however, most subphrenic infections subside spontaneously, with suppuration occurring in only about 25 per cent of cases.

Incision and drainage is just as necessary in the treatment of a subphrenic abscess as in suppurative processes elsewhere. The drainage of subphrenic infections, however, is unique in that the direct approach to the abscess frequently involves traversing uninvolved serous cavities such as the peritoneum or pleura. Subphrenic infections, like infections elsewhere within the peritoneal cavity, should be drained in such a way as not to contaminate an uninvolved serous cavity. The mortality following drainage of subphrenic abscesses was formerly high, frequently as high as 50 to 75 per cent. The high death rate was due to the associated contamination of an uninvolved serous cavity, the complication, rather than the originating abscess and its drainage, being responsible for the death. It is therefore imperative in the drainage of a subphrenic abscess to drain it in such a way that evacuation of the exudate can be obtained without contamination of uninvolved serous membranes.

An adequate knowledge of the anatomy of the subphrenic region is essential for the rational treatment of infections in this area. From a surgical standpoint, the subphrenic space should be considered as that area bounded above by the diaphragm and below by the transverse colon and transverse mesocolon (Fig. 290). This area is divided by the liver into two large spaces, the suprahepatic and the infrahepatic space. Although the infrahepatic space is not in direct contact with the diaphragm, infrahepatic infections above the colon and transverse mesocolon should be considered as subphrenic infections because they frequently are associated with infections above the liver.

The suprahepatic and infrahepatic areas are further divided into other spaces by peritoneal reflections. The suprahepatic space is divided into right and left areas. On the right side there are two spaces. One is a rela-tively small triangular space, posterior to the right prolongation of the coronary ligament, which is the reflection of the peritoneum from the undersurface of the diaphragm onto the upper surface of the liver. The other is a large space anterior to this peritoneal reflection (Figs. 290c and 291). The former is designated the right posterior-superior space and the latter, the right anterior-superior space. On the left side, because the peri-

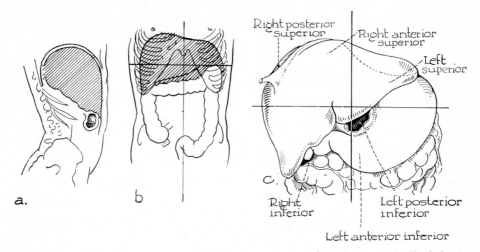

Fig. 290. Schematic drawings showing anatomy of subphrenic space. A. Shaded area represents the subphrenic space bounded above by the diaphragm and below by the transverse colon and the transverse mesocolon. B. Subphrenic (represented by shaded area) is subdivided by the liver into suprahepatic and infrahepatic portions. C. Locations of the various subdivisions of the subphrenic space.

toneal reflection from the undersurface of the diaphragm to the superior surface of the liver extends posteriorly along the posterior edge of the left side, there is only one space, the left superior space (Fig. 291a).

Above the liver there is also a relatively large space which is not intra-peritoneal but which lies between the reflections of the peritoneum; it is known as the extraperitoneal space (Fig. 291a). The area inferior to the liver is divided into right and left portions by the falciform ligament and the ductus venosus. To the right of these structures is one large space, the right inferior space, which is bounded above by the liver and below by the transverse colon and transverse mesocolon. The area to the left of the falciform and round ligaments and the ductus venosus is divided into two spaces by the stomach and its two ligaments, the gastrohepatic and gastro-colic ligaments. The space anterior to these structures, which is a part of the greater peritoneal cavity, is the left anterior-inferior space. The space posterior to the stomach, gastrohepatic and gastrocolic omenta, which com-prises the lesser peritoneal sac, is the left posterior-inferior space (Fig. 291b).

Although subphrenic infections may follow infection anywhere in the body, they usually develop as a complication of an intra-abdominal suppurative process. Well over half of all subphrenic infections or abscesses are the result of suppurative lesions of the appendix and perforative lesions of the stomach and duodenum. The next most frequent causes are lesions of the liver and biliary passages. The infection may, in very occasional instances, be of primary or metastatic origin or may result from extension of a thoracic lesion.

The mechanism of the spread of infection to the subphrenic space varies according to the original lesion. The simplest and perhaps the most frequent mode of extension is by local invasion from contiguous lesions, but extension may also take place through lymphatic routes or, less often, through vascular channels from neighboring or distant foci.

The most frequently involved space in subphrenic infection is the right posterior-superior space, probably because of its greater accessibility to inflammatory exudate extending upward from the iliac fossa along the paracolic groove. Associated with infection in this space of appendiceal origin there is not infrequently an infection below the liver on the right side involving the right inferior space. This space is most frequently involved also in infections originating in the gallbladder, duodenum and stomach. Less frequently encountered are infections of the right anterior-superior space. Infections on the left side, which are still more infrequent, may involve either the solitary space above the liver, the left superior space, or one of the two spaces below the liver, the left anterior-inferior or the left posterior-inferior space.

Accurate localization of a subphrenic abscess is essential for proper therapy because only by knowing the location of the space involved can incision and drainage be done in such a way as not to contaminate an uninvolved serous cavity. This is a particularly important consideration in subphrenic abscess because of the peculiar location of the lesion, *i.e.*, its proximity to two serous-lined cavities, the pleural and peritoneal, and the grave consequences of their contamination. It is therefore essential to institute a type of drainage which completely avoids the slightest possibility of contamination of the peritoneal or pleural cavities. This can be most effectively done by an extraperitoneal anterior or posterior approach, depending upon the location of the abscess.

In infections of the right anterior-superior, right anterior-inferior, left anterior-inferior, and the left superior spaces, drainage is best accomplished by utilizing the approach described by Clairmont. The incision is made anteriorly just beneath and parallel to the costal margin and is carried down through the abdominal parietes to the peritoneum (Fig. 292). The peritoneum is separated from the undersurface of the anterior abdominal wall and the inferior surface of the diaphragm until the abscess is reached. The abscess which lies intraperitoneally is then drained by plunging the finger through the pyogenic membrane and allowing the purulent exudate to escape through the tract which has been created and which is entirely

SUPRAHEPATIC

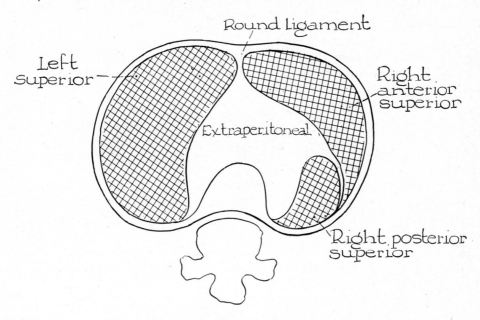

Round ligament

Left superior

Right anterior superior

Extraperitoneal

Right posterior superior

INFRAHEPATIC

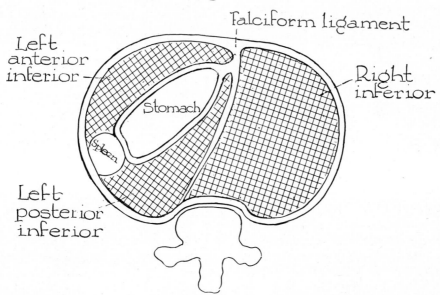

Falciform ligament

Left anterior inferior

Stomach

Spleen

Right inferior

Left posterior inferior

FIG. 291. Schematic drawings showing cross-sectional view of suprahepatic and infrahepatic subphrenic spaces and their various subdivisions represented by shaded areas.

extraserous (Fig. 292). This operation can be readily performed under local analgesia by infiltration of the abdominal wall with 0.5 per cent procaine hydrochloride solution. It can also be done satisfactorily under general anesthesia if this is considered preferable under the circumstances.

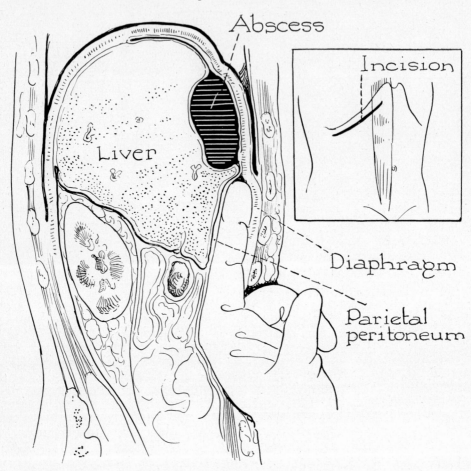

FIG. 292. Technic of extraperitoneal method of drainage of a subphrenic abscess in the right anterior-superior space. The incision shown in the inset is made below and parallel to the right costal margin. It is carried down through the abdominal muscle and transversalis fascia to the peritoneum. The parietal peritoneum is gently separated with the finger from the undersurface of the diaphragm until the abscess cavity is reached, thus permitting drainage of the cavity extraperitoneally.

For drainage of an abscess of the right posterior-superior space, which is the space most frequently involved, several methods of approach may be used but the extraperitoneal approach to be described is considered the most rational as well as the most effective because it avoids contamination of the pleural and peritoneal cavities. This method also permits the drainage of the co-existing abscess in the right inferior space which frequently accompanies right posterior-superior space abscesses.

The retroperitoneal operation is based upon an understanding of the anatomic relationships of the pleura to the twelfth rib and the spinous process of the first lumbar vertebra. As shown by Melnikoff, there is considerable variation in the relationship of the reflection of pleura to the twelfth rib; it may extend from completely above to completely below the rib (Fig. 293). In no case, however, and this is the significant fact, does the pleural reflection extend below the level of the spinous process of the first lumbar vertebra. Accordingly, if the opening into the retroperitoneal space by means of a transverse incision is made at this level, the possibility of contaminating the pleural cavity is completely avoided.

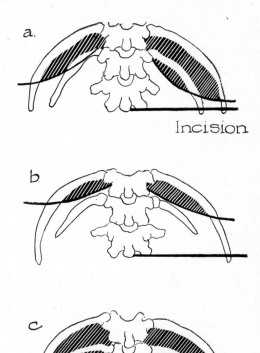

The operation can be performed under local anesthesia. Before the incision is made, the skin is marked at the level of the spinous process of the first lumbar vertebra so that this level can be readily ascertained during the course of the operation. With the patient in the lateral decubitus, the side to be operated upon being uppermost, an incision is made over and parallel to the twelfth rib (Fig. 294a), which is resected subperiosteally and removed in its entirety. A transverse incision is then made at the level of the spinous processes of the first lumbar vertebra, which has been previously marked on the skin (Fig. 294b). It is imperative that the incision be made transversely and that it does not parallel the original skin incision because, unless the incision is made at the level of the spinous

FIG. 293. Diagrammatic drawing modified after Melnikoff showing variations in the relationship of the reflection of the pleura (represented by the shaded area) to the twelfth rib, ranging from completely above to completely below the rib. In no case, however, does it extend down to the level of the spinous process of the first lumbar vertebra. Accordingly, a transverse incision made at the spinous process of the first lumbar vertebra will invariably miss the pleural reflection.

process of the first lumbar vertebra, there is danger of injuring the pleural reflection. This danger can be obviated by the transverse incision. The incision traverses the attachment of the diaphragm, the thickness of which varies considerably. In some individuals it is a rather strong muscular sheath, whereas in others it consists of only a few fibers. After incision through the diaphragm, the retroperitoneal space is entered (Fig. 294c). If a lesion is suspected in the right inferior space, its presence can usually be determined by palpation below the liver, where an induration is felt. By

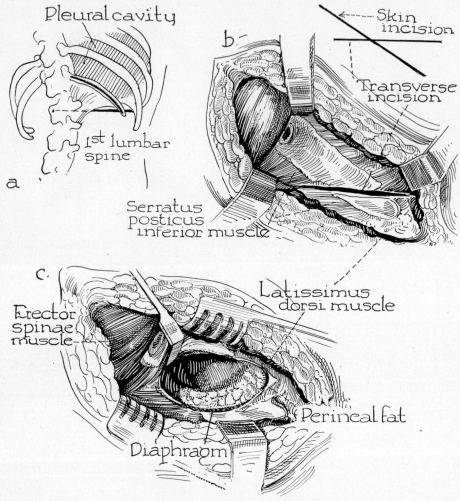

Fig. 294. Technic of extraperitoneal method of drainage of subphrenic abscess involving right posterior-superior space with or without associated abscess in the right inferior space. A. Skin incision is made over and parallel to the twelfth rib. The skin is marked at the level of the spinous process of the first lumbar vertebra. B. A transverse incision is made at the level of the spinous process of the first lumbar vertebra in the bed of the twelfth rib, which has been subperiosteally resected. C. The transverse incision is carried through the inserting fibers of the diaphragm, exposing the perirenal fascia and the liver retroperitoneally and below the diaphragm.

introducing an aspirating needle above the kidney into this area one can determine whether pus is present in this space. If it is present, the abscess can be opened extraperitoneally, without danger of contaminating the peritoneal cavity. If an abscess of the right posterior-superior space is suspected, the peritoneum from the under surface of the diaphragm is stripped away until the abscess is reached (Fig. 295a). The finger is then plunged through the wall and the abscess is evacuated through the tract

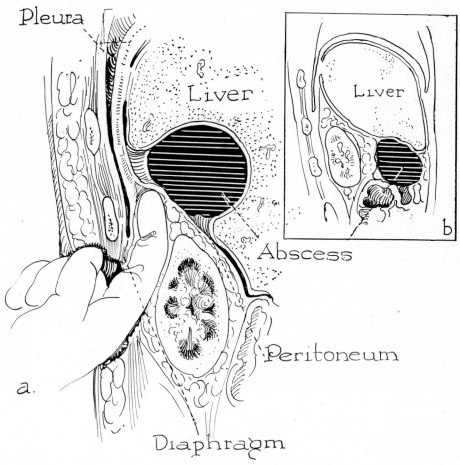

FIG. 295. Method of approaching and draining an abscess in the right posterior-superior space after entering the retroperitoneal area, as shown in figure 294. The peritoneum is gently peeled away from the undersurface of the diaphragm with the finger until the abscess cavity is reached. Inset shows location of subphrenic abscess in the right inferior space which may be drained simultaneously through this same incision.

thus made. In this way an extraperitoneal and extrapleural drainage is accomplished without danger of contamination of the pleural and peritoneal cavities. It is also possible through the incision described to drain concomitant abscesses in the right posterior-superior space and in the right inferior space. In cases in which an infection of the extraperitoneal space is suspected, the separation of the peritoneum from the undersurface of the diaphragm is continued upward until the extraperitoneal portion of the liver is reached and the abscess drained in this way.

Soft rubber tubes or a rubber tissue dam is placed in the abscess cavity and brought out through the wound, which is left open. Dry dressings are applied. Drainage is maintained until the tubes have been extruded, by which time the abscess cavity will have been almost completely obliterated.

LIVER ABSCESS

Although the treatment of hepatic infections and abscess is surgical, it may consist of either conservative or radical measures, depending upon the type and stage of the process. Thus in frank pyogenic abscess of the liver open drainage is essential, whereas in the amebic type of hepatic infections conservative or radical procedures may be indicated. In the latter form of hepatic disease conservative therapy consists of the administration of the specific drug emetine hydrochloride with or without aspiration depending upon the presence of indications for the latter. In early cases of amebic hepatitis the administration of emetine may be sufficient to prevent progression of the presuppurative stage to actual abscess formation. Even in cases in which early and very small abscess-formation has actually occurred, conservative measures are frequently sufficient to effect complete resolution. Generally, however, when the process has progressed to true abscess formation, evacuation of the contents by aspiration will be required in addition to the administration of emetine.

Evacuation of the abscess in noninfected cases by aspiration rather than by open drainage is essential in the management of this condition. The efficacy and superiority of this method of treatment have been well established. In previous publications it has been shown that the mortality rate in noninfected amebic abscesses of the liver treated by open drainage is approximately 21 per cent, whereas in similar cases treated by aspiration and the systemic administration of amebacides it is significantly lower, approximately 3 per cent.

The complications of hepatic abscess consist essentially of the development of generalized sepsis in the pyogenic type, the occurrence of secondary infection with pyogenic organisms in the amebic type, and in both types the occurrence of direct extension or rupture of the abscess into one of the adjacent viscera or serous cavities (Fig. 296). Other more infrequent complications are septic thrombosis and pulmonary infarction or embolism. Pleuropulmonary complications, especially of amebic hepatic abscesses, are not unusual, with the production of lung abscess, empyema or bronchohepatic fistula.

In cases of amebic hepatic abscess requiring aspiration the preliminary administration of emetine is important. It is generally given in the form of emetine hydrochloride, preferably subcutaneously, in daily doses of 0.065 gm. (1 gr.) for several days preceding the aspiration. Administration of the drug is continued in these daily doses until 0.39 to 0.65 gm. (6 to 10 gr.) have been given. Because of its toxicity in excessive dosage and its cumulative action, the noxious effects of this drug should be realized and considerable care should be exercised in its use. The maximum amount that should be given over any period of time should not exceed 10 mg. (⅙ gr.) per kg. of body weight, which for a patient weighing 150 pounds would be about 0.65 gm. (10 gr.) (Leake).

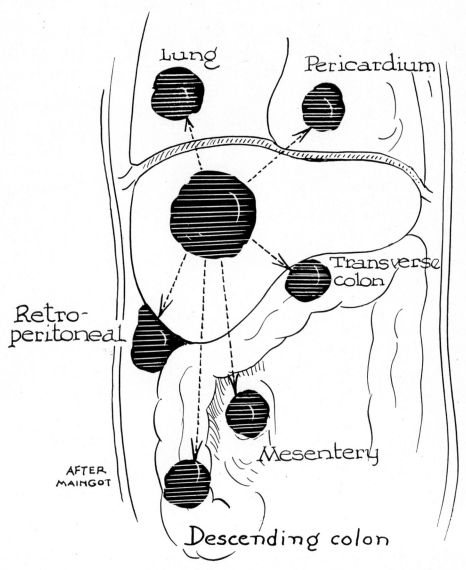

FIG. 296. Schematic drawing of liver abscess showing various sites of extension by rupture of the abscess.

The procedure of aspiration should be done in the operating room in order to minimize the danger of contamination of the abscess cavity with pyogenic micro-organisms, and because open drainage can be done immediately if the abscess is found to be secondarily infected. The cutaneous site of puncture and the direction of the introduction of the needle depend

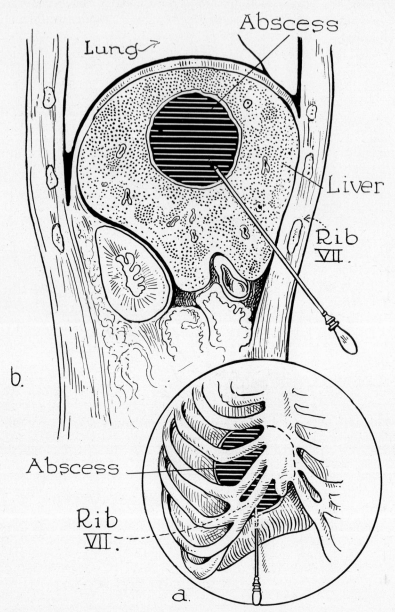

FIG. 297. Technic of aspiration of amebic hepatic abscess located in the anterior portion of liver. A. The needle is inserted just below the anterior costal margin about 4 to 6 cm. lateral to the midline. B. Diagrammatic representation of the sagittal section of the body at the level of the cutaneous puncture showing needle directed superiorly and posteriorly into the abscess cavity. (From Ochsner and DeBakey, *Surgery*, 13:460-493, [March] and 612-649, [April], 1943.)

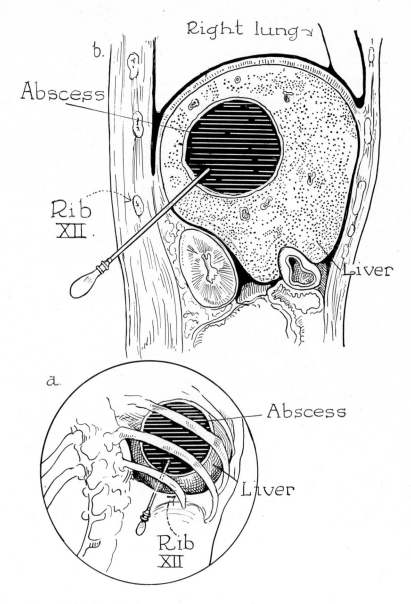

FIG. 298. Technic of aspiration of amebic hepatic abscess located in posterior portion of liver. A. The needle is inserted in the right lumbocostal angle. B. Diagrammatic representation of sagittal section at level of cutaneous puncture, showing needle directed superiorly and anteriorly into abscess cavity. (From Ochsner and DeBakey, *Surgery*, 13:460-493, [March] and 612-649, [April], 1943.)

largely upon the clinical and radiologic findings. In the presence of localizing signs and pointing of the abscess, the needle should be introduced
directly over the mass or at the site of greatest tenderness. If no localizing
signs are present, the roentgenograms may be useful in determining the
site and direction of the aspiratory needle. Accordingly, when the lateral

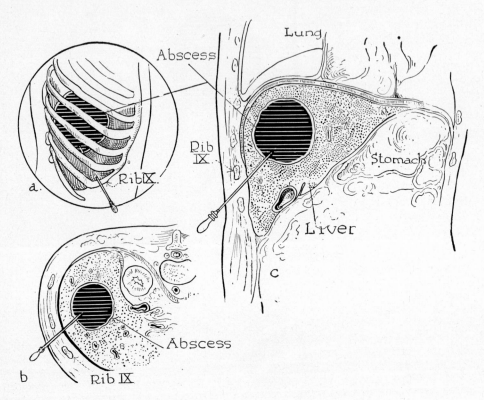

FIG. 299. Technic of aspiration of amebic hepatic abscess located near dome of liver.
A. The needle is inserted through the ninth or tenth intercostal space in the anterior
axillary line. B. Diagrammatic representation of horizontal flexion through liver abscess
and cutaneous puncture site showing posterior and medial direction of needle. C.
Diagrammatic representation of sagittal section of level of cutaneous puncture showing
superior direction of needle into abscess cavity. (From Ochsner and DeBakey, *Surgery*,
13:460-493, [March] and 612-649, [April], 1943.)

roentgenogram demonstrates an abscess in the anterior portion of the liver,
the needle may be inserted just below the right anterior costal margin,
about 4 to 6 cm. lateral to the midline, and directed superiorly and posteriorly (Fig. 297). Local analgesia with infiltration of 1 per cent procaine hydrochloride solution is adequate. Nicking the skin at the contemplated site of
puncture with a bistoury facilitates insertion of the needle. The needle
should be of short bevelled or, preferably, of the trocar type, with a short
fairly blunt point, about 15 cm. in length, with a caliber of 1 to 1.5 mm.
    It sometimes may be necessary to puncture the liver in several different

directions before encountering pus. Under these circumstances it is better to withdraw the needle entirely before reintroducing it in a different direction, rather than to change its direction while it is still in the liver. In this way unnecessary injury to the liver parenchyma can be prevented. It is also important to maintain suction during the introduction of the needle in order to determine when the abscess cavity is entered and to prevent passage of the needle through the abscess cavity into the liver beyond. As soon as the

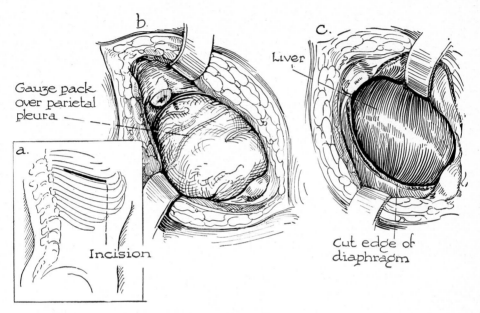

Fig. 300. Technic of transthoracic drainage of liver abscess. The incision is made (as shown in the inset) over the eighth or ninth ribs for a distance of 6 to 7 cm. and the rib is subperiosteally resected for the same distance, thus exposing the underlying pleura. The wound is then packed with gauze in order to produce sufficient reaction for development of adhesions between the visceral and parietal layers of the pleura, so that at a subsequent time, usually four or five days, an incision may be made through this area and into the liver without risk of contaminating the pleural cavity.

abscess cavity has been entered, as much as possible of the material within the cavity is aspirated. This may vary from a few hundred centimeters to as much as 2 liters.

In the occasional case of posteriorly located abscess, aspiration can be accomplished by introducing the needle in the right lumbocostal angle (Fig. 298). The needle is introduced just below and at about the midpoint of the right twelfth rib and then directed obliquely, anteriorly and superiorly, suction being maintained during the introduction of the trocar until the abscess cavity is entered. In a more laterally placed abscess near the dome of the liver, which is frequently observed, aspiration is best done by inserting the needle in the ninth or tenth intercostal space in the anterior axillary line and directing it superiorly, medially, and slightly posteriorly

(Fig. 299). In this way there is less likelihood of contaminating the pleural or peritoneal cavities.

In amebic abscesses of the liver that have become secondarily infected with pyogenic organisms, as well as in primary pyogenic abscesses, drainage is required. Here again it is imperative to institute that type of drainage which completely avoids the slightest possibility of contaminating the two virgin serous surfaces, *i.e.*, the pleural and peritoneal cavities. In general, the two types of drainage procedures which can be employed are transthoracic and transabdominal, either through a transserous or an extraserous approach. In the original form of the transthoracic procedure, suggested by Trendelenburg, in 1883, avoidance of contamination of the pleural cavity was attempted by suturing the costal and diaphragmatic layers of the pleura together.

Several modifications of this procedure were subsequently advocated, of which probably the most popular is that of Beck, who suggested a two-stage operation. The first stage consists of suturing the costophrenic pleural reflection and packing the wound for forty-eight hours with gauze impregnated with an irritative substance to produce adhesions. At the second stage incision is carried out through this area. Accordingly, in draining a laterally and posteriorly located pyogenic abscess, the incision is made over the eighth or ninth rib, following which resection of the rib over a distance of 6 to 7 cm. is accomplished (Fig. 300). The

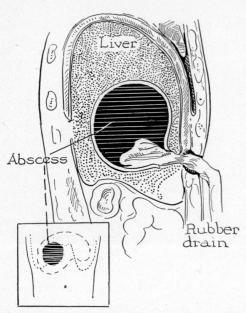

FIG. 301. Diagrammatic representation of method of extraperitoneal drainage of pyogenic abscess of liver located anteriorly. Depending upon whether adhesions are or are not present between the two layers of peritoneum, drainage may be instituted by a one- or two-stage procedure, by incising down to the peritoneum as in draining for a superior subphrenic space abscess. If no adhesions exist between the two layers of peritoneum, the wound should be packed until adhesions are formed; usually within several days an incision may be made through the bed of the wound between the two adherent layers into the abscess cavity. If adhesions are already present at the time of the original incision, a second-stage procedure is unnecessary.

underlying pleura is exposed and the wound is packed with gauze in order to produce sufficient reaction for adhesions to form between the visceral and parietal layers of the pleura so that subsequently incision and drainage through this area can be accomplished without danger of contamination of the pleural cavity. Several days later, usually four or five, the pack is removed and an incision is made through the two adherent layers of pleura and diaphragm exposing the underlying liver (Fig. 300). An aspirating needle is then introduced into the liver with the purpose of locating the abscess and after pus is encountered the liver substance is incised to provide open drainage of the abscess cavity.

While this type of drainage may occasionally be necessary for abscesses located in the posterior or posterior-lateral region of the liver, in most cases the extraserous retroperitoneal method of drainage similar to that described for subphrenic abscess is far more satisfactory. This has been repeatedly demonstrated by analysis of mortality and morbidity statistics which clearly reveal the superiority of the latter method.

Pyogenic abscesses located anteriorly in the liver can also usually be drained quite satisfactorily without the two-stage procedure through an incision down to the peritoneum, as in the drainage of an anterior-superior subphrenic abscess. If the abscess has progressed to the stage of pointing, it usually has become walled off from the peritoneal cavity by involvement of the abdominal parietes. Extraserous drainage in these cases may be done simply by incision over the point of greatest localization. If, however, there are no adhesions between the two layers of peritoneum, *i.e.,* the layer lining the parietes and that covering the liver, the wound should be packed until such adhesions are formed. Here, too, several days later an incision can be made between the two adherent layers and after determination of the site of the abscess by aspiration, the abscess is opened and drained to the outside (Fig. 301). Soft rubber tubes, or preferably several pieces of rubber tissue dam, are placed into the abscess cavity and brought out through the wound to secure adequate drainage. A dry dressing is applied and drainage is maintained until the cavity has become completely obliterated.

14

THE COLON AND APPENDIX

Roscoe R. Graham, M.D.* and Jessie Gray, M.D.

BASIC PRINCIPLES GOVERNING SURGICAL PROCEDURES ON THE COLON

Until relatively recent years the operative mortality in diseases of the colon was high. Two major factors were responsible for this mortality. The more important is the high incidence of infection following operations on the colon. The other factor is an anatomical one.

All vessels which supply the colon are terminal ones and enter the colon at right angles to its long axis. Good anastomotic arcades join the right colic with the ileocolic and middle colic arteries, thus giving the large bowel from cecum to midtransverse colon a very adequate blood supply. In contrast, the absence of any major arcades between the left colic and middle colic, and between the left colic and sigmoid vessels leaves the distal transverse colon and the descending colon dependent almost entirely on the blood supply derived from marginal arteries. Similarly the absence of major arcades between the last sigmoid branch and the superior hemorrhoidal artery leaves the rectosigmoid dependent also on a single marginal artery. Consequently the success of operations, particularly on the left colon, is going to depend upon recognition of and respect for these anatomical facts (Fig. 302).

The first requisite is that in division of the colon the clamps must be placed at an angle so that more of the antimesenteric border of the colon is resected than of the mesenteric border (Fig. 303). In this way we are insured, because of the terminal character of the vessels, of an adequate blood supply to the antimesenteric side of the anastomosis. Autopsy studies, contrary to the usually accepted statement, have shown in end-to-end anastomosis of the colon that failure of healing has occurred much more frequently at the antimesenteric than at the mesenteric border of the anastomosis. This is the result of the incorrect angle of division of the colon.

If a major vessel is divided in order to remove radically the lymphatic field, it is most important to recognize the length of colon dependent on this vessel for its nutrition. The resection must include all of this area in order that the remaining proximal and distal segments of bowel be adequately supplied from other sources.

Of recent years the mortality of colon surgery has been greatly reduced. This has been achieved by the appreciation and application of certain basic

* Deceased, after preparation of chapter.

552

principles. In reference to the role of infection in the morbidity and mortality, it is becoming increasingly apparent that patients die, not of contamination of the peritoneal cavity at the time of operation, but of continuous

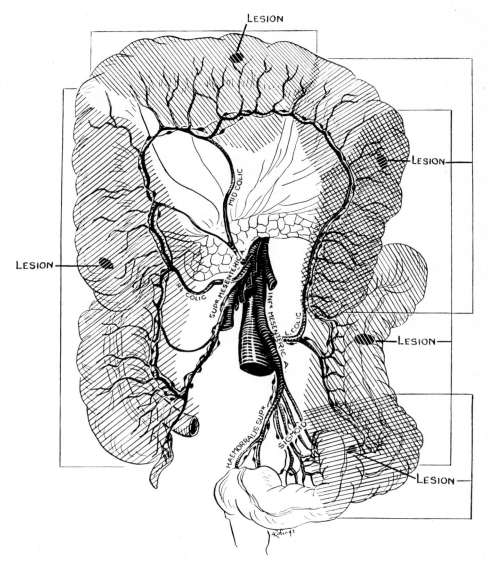

Fig. 302. The shading and brackets indicate extent of resection, determined by the blood supply and lymphatic drainage, for lesions in various areas.

leakage of infected material from anastomoses which fail to heal. Another important contribution is the recognition of the value of decompression in acute obstruction of the colon. Attempts primarily to resect the lesion and anastomose the edematous infected walls of an obstructed colon are almost invariably followed by disaster.

Even in the absence of prolonged large bowel obstruction, whenever resection of the colon has to be undertaken, the advisability of a preliminary defunctioning colostomy or cecostomy should be considered. This is particularly true in operations upon the left large bowel. Its blood supply, as discussed, is more precarious. The content of the left colon is solid or semi-solid, while that of the right colon is fluid or semi-fluid. When an efficient colostomy is done, the colon distal to it can be thoroughly irrigated and

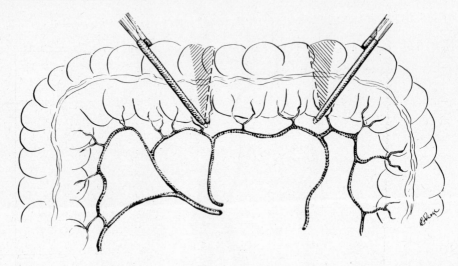

Angle of application of clamps to colon ensuring good blood supply to entire width of edges to be anastomosed.

FIG. 303. Showing correct angle of application of clamps for division of colon. If clamps are applied at dotted lines, shaded areas will slough because arteries supplying colon are terminal vessels running at right angles to the long axis of the bowel. The maximum area of necrosis would occur on the antimesenteric side of the bowel.

emptied of its content prior to an operative procedure. The segment of the bowel distal to the colostomy is at complete physiological rest. The edema and inflammatory induration always associated with a carcinoma of colon can be reduced to an amazing degree. A large fixed brawny colonic mass of questionable operability is very frequently reduced to a relatively small mobile tumor when the accompanying cellulitis has subsided, and an apparently inoperable lesion thus becomes operable provided the surgeon waits long enough. The defunctioning colostomy, therefore, not only increases the incidence of operability but reduces the incidence of infection following excision. It provides also complete physiological rest of the colon during healing of the anastomosis. A freshly completed anastomosis of colon which has immediately to carry the burden of physiological function will obviously be less likely to heal kindly than one which is completely defunctioned. The incidence of local abscesses, sinuses, fistula to neighboring organs and even peritonitis is much higher when a resection with immediate anastomosis is carried out without preliminary defunctioning unless such primary resections are confined to early, mobile, nonobstructing lesions. We are convinced that in a given series of left colon carcinomata, the percentage of lesions which are resectable will be greater when a defunctioning colostomy is used as indicated. As a defunctioning colostomy is practically devoid of any operative mortality, the only criticism which can be leveled at this type of multiple-stage operation rather than a primary resection with immediate anastomosis is the increase in hospital time and the prolongation of the patient's convalescence. Believing that a defunctioning colostomy decreases mortality as well as morbidity, we are convinced that any increase in time demanded by this type of management is thoroughly justifiable.

The development of chemotherapeutic agents has, of recent years, probably reduced the mortality from infection. The preliminary "moth-proofing" of patients by the preoperative administration of sulfonamides, streptomycin and penicillin reduces the incidence of postoperative infection. The local specific action of sulfasuxidine or sulfathalidine in rendering inert the bacterial flora of the colon is proven. These drugs, when given by mouth in adequate dosage over a long enough period of time, can tremendously reduce the number of pathogenic organisms in the stool. Ravdin and his coworkers have shown that the oral administration of streptomycin in $\frac{1}{4}$ gram doses a.c. and h.s. as a supplement to sulfonamide therapy almost completely eliminates pathogenic organisms from the colon.[8] When a preliminary cecostomy or defunctioning colostomy has been done these drugs must, of course, be introduced into the distal defunctioned colon or into the cecostomy. They may have a beneficial effect also upon the infection present in the cellulitis about the site of the lesion.

We believe it most desirable in colon surgery to secure accurate mucosa-to-mucosa apposition with end-to-end anastomoses. There is some debate as to the relative merits of open versus closed technics of anastomosis. The closed methods may result in less contamination of the field during the operation. They do not, however, permit accurate mucosa-to-mucosa suture as is possible with the open technic. It is our firm belief that a patient rarely dies of a peritonitis caused by contamination at the time of operation but rather from continuous infection resulting from a leak of an imperfect anastomosis. Consequently, we are of the opinion that the open anastomosis, with the accuracy of suture under direct vision which it permits, is the procedure of choice (Fig. 304). The most common cause of an anastomotic leak is a defect in the blood supply of the margins being united. The bleeding of the cut margins, which can be seen only with the open technic, is the surest evidence of the viability of the colon segments which are being anastomosed, and is one of the major additional advantages of the open method.

With a closed technic of anastomosis the lumen of the colon may be obstructed by a diaphragm of viable tissue. This accident has been known to occur even when the operation was carried out by an experienced surgeon. Variable degrees of edema always develop about the anastomosis irrespective

1. Stay sutures inserted and held tightly at each end of proposed suture line. Interrupted sutures unite serosa to serosa. Seromuscular coat incised to mucous membrane.

2

2nd row continuous catgut oversews seromuscular flap. Stay sutures make accurate approximation easy and are cut as catgut suture reaches them.

3. Lumen opened on both sides, showing on one side tissue crushed by forcep being cut away. This is done also on the opposite side.

Fig. 304(A). Open end-to-end anastomosis. Interrupted stitches are silk. (From Graham, Roscoe R., *Operative Surgery*, edited by F. W. Bancroft, J. B. Lippincott Company, Philadelphia.)

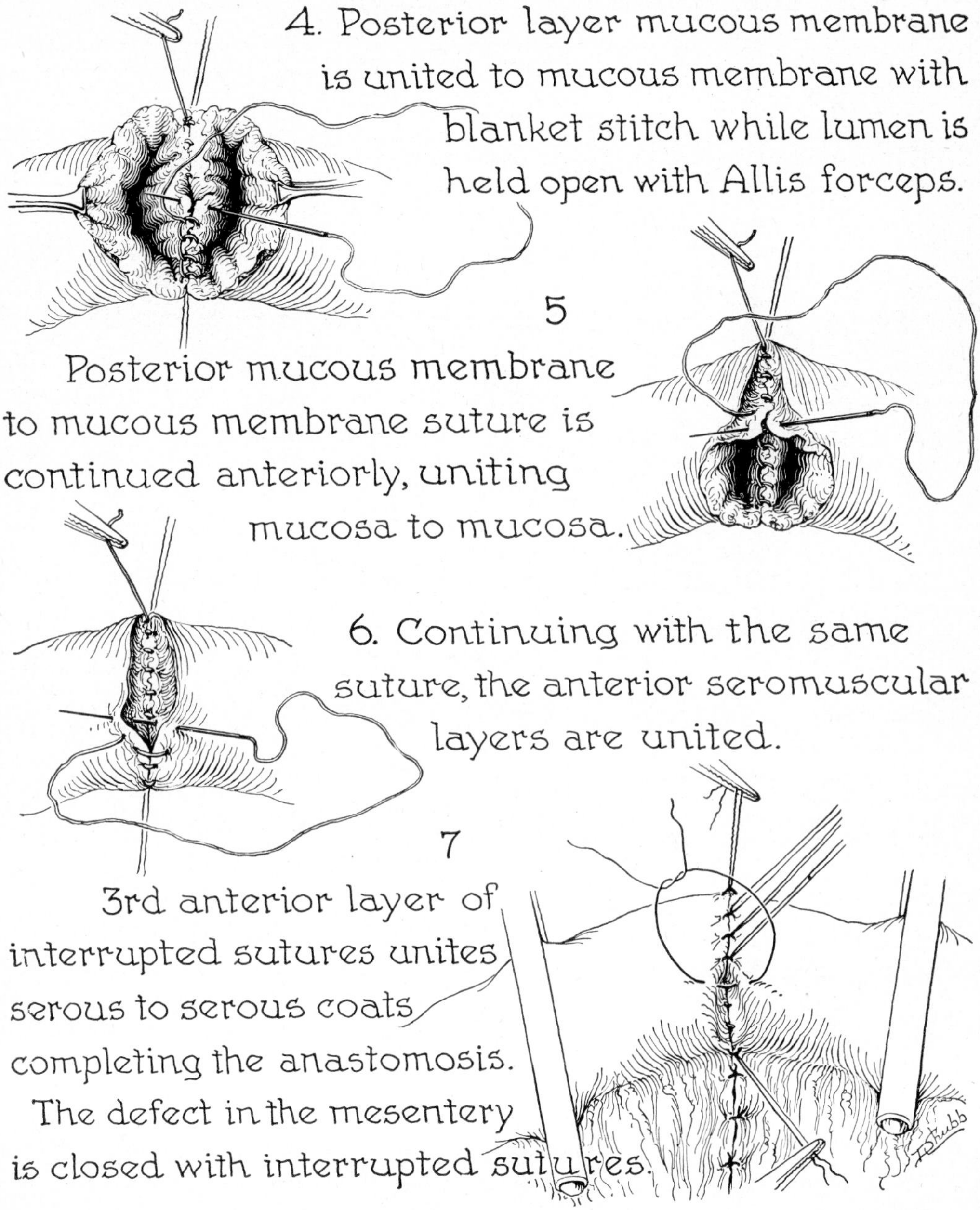

4. Posterior layer mucous membrane is united to mucous membrane with blanket stitch while lumen is held open with Allis forceps.

5

Posterior mucous membrane to mucous membrane suture is continued anteriorly, uniting mucosa to mucosa.

6. Continuing with the same suture, the anterior seromuscular layers are united.

7

3rd anterior layer of interrupted sutures unites serous to serous coats completing the anastomosis. The defect in the mesentery is closed with interrupted sutures.

FIG. 304(B). Open end-to-end anastomosis completed. Mesentery closed and anastomosis completed anteriorly by interrupted silk sutures. (From Graham, Roscoe R., *Operative Surgery*, edited by F. W. Bancroft, J. B. Lippincott Company, Philadelphia.)

of the technic used. One way of maintaining an adequate lumen during healing is to carry out the anastomosis over a rubber tube of suitable diameter (Fig. 305(4)). This maneuver is possible only when an open technic is used.

If a tube to maintain the lumen at the site of anastomosis is not being employed, some method of decompression proximal to the anastomosis is a

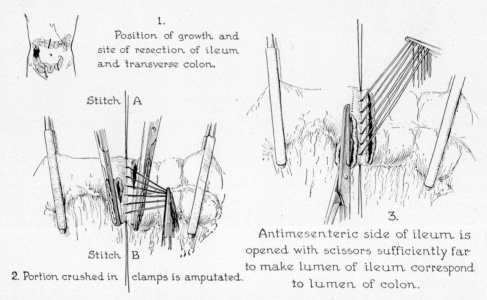

1.
Position of growth and site of resection of ileum and transverse colon.

Stitch A

Stitch B

2. Portion crushed in clamps is amputated.

3.
Antimesenteric side of ileum is opened with scissors sufficiently far to make lumen of ileum correspond to lumen of colon.

Fig. 305. Right colon resection. (1) Extent of resection. (2) Note that the approximation of seromuscular coats of ileum to transverse colon with interrupted silk sutures extends along the antimesenteric border of the ileum beyond its divided end to permit enlargement of the stoma of the ileum to equal that of the colon. (3) After cutting off the crushed edges held in clamps, the lumen of the ileum is increased by extending it along the antimesenteric border until the last silk stay suture is reached.

safety factor to tide over the period of edema. In the absence of a proximal defunctioning colostomy or decompressing cecostomy this result can be attained, as far as the small bowel is concerned, by use of the Miller-Abbott or preferably the Harris tube which should be passed well down into the terminal ileum prior to operation.

INDICATIONS FOR OPERATIVE THERAPY ON THE COLON

Trauma of the Colon. Certain fundamental principles in the handling of perforations of the colon have emerged from experience gained in the recent World War. It is now an accepted fact that, where the site of injury permits, perforated or seriously damaged areas of the colon excluding the cecum should be exteriorized rather than sutured and returned to the peritoneal cavity. This applies to lesions of the ascending, transverse, descending and sigmoid colons.

The technic of the exteriorization varies with the extent of the lesion, the patient's condition and the technical difficulties encountered. The simplest method is the rod colostomy, where the colon is exteriorized by passing a glass rod immediately beneath it at the site of the perforation to hold the colon outside the abdominal wall (Fig. 306(2)). Such colostomies are,

however, much more difficult to close subsequently than are colostomies of the Mikulicz type. Therefore, where possible, the two loops of colon leading to and from the perforation should be sutured together for a distance of 3 to 4 inches before fixing the emerging loops to the skin. This fixation may be accomplished either by the use of the glass rod as in a rod colostomy (Fig. 306) or by the application of clamps on either side of the perforation, between which the colon is divided, the clamps being left lying on the skin (Fig. 308(4)).

Holes in the cecum may also be exteriorized by suturing the cecum about the perforation to the skin as in a cecostomy. This, however, leads to the loss of large quantities of fluid and to skin excoriation about the cecostomy. For these reasons it is often advisable to close holes in the cecum with interrupted sutures and leave the sutured opening immediately beneath the skin in a right iliac muscle splitting incision. If the opening fails to heal and breaks down, it will then produce a cecal fistula in

4.
Catgut suture transfixes short rubber tube which is placed in lumen of ileum and colon across the anastomosis.

5.
Anastomosis is reinforced anteriorly with a layer of interrupted silk sutures.

FIG. 305. (Continued). (4) The continuous blanket stitch of catgut approximating the full thickness of the posterior edges has been inserted, and the short, wide, soft, rubber tube placed within the anastomosis is being transfixed by this suture. (5) The continuous catgut suture approximating the full thickness of the edges has been completed anteriorly, and inverted by a row of interrupted silk stitches.

the right lower quadrant. Under these circumstances fluid loss and skin excoriation can be reduced by the passage of a double lumened tube or a single lumened tube of the Harris type. The tube is passed through the small bowel until it presents at the cecostomy opening. It is then withdrawn a short distance into the terminal ileum and continuous suction applied to it. With this tube in place the patient can be fed a highly nourishing diet and plenty of fluids to maintain his state of nutrition and hydration until the skin about the cecostomy heals to the place where operative closure of the fistula can be undertaken. Because of the adequate blood supply and fluid or semi-fluid content of the cecum penetrating wounds of the cecum may be closed whereas a similar treatment of lesions in the colon would be disastrous. They should all be exteriorized if possible.

Sometimes the perforation of the colon occurs at a site that does not permit of exteriorization as, for example, in the lower sigmoid or rectosigmoid region. Or the multiplicity and extent of injuries to the bowel may make exteriorization inadvisable. Under these conditions suture of the perforations accompanied by a proximal colostomy which completely defunctions the damaged areas should be carried out.

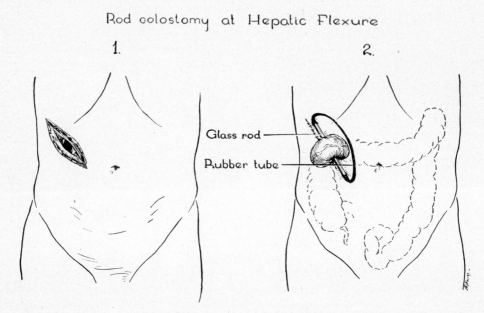

FIG. 306. Rod colostomy. (1) Incision for hepatic flexure colostomy. (2) Position of rod beneath emerging loop of colon, and rubber tube to prevent glass rod from slipping out.

Resections of traumatized colon are always open to grave question. These patients are completely unprepared for any operative procedure and almost invariably are in some degree of shock. The procedure of choice should be the simplest one which will safeguard the patient's life. It may be stated here again that it has been shown repeatedly that it is practically never infection resulting from contamination at the time of the injury when the bowel is open that proves lethal. Fatal infection almost invariably results from continuous leakage at the site of anastomoses or sutured openings left within the peritoneal cavity.

Mechanical Lesions of the Colon. INTUSSUSCEPTION. In an adult intussusception within the colon is a rare condition usually arising from the presence of a submucous lipoma or polyp. Because of the relative fixity of the colon, such intussusceptions are usually limited not only in extent but also as to site. Nevertheless they produce large bowel obstruction.

The operation of choice is reduction of the intussusception where possible with removal of the causative lesion. If the intussusception cannot be reduced manually, resection of the involved area may have to be carried out.

It is interesting to note that when colicky abdominal pain persists following a blind cecostomy for large bowel obstruction, the cause of the obstruction is almost invariably an unreduced intussusception of the colon.

VOLVULUS. Volvulus occurs in the sigmoid colon and cecum. In the sigmoid this accident depends upon the presence of a redundant colon with a long mesocolon. The x-ray diagnosis of this lesion has been described by Dr. M. R. Hall of the X-ray Department of the Toronto General Hospital. [1] When a volvulus of the sigmoid colon has been unwound, it is often possible to deflate safely the tremendously distended loop by the simple procedure of passing a long large rectal tube through the anus and milking the contents of the loop, which are frequently largely gas, downward to the tube to which suction can be applied. If this maneuver fails to empty the loop it may be necessary to open the distended bowel between mucosa forceps and thrust a suction tube into the lumen to deflate it sufficiently to facilitate the handling of the redundant twisted coil. This maneuver should be reserved for desperate cases only. On removal of the suction tube the opening should be oversewn and thoroughly washed, and instruments and gloves used during the procedure should be discarded. Exteriorization of this closure is imperative if the patient's condition precludes an obstructive resection.

Resection of the area of colon involved in the volvulus is advisable for two reasons. Its blood supply is already compromised, and the mesenteric arteries are very apt to become thrombosed even after the mesocolon is untwisted. Moreover, if the area is not resected the same conditions exist which made the volvulus possible and recurrence is frequent. When the volvulus involves the sigmoid an obstructive type of resection should be carried out (Fig. 307), the loops of the resultant colostomy emerging, where possible, through a separate muscle splitting incision. If the colon is too bulky to permit of passing it through a separate incision, the loops will have to emerge through the laparotomy wound which is closed about them.

When the cecum is the site of a volvulus the symptoms are those of low small bowel rather than large bowel obstruction. But tremendous abdominal distention develops with the same rapidity as in volvulus of the sigmoid. Here the operation of choice is to unwind the volvulus and fix the cecum to the right iliac fossa to prevent recurrence. Where the blood supply of the twisted loop has been so compromised as to make its removal imperative, a right colon resection with end-to-end anastomosis of terminal ileum to transverse colon over a tube should be performed (Fig. 305). If the condition of the patient and the changes which have occurred in the bowel wall make a resection with immediate anastomosis inadvisable, an obstructive type of resection is preferable.

Inflammatory Lesions of the Colon Requiring Operation. APPENDICITIS. The removal of the appendix is the commonest operative procedure to which the human abdomen is subjected and it is an operation which is very frequently relegated to the most junior member of the surgical staff. Yet appendectomy may be a very difficult operation requiring the most careful consideration of a mature surgical judgment.

SOLITARY DIVERTICULUM OF CECUM. Occasionally one encounters, usually mistakenly diagnosed as acute appendicitis, a solitary diverticulum of the cecum. Under these circumstances the diverticulum is very often acutely inflamed at the time of operation and the induration about it may

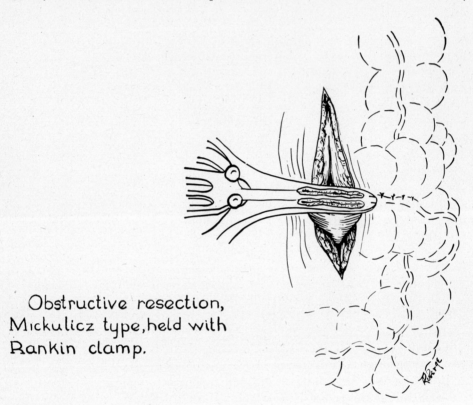

Obstructive resection, Mickulicz type, held with Rankin clamp.

FIG. 307. Rankin clamp applied to double-barreled colostomy resulting from obstructive resection.

make it simulate closely a carcinoma of the cecum. The absence of previous symptoms, particularly secondary anemia, suggestive of carcinoma of the cecum, and the presence of leukocytosis, fever and local signs of inflammation, may save the patient from a right colectomy if the surgeon is aware of the fact that solitary diverticula sometimes occur in this region.

If the diverticulum occurs on the free surface of the cecum and is not too indurated and inflamed the surgeon may be tempted to invert it and oversew its base from the serosal surface. This is a mistake as the diverticulum almost invariably recurs. The operation indicated is a wedge resection of the diverticulum after mobilizing the cecum. The operative area should be decompressed by the passage of a tube. Should the ileocecal junction be involved by the induration about the diverticulum, the entire cecum may have to be removed.

PERFORATED SOLITARY DIVERTICULUM OF THE ASCENDING COLON. The ascending colon is also not infrequently the site of a solitary diverticulum which is usually symptomless unless it becomes the site of an acute inflammatory process which may even result in perforation and abscess formation.

Under these circumstances the perforation should be drained as suggested in appendical abscesses. No attempt should be made to close the perforation or remove the diverticulum. Should a fecal fistula persist it may be dealt with as discussed under "Fecal Fistulae."

DIVERTICULITIS OF COLON. *Acute Perforation of Colon.* Acute diverticulitis is not a surgical problem unless some complication develops. Not infrequently, however, when operating upon a patient for erroneously diagnosed acute appendicitis, the surgeon is confronted with an acute diverticulitis of a loop of sigmoid colon lying in the right iliac fossa and often presenting a local perforation which has given rise to the symptoms and signs of appendicitis.

Any radical procedure, such as resection of the involved loop of colon, is, of course, completely contraindicated at this stage. The perforation should not be sought and, if apparent, is impossible to close by suture. The inflamed colon should be isolated as well as possible and drainage instituted as later described for acute intraperitoneal infection. A fecal fistula usually develops and will have to be dealt with subsequently as, in our experience, it never heals spontaneously.

With Obstruction. Obstruction of the sigmoid colon is a not infrequent complication of diverticulitis and it may be impossible to exclude carcinoma as the cause. Under these circumstances the lesion requires resection. When the diverticulitis does not extend too low in the sigmoid an obstructive resection may be carried out (Fig. 307). The resulting colostomy must be left for sufficient time for all adjacent inflammatory reaction to subside before closure is attempted. If, however, the involvement of the colon extends so low as to make an obstructive resection impossible, it is our practice, because of increased safety, to defunction the left colon completely by a transverse colon colostomy (Fig. 308). Sufficient time must elapse following the defunctioning colostomy to permit of complete subsidence of the inflammatory reaction before undertaking resection of the involved area with immediate anastomosis.

With Abscess Formation. When diverticulitis results in perforation and the development of a tender palpable inflammatory mass it has been found unwise to approach the site of the lesion directly as a primary surgical procedure. Such interference can only result in the spread of infection, possibly to a fatal peritonitis, and to the certain development of persistent fecal fistulae. Usually the mass responds to chemotherapy and supportive measures as do appendical masses. However, when it continues to enlarge and is accompanied by a persistent fever and leukocytosis, the procedure of choice is to avoid completely any local operation, and instead perform a defunctioning transverse colon colostomy (Fig. 308). This places the diseased colon completely at rest and makes possible irrigations of the defunctioned segment with saline introduced into the distal stoma of the colostomy. The infection responds to the local administration of sulfasuxidine or sulfathalidine through the distal colostomy opening. Abscesses about an area of diverticulitis have a strong tendency to drain spontaneously into the lumen of the colon once the bowel has been put at rest. In this way operative drainage of abscesses with the subsequent development of fecal fistulae may be avoided.

If sigmoid diverticulitis has been so serious as to necessitate a defunctioning colostomy, our experience has shown that the residual damage is so great that it is necessary to resect the involved colon in order to safeguard the patient's future. Closure of the colostomy without such a resection is too apt to be followed by obstruction or recurrent exacerbations of the disease. The resection, however, should rarely be carried out until at least six months have elapsed following the colostomy. Occasionally a much longer interval is desirable, often a year or more, to allow of complete subsidence of infection and make resection safe. Contrary to many statements a transverse colon colostomy can be regulated with as little inconvenience as one in the sigmoid colon. It cannot be too strongly urged that diverticulitis requiring surgical interference is a very serious disease and demands considered judgment in its management. Sometimes the mere injection of barium into the distal limb of the colostomy in an effort to determine the progress of the disease produces sufficient irritation to initiate an acute exacerbation. Furthermore, x-ray studies, apart from determining the site of the lesion, give little valuable information as to the seriousness or progress of the disease.

When, however, a sufficiently long interval of complete defunctioning has been allowed, resection of the diseased colon with end-to-end anastomosis may be performed with safety. Following resection several weeks must be allowed to elapse before the colostomy is closed.

With Fistulae. A local perforation or abscess associated with diverticulitis not infrequently results in fistulae between the colon and small bowel, vagina, bladder or skin. Here again a direct surgical attack upon the diseased colon in an attempt to extirpate it and thus cure the fistulae is courting disaster. The wise and safe way to deal with this problem is the same as that employed for acute diverticulitis with a persistent inflammatory mass, namely to defunction the colon completely by a transverse colon colostomy. The sigmoid colon with its fistulae is then treated by repeated irrigations of saline into the distal stoma for at least six months before resection of the lesion is undertaken. In some instances the fistulae may close spontaneously on this management. The resection may be deferred indefinitely, particularly in elderly, debilitated or tremendously obese individuals with a very extensive or very low lying lesion. Under these conditions resection to enable the subsequent closure of the colostomy might entail a prohibitive operative risk.

1. Opening in omentum through which loop of transverse colon is to be drawn.

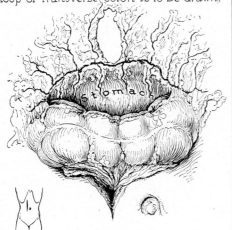

Site of incision.　Greater omentum separated from mid transverse colon.

2. Rubber tube through opening in mesentery enables colon to be drawn through opening in omentum shown in figure 1.

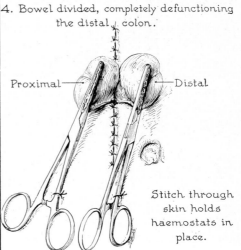

Proximal

Distal

Proximal and distal limbs of transverse colon sutured together as in Mickulicz procedure.

Cautery divides the exteriorized loop of colon.

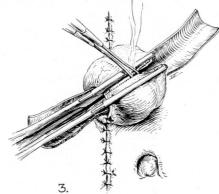

3.

Opened rubber tube enables Kocher haemostats to grasp bowel without wounding mesentery and also protects bowel and mesentery from cautery.

4. Bowel divided, completely defunctioning the distal colon.

Proximal

Distal

Stitch through skin holds haemostats in place.

FIG. 308. Mikulicz type of colostomy in transverse colon. (1) Omentum dissected off colon and aperture made in gastrocolic omentum. (2) A loop of colon suspended by rubber tube. Two limbs of bowel sutured together for four inches and brought out through aperture in gastrocolic omentum. (3) Complete transection by cautery of clamped exteriorized loop of colon with protection by opened rubber tube. (4) Fixation by skin stitches of clamps holding two ends of divided transverse colon. Proximal clamp may be removed in 24 hours or sooner, if necessary. Distal clamp remains in situ for 60 hours.

FECAL FISTULAE. Colonic fistulae result either from traumatic lesions, extensive neoplasms or inflammatory disease such as diverticulitis and actinomycosis, and the treatment varies with the cause. It may, however, be stated that the colon which is the site of a fistula, irrespective of etiology, must be decompressed, defunctioned or excluded before any local operation designed to cure the fistula is undertaken.

Fecal fistulae that result from trauma will necessarily occur either in exteriorized or in already defunctioned bowel. The principles and details of their management are those previously discussed under trauma of the colon or those which will be discussed subsequently under closure of colostomy stomata.

If a fistula of the left colon opening into an adjacent organ or externally has resulted from a perforating carcinoma, a proximal defunctioning colostomy is the essential preliminary procedure. If the disappearance of the inflammatory reaction should reveal a lesion which is resectable, a much more extensive removal can be carried out safely after an adequate period of absolute physiological rest. Colonic fistulae that result from perforating carcinomata are, however, rarely amenable to radical extirpation, and those that are almost invariably occur in the region of the cecum. When they arise from the left colon a proximal defunctioning colostomy will give great comfort to the patient. The penetration of a carcinoma of the cecum producing a pericecal abscess which is mistaken for and drained under the diagnosis of appendical abscess always results in a fecal fistula which will not heal. For such a fistula an operation which excludes the right colon and restores gastro-intestinal continuity is the operation of choice (Fig. 309).

A cecal fistula as a complication of an acute pyogenic appendicitis tends to heal spontaneously. Cecal fistulae secondary to actinomycosis are dealt with in exactly the same manner as if they were due to carcinoma. Perforated diverticulitis is almost invariably the basis of all other colonic fistulae.

ACTINOMYCOSIS. Actinomycotic infection of the gastro-intestinal tract involves most commonly the ileocecal area and produces the well known abscess riddled lesion directly invading all surrounding tissues with no regard for fascial planes, anatomical layers or lymphatic drainage. Cure of this disease depends upon thorough local excision and drainage accompanied by radiation treatment and chemotherapy. In ileocecal actinomycosis the operation indicated is a right colon resection with block excision of involved tissues in the area of the disease, saving only such important structures as the right ureter and right common iliac vessels.

HYPERTROPHIC ILEOCECAL TUBERCULOSIS. Gastro-intestinal tuberculosis is primarily a medical problem. Sometimes, however, the disease takes the form of a well localized hypertrophic lesion in the ileocecal region. When this occurs resection of the cecum or possibly the whole right colon is indicated.

ULCERATIVE COLITIS. Of recent years the experience of the Roosevelt Hospital group in New York has led to greater clarification of the role of surgery in the management of patients with this serious disease. Certain fundamental principles of treatment have been established. One is that the patient's condition should not be allowed to deteriorate until an ileostomy is being done as an emergency operation for hemorrhage or sepsis. The operative mortality of such urgently performed ileostomies is prohibitive. The next established principle is that proximal defunctioning is an absolute requisite as a preliminary to surgical excision. This takes the form of an ileostomy in most cases, but may be a transverse colon colostomy if the disease is limited to the left colon. Further, it has been shown that the time interval between defunctioning and resection should be that required to attain the maximum improvement of nutrition and quiescence of infection.

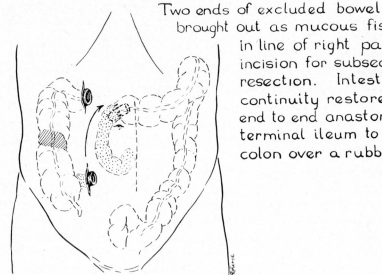

Two ends of excluded bowel brought out as mucous fistulae in line of right paramedian incision for subsequent resection. Intestinal continuity restored by end to end anastomosis of terminal ileum to transverse colon over a rubber tube.

FIG. 309. Right colon exclusion.

Resection should then be carried out before another exacerbation of this rhythmically recurring disease develops. The interval required is usually in the neighborhood of four to six months.

The entire area of involved colon must be excised. Where this necessitates a total colectomy it must be done in stages to suit the patient's ability to withstand operation. Often the right, transverse and descending colons can be resected at one stage, and the abdominoperineal resection of sigmoid and rectum is deferred until the patient has adequately recovered from this procedure. Another important fact now recognized is that the stumps of unresected portions of the colon should, in this disease, never be closed and returned to the peritoneal cavity. If this is done a flare up of infection very frequently results in failure of healing of the stump giving rise to fatal peritonitis. These stumps should always be brought out of the abdominal wall as mucous fistulae, preferably at the site of a subsequent incision to resect the rest of the diseased colon. This applies to the distal cut surface of the ileum when an ileostomy has been done, as well as to the sigmoid stump following a subtotal colectomy. Through these mucous fistulae the residual diseased bowel can be irrigated and exposed to local chemotherapy.

A last important principle is that when the rectum and lower sigmoid seem to be free of disease, a very long interval, at least two years, must be allowed to elapse before the reestablishment of intestinal continuity is considered. The condition of the rectum and sigmoid must be very carefully assessed by x-ray and sigmoidoscopic studies to be absolutely sure they are free from disease before they are subjected to the stress of exposure to irritating ileal content following the anastomosis of the ileum to the rectosigmoid stump. The same is true when a transverse colon colostomy has been performed for disease apparently localized to the descending colon and upper sigmoid.

Neoplasia of the Colon. BENIGN. *Submucous Lipoma.* The presence of a submucous lipoma produces no signs or symptoms as a rule unless it gives rise to an intussusception of the colon. Then large bowel obstruction with pain which is unrelieved by a blind cecostomy develops. The operations indicated for this condition were discussed previously.

Benign Polypi. Polypi of the colon present the two outstanding features characteristic of all polypi, namely bleeding and a strong tendency to undergo malignant change. It is usually the bleeding which brings about the investigation of the patient. The polypus may be discovered either by radiological examination, or by direct vision through a sigmoidoscope, or by careful manual palpation of the colon in cases subjected to laparotomy because of large bowel bleeding of undetermined origin.

The malignant change in these polypi begins at their apices and produces a carcinoma which has a tendency to be only locally malignant for quite a long period of time. Therefore it is advisable to treat these lesions by conservative local resection rather than by the extensive surgical procedures usually carried out for carcinoma. Subsequently x-ray and sigmoidoscopic investigation should be repeated at frequent intervals over a prolonged period for evidence of any recurrence.

The colon is opened at the site of the polypus which is then examined under direct vision. If the polypus is solitary and presents no firm induration or fixation of its base suggesting malignant change with extension into submucosa, a local resection of the polypus with subsequent careful closure of the colon is justified. The pathological report in these lesions is almost always "malignant polypi." This should not alarm the surgeon, but emphasizes the necessity of reinvestigation of the patient by sigmoidoscopic and radiological methods at three month intervals for a year or two seeking evidence of any recurrence.

Multiple Polyposis. Sometimes polypi of the colon are extremely numerous and may be scattered throughout the entire extent of the large bowel. This condition of multiple polyposis may be a primary one. Although there is a strong hereditary trend in these cases, the polypi are apparently not congenital as they usually do not appear until the patient reaches his teens. Other cases are really a pseudopolyposis, the polypi having developed from the hypertrophy of little islands of intact mucosa surrounded by the scarring of multiple healed ulcers of the colon. Under these circumstances the lesion develops as a late complication of ulcerative colitis or amoebic dysentery.

Whatever their origin these polypi all present a strong tendency toward malignant change. It is a common occurrence to find several early polypoid carcinomata in a colon resected for multiple polyposis. For this reason radical surgical excision of all the large bowel containing multiple polypi is indicated. This sometimes necessitates total colectomy in stages, leaving the patient with a permanent ileostomy. If not treated in this way these patients almost invariably die of large bowel carcinoma, and, especially in young people for whom life holds much, such a radical approach is justified.

If there are a few small polypi in the rectum and lower sigmoid, it is justifiable to be conservative, fulgurizing the polypi through a sigmoidoscope. This implies sigmoidoscopic examinations at three month intervals.

MALIGNANT. The presence of a large bowel carcinoma is the cause, either directly or indirectly, of the majority of operations upon the colon. All patients with colon neoplasm present problems in nutrition. In right colon carcinomata the nutritional defect results from the bleeding and diarrhea almost invariably associated with these lesions, frequently resulting in a profound anemia. In the left colon, the nutritional defect is caused and overshadowed by chronic or subacute intestinal obstruction. It is disastrous to concentrate our treatment on the local malignancy forgetting to assess the associated disturbance occurring in the individual. The nutritional defect must be recognized, evaluated and, as far as possible, corrected before radical surgical extirpation of the disease is undertaken. This will be discussed in greater detail in the section on preoperative preparation of patients.

Carcinomata of Cecum and Ascending Colon. Generally speaking malignant growths of the colon proximal to the hepatic flexure tend to be of the polypoid variety. These tumors bleed continuously and stimulate an increased frequency and fluidity of stools, but rarely produce obstructive symptoms.

The operation of choice in resectable lesions is a one stage removal of the right colon (Fig. 305). If the lesion is not removable the surgeon may be tempted to perform a side-to-side anastomosis of the terminal ileum to the transverse colon, thus short circuiting the lesion without interruption of the bowel continuity. Although this is the simplest procedure to carry out under these circumstances, it is inadequate. It does not completely defunction the colon and the content of the terminal ileum may be driven into the right colon to meet a reflux from the transverse colon thus giving rise to persistent symptoms of obstruction.

Another alternative is to transect the terminal ileum and do an end-to-side anastomosis of its proximal end to transverse colon. The distal transected end of ileum may then be closed and dropped back into the abdomen. Such a procedure, however, violates one of the basic principles of colon surgery insofar as it leaves a long blind diverticulum off the intestinal canal.

Transverse colon content may travel proximally as well as distally from the end-to-side anastomosis and often causes impaction in the ascending colon. Consequently, it is necessary to make a separate stab wound through which to draw the distal cut end of the ileum. One then has a mucous fistula as a safety valve for the defunctioned right colon and through which the ascending colon may drain and be irrigated.

If the extent of the local lesion renders it at the moment inoperable but permits consideration of subsequent resection of the right colon it is advantageous to exclude it completely by transection of the transverse colon as well as of the terminal ileum (Fig. 309). The proximal end of terminal ileum is then anastomosed to the distal stump of transverse colon thus restoring the continuity of the intestinal tract. The remaining ends of ileum and colon are brought out through separate stab wounds as mucous fistulae. Through these stomata the excluded colon may be irrigated and the inflammatory reaction is reduced to a minimum by this as well as by the complete physiological rest.

An apparently nonresectable lesion may become removable as a result of this complete defunctioning and frequent lavage. For this reason, whenever the feasibility of resecting a right colon carcinoma is questionable, the primary approach should be through a left paramedian incision. If the lesion necessitates a right colon exclusion, the divided ends of the colon and ileum of the excluded segment can then be exteriorized through stab wounds in the line of a subsequent right paramedian incision made for excision of the segment.

Carcinomata between Hepatic Flexure and Rectosigmoid. Most carcinomata of the transverse and left large bowel are of the stenosing type producing progressive obstruction with its inevitable clinical syndrome. These are the tumors which most often produce the acute large bowel obstruction which demands cecostomy as a life-saving procedure.

When the obstruction is not so acute as to demand cecostomy, one is faced with a decision as to whether preliminary operative decompression might not still be desirable. There is increasing evidence of the efficacy of the sulfonamides, streptomycin and penicillin in controlling infection. The addition of parenteral therapy combined with the use of an in-dwelling Miller-Abbott or Harris tube can often control the biochemical and pathological disasters of obstruction. The combined use of these drugs and tube decompression is increasing the incidence of one stage primary resection of transverse and left colon. However, such a procedure demands the most careful preoperative preparation and mature clinical judgment to achieve as high a resectability rate with as low a mortality and morbidity as is obtained when a preliminary cecostomy or transverse colon colostomy is carried out.

If the tumor occurs in the segment of colon supplied by the middle or left colic artery, a cecostomy is the operation of choice if operative decompression is decided upon. Even if the carcinoma is situated in the distal portion of the area of colon supplied by the left colic artery, this vessel must be sacrificed at its origin in order to remove the entire field of lymphatic drainage. This deprives the distal transverse colon of all blood supply except the small marginal vessel arising from the middle colic artery. Thus it is not possible, even under these circumstances, to do a defunctioning transverse colon colostomy as a preliminary procedure, because such a colostomy would lie within the anatomical scope of the resection demanded for reasons of blood supply.

The transverse colon, splenic flexure, descending and upper sigmoid colons lend themselves so well to mobilization that carcinomata in these regions can very often be removed by a primary obstructive resection as described by Rankin. This type of resection is an unusually safe operation because no anastomosis of the bowel is left within the peritoneal cavity, and the dangerous area is entirely exteriorized. It is, however, a slightly more limited resection than can be accomplished by removal of the lesion with end-to-end anastomosis. Sufficient slack must be left to allow of the approximation of two loops of colon, 3 inches in length, coming up to the skin surface (Fig. 307). Therefore, the length of bowel that can be removed is 6 inches shorter than the resection possible when an end-to-end anastomosis is performed within the peritoneal cavity. The removal of the lymphatic field is similarly more limited. For this reason the obstructive resection of the colon may better be reserved for inflammatory, mechanical and traumatic lesions. In carcinoma, where the removal of the area of lymphatic drainage with an adequate length of bowel on either side of the lesion is of paramount importance, resection with immediate anastomosis is usually to be preferred. This argument is supported by the frequent occurrence of metastases in the region of the colostomy closure following obstructive resection. However, in patients whose general condition is poor, or who have hepatic secondaries, multiple stage operations are inadvisable. Then if obstruction or inflammatory edema make primary resection with immediate anastomosis unsafe, the obstructive resection offers a relatively simple and rapid means of removing the primary growth in a very safe manner. The resultant colostomy may even be permanent, but if the patient's condition improves it is quite easily closed at a later date.

Primary resection with immediate anastomosis of a lesion which demands division of the superior hemorrhoidal artery for its adequate removal presents a new problem. In order to ensure an adequate blood supply of the rectal stump the resection must be carried distally to the level of the levator ani muscles. This exposes the widely dissected and vulnerable retroperitoneal space to infection from the colon. Even slight obstruction with its inevitable accompaniment of some degree of edema and pericolic cellulitis makes primary resection with immediate anastomosis hazardous and therefore inadvisable. Only in the complete absence of any obstruction whatsoever should primary resection with restoration of continuity be considered in carcinomata of the distal sigmoid colon. The great majority of these lesions will be more safely handled by a preliminary defunctioning transverse colon colostomy.

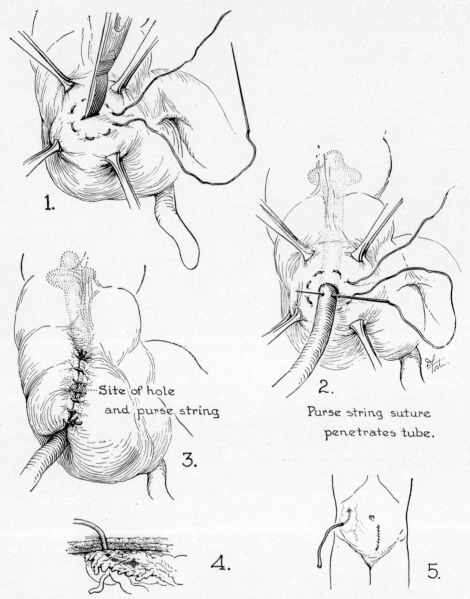

1.

2.
Purse string suture
penetrates tube.

3.
····Site of hole
and purse string

4.
Tube pulled through omentum which is placed
between cecum and parietal peritoneum.

5.
Tube brought through
stab wound – abdominal wall.

FIG. 310. Stab cecostomy from within the abdomen. (1) Incision of cecum within
purse-string suture with cecum held high by four Allis clamps to prevent soiling. (2)
Transfixion of retention catheter by purse-string suture. (3) Catheter buried in wall of
cecum by Witzel method. (4) Interposition of omentum between cecum and abdominal
wall. (5) Location of cecostomy stab wound. (From *Am. J. Surg.*, 46(No. 1):135-142, [Oct.],
1939.)

When a primary resection with immediate anastomosis has been decided upon and performed, if at the completion of operation any doubt exists as to the security of the anastomosis, decompression may be provided by doing a simultaneous stab cecostomy from within the abdomen (Fig. 310).

It is always advisable to bear in mind the great advantages of some preliminary defunctioning or decompressing procedure, particularly in carcinomata of the lower sigmoid region. Here the tumor lies below the supply of the left colic artery so that a transverse colon colostomy is possible. To recapitulate, this colostomy: (1) completely defunctions the bowel; (2) allows of irrigation hastening the disappearance of the edema, infection and induration about the tumor; (3) permits the direct application of sulfonamides and streptomycin; (4) with this, many a seemingly unresectable lesion becomes operable; (5) permits the extensive removal of all retroperitoneal, areolar and lymphatic tissue with comparative safety; (6) keeps the anastomosis at rest until healed; and (7) should perianastomotic suppuration occur it will drain into the lumen of the bowel without disastrous sequelae. We believe that almost all cases of fatal peritonitis result from continuous leak due to failure of healing of intraperitoneal anastomoses, rather than from contamination at the time of operation. Therefore, when any doubt exists as to the risk of primary resection, the safety factor resulting from a preliminary colostomy more than justifies the time consumed by the multiple stage procedure.

PREPARATION OF PATIENTS WITH CHRONIC LESIONS OF COLON

Cleansing of Colon and Administration of Antibiotics. Unless obstruction is of such degree as to contraindicate catharsis, the preliminary administration of laxatives as well as enemata is indicated to empty the gastrointestinal tract and clear the colon of scyballous masses. The administration of streptomycin requires an empty colon to produce its maximum effect on the bacterial content.

An ounce of liquid paraffin is given each night. In the morning two drachms of concentrated (50 per cent) magnesium sulfate are administered and this dose is modified so that the patient has at least two stools daily. Enemata are given in the afternoon only if two stools are not obtained. Salts and oil are administered until the colon proximal to the lesion has been thoroughly emptied, and this will require from three to five days, depending upon the degree of obstruction present.

Catharsis and enemata are then discontinued and oral administration of streptomycin is begun in $\frac{1}{4}$ gram doses a.c. and h.s. This is carried on for three days during which the patient remains on a very low residue diet. Twenty-four hours before operation the dose of streptomycin is doubled and the route of administration changed from oral to intramuscular injection, $\frac{1}{2}$ gram being given every 6 hours. During the 24-hour period immediately before operation, penicillin also is given intramuscularly in 50,000 unit doses every three hours. There is some evidence to show that penicillin and streptomycin should be given separately in order for each to achieve its maximum effect. The appearance of tinnitus is, of course, an indication for the immediate cessation of streptomycin administration. Postoperatively the administration of streptomycin is continued for 72 hours and of penicillin for as long as 5 days in the same dosage as was used in the 24-hour period immediately before operation. It should be remembered that these drugs may cause and maintain fever.

In the presence of any distention or crampy abdominal pain a Miller-Abbott or Harris tube should be put down at the start of preparation to decompress the entire small bowel. In the absence of such symptoms a tube is started down 24 hours before operation and the patient may be fluoroscoped the night before operation to determine the position of the tube. In the late afternoon of the day before operation saline enemata are given until the return is clear.

Chemotherapy. In the absence of a colostomy or cecostomy, sulfasuxidine is given by mouth. The dosage we have employed is 8 to 10 grams in 24 hours divided into 4 doses. This is begun at the start of preparation and carried on throughout both the mechanical cleansing and the streptomycin phases. In our experience sulfasuxidine has a mildly laxative effect.

Correction of Nutritional Defects. The patient's nutritional state is carefully assessed. Hematological studies are made including estimations of the plasma proteins and plasma chlorides. Kidney function is evaluated and estimation of the nonprotein nitrogen is always done. Whole blood transfusions are employed to correct secondary anemia, and these may be supplemented by plasma where hypoproteinemia exists although the oral administration of protein is the most effective method of attaining a normal plasma protein level. Rarely the intravenous administration of fluids may be necessary to combat dehydration, and hypertonic saline may be given if the plasma chlorides are below normal levels.

A low residue, high protein diet is desirable in the preoperative preparation of the patient. The lack of residue from the diet is essential to the maximum efficiency of streptomycin therapy. Large quantities of fluid are given by mouth. The caloric value of the diet should be high and its protein content may be increased by the addition of skimmed milk powder. Avitaminosis is also corrected and vitamins are added to the diet freely. Synthetic vitamin C is administered in doses of 100 milligrams three times daily.

INCISIONS

John B. Deaver made the epigrammatic remark, "Only cut what you can see and always see what you cut!" In no field of surgery is this more essential than in the abdomen. This implies perfect exposure on all occasions. Such is achieved only through the use of an adequate incision properly placed. As Ogilvie has stated, "The use of stalked lights and long instruments working through a small incision is merely an example of perverted ingenuity!"

We must never lose sight of the fact that incisions heal from the sides, not from the ends. A long incision will heal as promptly as a short one, minimizing the trauma not only to the abdominal wall but to the whole operative field and, as a corollary, must be safer.

McBurney Incision. It is our practice, except in very unusual circumstances, to expose the appendix via the right lower quadrant muscle splitting incision first described by McBurney (Fig. 311). A right paramedian incision is only justified where the diagnosis is in doubt or where a co-existing lesion

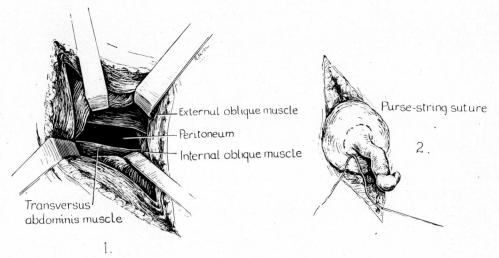

FIG. 311. (1) The McBurney or gridiron muscle-splitting incision. (2) Purse-string suture for appendectomy inserted ready to tie.

in the female pelvis is suspected. Even when the diagnosis is in doubt it is amazing how accurately one can assess the intraperitoneal lesion through this incision with minimal trauma and no increased risk. If the patient is found to have some other condition necessitating a more adequate exposure, the gridiron incision may be abandoned and a paramedian one made. No apology need be made for this change of incision. The muscle splitting wound will heal just as rapidly as the larger one, and it is surprising how frequently a McBurney incision will be adequate. It has the advantage of cutting no muscle fibers and no important nerves and there is a tendency for this wound to draw together rather than apart when the patient strains. Moreover, in acute appendicitis the inflamed organ is not dragged across the peritoneal cavity as it is when approached by a paramedian incision, but is picked out of the peritoneal cavity through an incision which immediately overlies it. The general peritoneal cavity can be completely protected from contamination by the use of this atraumatic direct approach, which weakens the abdominal wall less than any other type of incision providing it is properly closed. Particularly important in closure is the accurate apposition of the aponeurosis of the transversus. This incision is described under appendectomy.

Split Muscle Incisions in Other Quadrants. Muscle splitting incisions are very frequently indicated in quadrants of the abdomen other than the right lower. In the right upper quadrant this incision is employed for the hepatic flexure colostomy (Fig. 306), used to defunction the transverse colon in the presence of a gastro-jejuno-colic fistula. In the left iliac region it is used for sigmoid colostomies. Whenever the colon is being brought out through the abdominal wall as a temporary or permanent colostomy, a grid-iron incision will weaken the abdominal wall least, can be closed with fewest herniae and should be employed whenever possible. There are three exceptions to this rule. One is in the transverse colon colostomy when an upper right rectus muscle splitting incision is employed. Two is where we wish to place a colon stump in the line of the incision for a subsequent resection. Three is where an obstructive resection is being performed and the loop being resected is too bulky to be delivered through a muscle splitting incision in the flank. The colostomy may then have to be left in the laparotomy wound which is closed about it.

The muscle splitting incision is of great value also in the drainage of abscesses from any cause. Sometimes the inflammatory lesion is directly approached through a suitably situated gridiron incision. At other times the necessity for drainage becomes evident after the abdomen has been opened through a paramedian incision. Under these circumstances the packing and drainage tubes should be brought out via a separate muscle splitting incision. In this way infection of the laparotomy wound may be avoided and the incidence of subsequent incisional hernia is reduced.

Paramedian Incisions. Our experience with transverse incisions across the abdomen has not been happy. Consequently for extensive exposure of the peritoneal cavity we employ the vertical paramedian incision.

DISPLACING RECTUS. Whether the rectus muscle is displaced laterally or split longitudinally depends largely upon the suture material we intend to use for closure. The distance of the skin incision lateral to the umbilicus depends upon the patient's obesity and the degree of diastasis recti present. It should be placed just lateral to the medial margin of the rectus muscle. Great care should be taken to make the incision through the skin at exactly right angles to the skin surface, as skin healing and the subsequent scar will then be much better. Other scars present within range of the planned incision should be excised, even though this necessitates the displacement of a skin and subcutaneous fat flap to gain access to the midline of the rectus muscle. The presence of a previous operation scar in close proximity to the incision being made interferes with the blood supply of the skin on the side of the incision bordering on the old scar and therefore prevents perfect wound healing.

The incision is deepened to expose the anterior sheath of the rectus muscle which must be well cleared to facilitate subsequent accurate closure of sheath margins without the interposition of fat. If it has been decided to displace the rectus muscle, the anterior sheath of the muscle is incised in its midline for the full length of the incision. The medial portion of the anterior sheath is then dissected up from the muscle which is retracted laterally. The peritoneal cavity is now opened by an incision through the posterior fascial sheath of the rectus. This incision in the posterior sheath should be behind the midline of the rectus muscle so that, on closure, the replaced muscle lies between the scars in its posterior and anterior sheaths.

SPLITTING RECTUS. If the rectus muscle is to be split longitudinally we have found that it is technically easier to incise the anterior sheath of the rectus and split the muscle fibers simultaneously as one layer. The incision of the anterior sheath with scalpel should precede by half an inch the splitting of the muscle fibers. In this way vessels in the muscle crossing the line of division are rendered visible and can be caught by hemostats before being cut or torn. The posterior fascia and peritoneum are then opened in the same manner as in the muscle displacing incision.

METHODS OF WOUND CLOSURE

The fundamental principles upon which sound wound healing depends are now well recognized. Of recent years particular appreciation has been accorded the importance of hypoproteinemia and avitaminosis in the incidence of wound disruption. This applies not only to wounds in the abdominal wall but also to the speed and soundness of healing of intestinal anastomoses. The necessity of adequate preoperative preparation of patients, to correct nutritional defects, particularly low plasma protein levels and vitamin deficiencies, especially of vitamin C, cannot be overemphasized. The most meticulous technic of wound closure will fail if the physiological requisites for tissue repair are neglected.

It is our belief that more wound infections result from poor hemostasis than from contamination of the wound during operation. A yearly analysis of our own wound infections has repeatedly confirmed this statement. Perfect hemostasis can be achieved, and wound trauma minimized only by handling tissues with the utmost gentleness. Great care must be taken to minimize wound contamination. But an absolutely dry wound is, in our opinion, the prime requisite to healing by first intention.

Accurate anatomical apposition of the various layers of the abdominal wall is essential. Tension sutures across the line of the incision we have discarded completely. These sutures cause wound pain and are the source of many abscesses. Moreover they do not prevent the disruption of wounds. We prefer now to depend on closely placed interrupted stitches of nonabsorbable suture material.

We are greatly impressed with the value of stainless steel wire, as advocated by Jones,[2] for abdominal wound closure. A rectus muscle splitting incision is preferable for this technic (Fig. 312). Such wounds show an almost complete absence of tissue reaction. Wire closure has been found to be particularly advantageous in abdomens which are being reopened through an old scar, and in patients suffering from carcinoma, nutritional deficiency or old age. It withstands infection extremely well and a wound closed with wire may suppurate for weeks without either disruption or extrusion of the wires. When wounds are sutured with wire early ambulation may be practised with complete confidence.

Silk does not withstand infection well and should not be used where contamination has occurred or where infection is anticipated.

Gridiron incisions, performed for acute appendicitis or colostomies, are closed with o or oo chromicized catgut. Special care must be taken to approximate accurately the transversalis fascia, as closure of this layer is most important in the prevention of postoperative herniae.

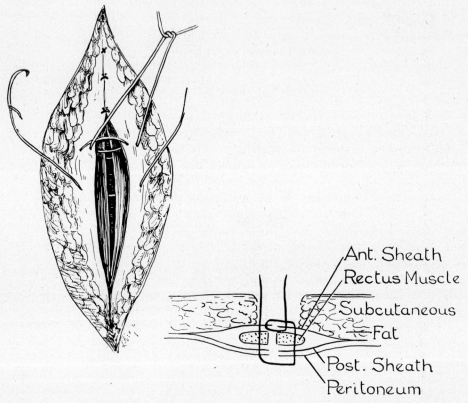

Ant. Sheath
Rectus Muscle
Subcutaneous
Fat
Post. Sheath
Peritoneum

FIG. 312. Wire closure of paramedian rectus splitting incision. Interrupted figure-of-eight stitches through, first, full thickness of rectus with both sheaths and peritoneum, and second, margins of anterior sheath only.

TECHNIC OF OPERATIONS UPON COLON

Appendectomy. THE INTERVAL APPENDIX. A gridiron incision (Fig. 311(1)) is employed for appendectomy except under rare circumstances. The skin incision should traverse a point approximately one third of the distance from the anterior-superior spine of the ilium to the umbilicus. It should be placed well lateral to the lateral border of the rectus muscle. Most commonly about half of the incision lies above and about half below a line drawn from the anterior-superior spine of the ilium to the umbilicus. In acute appendicitis the midpoint of the incision is determined by the location of the point of maximum tenderness. It is wise to divide the internal oblique and transversus as separate layers although the directions of their fibers are almost parallel. The margins of the separated transversus should be identified by the application of hemostats because the careful closure of this layer is a most important factor in the prevention of incisional hernia.

On opening the peritoneal cavity, before disturbing its contents, an attempt should be made to ascertain the exact location and condition of the appendix by palpation. The right side of the pelvis and whole right lower portion of the abdomen can be digitally palpated through this wound. The terminal ileum may be recognized by the direction of its blood vessels which run parallel to the long axis of the bowel.

The ileocecal junction is now gently delivered into the wound and drawn upward. The base of the appendix can be located close to this junction where the longitudinal muscle striae of the cecum converge. The entire appendix can very frequently be delivered and exposed. In high lying retrocecal appendices, it is on occasion necessary to draw the cecum downward and laterally and then fold it upward toward the umbilicus in order to expose the complete appendix. In these cases very commonly a fold of peritoneum binds the lateral border of the appendix to the posterior surface of the cecum. By incising this fold the appendix can be freed often without bleeding. Occasionally about the middle of the appendix there is a thick strand of peritoneum which fixes it firmly to the posterior aspect of the cecum. This strand also has to be incised in order to deliver the appendix.

The mesentery of the appendix is transfixed and ligated in segments. In acute appendicitis fine absorbable ligature material or cotton should be used. In the interval appendix only, is silk permissible. The base of the appendix is ligated with oo chromicized catgut after being crushed by a hemostat. The appendix is then delivered from its mesentery.

A purse-string suture is now inserted in the wall of the cecum about the base of the appendix (Fig. 311 (2)). The needle carrying this suture is inserted deep enough that when it is emerging the tissues overlying the point are blanched. This blanching indicates that the suture has included the submucous layer of the bowel (the strong "sausage casing" layer). An atraumatic intestinal suture is employed for this. A hemostat is placed across the appendix just distal to its ligated base, and the base is held by a second pair of forceps. The appendix is divided between these two forceps distal to the ligature by a scalpel or preferably by the cautery. If a scalpel is used the stump is cauterized by pure carbolic acid followed by alcohol. The stump is depressed and the purse-string suture is drawn tight and tied. Very often it is possible to draw up the ligated mesentery and hold it over the buried stump of the appendix with two more knots of the purse-string suture.

The omentum can usually be found under the anterior abdominal wall toward the umbilicus and this is drawn down and placed in the right iliac fossa. The peritoneum is closed with a continuous suture of double oo chromicized catgut. The transversus abdominis and internal oblique muscles are then approximated separately with interrupted stitches, particular care being taken with the transversus abdominis which can so readily retract. Suture of only the anterior fascial sheath of the internal oblique muscle secures adequate approximation without strangulation of muscle fibers. The external oblique aponeurosis may be closed with a continuous suture of the same catgut. A few interrupted ooo plain catgut stitches close the Scarpa's fascia. This will often protect the deeper layers of the wound from mild skin infection. The skin is approximated with interrupted silk sutures with or without the use of Michel skin clips. We are convinced of the value of interrupted as opposed to continuous suture in skin closure.

ACUTE APPENDICITIS. In all operations for acute appendicitis, just before opening the peritoneal cavity the wound is smeared with some oily and mildly antiseptic material. We use bismuth iodoform paraffin paste (BIPP) wiping it carefully into all the recesses of the muscular, fascial and fatty surfaces leaving no excess. If seropurulent fluid wells up into the wound on opening the peritoneal cavity, the incision is at least in part protected by this thin film of oily antiseptic.

The more acutely involved the appendix the more adequate must be the exposure. Rough handling will often rupture an acute appendix. Increased exposure of an appendix lying in the pelvis may be obtained by splitting the internal oblique and transversus muscles medially into the lateral border of the rectus sheath. Great care must be taken in closing such an incision to approximate the layers of the rectus sheath accurately at the medial end of the wound.

If there is difficulty in the exposure of a high lying retrocecal appendix, extend the splitting of the external and internal oblique. If this proves inadequate the internal oblique and transversus muscles should be cut at right angles to the direction of their fibers. The increased risk of an incisional hernia is more than justified by the decreased incidence of rupture of an acutely inflamed appendix which often results from rough retraction and manipulation unavoidable with inadequate exposure.

When the appendix is difficult to expose in spite of these changes in the incision, it may be advisable to resort to the retrograde removal of the appendix (Fig. 313). An opening is made in the mesentery of the appendix isolating its base, which is crushed and ligated. A forcep is placed across the appendix just distal to the ligature. The appendix is divided between this forcep and the ligature. A purse-string suture is inserted and tied over the inverted stump. The mesentery of the appendix is divided piecemeal between hemostats. Traction on the segments attached to the appendix gradually delivers the appendix and exposes its mesentery throughout this maneuver. The removal of a well buried appendix is very remarkably facilitated by this retrograde technic.

If at the conclusion of an operation for acute appendicitis the peritoneum, parietal and visceral, is still intact so that the retroperitoneal tissues have not been contaminated, drainage of the peritoneal cavity is superfluous. Using this principle to guide our drainage of the peritoneal cavity, where the appendix has been perforated a percentage of such patients will develop local intraperitoneal abscesses. We believe that drainage instituted at the time of operation would not have prevented these. Fortunately most of these abscesses will occur in the pelvic cul-de-sac and can be drained safely through the rectum or vagina.

When a contaminated peritoneal cavity with an intact peritoneum has been closed without a drain it is wise to place a soft rubber drainage tube down to the peritoneal closure. The abdominal wall is much more intolerant of infection than is the peritoneal cavity.

If the appendix has actually perforated with gross contamination of the peritoneal cavity, drainage should be instituted. Our method of accomplishing this is by the use of so-called "curtain drainage" advised by Gurd,[3] employing well oiled gauze packing. Two drachms of bismuth iodoform paraffin paste added to 8 ounces of sterile liquid paraffin makes a very good medium with which to impregnate the gauze for drainage. Three strips of 8-inch gauze folded to 2-inch width, soaked in this material, are placed in the peritoneal cavity about a fairly large rubber drainage tube. The drainage tube is introduced

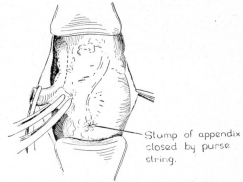

Stump of appendix closed by purse string.

FIG. 313. Retrograde removal of high retrocecal appendix. The appendix is divided at its junction with the cecum and the stump closed. Then the mesentery is doubly clamped and divided in segments. Traction on each successive forcep on the mesentery attached to appendix permits its delivery without direct traction on the gangrenous appendix, thus lessening likelihood of rupture during removal.

with long forceps to the bottom of the pelvis. One strip of gauze is shoved into the pelvis around the tube. The second is placed in the right colic gutter. The third strip lies medial to the cecum and packs off the terminal ileum and small bowel from the region of the perforated appendix (Fig. 314). If an abdominal pack has been introduced during the operation, this third piece of gauze should be introduced as the pack is removed in order to maintain the protection of the general peritoneal cavity. All three gauze strips emerge from the McBurney wound about the drainage tube. The wound is very loosely closed about the drains, using interrupted sutures. This minimizes pocketing of infection in the layers of the abdominal wall. The gauze packing and tube are left in situ for five days and are then removed as a whole under light anesthetic. The drainage tube may or may not be replaced at this time depending upon the amount of discharge from the wound. In our experience there is very profuse discharge for thirty-six to forty-eight hours only.

APPENDICAL ABSCESS. An appendical abscess may be drained either through the rectum, or the abdominal wall depending upon its location.

If the abscess is situated in the pelvis and a point of definite softening can be felt on digital rectal examination, it has localized sufficiently to warrant rectal drainage. Under general anesthesia, with the examining finger at the softened area in the induration, a closed uterine dressing forcep is

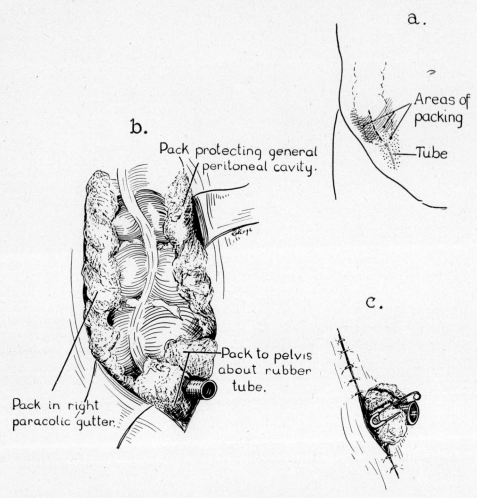

FIG. 314. Method of insertion of packing for perforated appendicitis. (a) Diagram of the location of the skin incision and the position of the three packs and tube. (b) The relation of the three packs to the cecum, one protecting the general peritoneal cavity, one into the pelvis and one in the right paracolic gutter. (c) The ends of the three packs and tube, fixed by a safety pin, after skin closure.

pushed through the rectal wall at this point. The forcep enters the abscess cavity with an alarming suddenness as its point penetrates the resistant submucous layer of the rectum. The forcep is opened on withdrawal to enlarge the drainage opening and a finger is immediately thrust through the opening in order not to lose it in the redundant folds of rectal mucosa. A soft rubber drainage tube 1 to 1.5 cm. in diameter is guided into the abscess cavity along this finger. The drainage tube should be long enough to protrude through the anal orifice where it is fixed by a suture to the perianal skin.

A properly placed muscle splitting incision is ideal for the drainage of a retrocecal appendical abscess. Through such an incision adequate drainage is accomplished without opening the peritoneal cavity. The protection of the wound, as previously described, by a thin film of oily antiseptic before entering the abscess is particularly valuable here.

No search should be made for the appendix. The old adage that the surgeon should run when the pus runs is very pertinent here. We must remember we are now operating upon an intraperitoneal abscess which is the result of appendicitis and not operating for appendicitis itself. When pus is encountered a soft rubber drainage tube is introduced into the abscess cavity. Oiled and BIPPed gauze, previously described, is packed into the cavity around the tube in a quantity sufficient to fill the cavity completely and thus prevent any pocketing. The wound is sutured loosely with interrupted stitches. The gauze should not be removed for five days and then always under light anesthesia. A surprisingly clean granulating wound is left. The drainage tube remains in situ until the discharge diminishes.

Oiled and BIPPed gauze used in this way for the drainage of appendical abscesses has distinct advantages over simple drainage with a rubber tube: (1) Profuse drainage which is so desirable occurs for the first thirty-six to forty-eight postoperative hours; (2) painful dressings and repeated wound packing are eliminated; (3) wound reaction is minimized and sloughing is very rare; (4) the incidence of secondary abscess formation is distinctly low; (5) the wounds heal more promptly, and (6) the incidence of incisional herniae is surprisingly low because of the absence of wound sloughing.

Cecostomy. In acute large bowel obstruction decompression of the distended colon is absolutely imperative. A laparotomy to determine the site and extent of the obstructing lesion is unnecessary and dangerous unless the lesion is a volvulus of the cecum or sigmoid colon. The edema which is an inevitable accompaniment of obstruction permits the egress of organisms from the lumen into the bowel wall and mesentery. The manipulation of such an edematous colon incidental to an exploratory laparotomy invites peritonitis. Therefore a "blind" cecostomy, that is a cecostomy performed without exploration of the abdomen, is the optimum procedure. It may be superfluous to state that the double lumened tube will not decompress the obstructed colon but is useful in relieving the small bowel distention which is often associated with prolonged obstruction of the colon.

A short muscle splitting incision in the right lower quadrant about 2 inches from the anterior-superior spine of the ilium should be employed for a cecostomy (Fig. 315). Even in the presence of prolonged large bowel obstruction, the distention of the cecum rarely prevents its being delivered into the wound. A knuckle of cecum about 3 cm. in diameter should remain superficial to the skin closure. A few interrupted oo chromicized catgut sutures are employed to close the muscular layers of the abdominal wall about the protruding cecum. No sutures are ever placed in the cecal wall deep to the skin. Such sutures are not only unnecessary but invite peritonitis and wound infection from leaks. Fine interrupted catgut stitches attach the four quadrants of the protruding cecum to the skin (Fig. 315). The remainder of the skin incision is then closed with interrupted silk sutures. The protruding cecum is dressed with vaseline gauze and it may be opened with the cautery at any time from a few hours to two days following operation. The degree of obstruction determines the urgency of opening the cecum.

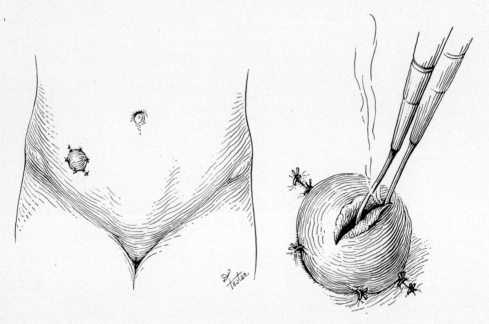

FIG. 315. Location and opening by cautery of blind cecostomy. Note interrupted catgut stitches fixing angles of protruding cecum to skin. N.B. No stitch placed deep to skin enters cecal wall. (From *Am. J. Surg.*, 46(No. 1):135-142, [Oct.], 1939.)

Sometimes difficulty is experienced in holding the cecum to the anterior abdominal wall with a small portion protruding above the skin level. This is particularly so in obese patients or in those in whom the cecum is greatly distended. In the latter group a larger knuckle of cecum must be exteriorized in order to compensate for the shrinkage that follows decompression of the cecum.

Incredible as it may seem it is possible to mistake a distended sigmoid with an elongated mesentery for the cecum. Both have longitudinal bands, and in the desperately ill patient, unless one is alert to this possibility, the desire to minimize the operative interference may lead to this error. However, realizing that such is possible, very gentle manipulation can determine the presence or absence of appendices epiploicae which are the hallmark of sigmoid colon.

When the obstruction has been so prolonged and complete that the cecum is tremendously distended and it is unwise to deliver it, some method of decompression in situ must be carried out. It has been suggested that in these cases a hypodermic needle on a syringe may be thrust into the cecum to suck off gas and relieve the distention. In our experience this is dangerous and useless. It very frequently results in a tear of the cecal wall radiating from the site of the needle puncture, and furthermore the lumen of the needle is too small to empty the cecum. A better method is to isolate the cecum with abdominal packs and then thrust into it a large trocar, to which suction is already applied. When the distended cecum begins to deflate the assistant promptly picks up the cecal wall with Allis forceps placed on either side of the point of entrance of the trocar. This area of cecum is rapidly delivered from the abdomen. On withdrawing the trocar a Kelly forcep placed across the cecum closes the opening. The cecum can then be opened when advisable by amputating the small segment beyond the forcep which is then removed.

On the second or third day after operation 4 ounces of boiled linseed oil, which is cheap and readily available, are instilled into the cecostomy night and morning. Subsequent saline irrigations will empty the large bowel proximal to the obstructing lesion. This regimen should be continued until the linseed oil appears spontaneously per rectum and the saline irrigations also pass freely through the colon. At least three weeks should elapse before concluding that the obstruction is due to structural disease and not to associated edema. If at the end of three weeks it is impossible for the patient to pass per rectum saline introduced through the cecostomy, a defunctioning transverse colon colostomy should be the next operative procedure, provided, as previously discussed, it will not interfere with an adequate subsequent resection, in which case an obstructive resection is advisable.

The cecostomy here described is life saving in that it functions and decompresses the colon at the time when this is needed most urgently. The penalty of this great asset is the necessity of operative closure. Cecostomies made with a technic providing for spontaneous closure do not function adequately at the time decompression of the colon is imperative.

Rod Colostomy. If a colostomy is to be temporary the Mikulicz type is preferable because of the ease of its closure. When the colostomy is to be permanent, when the poor condition of the patient demands the very minimum of operative trauma, or when it is technically not possible to perform a Mikulicz type, a rod colostomy may be mandatory.

The rod colostomy here described is of the hepatic flexure although the same technic may be applied to any portion of the colon. Damon Pfeiffer first utilized defunctioning of the transverse colon as a preliminary to gastric resection in patients suffering from gastro-jejuno-colic fistula.

An upper right abdominal muscle splitting incision paralleling the fibers of the external oblique muscle is made lateral to the outer border of the rectus (Fig. 306 (1)). The incision should be placed sufficiently below the costal margin to allow of the comfortable application of a colostomy irrigation cup, and need not be more than 3 inches in length unless the patient is very obese. On opening the peritoneum the first loop of colon encountered is delivered into the wound. This will usually be a portion of the proximal transverse colon.

It is always desirable to make a colostomy as far from the cecum as is compatible with the location of the lesion. The more distally placed the colostomy, the more readily it is controlled. The colon is freed from omentum and adherent fat for about 2 inches at the site selected for the colostomy. An opening sufficiently large to admit the rod is made in an avascular spot in the mesentery of this segment. This rod rests on the abdominal wall at right angles to the long axis of the bowel (Fig. 306 (2)). It supports the colon beneath which it has been passed so that a loop lies superficial to the skin.

The incision is now closed about the protruding colon using interrupted double oo chromic catgut or cotton sutures. None of these stitches enter the wall of the colon. The fixation of the colon depends entirely on the glass rod. The two ends of a short piece of rubber tubing are threaded over the two ends of the glass rod to prevent it from slipping out from beneath the colon and a vaseline dressing is applied. This colostomy is opened in twenty-four to forty-eight hours by incising with the cautery the anterior wall of the colon at right angles to its long axis. The division of the deep wall of the colon and removal of the glass rod are deferred for at least two weeks. This permits firm fixation of the colon to the abdominal wall before removing the rod. If this precaution is not observed retraction of the colostomy is very apt to occur.

Transverse Colon Colostomy (Mikulicz Type). The Mikulicz type of colostomy has several advantages over the rod type. It is much easier to close subsequently and is less apt to retract into the abdomen. It also allows of immediate complete division of the colon, thus avoiding any theoretical possibility of fecal material entering the distal loop of colon. Consequently the Mikulicz type of colostomy immediately and completely defunctions the colon distal to it.

The colostomy here described is of the transverse colon, although the same technic may be applied to any portion of the large bowel that can be sufficiently mobilized.

An upper right paramedian incision about 4 inches in length is made, the rectus muscle being split longitudinally. This incision is adequate to admit a hand to explore the peritoneal cavity. In cases of carcinoma palpation of the liver for secondaries should be carried out at this time, because the presence of the colostomy makes this almost impossible or at least dangerous at the time of the subsequent resection. The exploration of the peritoneal cavity must be extremely gentle because rough handling increases edema and spreads infection.

The transverse colon and its attached omentum are delivered into the wound and the site of the colostomy is selected at the apex of the delivered loop. By sharp dissection the omentum is separated from the transverse colon for about 4 inches (Fig. 308(1)). An opening is made at an avascular spot in the transverse mesocolon immediately adjacent to the colon at the site selected for the colostomy. A rubber tube split down one side is inserted into this opening. The two ends of this rubber tube are clamped together with a Kocher forcep through which traction can be made so that the afferent and efferent limbs of the colon fall together.

The longitudinal taeniae of these two limbs are sutured with a fine intestinal suture for a distance of about 4 inches. The rubber tube which suspends the apex of the colon is now passed through the detached omentum which is laid down over the line of suture approximating the two barrels of the colon, completely isolating the peritoneal cavity from the region of the colostomy (Fig. 308(2)). This becomes an excellent safeguard for the peritoneal cavity at the time of closure of the colostomy.

With double oo chromic catgut suture the closure of the wound is begun at its upper end. The peritoneum and posterior fascia of the rectus are approximated from the upper angle downward until the point is reached where the loop of colon seems to emerge naturally from the abdominal cavity. The suture is then locked and is brought out through the rectus muscle into the anterior sheath of the rectus. The closure of the anterior sheath can then be continued with the same stitch to the upper angle of the wound again. A similar closure of the posterior and anterior sheaths of the rectus can now be carried out in the lower end of the wound up to the place where the colon comes through the abdominal wall. The closure of the wound about the colon must not be so tight as to embarrass circulation. On the other hand it must be sufficiently snug to prevent herniation of the colon.

By opening up the split rubber tube which lies beneath the exposed loop, two Kochers can be passed through the opening in the transverse mesocolon and clamped across the bowel parallel to one another. These Kochers should be applied so that their handles lie downward. The colon is then divided completely with the cautery between the two Kochers (Fig. 308 (3)). The handles of the Kochers are sutured to the abdominal wall (Fig. 308 (4)). A vaseline dressing is applied to the colostomy. The clamp on the proximal lumen can be removed in twenty-four to forty-eight hours to relieve obstruction, but the distal clamp should be left in situ for forty-eight to sixty hours to prevent retraction of the colostomy. Irrigations are started on the fourth or fifth day.

Obstructive Resection. When the lesion to be resected lies between the transverse and the sigmoid colon, if resection with immediate anastomosis is not advisable, an obstructive resection may be undertaken. The splenic flexure of the colon is most difficult to mobilize and therefore a left paramedian incision is indicated. The abdomen should always be explored for secondaries in the liver, other pathological lesions, and secondary implants in the rectovesical pouch. The primary lesion itself is then examined and its resectability determined.

The colon must be mobilized. This mobilization is begun by incising the lateral peritoneal reflection of the descending colon. The greatest difficulty in mobilization will be encountered at the region of the splenic flexure where the lieno-colic ligament has to be divided. The anterior layer of the lesser peritoneal sac is also divided. If the lesion lies in the mid or left trans-

verse colon the full extent of the gastrocolic mesentery must be divided and
the entire descending colon with the splenic flexure is mobilized. The attached omentum is removed with the colon. Having mobilized the colon
thoroughly on its lateral aspect it is dissected up from the posterior abdominal wall, care being taken to isolate and protect the left ureter.

In this obstructive resection provision must be made for the resection of
an adequate length of bowel on either side of the lesion. The limbs of the

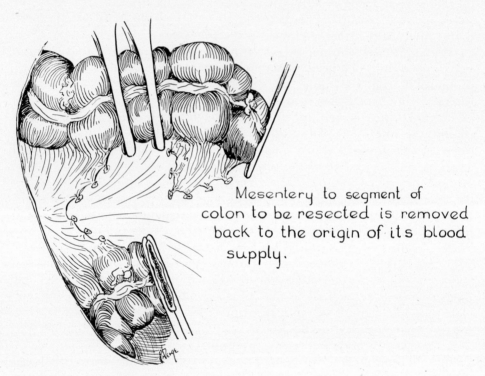

Mesentery to segment of
colon to be resected is removed
back to the origin of its blood
supply.

FIG. 316. Resection of colon with wedge of mesentery. The mesentery must be radically
removed in all resections of the colon for carcinoma.

colon proximal and distal to the segment to be resected must be approximated by suture for a distance of 4 inches. Consequently, in selecting the
sites for division of the bowel sufficient slack must be left to allow for this
approximation of the afferent and efferent limbs. If this principle is not
observed there will be disastrous tension on the colostomy.

The sites for division having been selected with regard for this necessary
slack, incisions are made through the peritoneum only on the medial aspect
of the mesentery beginning at each of the selected points of division and extending to meet at the root of the mesentery. In this way a wedge of mesocolon is outlined whose base consists of the length of colon to be resected
and whose apex lies at the root of the mesocolon (Fig. 316). The mesentery
is now divided along the preliminary incisions of the peritoneum. The
vessels are divided between clamps as they are encountered. The main artery

of supply at the posterior apex is doubly clamped and doubly ligatured. A wedge-shaped section of mesentery containing the lymphatic drainage is thus resected along with the length of colon. The divided mesenteric vessels are now ligated.

With the selected sites of division of the bowel approximated, the afferent and efferent limbs of colon are sewn together with continuous intestinal suture for a distance of 3 to 4 inches. The defect in the mesentery is then closed by approximating the cut margins with interrupted sutures.

Whenever possible the lesion should be exteriorized through an independent incision, preferably of the muscle splitting type, sufficiently removed from bony prominences to permit the comfortable application of a colostomy irrigation cup. Sometimes it is necessary to utilize the operation wound for this procedure. In the muscle splitting incision for the exteriorization of the lesion the split margins of the external oblique are nicked half an inch deep at right angles to the direction of their fibers in the middle of the wound to prevent pressure necrosis of the limbs of the colostomy.

If the segment of colon to be resected is too bulky to be delivered through the independent incision, a Rankin clamp (Fig. 307), two Peyer's clamps or large Kocher forceps are introduced into the abdominal cavity through this independent incision and are placed transversely across the colon, one at the proximal and the other at the distal proposed site of division. Two other forceps are now applied across the colon parallel and close to each of these. These latter forceps are introduced through the paramedian incision and are applied on the lesion side of the first two forceps. The colon is now divided with the cautery between the clamps at either end of the portion to be resected, and the specimen is removed. The ends of colon are now withdrawn through the independent incision as a double-barreled colostomy (Fig. 307).

Sometimes it is possible to deliver the lesion and entire area of bowel to be resected through the independent incision. The lesion should be withdrawn from the abdomen until the point of approximation of the two limbs of the colon is at skin level. The original incision can then be closed before the amputation of the isolated segment.

The clamp on the proximal limb of protruding colon can be removed in twenty-four hours if necessary. It is preferable, however, to defer this for forty-eight to sixty hours if possible, to allow sealing of the colostomy wound with fibrin before exposing it to gross fecal contamination. The clamp should be left on the distal limb of colon for sixty hours. Irrigations of the colostomy may be started on the fourth or fifth day.

Aseptic Anastomosis. The development of technical procedures for the so-called aseptic anastomosis in the gastro-intestinal tract, long championed by Harry Kerr [4] and Wayne Babcock,[5] and recently advocated by Wangensteen [6] and Holman,[7] is stimulated by the thought that contamination of the peritoneal cavity by contents of the tract during an open anastomosis is to be prevented at all costs. While we do not deny this ideal, bacteriological studies show that it is almost impossible of achievement irrespective of the technical procedure employed. Too often we have cultured organisms from the retroperitoneal tissue in the neighborhood of the lesion. To be certain of an adequate blood supply to the segments of bowel to be anastomosed is the most important single factor in securing sound healing. It

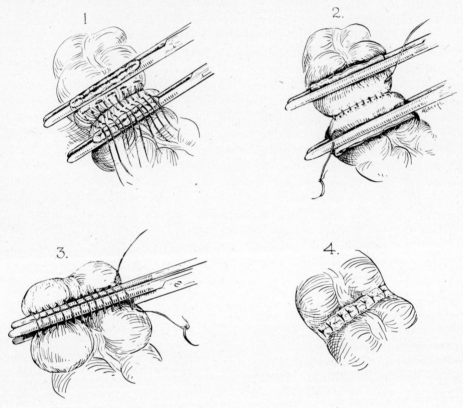

Aseptic Anastomosis

FIG. 317. Aseptic anastomosis. (1) Outside layer of interrupted mattress sutures of silk in posterior seromuscular coats ¼-inch from clamps and ⅛-inch apart. (2) Inside layer of continuous catgut suture in posterior seromuscular coats ⅛-inch only from clamps. (3) Clamps rolled together to permit continuation of continuous inside layer of catgut suture in anterior seromuscular coats, also ⅛-inch from clamps. (4) Interrupted silk sutures in anterior seromuscular coats complete outside layer of the anastomosis after removal of clamps. The diaphragm at the site of the anastomosis is then thoroughly opened up by pressure of the thumb and finger.

is not as easy to be certain of this in a closed as in an open anastomosis where bleeding can be seen. The tissue which is inverted, no matter what technic is used in the performance of an aseptic anastomosis, may act as a diaphragm producing stenosis.

The ends of colon to be anastomosed, each held in thin bladed crushing forceps, are laid side by side in such manner as to approximate the posterior serosal surfaces. These surfaces are united by interrupted silk stitches placed never more than one quarter of an inch from the clamped borders of the colon and about one eighth of an inch apart (Fig. 317(1)). The posterior seromuscular coats of colon are then sewn together with continuous catgut starting at the mesenteric border. This suture should be placed one eighth of an inch from the crushing clamps and deep enough to catch the resistant and vascular submucosal layer of both limbs of colon (Fig. 317(2)).

The forceps are now rolled to approximate the anterior serosal surfaces. The intestinal suture is then continued to unite the anterior seromuscular layers. It can then be tied to the beginning of the suture originally left long for this purpose (Fig. 317(3)).

The crushing forceps are now opened and slid from between the layers of sutures on the anterior and posterior aspects. Interrupted silk stitches then complete the approximation of the anterior serosal surfaces (Fig. 317(4)). The anastomosis is now complete without the lumen of the bowel having been open. The patency of the anastomosis is established by grasping it with thumb and finger approximated through its lumen from outside the serosal surface. In this way the adherence of anterior and posterior walls resulting from being crushed by the clamps is broken down. It is tremendously important to do this thoroughly in order to avoid an obstructive diaphragm.

Open Anastomosis. When an open anastomosis is to be carried out rubber covered intestinal clamps are applied to each segment of the colon to prevent spilling. These clamps should be placed sufficiently proximal and distal to the site of the anastomosis that their presence will not compromise the performance of the anastomosis.

In order that contamination during the operation may be reduced a scheme of draping has been evolved. Just before it is necessary to open the lumen of the bowel the usual drapes are covered by a red cotton sheet 3 feet square, one end of which is slit for a distance of 18 inches so that it may incorporate and isolate the local operative field. The red color, so universally used to indicate danger, is a vivid reminder to all that anything which comes in contact with this red drape is contaminated. The nurse does not touch any instruments or wipes on this red drape with gloved hands but always uses instruments as in the "no touch" technic. When the lumen of the bowel is finally closed so that further contamination is unlikely, the red drape and all instruments, gauze and wipes which have come in contact with it are discarded. The surgeon then changes his gloves before proceeding with the anastomosis. This draping has become known locally as the "Red Flag" Technic and as such it will be referred to subsequently (Fig. 318).

The details of all gastro-intestinal anastomoses have common essentials. Figures 304 A and B, illustrate the steps of an end-to-end anastomosis in the small bowel for the sake of clarity, but the same detail is applicable to end-to-end anastomoses of colon. A three layer anastomosis is used in all instances. All anastomoses are begun by inserting stay sutures at either end of the proposed stoma (Fig. 304A(1)). The tension on these makes easy the accurate spacing of the interrupted sutures which unite serosa-to-serosa. We use fine silk for all interrupted sutures indicated in the operative detail. The first row of interrupted sutures is then held taut while the seromuscular coats of both segments are incised down to the mucosa above and below this suture line forming definite seromuscular flaps as indicated in figure 304A(1). With continuous fine chromic catgut on an atraumatic needle, the seromuscular flaps are united by a continuous over-and-over suture (Fig. 304A(2)). The suture is then wrapped in gauze in readiness to complete a second row anteriorly. The lumina are opened and any excessive content wiped out with gauze soaked in 1:1000 acriflavine. The crushed tissue is excised (Fig. 304A(3)). A second continuous chromic catgut suture on an atraumatic needle unites the posterior layer of mucosa-to-mucosa with a blanket suture. This secures accurate apposition and perfect hemostasis (Fig. 304B(4)). The suture being continued along the anterior portion of the stoma unites mucosa-to-mucosa by means of an over-and-over suture. If there should be a discrepancy in diameter of the lumina, this can be compensated for by taking two needle bites of the redundant mucosa for every single bite on the opposite side. This anterior mucosa-to-mucosa suture being completed, the suture is tied to the loose end of the origin of the posterior mucosa-to-mucosa suture. The suture which was used to unite the posterior seromuscular flaps and which has been wrapped in gauze, now unites the anterior seromuscular flaps (Fig. 304B(6)). The third and final anterior layer is completed by means of interrupted sutures (Fig. 304B(7)).

A rubber tube as described in resection of the right colon (Fig. 305(4)), may be fixed in the lumen of the colon across the anastomosis to maintain with certainty its patency until all postoperative edema has subsided. It is passed usually between the seventh and twenty-first postoperative day. Occasionally it may require digital removal from the rectum.

If an end-to-side or side-to-side anastomosis is to be carried out, either one or both ends must be closed. This is most easily accomplished if the bowel is divided by the three forcep method, two forceps being left on the end of colon to be closed. This method is illustrated in figure 319 as employed for cecostomy closure. The superficial of the two forceps is removed and the frill oversewn. The remaining forcep is removed and the crushed tissue is invaginated by a further layer of catgut suture, the corners being inverted by means of an adaptation of the principle of the purse-string suture. A third layer of interrupted silk sutures completes the closure. One can then proceed with restoration of continuity using either an end-to-side or side-to-side arrangement of the segments, the details of the anastomosis being identical with that described for the end-to-end procedure.

Resection of Right Colon. After opening the abdomen, 12 inches of the terminal ileum, the cecum, the ascending and proximal transverse colon are isolated by abdominal packs. The lateral peritoneal reflection of the cecum and ascending colon is divided. This permits the mobilization of the entire

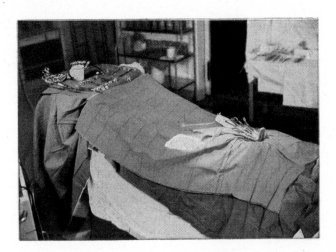

Fig. 318. Details of colored draping to prevent contamination. This shows the use of colored drapes in isolating potentially infected instruments and swabs during the course of an anastomosis. On the instrument stand is the enamel cup containing 1 in 1000 aqueous solution of acriflavine. All instruments and swabs which come in contact with the "Red Flag" are discarded after the lumen of the gastro-intestinal tract is closed. (From Graham, Roscoe R., *Operative Surgery,* edited by F. W. Bancroft, J. B. Lippincott Company, Philadelphia.)

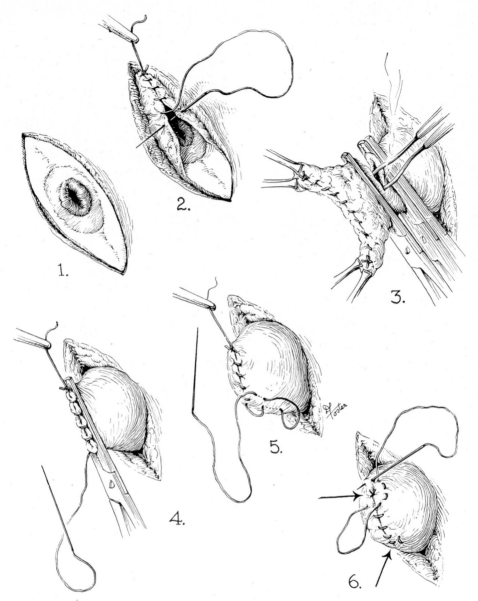

FIG. 319. Closure of cecostomy. (1) Elliptical skin incision. (2) Oversewing skin to close temporarily the cecostomy stoma. (3) After adequate mobilization of cecum the stoma is excised using the three clamp method and the cautery. (4) Oversewing of fringe of crushed wall of cecum remaining after removal of one clamp. (5) Note stitch used to invert the lower angle in the inversion of the oversewn crushed tissue. (6) Note purse-string suture used to close upper angle of inversion suture. (From *Am. J. Surg.*, 46(No. 1):135-142, [Oct.], 1939.)

right colon (Fig. 320). In dissecting the right colon from the posterior abdominal wall it is always a surprise to find the third part of the duodenum lying much lower than one expects. Unless this anatomical arrangement is appreciated and recognized it is very easy unwittingly to wound the duodenum with disastrous consequences. The right ureter should be identified and protected. It is often carried medially with the mobilized colon and can easily be damaged if it is not definitely identified. The site of division of the terminal ileum is then selected. Similarly the point of division of the colon beyond the lesion is determined. If the right colic artery has to be sacrificed in order to eradicate the disease, the resection must be carried well into the transverse colon to ensure an adequate blood supply from the middle colic artery (Fig. 305(1)).

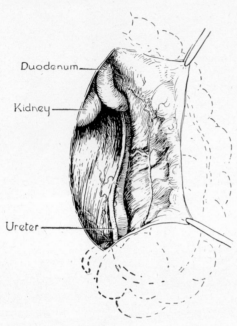

Duodenum

Kidney

Ureter

FIG. 320. Mobilization of right colon showing relationship of duodenum and ureter posteriorly.

A V-shaped incision is now made in the peritoneum only on the medial aspect of the ileocecal mesentery from the selected site of division of the terminal ileum to that of the colon, extending posteriorly to the root of the mesentery. As the colon has been dissected completely free posteriorly, it can be lifted up and the blood vessels extending to the terminal ileum, cecum and ascending colon are readily visualized. These vessels are divided between hemostats along the line of the incision in the peritoneum.

Two Kocher forceps are placed obliquely across the terminal ileum, parallel to one another, at the site selected for its division. The obliquity of the application of these forceps, as previously discussed, is to ensure a more radical excision of the antimesenteric than of the mesenteric border of the ileum. This will ensure a good blood supply to the entire width of the cut margin of the ileum at the line of the anastomosis (Fig. 303). Two large Kocher forceps are placed in a similar manner across the colon at the site selected for resection. The terminal ileum and colon are divided with the cautery between each pair of Kocher forceps. The specimen is removed and the clamped vessels in the margins of the mesentery are ligatured with silk. The defect in the mesentery on the medial aspect of the anastomosis is repaired by approximating the mesenteric margins with interrupted silk sutures.

An end-to-end anastomosis of terminal ileum to the colon is now carried out using the technic described under "Open Anastomosis" and always remembering to apply the rubber covered clamps to the ileum and colon before opening the lumen. As there is discrepancy between the widths of the two ends of bowel to be anastomosed, that of the ileum can be increased to equal the diameter of the colon by enlarging the opening in the ileum by incising its antimesenteric border. When the first row of interrupted silk sutures is inserted into the seromuscular coats of the two limbs of bowel it is carried along the antimesenteric border of the ileum to permit this (Fig. 305(2)). When the crushing forceps are cut off and the lumina laid open, the opening in the terminal ileum can be enlarged along its anti-mesenteric border until the point of the last seromuscular interrupted silk suture is reached (Fig. 305(3)).

After the posterior edges of the two lumina have been approximated by a continuous stitch of intestinal catgut, a piece of soft rubber tubing, about one and a half inches long and with a lumen as wide as the diameter of the ileum will permit, is selected. The stitch is then passed through the center of one lateral border of the short wide rubber tube, and the tube is threaded down the suture to the anastomosis where one end of it is introduced into each open lumen of bowel (Fig. 305(4)). The same intestinal suture is then brought out to the serosal surface of the bowel and used to continue the approximation of the anterior edges of the lumina.

After completing the anastomosis (Fig. 305(5)), if additional protection is desired, a piece of omental fat can be laid along the anastomosis so as to surround it completely like a collar. This is held by tying the tails of the last row of interrupted silk stitches about it.

Drainage of the retrocolic space should be established by a rubber tube emerging from a stab wound in the right flank. The raw surface of the bed of the colon is now covered by suturing the lateral parietal peritoneum to the mesentery of the colon and ileum.

Postoperatively there is often a profuse discharge of clear fluid from the drainage tube in the right flank which may cause the surgeon concern as to the integrity of the right ureter. In a few days, however, this diminishes, and the tube may then be shortened and ultimately removed.

Right Colon Exclusion. This procedure (Fig. 309) is applicable to lesions of the right colon which do not permit of immediate resection such as extensive carcinomata or inflammatory lesions with or without fecal fistulae. The abdomen is opened through a paramedian incision on the left side for reasons previously discussed (page 570). The peritoneal cavity is carefully explored, the extent of the local lesion is assessed and the decision to exclude it rather than attempt its removal is confirmed.

The terminal ileum is divided by the cautery between two Kocher forceps at an appropriate site. The mesentery of the terminal ileum must be divided parallel to its vessels for a sufficient distance to permit exteriorization of the distal cut end and approximation of the proximal end to the transverse colon.

The point for division of the transverse colon proximal to the middle colic artery is now selected and the omentum is detached from this area. This opens the lesser sac of peritoneum. The transverse colon is divided by the cautery between two large Kocher forceps or Peyer's clamps. The transverse mesocolon must also be split toward its abdominal attachment for a sufficient distance to permit exteriorization of the proximal cut end and approximation of the distal end to the terminal ileum. This division of the transverse mesocolon must be performed with care to identify and protect the main trunk of the middle colic artery.

The stumps to be exteriorized are brought out through two independent stab wounds in the right rectus muscle so that, should subsequent resection be attempted, they can be included in the operative incision. A Kocher forcep inserted through each stab wound can be applied to the stump and the original Kocher placed on the bowel for division is removed. It is then possible to pull each stump at least 1 to 2 inches outside the skin level. These Kocher forceps should remain on the bowel for forty-eight to sixty hours. An end-to-end anastomosis of the terminal ileum to the transverse colon is now carried out over a tube (Fig. 305(2)-(5)).

This maneuver is followed in most cases by an amazing improvement in the general condition and comfort of the patient. Very frequently a desperate situation with what appears to be a hopeless lesion is transformed into one in which an elective operation may be undertaken successfully, so great is the reduction of edema and cellulitis.

Resection of Transverse or Left Colon with Immediate Anastomosis. Any lesion of large bowel situated between distal transverse colon and rectosigmoid junction may be resected with immediate anastomosis. As pointed out in the previous discussion, such a resection with anastomosis is always anatomically more extensive than an obstructive type of removal. However, a resection with immediate restoration of continuity is justifiable only in the absence of obstruction or when there is a previous or coincidental cecostomy or defunctioning colostomy.

The splenic flexure is the least accessible portion of the large bowel and the most difficult to mobilize. For this reason a left paramedian incision is indicated. If there is much fixation of the lesion by inflammatory induration or if obstruction has resulted in dilatation and edema of the proximal colon, resection with immediate anastomosis should be abandoned as a primary procedure. A proximal defunctioning colostomy or a cecostomy would have been ideal but as the abdomen is open an obstructive type of resection may be justifiable. If, however, the lesion is readily mobilized and the colon proximal to it seems to be completely free from evidence of obstruction, resection with immediate restoration of continuity may be performed.

If there is even slight edema of the colon and a primary resection with immediate anastomosis has been done, decompression of the colon can be secured by performing a simultaneous stab cecostomy from within the abdomen (Fig. 310). This is an excellent safeguard for the anastomosis even though the preoperative preparation has been as thorough as outlined in the discussion on page 573.

TRANSVERSE COLON. If the lesion is so situated that its adequate removal demands the sacrifice of the middle colic artery, the resection must extend from the region supplied by the right colic artery well into that supplied by the left colic artery. Such a resection necessitates the thorough mobilization of the splenic flexure and the division of the full extent of the gastrocolic ligament.

Tension on any colon anastomosis is irrefutable evidence of inadequate mobilization. If the colon is thoroughly mobilized any part of it can be approximated to any other part without tension. Therefore the length of the resected segment need never be limited because of fear of tension. In carcinoma the sites of transection of the colon are determined by the lymphatic drainage of the segment involved by the lesion (Fig. 302). The lymphatics accompany the blood vessels. Thus it is important to ensure that the remaining parts of the colon have adequate circulation after thorough removal of the lymphatic field.

Removal of the lymphatic field is accomplished by the excision, along with the segment of colon, of a triangular area of mesentery, the base of which extends between the two points of division of the bowel and whose apex is at the root of the mesentery (Fig. 316).

The bowel is divided with the cautery between forceps applied at the proximal and distal points of division of the colon. The specimen is removed and hemostasis secured by ligation of the vessels in the borders of the mesentery.

The wedge-shaped defect in the mesentery is closed by approximating its cut borders with interrupted silk sutures from the apex at the doubly ligated stump of the middle colic artery up to the site of the proposed anastomosis. A three layer type of anastomosis is performed over a tube between the ends of colon as previously described (Fig. 304, A and B).

DESCENDING COLON. If the lesion is situated in the descending colon the left colic artery must be sacrificed in the adequate removal of the lymphatic field. The resection extends from the area supplied by the middle colic artery down to the region supplied by the sigmoid branches arising from the inferior mesenteric artery (Fig. 302). The splenic flexure must be completely mobilized and the descending colon freed laterally by the division of its peritoneal reflection onto the left lateral abdominal wall. The gastrocolic ligament requires division to the middle of the transverse colon and the sigmoid colon also must be well mobilized to permit its approximation to the transverse colon without tension.

The sites of division of the bowel are now determined. A wedge of mesentery similar to that described for resection of the transverse colon is freed from its vascular and peritoneal attachments. In this instance the apex of the wedge is at the source of the left colic artery. Hemostasis is secured and the left colic artery is doubly ligatured. The segment of colon to be resected is divided by the cautery and removed. The ends of the colon are then anastomosed over a tube. The defect in the mesentery is closed with interrupted sutures. Often an adjoining piece of omentum can be used to reinforce the anastomosis by laying it along the line of anastomosis and tying it loosely in place with the long ends of the interrupted inverting silk stitches in the seromuscular coat.

Sometimes the anastomosis can be placed extraperitoneally by dissecting up a flap of parietal peritoneum, laying the anastomosis beneath it and suturing the edge of this peritoneal flap to the surface of the reconstructed mesentery of the colon medial to the anastomosis. If the anastomosis is not placed extraperitoneally the retrocolic space should be covered by suturing the lateral peritoneal flap to the colon proximal and distal to the anastomosis. Stab drainage of the retrocolic space never does any harm.

Stab Cecostomy from within the Abdomen. This procedure is carried out as an accompaniment of resection of the left colon to safeguard the immediate anastomosis. Occasionally it is useful if the colon has been seriously involved by inflammatory processes of the pelvic viscera or traumatized during operations for such lesions.

The cecum is exposed and a purse-string suture of oo chromic catgut is inserted into the seromuscular layers of its anterior aspect, the circle of the purse string being about three quarters of an inch in diameter (Fig. 310(1)). With the area well isolated by abdominal packs four Allis forceps elevate the region outlined by the purse-string suture. A stab opening is now made into the circle of this purse string. A Pezzer catheter is inserted into the cecum and the purse string passed through the catheter before it is tied tightly about it (Fig. 310(2)). A second purse string of the same suture is now inserted and tied again about the catheter inverting the first circular suture or, as illustrated (Fig. 310(3)), the catheter is "Witzeled" into the caput coli. The omentum is drawn down over the region of the cecum and the tube is drawn through it so that the omentum lies over the cecostomy (Fig. 310(4)). A stab wound is now made through the abdominal wall in the right iliac fossa and a forcep passed through this opening into the abdomen grasps the end of the catheter and withdraws it from the abdomen (Fig. 310(5)). The catheter is withdrawn until the cecum with the interposed omentum is snugly against the anterior abdominal wall. Two silk sutures in the skin at the edge of the stab wound are tied firmly about the catheter so as to prevent the cecum from falling back from the anterior abdominal wall.

This stab cecostomy provides a reassuring safety valve in patients who have had a resection with immediate anastomosis as a primary operation for a lesion situated between the midtransverse and the upper sigmoid colon. It relieves the tension on the anastomosis until healing occurs and has the great advantage of healing spontaneously. When the tube over which the anastomosis was performed has been passed and the patient is having bowel movements per rectum the cecostomy is no longer needed. The Pezzer catheter then can be cut off at the level of the skin and its tip falls into the cecum. The end of the catheter within the cecum is readily passed by the colon and the resultant cecal fistula will shrink down and disappear spontaneously if there is absolutely no obstruction of the large bowel. No attempt should be made to push the remaining tip of the catheter into the cecum as this may separate the cecum from the abdominal wall and result in peritonitis.

Closure of Mikulicz Colostomy. Before considering the closure of any colostomy, the adequacy of the colonic lumen in the distal segment is confirmed by a barium enema, supplemented by a sigmoidoscopic examination when necessary.

The preliminary step to the closure of a colostomy of the Mikulicz type is crushing the spur. A Mikulicz clamp, or some modification of it, is applied to the spur by slipping one blade down each limb of the double-barreled colostomy for a distance of 2 to 3 inches (Fig. 321). The clamp is tightened firmly and a thick "doughnut" made of dressings is applied about the emerging handle of the clamp to prevent it from being rocked from side to side with resultant pressure on the colon at the tip of the clamp. A bath towel rolled up longitudinally and wrapped around the handle makes a good stabilizer. The handle of the clamp and dressings holding it are then retained by an abdominal binder so that the patient may be ambulatory. The clamp has to remain on five days before we are certain that ischemic necrosis of the spur within its blades has occurred. Each day the screw should be further tightened if possible to maintain the pressure. At the end of five days, if the clamp has not fal-

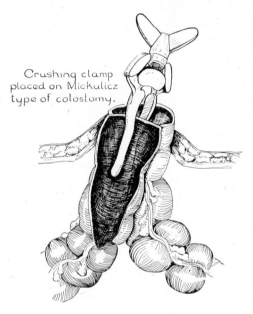

Crushing clamp placed on Mickulicz type of colostomy.

FIG. 321. Crushing clamp is left on spur for five days to ensure its complete necrosis. The line of necrosis must be broken down by finger after removal of clamp to obviate revascularization.

len off, it should be removed and a gloved finger inserted into the colostomy opening breaks down the spur along the line of necrosis. The spur need be crushed and broken for a distance of only half the diameter of the colon in order to have an adequate lumen subsequent to closure.

Ten days to two weeks should elapse between the breaking down of the spur and the actual closure of the colostomy. This time interval allows the edema to subside completely. During this interval the patient continues to irrigate the colostomy although now the differentiation between proximal and distal loops is somewhat more difficult.

The proximal loop of the colostomy should be irrigated thoroughly the day before it is to be closed, and the patient is placed on clear fluids with paragoric for twenty-four hours prior to operation. The two main factors

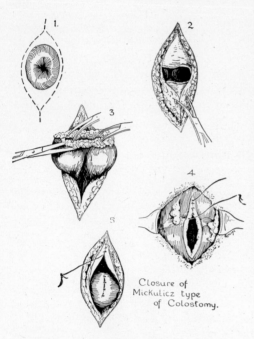

Closure of
Mickulicz type
of Colostomy.

FIG. 322. Closure of Mikulicz type of colostomy. (1) The spur having been crushed ten days to two weeks previously, an elliptical incision in the skin encompasses the stoma. (2) The borders of the ellipse of skin are approximated by towel clips to close the stoma temporarily. Using these as a handle for traction, the bowel is mobilized by excising the peristomal scar and fat exposing the layers of the abdominal wall. (3) The muco-cutaneous margin with the edematous mucous membrane, fat and scar is excised, leaving pliable vascular bowel edges free from scar and induration. (4) The colon is closed in layers by the open technic, the line of closure always being at right angles to the long axis of the bowel to obviate stenosis. In the closure of a transverse colon colostomy this may be done without fear of contaminating the general peritoneal cavity which is protected by the omentum through which the loop of bowel was drawn in the original making of the colostomy. Successful closure depends upon adequate mobilization and complete excision of the scarred indurated margins of the stoma permitting accurate suture without tension. (5) Abdominal wall closure may be in layers or by through-and-through interrupted sutures of catgut or stainless steel wire.

essential in securing primary healing of the colostomy closure are, first, the complete excision of all edematous mucous membrane and scar tissue about the stoma and, second, the thorough mobilization of the colon which is only possible if the first factor has been accomplished. The entire colostomy scar is outlined by an elliptical incision (Fig. 322(1)). The incision is deepened to expose the anterior sheath of the rectus, well lateral to the borders of its aperture and wide of all scar in the subcutaneous fat. Hemostasis is now secured, skin towels are applied and the two lateral margins of the ellipse of skin about the mucocutaneous border of the colostomy can be oversewn or approximated with Allis or Kocher forceps so as to invert and close the colostomy opening (Fig. 322(2)).

All the scar tissue and fat are now dissected off the anterior sheath of the rectus from all sides toward the aperture through which the colon emerges. This is facilitated by steady traction on the colostomy itself in an upward direction. The borders of the opening in the anterior sheath of the rectus are finally identified and carefully freed from the colon. Tension meanwhile is maintained on the colostomy to draw it upward. Under this steady traction the rectus muscle and its posterior sheath are similarly separated from the walls of the emerging colon by sharp dissection. In this way the colon is completely mobilized from the abdominal wall. The peritoneal cavity is almost invariably opened in this mobilization, but general peritonitis need not be feared because in the original operation the area was well isolated by the omentum, through which the loop of bowel was drawn.

Having mobilized the colostomy from the abdominal wall in this way all the fat and fibrous tissue adherent to the walls of the colon must be dissected off the bowel (Fig. 322(3)). The mucocutaneous junction, including edematous mucosa and all the adherent scar, is trimmed away from the colon leaving soft vascular non-edematous mucosal edges which can be closed without tension. This is in marked contrast to attempting to close the firm indurated rolled margin that persists if fibrous tissue is left adherent to it.

The scar marking the site of the old spur is identified and grasped at either end with Allis forceps. The approximation of the freshened cut edges is now begun with a continuous mucosal stitch of ooo chromic intestinal suture (Fig. 322(4)). This is begun at the upper margin of the opening and continued in an anterior and downward direction until the lower margin of the crushed spur is reached. The same suture can then be employed to retrace one's steps with an inverting catgut suture in the seromuscular coat. A third layer of catgut suture is now inserted in the form of several interrupted inverting seromuscular stitches. This closure of the colon is and must be in a direction transverse to the long axis of the bowel in order not to compromise the lumen and produce obstruction.

The closed colon drops back into the peritoneal cavity. The abdominal wall is then closed with interrupted sutures of catgut, cotton or wire (Fig. 322(5)). It is advisable to place a soft rubber drainage tube down to the anterior sheath of the rectus. This tube allows the escape of serum and may be removed completely in forty-eight hours.

Closure of Cecostomy. The same principles must be applied in cecostomy closure as have been emphasized in closure of the Mikulicz colostomy, namely, the complete excision of all scarred tissue from the abdominal wall and from the margins of the bowel opening, as well as the thorough mobilization of the cecum so that it can be closed without tension.

The entire scar of the cecostomy is outlined by an elliptical incision which passes as close to the mucocutaneous junction on either side as is compatible with being wide of all scar tissue (Fig. 319(1)). This incision is deepened to expose the fascia of the external oblique aponeurosis on all sides of the cecostomy. Hemostasis is secured and skin towels are applied. Then the opening of the cecum can be closed by rolling the margins of the ellipse of skin to be excised together and holding them approximated with Allis or Kocher forceps or, as illustrated in figure 319(2), by a running suture. By traction upward on the cecostomy the fat and scar tissue are dissected from the surface of the external oblique aponeurosis toward the opening through which the cecum emerges. The margins of the external oblique about the cecum are completely freed and the cecum is pulled up until the internal oblique and transversus muscles can be similarly identified and separated from its walls.

The cecum is now so well mobilized that it is a simple procedure to use the three forcep method in excising the stoma. The scarred cecostomy opening with its ellipse of skin is then excised by the cautery superficial to two of the clamps and the more superficial of the Kochers left on the cecum is removed (Fig. 319(3)). This leaves a crushed fringe of bowel wall which can be rapidly oversewn with a running intestinal suture of fine catgut (Fig. 319(4)). The remaining Kocher is then removed and using the same intestinal suture the crushed tissue is inverted with a line of seromuscular continuous suture (Fig. 319(5)). Several interrupted catgut sutures are then employed in the seromuscular coat to form another inverting layer (Fig. 319(6)). The cecum is now returned to the peritoneal cavity. The abdominal wall is closed in layers using interrupted sutures of double oo chromic catgut. The approximation of the internal oblique and transversus muscles deep to the external oblique must be performed with accuracy to prevent a subsequent hernia. A soft rubber drainage tube may be inserted to the external oblique if hemostasis has been difficult or the abdominal wall is obese and serum is anticipated, but this is rarely necessary.

Closure of Rod Colostomy. As the afferent and efferent limbs of a rod colostomy have not been sutured together for several inches as in the Mikulicz type, there is no spur to be crushed. For this reason there is greater danger of compromising the lumen of the colon in the closure of a rod colostomy. This, however, can be avoided. The same adequate mobilization of the colonic stomata from the layers of the abdominal wall must be carried out as described in the closure of a cecostomy and Mikulicz colostomy. The scar about the stomata and the edematous mucous membrane must also be excised. This can be safely accomplished maintaining an adequate blood supply to the colon if more of the antimesenteric portion of the bowel is excised than of the mesenteric side. This has the further advantage of increasing the lumen at the anastomosis.

The closure of this stoma is then carried out as an open end-to-end anastomosis. It may even be wise to fix a tube across the anastomosis as described for an end-to-end ileocolic anastomosis following right colon resection (Fig. 305(4)).

The closed colon is then dropped back into the abdomen. The abdominal wall is closed with interrupted stitches of catgut, cotton or steel wire. A drain may be placed down to the fascia if indicated. The skin is closed with interrupted sutures.

Subtotal Colectomy. Removal of the colon from cecum to lower sigmoid in one stage is sometimes indicated for ulcerative colitis or multiple polyposis. An ileostomy should be performed as a preliminary step to subtotal colectomy, the proximal end of the divided ileum being brought out through a wound in the right lower quadrant and the distal end being brought out on the left side of the abdomen in the line of the proposed left paramedian incision for the colectomy. The patient suffering from multiple polyposis may be in sufficiently good condition to permit the ileostomy and subtotal colectomy being done at one operation. In the presence of ulcerative colitis the ileostomy should be a preliminary rather than a coincidental procedure except in carefully selected cases and after adequate preoperative preparation.

The colectomy itself comprises a combination of right and left colon resections. The whole right colon must be mobilized, due care being taken for the protection of the right ureter and duodenum (Fig. 320). The entire gastrocolic omentum must be divided. Both splenic and hepatic flexures must be completely mobilized as well as the descending and sigmoid portions of the bowel with protection of the left ureter. The distal sigmoid colon is transected between clamps. The mesentery of the terminal ileum distal to the site of its division and the mesentery of the mobilized colon right around to the site of transection of the sigmoid are then divided so as to allow removal of the whole of the ascending, transverse and descending colons. All the vessels in the mesentery are divided between forceps and the right, middle and left colic arteries are doubly ligatured.

The distal cut end of sigmoid is brought out through the lower end of the incision as a mucous fistula. This prepares the way for its subsequent excision in an abdominoperineal resection of lower sigmoid and rectum if total colectomy is necessary. It is never permissible to close and return to the peritoneal cavity the proximal end of the remaining colon if the patient is suffering from ulcerative colitis because of the danger of peritonitis.

After such a subtotal colectomy it is not usually possible to reperitonealize the entire posterior wall of the abdominal cavity. However, such peritoneal edges and folds as can be approximated, to keep the small intestine away from contact with unperitonealized surfaces, should be sutured together with interrupted silk stitches. Both colic gutters should be drained by tubes drawn through stab wounds in the two flanks.

This operation is greatly facilitated by the preliminary passage of a double or single lumened tube into the terminal ileum. The collapsed small intestine becomes shuffled up on the tube and comprises a much smaller bulk of bowel to be packed off, first to the left and then to the right as the mobilization of the colon proceeds from the cecum distally.

The advances which have recently been made in the preoperative and postoperative care of patients, together with refinement in surgical technic, have made this formidable operative procedure possible without prohibitive mortality even for patients who are desperately ill from ulcerative colitis.

CONCLUSION

The present status of surgery of the colon is in sharp contrast to that of a decade ago when the mortality was great, the morbidity was distressing to the patient and the whole problem a discouragement to the surgeon. However, the appreciation of the contributions of the fundamental scientists and the application of these to the clinical problem have in no department of surgery been responsible for greater advances. The recognition and correction of the nutritional and biochemical disturbances which are an almost inevitable accompaniment of all diseases involving the colon have led to adequate preoperative and postoperative management. The increased time consumed in preparing such patients for operation is reflected by a decreased mortality, a reduction in the postoperative morbidity and a shorter convalescence. This appreciation of the factors responsible for the patient's illness and their treatment in a proper sequence has probably been responsible to a greater degree than any refinement in surgical technic for the improvement and extension of surgical therapy in diseases of the colon. While chemotherapy has undoubtedly been of inestimable value in controlling infection, it in no way lessens the necessity for meticulous care in the management of these patients either during the operation or in their preoperative or postoperative care. It is no longer possible to treat diseases of the colon adequately if one's sole equipment is but a brilliant technical skill.

REFERENCES

1. HALL, M. R. *Am. J. Roentgenol.,* 39[No. 6]:[June], 1938.
2. JONES, T. E. *Surg., Gynec. & Obst.,* 72:1056, 1941.
3. GURD, F. B. *Ann. Surg.,* 113:987-1000, [June], 1941.
4. KERR, H. H. *J.A.M.A.,* 81:641, 1923.
5. BABCOCK, W. W. *Surg., Gynec. & Obst.,* 75:485-489, [Oct.], 1942.
6. WANGENSTEEN, O. H. *Surg., Gynec. & Obst.,* 70:59-70, [Jan.], 1940.
7. HOLMAN, E. *Surg., Gynec. & Obst.,* 74:146, 1942.
8. ZINTEL, H. A. *Am. J. Med.,* 2:443-448, [May], 1947.

15

THE LOWER PART OF THE SIGMOID, THE RECTUM AND ANUS

Claude F. Dixon, M.D. and A. Lee Lichtman, M.D.

Most of the procedures for resection of cancer of the colon were outlined at the turn of the century. So many variations were described that it is difficult to perform any procedure that was not recorded in that period. However, in most instances they were applied in a few cases and with a rather high mortality rate. In the past five years such great improvement has occurred in colonic surgery that it is now possible to perform most procedures with a mortality rate per patient of less than 5 per cent.

There is a great deal of variation in the limits and relations of the rectum and sigmoid. The shape of the pelvic outlet, obesity of the patient, mobility of the sigmoid, the lowest reflection of the pelvic peritoneum and, if the patient is a woman, the presence of adnexal inflammation, cystocele and rectocele affect the application of operative methods. Because the limits of the rectosigmoid and the ampulla of the rectum are so poorly defined we prefer to locate lesions of these regions in terms of the distance of the lower edge from the dentate (pectinate) line as measured through a proctoscope. In proctologic procedures failure to define landmarks clearly has led occasionally to unfortunate results. Inadequate specification of the anomucosal juncture in Whitehead's radical hemorrhoid operation, with the use of the indefinite term "free skin margin," has produced unfortunate postoperative deformity. In this chapter we shall consider the surgical treatment of lesions within 20 cm. of the dentate line.

PREOPERATIVE PREPARATION OF THE COLON

In any procedure in which there is possibility of opening into, or resecting a part of, the large intestine, the colon should be prepared, if practicable, to reduce soiling and infection. In emergency procedures, in which there is no response to conservative methods of decompression or in which they are contraindicated, the risk is greatly increased and no measure can be taken to reduce the bacterial content of the stool. But in all other cases there should be a preparatory period of three to five days during which the patient is fed a non-residue diet, high in protein, carbohydrate and vitamins. Sodium phosphate is administered and the colon is irrigated twice daily up to the day before operation. Camphorated tincture of opium is given the day before operation. Anemia is corrected by blood transfusions. Sixty grains (4 gm.) of sulfasuxidine or sulfathalidine is given every four hours the first day and 30 grains (2 gm.) is given every four hours thereafter. The patient should receive a minimum of 720 grains (48 gm.) in seventy-two hours. One milligram of vitamin K is given daily. While the use of sulfasuxidine has not met the favor of all surgeons we feel that the resulting reduction of coliform bacteria in the stool has greatly reduced the incidence of postoperative peritonitis. The value of preparation with sulfasuxidine has been appreciated most by surgeons who perform open anastomoses. Furthermore the postoperative course is improved, since the poor solubility of the drug permits it to remain in the intestine to prevent effects of the physiologic or mechanical obstruction that follows all operations in which the intestines are manipulated.

Table 4 presents the operative mortality rates for all operations on the sigmoid, rectosigmoid and rectum performed at the Mayo Clinic during certain years. It can be seen that the mortality rate following operations on the sigmoid in 1944 was 8 per cent of what it had been in 1907 to 1936, inclusive, while that of the rectum was 40 per cent of what it had been in the earlier period. It is our impression that operations on both the sigmoid and the rectum were aided by the parenteral and intraperitoneal administration of soluble sulfonamides. The additional use of sulfasuxidine, as previously suggested, has further improved the results of removal of lesions above the pelvic peritoneal fold. Whereas formerly operations on lesions of the lower part of the rectum were attended with the least risk, they now have the highest mortality rate.

TABLE 4. *MORTALITY RATES FOLLOWING ALL OPERATIONS PERFORMED ON THE SIGMOID, RECTOSIGMOID AND RECTUM*

SEGMENT		1907-1936	1941	1944
Sigmoid	Cases	829	191	218
	Mortality rate, per cent	22.1	6.3	1.8
Rectosigmoid	Cases	779	73	111
	Mortality rate, per cent	24.0	4.2	3.6
Rectum	Cases	2,000	213	246
	Mortality rate, per cent	13.2	5.1	5.3

SURGICAL TREATMENT OF MALIGNANT LESIONS OF THE RECTUM AND LOWER PART OF THE SIGMOID

Choice of Procedure. Since most surgeons strive for technical improvement in the procedure that affords the best result in their hands, few studies are available that compare applicability, mortality and survival rates under similar conditions. Progressive improvement has permitted more radical resections and excision of the lesion when the small intestine, uterus and adnexae, bladder or prostate is involved. In many surgical clinics, resection is performed even in the presence of small metastatic lesions in the liver, since the patients derive temporary benefit from the procedure. One can expect to find hepatic metastatic lesions in 12 to 14 per cent of the cases. Recent reports show resectability rates varying from 70 to 95 per cent. Attention of many surgeons has now been turned toward evaluating the possibility of preserving the sphincter mechanism of the anus since it has been shown that retrograde spread of cancer in this region is limited and surgical procedures can be performed without added risk.

At present the one-stage combined abdominoperineal procedure is considered the method of choice in the majority of the surgical clinics. It is the most generally applicable procedure. It has been demonstrated, however, that carcinoma of the rectum does not spread distally for more than 2 to 3 cm. unless the proximal lymphatic channels are blocked.[1] It is questionable whether any procedure is radical enough in the few cases in which there is such retrograde lymphatic invasion. By a study of survival rates following the application of the various methods in different segments of the rectum one can determine at which point it is necessary to sacrifice the anus. One must remember also that following perineal resection, in addition to losing the sphincter mechanism the patient may suffer loss of sexual function and occasionally has temporary difficulty with vesical function.

Anterior resection with preservation of the sphincter muscles can be performed for most lesions more than 8 or 10 cm. from the dentate line. One occasionally encounters cases in which the lesion is as low as 6 cm. from the dentate line but in which the situation of the pelvis permits resection and anastomosis of the sigmoid to the rectal stump. On the service of the senior author, this procedure has been applied for the past fifteen years. Figure 323 shows the distribution, grade and nodal involvement of the lesion in 340 cases in which the operation was not of a palliative nature. The resectability rate was 86 per cent for lesions more than 10 cm. from the dentate line. The survival rates are given under the description of the operation. The impression gained from these cases is that resection of the lesions together with 3 to 4 cm. of normal rectum distally produces satisfactory results. Anterior resection when the lesion is less than 8 cm. from the dentate line is, we believe, usually inadvisable. When the lesion lies between 8 and 10 cm. from the dentate line, often the decision as to which procedure to apply depends on the extent of the lesion, which in turn can be determined only after laparotomy has been performed and the rectum has been partially mobilized.

Lesions not resectable through an anterior abdominal incision are removed through an abdominoperineal approach. As has been mentioned, the one-stage operation has met with favor among the majority of surgeons. Frequently the procedure is attended with a good deal of shock, especially if the patient is elderly. Since the dissection in the region of the process in the case of a low-lying tumor is done at the last part of the operation with an intervening change of position of the patient, the surgeon may be pressed for time and sacrifice the extent of the radical perineal excision. The

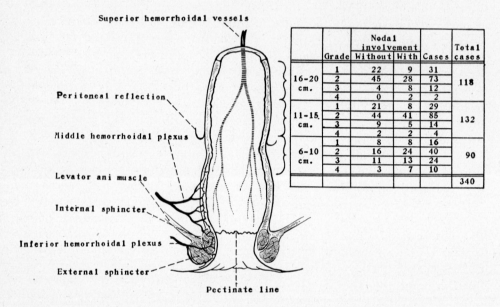

	Grade	Nodal involvement		Cases	Total cases
		Without	With		
16-20 cm.	1	22	9	31	118
	2	45	28	73	
	3	4	8	12	
	4	0	2	2	
11-15 cm.	1	21	8	29	132
	2	44	41	85	
	3	9	5	14	
	4	2	2	4	
6-10 cm.	1	8	8	16	90
	2	16	24	40	
	3	11	13	24	
	4	3	7	10	
					340

Labels on figure: Superior hemorrhoidal vessels; Peritoneal reflection; Middle hemorrhoidal plexus; Levator ani muscle; Internal sphincter; Inferior hemorrhoidal plexus; External sphincter; Pectinate line

FIG. 323. The distribution, grade and nodal involvement of the lesions in 340 cases of nonpalliative anterior resection.

survival rate after resection of lesions in the terminal 6 cm. of the rectum is much poorer than after resection of lesions in the upper half of the rectum by any method. There are many reasons for this. The grade of malignancy of the lower-lying malignant processes tends to be higher, the nodal involvement more extensive, and the pathways of local spread tend to be more difficult to eradicate. The closer a lesion is to the dentate line, the poorer the prognosis, and lesions that spread past the mucocutaneous line have a poor prognosis indeed. Lesions of the lower part of the rectum are more difficult to cure because they are in a very strategic position from the standpoint of possibilities for dispersion of cancer cells. The veins of the region drain into both the portal and the systemic circulation and the lymphatics drain not only in the direction of the mesosigmoid but also along the middle hemorrhoidal vessels and endopelvic fascia investing the levator ani muscle.[2] Therefore, it is not sufficient to be radical in the removal of the mesosigmoid, and there must be a wide excision of the perianal skin, ischiorectal fat, levator ani muscle and its investing fascia, the perirectal tissues and pelvic peritoneum. This can better be performed with the patient in the prone position at a separate sitting than during the abdominal phase of the surgical care.

Babcock and Bacon are advocates of abdominoperineal proctosigmoid-ectomy with preservation of the sphincter muscle.[3] They have applied this procedure to lesions as low as 3 cm. from the dentate line, which include 80 per cent of cancers of the sigmoid, rectum and anus. In the experience of some surgeons, however, this method has found a much more limited application, being reserved for freely movable, small lesions between 4 and 10 cm. from the dentate line. It should be remembered, however, that following this operation the sphincteral function is satisfactory in 60 to 80 per cent of the cases and that when the sigmoid is drawn down, its vascular supply must permit 10 cm. more extension than is necessary in the procedure of anterior resection. Furthermore there is a very limited resection of perianal and perirectal tissue. We believe this is important in the consideration of lesions of the lower half of the rectum.

While the modified Mikulicz type of operation is the subject of extensive criticism, satisfactory survival rates have been secured by many surgeons. Adequate mobilization of the rectum permits removal by the Mikulicz operation of lesions as low as 14 cm. from the dentate line if the patient is slender. Subsequent resection of the exteriorized lesion down to the fascia permits removal of some of the mesosigmoid. The operation of exteriorization in which an intraperitoneal resection is performed in the first stage can be applied to lesions as low as 18 cm. from the dentate line. These procedures are applicable to the lower part of the sigmoid when the degree of dilatation of the sigmoid or the condition of the patient does not permit end-to-end anastomosis. There is thus, at least to a certain extent, a choice of procedures under the particular conditions just mentioned.

The introduction of sulfonamides and development of methods of decompression have warranted reinvestigation of the possibility of performing anterior resection without temporary proximal colostomy.[4,5] At present, this omission of colostomy adds, we think, materially to the mortality rate but it is possible that with future development of chemotherapeutic and antibiotic substances effective against coliform organisms the plan may be feasible in the removal of lesions down to about 14 cm. from the dentate margin. However, the resection of lesions at a lower level involves suture of a portion of the rectum which is devoid of serosa. The posterior wall of the rectum is very thin and the blood supply is just adequate for healing if no stress is placed on the suture line. There is a large dead space in the hollow of the sacrum that is a potential site for infection. Fistulas occur in about 5 per cent of the cases and, if proximal colostomy is performed, healing merely entails a delay of one to three weeks. Experience gained from 220 cases in which a large rectal tube was passed through the anus beyond the anastomosis (Fig. 324) revealed that this procedure is not as dependable as colostomy. Therefore, under present conditions, temporary proximal transverse colostomy seems advisable in the performance of anterior resection.

Table 5 gives the mortality rates for operations on the sigmoid and rectum performed at the Mayo Clinic from 1930 through 1944. In order to present the present-day picture the mortality rates for 1943 and 1944 are also given separately.

TABLE 5. *MORTALITY RATES FOLLOWING PROCEDURES ON THE SIGMOID AND RECTUM PERFORMED AT THE MAYO CLINIC*

OPERATION	APPLICA-BILITY*	1930-1944			1930-1942			1943-1944		
		CASES	HOS-PITAL DEATHS	MORTAL-ITY RATE, PER CENT	CASES	HOS-PITAL DEATHS	MORTAL-ITY RATE, PER CENT	CASES	HOS-PITAL DEATHS	MORTAL-ITY RATE, PER CENT
Anterior resection	6-20	308†	30	9.7	200	29	14.5	108	1	0.9
Posterior resection	0-10	761	37	4.9	654	35	5.4	107	2	1.9
Combined abdomino-perineal resection	0-24	902	62	6.9	651	50	7.7	251	12	4.8
Proctosigmoid-ectomy with preservation of sphincter	4-10	109‡	12	11.0						
Mikulicz	More than 14	255	27	10.6	194	24	12.4	61	3	4.9
Exteriorization	More than 18	436	63	14.4	372	62	16.7	64	1	1.6

* Distance in centimeters from dentate line of lesions to which the respective operation is applicable.

† In a more recent compilation the nonpalliative operations of anterior resection were selected. The operation was performed in 340 cases with twenty deaths (5.9 per cent). In the five year period, ending October 1, 1945, 184 of these operations were performed with two deaths (1.1 per cent).

‡ Operation was performed before 1930 in some of these cases.

Colostomy. Emergency proximal colostomy is performed in the presence of obstruction of the terminal portion of the colon when conservative efforts at decompression fail. Digital examination will identify lesions in the lower part of the rectum for which sigmoidal colostomy can be performed. It is advisable to place the stoma as far distally as expedient, but if subsequent anterior resection is possible, the incision is best made over the transverse colon in order to permit mobilization of the left portion of the gut at the second operation. Simple colostomy is adequate. More elaborate forms of colostomy entail added risk and disposition of the loops sometimes causes embarrassment of the blood supply to the loops.

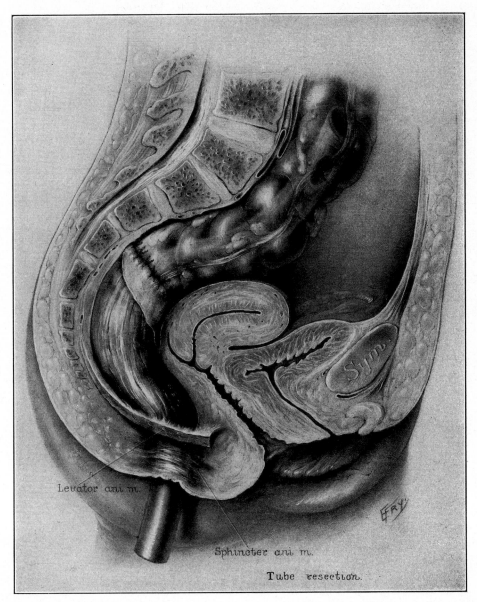

FIG. 324. Anterior resection and large rectal tube inserted for decompression.

The transverse colon is conveniently situated for the performance of colostomy. It is mobile enough to be brought through the omentum and out of the abdomen without tension even if the patient is obese. Herniation of the small intestine, prolapse and retraction seem to be rare as complications of transverse colostomy. Obese patients can manage a transverse colonic stoma perhaps with more ease than a sigmoidal stoma.

In the performance of transverse colostomy a short upper left rectus muscle-splitting incision is made. An exploration should not be carried out if distention is extreme but occasionally the surgeon can gently examine the liver, peritoneum, and colon to determine the limits of the lesion and involvement of lymph nodes and evaluate resectability. The distended transverse colon is identified and the omentum is dissected free from its anterior wall for a short distance. The loop of transverse colon is drawn through an avascular region of the omentum. A rubber tube is then passed through the mesentery under the colon. Five grams of sulfathiazole is scattered in the peritoneal cavity. The abdominal incision is closed in layers loosely around the emerging loop. The rubber tube is reinforced by a glass or plastic tube inside it and tied in position. The incision in the skin is protected by heavy petrolatum gauze. If distention is extreme some of the gas can be tapped by inserting an 18 gauge needle in the exteriorized loop and the colon can be opened by cautery incision in six hours. Otherwise, the colon should be opened by a transverse cautery incision carried out twenty-four hours later in the patient's room.

If the lesion is too low for anterior resection, a low left rectus incision is made for sigmoidal colostomy, as is described under posterior resection. Difference of opinion exists about the performance of palliative colostomy in cases in which obstruction is not present but hepatic metastatic lesions are demonstrable. The surgeon must judge whether obstruction will occur before the distant metastatic lesions overcome the patient. Palliative colostomy reduces infection and hemorrhage from the lesion. It checks diarrhea and occasionally relieves some of the pain accompanying low, inoperable lesions.

Technic of Mobilization of the Sigmoid and Rectum. To avoid repetition the fundamental approach to the mobilization of the sigmoid and rectum will be presented separately here. With this basic method, any of the innumerable variations in the procedures can be applied. In combined operations it is advisable to do as much through the abdominal incision as is possible. The shape of the pelvic bowl, the fat content of the mesentery and the local relations of the lesions are apparent only after the abdomen has been opened. These things determine how much can be done by the abdominal approach and how much should be left for the perineal phase.

THE ANTERIOR ROUTE. The bladder should be emptied before the operation is begun. To permit emptying of gas a rectal tube is left in the anus until just before the operation. The left rectus muscle-splitting incision is made to extend from the pubic bone to a short distance above the umbilicus. The liver, peritoneum and omentum are examined for metastatic lesions. Note is made of the condition of the gallbladder, appendix and stomach. The entire colon is palpated, for synchronous malignant lesions are found in 5 per cent of the cases. The local relations of the lesion are determined and the procedure to be followed is decided tentatively.

With the sigmoid drawn medially and upward, the peritoneum to the left of the sigmoid, which marks the fusion of the posterior leaflet of the primitive mesocolon to the posterior parietal peritoneum, is dissected away

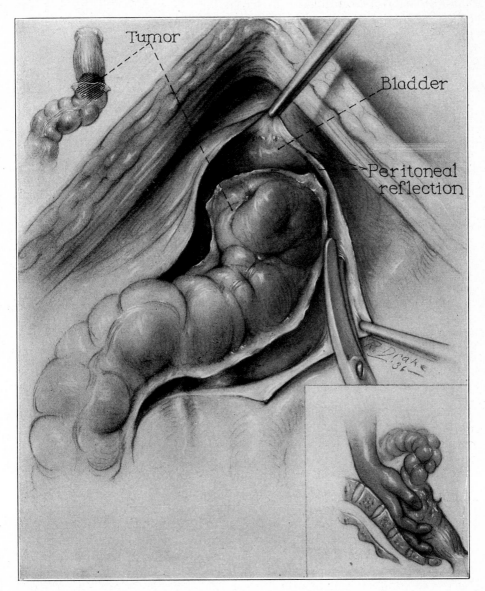

FIG. 325. Peritoneal incision for mobilization of the rectum. Inset shows separation of the rectum from its posterior attachments. (From Dixon, C. F., *Surgery*, 15:367-377, [Mar.], 1944.)

from the mesosigmoid. The patient is placed in extreme Trendelenburg position and the small intestine is walled off by moist abdominal pads. An abdominal retractor is adjusted and, if the patient is a woman, a long, flat, pliable blade is used to retract the uterus and adnexae. The sigmoid is freed until the root of the mesentery is visible and the left ureter is identified and marked. It is occasionally necessary to ligate the spermatic or ovarian vessels. The sigmoid is then shifted to the left and the peritoneum of the right side of the mesosigmoid is incised. The right ureter is identified. The two peritoneal incisions are then joined by a curved incision in the pouch of Douglas (Fig. 325). If the lesion lies at the peritoneal reflection or below, an adequate cuff of peritoneum must be left attached to the rectum. While gentle traction is exerted on the rectum the right hand is passed along the hollow of the sacrum (Fig. 325, inset), bluntly separating the rectum from its posterior attachments. Care must be observed to avoid bruising the sacral veins. In this manner the ampulla of the rectum can be freed as far as the coccyx. If the patient is male, the ureters and bladder are pushed back and the anterior wall of the rectum is freed from the seminal vesicles, vas deferens and prostate. If the patient is female, the anterior wall of the rectum is freed from the vaginal wall. The lateral stalks of the rectum, in which the middle hemorrhoidal vessels run, must occasionally be ligated well out from the rectum. If more mobility of the sigmoid is needed, the left peritoneal incision can be extended toward the spleen and the splenic flexure can be mobilized.

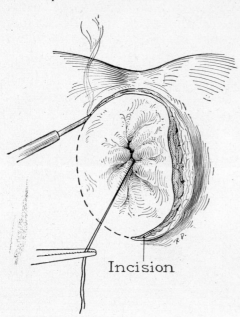

Incision

FIG. 326. Incision for posterior resection.

THE POSTERIOR ROUTE. Greatest accessibility for radical posterior resection is secured with the patient in the prone position and the pelvis elevated by a padded kidney rest. A diathermy knife can be used to advantage in most of the dissection because the tissues are so vascular. Some surgeons place a catheter in the urethra to prevent injury to that structure.

The anus is closed by a purse-string suture which can also be used as a tractor. An elliptic incision is made around the anus, extending from the coccyx to the central point of the perineum (Fig. 326). If the lesion is low in the rectum, a wide oval of skin should be excised. The ischiorectal fat is incised wide of the anus, the inferior hemorrhoidal vessels being ligated as they are encountered. The incision is then deepened until the origin of the levator ani muscles is encountered. Then the anococcygeal ligament is cut transversely and the coccyx is isolated. It is grasped with a towel clip and disarticulated from the sacrum. The fascia propria of the rectum is then separated from the sacrum by sharp dissection and the rectum is freed as far as the promontory of the sacrum. The midsacral vessels are touched with the cautery if bleeding is encountered. A narrow gauze pad is used to fill the posterior space. Beginning posteriorly, the coccygeus and levator ani muscles are resected as close to their origins as possible together with the investing visceral endopelvic fascia (Fig. 327). The anterior attachments of the rectum must be divided by sharp dissection. Incision is made anterior to the transversi perinei muscles and the attachments of the external sphincter to the bulbocavernosus are cut between clamps. Large venous sinuses may be encountered here. The rectum is then pulled straight up to demarcate the plane of dissection.

If the patient is female, two fingers of the left hand are placed in the vagina so that the dissection can be carried along its posterior wall. If the vaginal wall is involved a section may be excised. Vascular connections should be clamped before they are cut. The peritoneum soon comes into view. It is incised. It should be remembered that the ureters run close to the cervix at this point. (The uterus and adnexae can be removed at this stage, if necessary.) Next the peritoneal incision is extended around the rectum, an adequate cuff being resected.

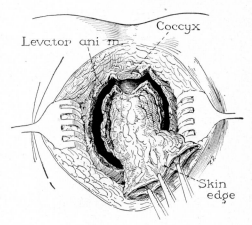

FIG. 327. Levator ani muscle is incised widely.

If the patient is male, the dissection is carried over the bulb of the corpus spongiosum and the membranous urethra. When the prostate comes into view the dissection is continued up between the two layers of Denonvillier's fascia, but if a perforating lesion of the anterior wall of the rectum is found, it is best to remove the capsule of the prostate. When prostatic involvement is encountered, part or all of that organ can be removed as indicated. Dissection is then carried over the seminal vesicles. If they are involved, they are to be excised, but carefully, since the ureters cross the vas deferens above them. The lateral attachments of the rectum should be ligated and cut well away from the rectum if this has not been done by the abdominal approach. The peritoneum is incised (Fig. 328) and the bladder then comes into view. Occasionally, a segment of its wall must be excised from below because of malignant involvement. The vesical wall can then be closed by two rows of sutures.

If the sigmoid has been freed in the abdominal approach, a large part of it can be drawn into the posterior incision at this stage in the operation. The mesosigmoid can be mobilized from below if necessary. It is possible to ligate the superior hemorrhoidal vessels well up in the abdomen (Fig. 329).

Resection through the perineal approach alone has several disadvantages. While it is possible to ligate the superior hemorrhoidal vessels high up, one cannot determine the state of the liver and peritoneum or whether there is an involved node above the point of ligation.

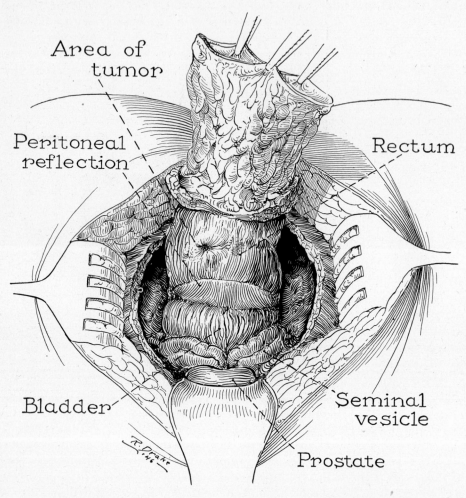

FIG. 328. Incision in the peritoneum, which has been reflected off the bladder.

Anterior Resection for Malignant Lesions of the Upper Part of the Rectum and Lower Portion of the Sigmoid with Preservation of Intestinal Continuity by Colorectostomy.[6] The abdominal incision is made and the left part of the colon is mobilized as has been described under "The Anterior Route," (Fig. 325). The site for proximal transection is selected well up on the sigmoid so that the distal end will reach the lower part of the rectum without tension. The superior hemorrhoidal vessels or inferior mesenteric vessels are ligated above any palpable nodal involvement (Fig. 330). It is not necessary to observe any "critical point." One strives for a radical excision of the lymphatics in the pelvic mesocolon, while the marginal vessels provide circulation to the distal end of the proximal segment of bowel. The mesentery of the sigmoid is omegoid and the sigmoid can be made to reach further into the pelvis by ligating the inferior mesenteric vessels higher up (Fig. 331). This fact insures adequate removal of the mesosigmoid in low resections. With these points in mind, the mesosigmoid is resected between clamps, the

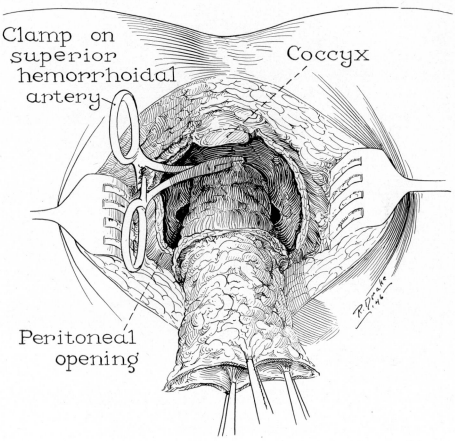

Clamp on superior hemorrhoidal artery

Coccyx

Peritoneal opening

FIG. 329. The superior hemorrhoidal vessels are ligated as high as possible.

marginal vessels being preserved up to a point just under the site selected for transection of the sigmoid. The sigmoid is then divided between Payr clamps that have been placed so that more of the antimesenteric border than of the mesenteric border is resected. Arterial pulsation should be visible in small fat tags close to the clamp. If these fat tags are stripped away too vigorously to provide a clean serosal surface the blood supply may be impaired since these small vessels are end arteries. The rectum and distal portion of the sigmoid are then wrapped in a pad and reflected over the pubis.

By gentle steady traction on the rectum with a hand in the hollow of the sacrum, the curves, valves and folds of the rectum can be stretched to give added length. The vascular stalks of the lower part of the rectum are grasped with long curved clamps, cut and ligated. With the relaxation of the patient provided by anesthesia, the levator ani muscles are funneled into the pelvis and the lesion which was 8 cm. from the dentate line during proctoscopy

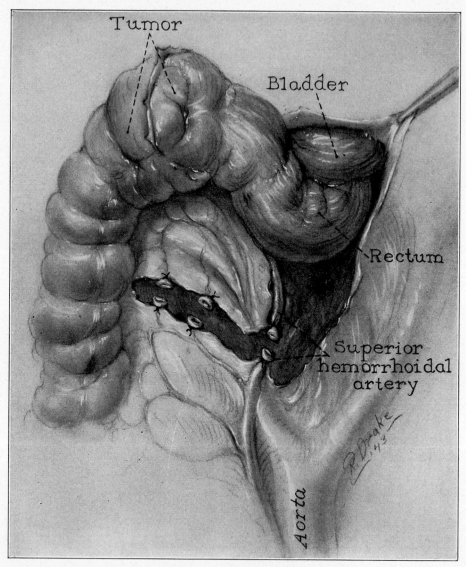

FIG. 330. The superior hemorrhoidal vessels or inferior mesenteric vessels are ligated as indicated. (From Dixon, C. F., *Surgery*, 15:367-377, [Mar.], 1944.)

now lies 12 to 14 cm. from that line. A specially constructed rubber-guarded curved clamp is placed well below the lesion so that at least 4 cm. of normal rectum can be resected below the lesion (Fig. 332). A second clamp is placed proximal to the first and the sigmoid and upper part of the rectum are resected with a cautery. A second curved clamp is placed across the distal portion of the sigmoid at right angles to the Payr clamp so that the sigmoid will be turned 45 degrees when it is anastomosed to the rectum. The Payr clamp is removed and the crushed segment of sigmoid is excised. A pad is placed in the hollow of the sacrum and the sigmoidal clamp is placed beside the rectal clamp deep in the pelvis to permit end-to-end anastomosis (Fig. 332, inset).

Open anastomosis permits visualization of the blood supply, better hemostasis and a larger lumen, and less crushed tissue is turned in. The so-called aseptic anastomosis of the rectum requires difficult maneuvers deep in the pelvis and there is danger of creating a diaphragm by catching the mucosa of the opposite side in the sutures. Closely placed interrupted sutures in one

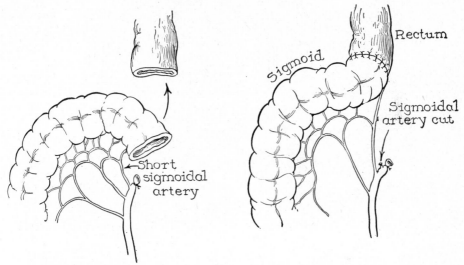

FIG. 331. Ligation higher on the inferior mesenteric artery provides greater mobility of the sigmoid. (From Dixon, C. F., *Surgery*, 15:367-377, [Mar.], 1944.)

row suffice for the posterior portion since there is no serosal covering for the thin rectal wall. Two rows can be placed in the anterior half. After the first row has been placed, the clamps are removed and a reinforcing row of interrupted inverting Halsted mattress sutures is added (Fig. 333). Then 5 gm. of sulfathiazole is dusted over the anastomosis and in the hollow of the sacrum after it has been verified that hemostasis has been obtained. A Penrose cigaret drain is placed in the hollow of the sacrum and is brought out through the lower angle of the incision. The pelvic peritoneum is sutured, the anastomosis being placed retroperitoneally (Fig. 333, inset). All pads are removed and the table is leveled. A convenient loop of the transverse segment of colon is brought through the omentum to emerge from the upper angle of the incision in order to provide for a temporary colonic stoma. The abdominal incision is closed in layers, tension being avoided around the limbs of the loop of colon, which are supported by a rigid tube passing through the mesentery.

The exteriorized loop of colon is opened twenty-four hours later by a longitudinal incision 4 cm. long made with a cautery. A rubber dam is sealed to the skin below the colonic stoma to protect the Penrose drain from contamination. About thirty-six hours after operation the patient usually can begin to take liquids by mouth and the intake may be increased slowly.

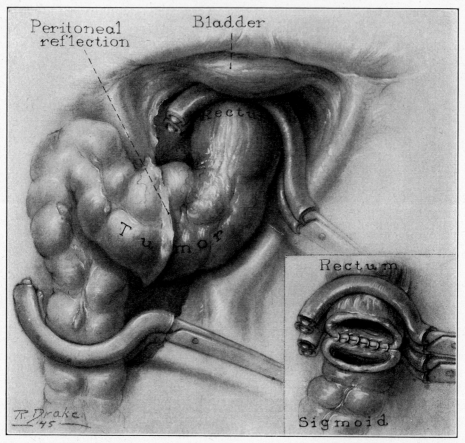

FIG. 332. Application of the curved, rubber-covered clamps. Inset shows the posterior row of sutures.

Gentle withdrawal of the drain is begun on the eighth postoperative day. When all rectal and suprapubic drainage stops, usually on the tenth or eleventh day, the tube under the transverse colonic stoma can be removed. During the third postoperative week, patency of the anastomosis and absence of fistula are determined by passage of 250 cc. of water down from the distal limb of the exteriorized loop of colon and upward from the rectum. Free passage of water in five minutes without leakage through the former drainage site is evidence of a satisfactory anastomosis. Clamps are then applied to the colostomy spur and left in situ for six or seven days. After induration from the clamps has receded the colon is prepared for closure of the stoma by giving three-way irrigations and the administration of sulfa-suxidine as indicated previously.

CLOSURE OF THE COLONIC STOMA. A short incision is made through the old scar encircling the stoma. The colon is freed from the abdominal wall,

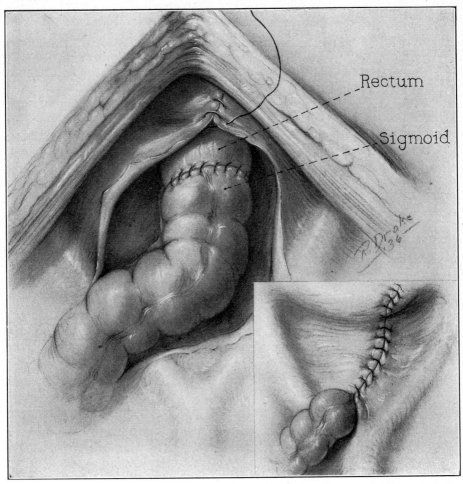

FIG. 333. The anastomosis is completed and then (inset) is placed retroperitoneally. (From Dixon, C. F., *Surgery*, 15:367-377, [Mar.], 1944.)

each layer being dissected out to provide fascia and peritoneum for closure. The peritoneum is opened and all tissues encircling the stoma are dissected away. The mucosal lip is unrolled and scar tissue is removed. The opening in the colon is closed transversely by a Connell suture of catgut which is reinforced by interrupted Lembert sutures. Omentum or fat tags are used to cover the suture line and 5 gm. of sulfathiazole is scattered in the abdominal cavity. The abdominal wall is closed in layers with a small Penrose drain in the subcutaneous space.

Three hundred and twenty-four closures performed by the foregoing technic resulted in a mortality rate of 0.3 per cent. In six of the cases (1.9 per cent) there was fecal drainage for a short time. In all but one of the six cases the fistula healed spontaneously within a few months.

Survival rates following 272 nonpalliative anterior resections are given in figures 334 and 335.

Posterior Resection in Two Stages. [7,8,9] FIRST STAGE. The abdominal incision is made and the sigmoid is mobilized as described under "The Anterior

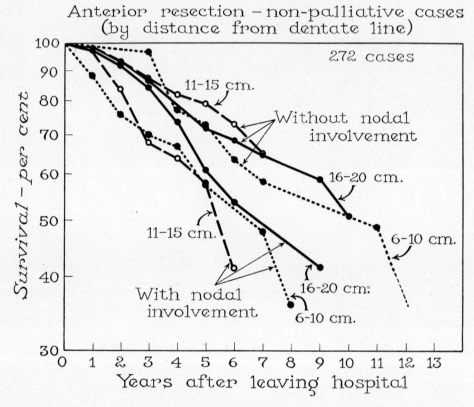

FIG. 334. Survival rates after 272 nonpalliative anterior resections. The rates are figured according to distance of the lesion from the dentate line.

Route." The pelvic peritoneum is not opened. The superior hemorrhoidal vessels are ligated. Next the mesentery is transected and its vessels are ligated. The sigmoid is then divided by cautery between two Payr clamps. If the distal portion of the sigmoid is redundant a convenient segment is excised. The distal stump is then sutured shut over the Payr clamp and closure is reinforced with a second row of inverting sutures. This stump is allowed to remain free in the abdomen. The circulation from the middle and inferior hemorrhoidal vessels is sufficient to support this stump. Examination of the lesion after resection will show, however, that the diminished circulation has caused degenerative changes in the lesion.

The proximal stump of the sigmoid is then brought out as a single-barreled permanent colonic stoma through a left McBurney incision. A short incision is made through the abdominal wall to the left of the original incision and a Payr clamp is passed through it from the outside. The sigmoid is transferred to it from the original clamp aseptically. No stitches are placed in the wall of the sigmoid to hold it to the abdominal wall and the Payr

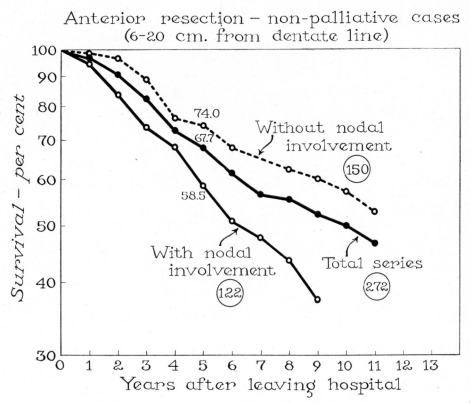

FIG. 335. Survival rate, same cases as in figure 334, on basis of absence or presence of nodal involvement.

clamp is used to keep the end of the sigmoid elevated a few centimeters away from the abdominal wall. It is occasionally necessary to attach the mesentery to the lateral abdominal wall to prevent herniation. The stoma is opened in twenty-four hours by cautery incision under the clamp and the clamp is left on to support the stoma for seven days.

Since a large majority of the patients who have low rectal lesions may be poor risks the foregoing procedure would be too much for them and simple sigmoidal loop colostomy is all that can be performed in the first stage. After mobilization of the sigmoid a rubber tube is passed through the mesentery under the colon. The site selected is the most proximal fixed portion of the sigmoid that can be brought out of the abdominal wall. This will prevent future prolapse and will provide the maximal amount of re-

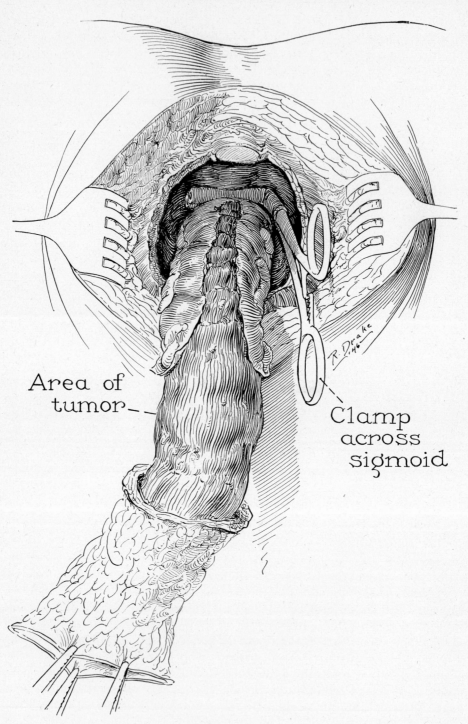

Area of
tumor—

Clamp
across
sigmoid

FIG. 336. A clamp is placed across the sigmoid near the promontory of the sacrum.

dundant sigmoid for resection through the posterior incision, permitting high ligation of the superior hemorrhoidal vessels in the pelvic mesocolon. The loop of sigmoid is brought out of the incision and the abdomen is closed in layers around it. A glass or plastic tube is passed through the rubber tube to support the loop. A rubber tube may be substituted after a week but the latter should not be removed until the posterior operation is carried out so that the loop is firmly fixed and will not retract.

After two weeks the patient is ready for the posterior procedure. The colon is prepared by irrigations and sulfasuxidine. Sulfasuxidine paste is instilled into the rectum. Remarkable reduction of the size of the lesion results from the reduction of infection due to diversion of the fecal stream. Many lesions originally beyond resectable limits can be removed after this reduction of size. If the superior mesenteric vessels have been ligated in the abdominal phase there is additional retrogression in the lesion. If there are no distant abdominal metastatic growths, very few lesions are left untreated. If the lesion is too large for removal at the time of examination intensive radium therapy may be applied and the lesion may be examined again in three months. This often reduces the lesion to resectable limits. After such

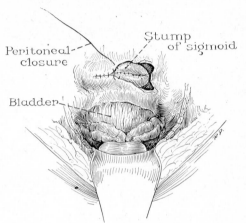

Fig. 337. As the peritoneum is closed the sigmoidal stump is fixed to it by a few sutures.

treatment the senior author has resected lesions that involved the posterior vaginal wall, cervix, vulva and urinary bladder. In some cases the entire prostate was removed with a rectal lesion. Although a cure may not be obtained the patient is made much more comfortable. Large, low-grade lesions of the lower part of the rectum are complicated by hemorrhage, severe tenesmus and foul, purulent drainage.

SECOND STAGE. While the patient is under spinal anesthesia, posterior resection is performed as described under "The Posterior Route," (Figs. 326, 327 and 328). If a single-barreled colonic stoma was established and the superior hemorrhoidal vessels were ligated in the abdominal phase, the sigmoid stump and rectum can be removed as soon as the peritoneum is opened. The peritoneum is closed after 2.5 gm. of sulfathiazole has been scattered in the peritoneal cavity. If a double-barreled sigmoidal stoma [10,11] has been established previously, the superior hemorrhoidal vessels must be ligated from below. After the peritoneum has been incised around the rectum the sigmoid and its mesentery can be mobilized from below. If mobile redundant sigmoid has been prepared during the abdominal phase a high ligation of the superior hemorrhoidal vessels and radical excision of the mesosigmoid

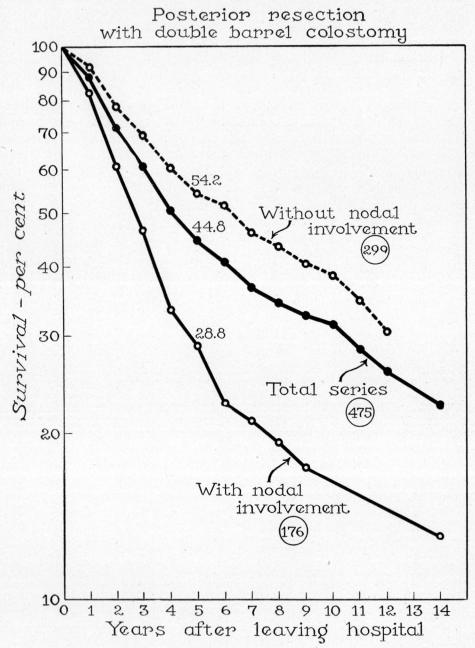

FIG. 338. Survival rates after posterior resection showing the poor prognosis following resection of low rectal lesions if the nodes are involved.

can be performed with the aid of long curved clamps (Fig. 329). A major part of the sigmoid can be delivered into the posterior incision. By using a long, heavy right-angled clamp the sigmoid can be grasped and transected high up so as to leave a very short distal loop (Fig. 336).

The sigmoidal stump is sutured shut and 2.5 gm. of sulfathiazole is scattered into the peritoneal cavity. The peritoneum is closed, a few of the

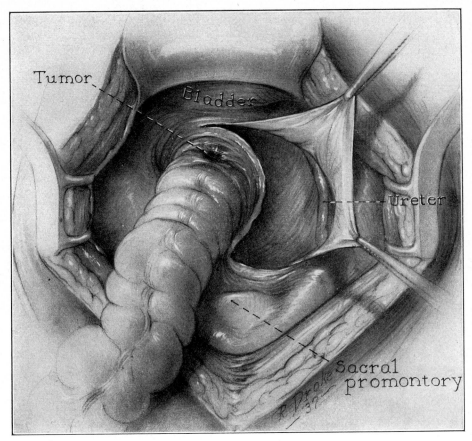

FIG. 339. The peritoneum is incised and the ureter is identified.

sutures being passed through the line of closure of the sigmoidal stump in order to keep it in contact with the newly formed pelvic floor (Fig. 337). Hemostasis in the posterior incision is verified and 5 gm. of sulfathiazole is scattered in the incision. A pliofilm lining is inserted in the cavity and is packed firmly with gauze to provide hemostasis and support the pelvic floor. The skin is closed around the pack, a 5 cm. opening being left in the most dependent part.

The posterior pack is removed in three days and the incision is irrigated twice daily. The patient must be watched for bleeding from the posterior incision from the fourth to the twelfth day. Diligent care of the posterior incision is essential and it is examined digitally to prevent pocketing and formation of abscess. Initial emptying of the bladder may be temporarily impaired and frequently a catheter must be left in place for nine to twelve days. Since the patients are usually aged, transurethral prostatic resection

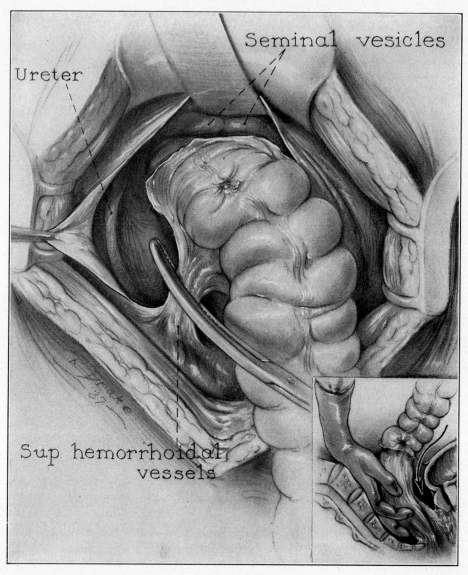

FIG. 340. Ligation of the superior hemorrhoidal vessels. Inset shows separation of the rectum from its posterior attachments.

must occasionally be performed if the patient has had urinary difficulty before operation because the removal of support that has been given to the bladder by the presence of the rectum may increase the urinary difficulty. If a distal blind sigmoidal stump is left, it must be irrigated weekly to prevent accumulation of debris.

The survival rate in 475 cases in which posterior resection was performed after previous double-barreled colostomy is given in figure 338. The lesions were in the lower part of the rectum and it should be recalled that the

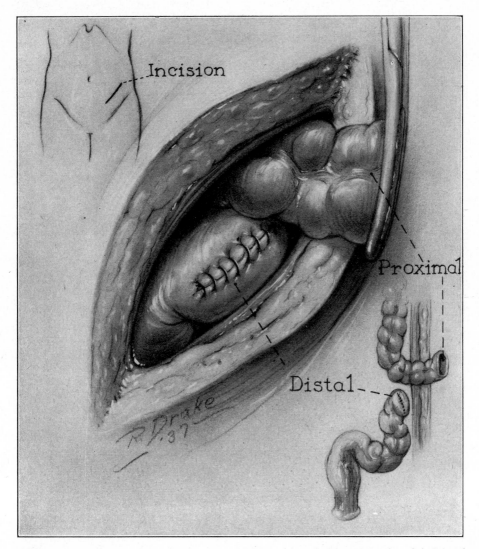

FIG. 341. The distal stump of the sigmoid is closed and the proximal end is brought out through a left McBurney incision as a single-barreled colostomy.

prognosis of these lesions is not as good as that of the lesions above the pelvic peritoneal fold.

The One-stage Combined Abdominoperineal Resection.[12,13,14] THE ABDOMINAL PHASE. Abdominal incision is made and the sigmoid and rectum are mobilized as described under "The Anterior Route," (Fig. 339). Occasionally, if the patient is obese, one cannot free the rectum as far as the coccyx but every effort should be made to do so. The superior hemorrhoidal vessels are ligated (Fig. 340) and the mesosigmoid is resected, observing the precautions described in the anterior resection operation. A site for transection of the sigmoid is selected that will make it possible for the proximal stump to be brought out of the abdominal wall as a single-barreled stoma with neither tension nor redundancy. This site is usually somewhere in the

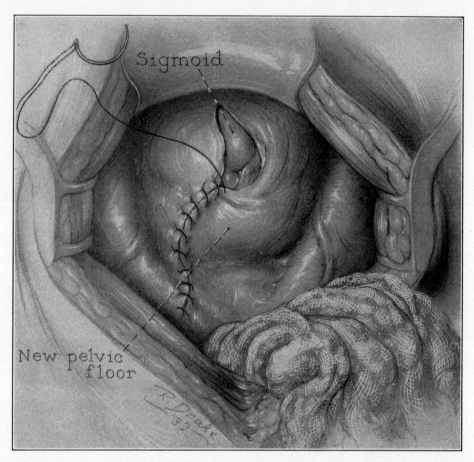

FIG. 342. A new pelvic floor is formed by suturing the peritoneum.

proximal portion of the sigmoid. The sigmoid is transected between Payr clamps. The distal stump is closed and inverted (Fig. 341). The sigmoid and rectum are placed in the hollow of the sacrum. The pelvic peritoneum is approximated, reforming the pelvic floor near the pelvic brim (Fig. 342). The proximal end of the sigmoid is brought out of a left McBurney incision as described under "First Stage," (Fig. 341). Five grams of sulfathiazole is inserted and the closure of the abdominal cavity is carried out in layers.

PREPARATION FOR THE PERINEAL PHASE. This stage of the operation is performed with the patient in the lithotomy position since it would be too time consuming and productive of shock to place the patient in the prone position. The change to the lithotomy position must be performed with dispatch, with each member of the surgical team schooled in the part he plays in dressing the abdominal wound, moving the patient and adjust-

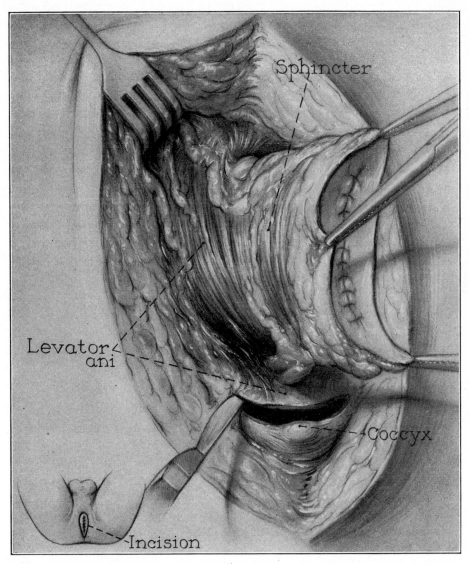

FIG. 343. Incision in skin and levator ani muscle.

ing the stirrups, placing the purse-string suture in the anus, preparing the field, draping, using fresh gowns and gloves, and setting up a new instrument table. The buttocks must be well over the edge of the table and the head of the table must be slanted downward to about 30 degrees. If the patient is male an indwelling urethral catheter should be in place and the scrotum should be drawn away from the field. If the patient is female the vagina should be prepared carefully.

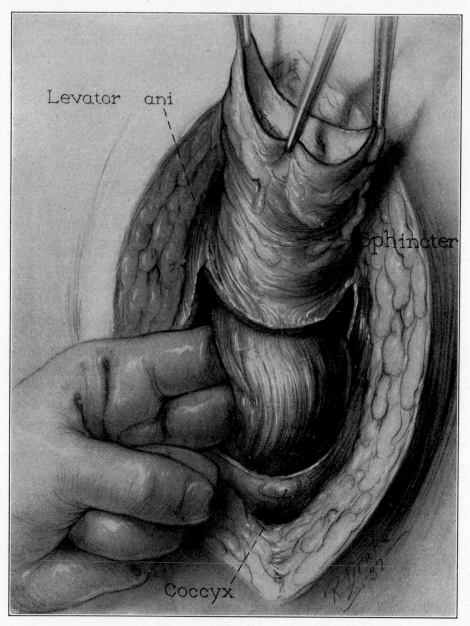

Fig. 344. The rectum and sigmoid are drawn out of the sacral hollow.

Intravenous administration of fluids may occasionally be necessary in this phase of the procedure, for the patient's blood pressure occasionally falls during the change of position. The surgeon must not be hurried for there is no reason in being very radical in the abdominal part of the operation and then coring the rectum out as a tube, missing the lateral spread in the levator ani muscles and perirectal tissues.

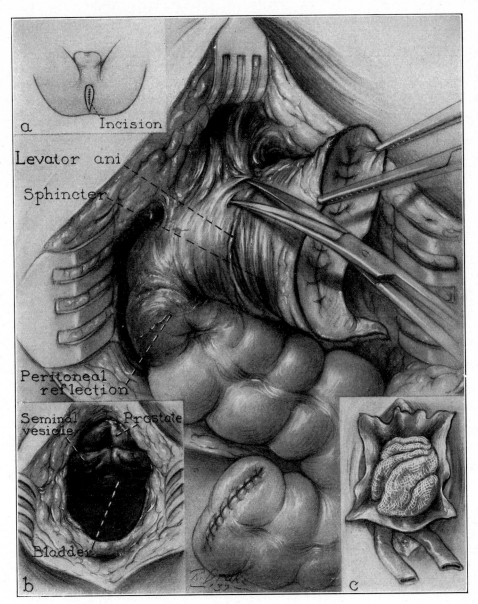

a. Incision

Levator ani

Sphincter

Peritoneal reflection

Seminal vesicle Prostate

Bladder

b

c

FIG. 345. The rectum is dissected away from the structures anterior to it. a. Incision in skin. b. Structures anterior to the rectum in the male. c. The pack has been inserted.

THE PERINEAL PHASE. An elliptic incision is made around the anus from the coccyx to the midpoint of the perineum (Fig. 343, inset). An effort is made to remove the structures as described under "The Posterior Route."

When the lesion is low the perianal skin and ischiorectal fat should be excised widely. The anococcygeal ligament is incised transversely and the coccygeus muscle is cut toward the sacrosciatic ligaments. The levators are incised near their origin (Fig. 343). After blunt dissection in the hollow of the sacrum the sigmoidal stump and the rectum are drawn out of the pelvis

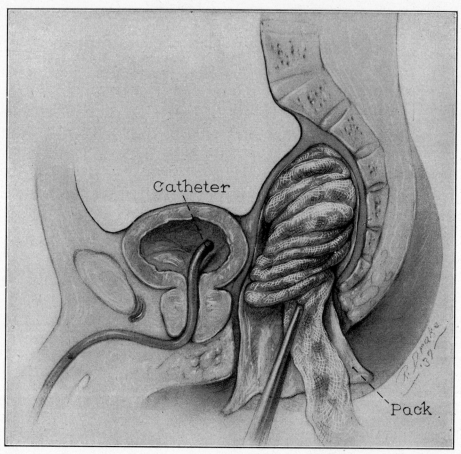

Catheter

Pack

Fig. 346. Side view of the pack in position.

(Fig. 344). If the abdominal mobilization of the rectum has been adequate, only part of the anterior attachments of the rectum remain to be separated. If the patient is male the dissection is carried along the posterior surface of the membranous urethra, prostate and seminal vesicles (Fig. 345). If the patient is female the rectum is dissected from the vagina. The rectum and sigmoid are then removed. Since the peritoneum has been closed abdominally the procedure is completed by verifying that hemostasis has been obtained, inserting 5 gm. of sulfathiazole, packing the cavity with gauze lined with pliofilm (Figs. 345c and 346) and partially closing the cutaneous edges.

The care and precautions are the same as those described under posterior resection. The colonic stoma should be opened twenty-four hours after operation. If the patient is anemic transfusion of blood may be necessary during or after the procedure. The survival rates in cases in which the

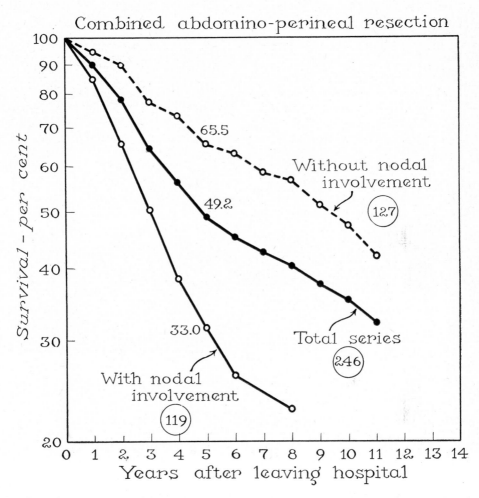

FIG. 347. Survival rates after combined abdominoperineal resection, showing the poorer progress when there is nodal involvement than when the nodes are not involved.

combined abdominoperineal procedure was applied are given in figures 347 and 348.

Exteriorization Operations with Extraperitoneal or Intraperitoneal Resection.[15] If the patient is of suitable body build it may be possible to resect lesions as low as 14 to 18 cm. from the dentate line by a modified Paul-Mikulicz procedure. To deliver the lesion into the incision when it is so low one must free the rectum down to the levator ani muscles as described under "The Anterior Route." A tube is passed through the mesentery and

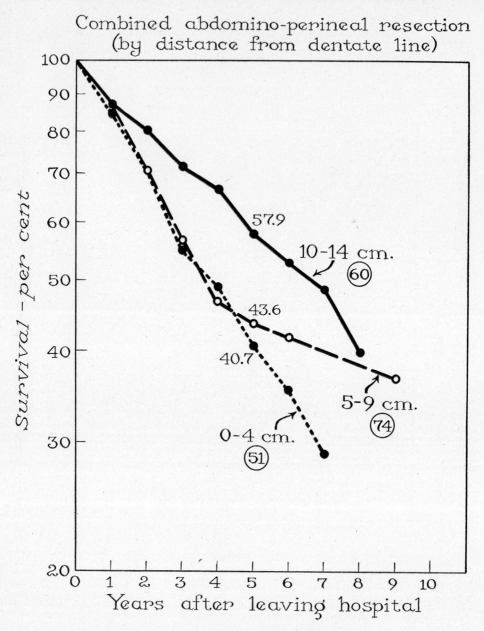

Combined abdomino-perineal resection (by distance from dentate line)

Survival - per cent (vertical axis)

57.9

10-14 cm. ⓐ60

43.6

40.7

5-9 cm. ⓐ74

0-4 cm. ⓐ51

Years after leaving hospital (horizontal axis)

FIG. 348. Survival rates for combined abdominoperineal resection of lesions below the pelvic peritoneal reflection. Poorer prognosis is revealed for cases in which the lesions are near the dentate line than for those in which the lesions are farther from the dentate line.

after the two loops are sutured together the peritonium and fascia are closed about the protruding loop (Fig. 349). Iodoform gauze is packed around the loop, keeping the skin open. This permits resection of the lesion down to the fascia seven to ten days later. Thus an extra 2 to 3 cm.

of mesentery and distal loop can be resected. At this time a large clamp is placed on the spur and the skin is partially closed around the clamp (Fig. 350). The resulting fistula may be given a trial at spontaneous closure.

The obvious criticism of this procedure is that the lymphatic drainage along the inferior mesenteric vessels is not resected. The survival rate after applying the foregoing modified Mikulicz procedure is given in figure 351.

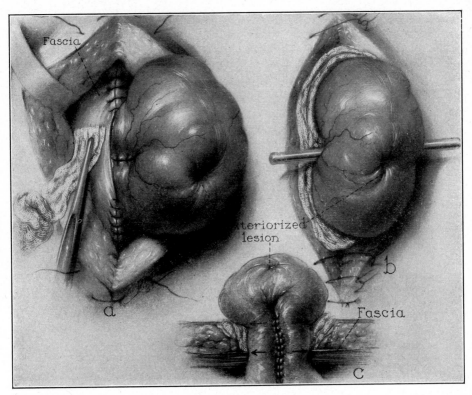

FIG. 349. Modified Mikulicz resection showing how the skin is kept out of the field by packing, making it possible to remove sigmoid down to the fascia.

Better results are obtained from the exteriorization procedure in which an intraperitoneal resection is performed and a wedge of adjacent mesentery is excised, but it rarely can be applied to lesions less than 14 to 18 cm. from the dentate line. The segment of bowel is resected between clamps and the mesenteric defect is closed. The two limbs of the segment are studied with reference to blood supply. If this is adequate they are included in a three-bladed clamp. Five grams of sulfathiazole is scattered in the peritoneal cavity and the abdominal wall is closed around the emerging limbs of the segment. In twenty-four hours the proximal limb is opened by cautery puncture beneath the proximal blade of the clamp. The clamp is removed in seven days. The spur may be clamped immediately or in two to three weeks and the colonic stoma may be closed, see "Closure of the Colonic Stoma," as soon

as induration has subsided. The survival rate after application of this exteriorization operation is given in figure 351.

**Abdominoperineal Proctosigmoidectomy with Preservation of the
External Sphincter** [3,16] (**The Pull-through or Hochenegg's Operation**).
ABDOMINAL PHASE. The mobilization of the colon is described under "The
Anterior Route," with liberation of the rectum as far as the levator ani
muscle. In selecting the site of ligation of the superior hemorrhoidal or in-

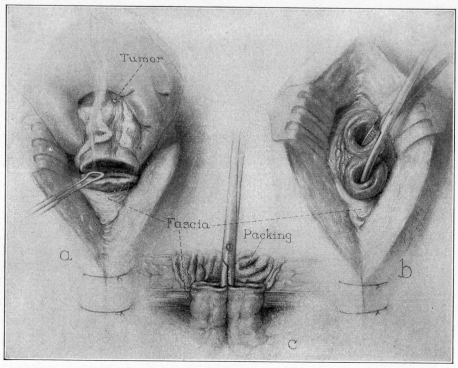

FIG. 350. a. Excision of the sigmoidal loop down to the fascia. b. and c. Application
of a clamp to crush the spur.

ferior mesenteric vessels and the point of the sigmoid that is to pass through
the external sphincter the same precautions are observed as described under
the anterior resection operation. There is this difference, however. The
point selected on the sigmoid must reach about 10 cm. farther than in the
anterior resection operation. After the superior hemorrhoidal vessels have
been ligated and the segment of mesosigmoid has been resected with preservation of the marginal vessel, the lowest point on the sigmoid in which
good arterial pulsations are seen is marked by a suture. The peritoneal floor
is reconstructed high on the sigmoid and 5 gm. of sulfathiazole is scattered
in the peritoneal cavity. While temporary transverse colostomy performed
at this point is not advocated by a majority of surgeons, it will insure better
healing of the perineal wound and we believe will give better sphincteral
control. The abdomen is closed in layers.

THE PERINEAL PHASE. The remarks made about changing to the extreme lithotomy position in the abdominoperineal resection are applicable here. Because dissection is carried between the external and internal sphincter in this operation, the purse-string suture closing the rectum should be placed just inside the dentate line. Again this suture is left long as a tractor. Incision is made from the coccyx to the perineal body encircling the rectum just at the dentate line. The external sphincter is dissected away from the rectum

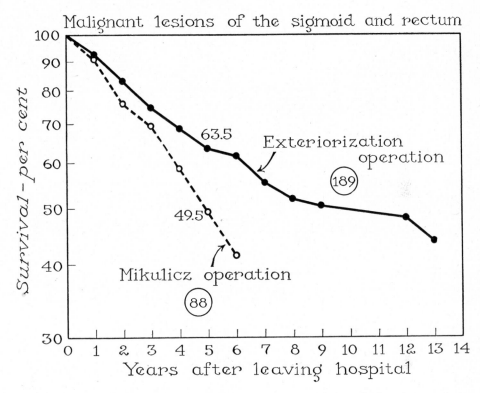

FIG. 351. Survival rates after the modified Mikulicz procedure and after the exteriorization procedure with intraperitoneal resection.

and split posteriorly. The anococcygeal ligament is incised, the fascia propria of the rectum is separated from the sacral hollow and the dissection is continued until one arrives at the point prepared from above.

While traction is exerted on the purse-string suture, the external sphincter is dissected back and retracted. This brings the insertion of the levator ani on the rectum into view (Fig. 352a) so that it can be incised around the rectum. Elevation of the external sphincter and transversi perinei muscles permits separation of the anterior attachments of the rectum. By sharp dissection the rectum is separated from the prostate and seminal vesicles in the male and the vagina in the female. The dissection is completed and the rectum and sigmoid are delivered through the posterior incision (Fig.

352b). The marked point of viability should extend at least 6 cm. beyond the cutaneous edges; otherwise retraction may produce a sacral fistula.

Five grams of sulfathiazole and a Penrose cigaret drain are placed in the sacral hollow. The levator ani muscles are approximated and the pelvic

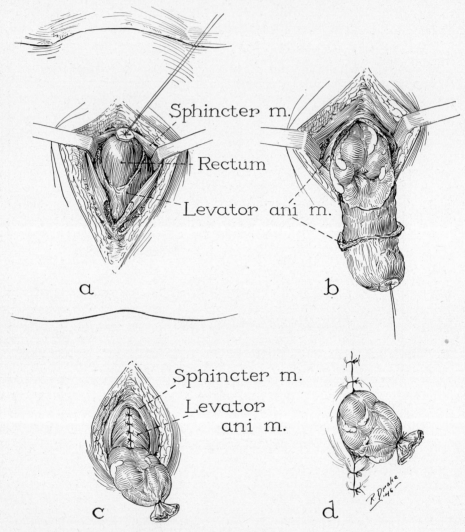

FIG. 352. The perineal phase of abdominoperineal proctosigmoidectomy with preservation of the external sphincter muscle.

diaphragm is reconstructed (Fig. 352c). Some surgeons bring the ends of the sphincter together at this time while others close the ends in ten days. The skin is closed with the drain emerging in the region of the coccyx. Clamps are placed across the sigmoid about 6 cm. from the incision. The lower part of the sigmoid and the rectum are resected (Fig. 352d). After three days the drain is removed and an opening is made in the sigmoid proximal to the clamp. On the tenth day part of the redundant sigmoid is resected leaving about 2 cm. protruding to insure against stricture. The patient is instructed in voluntary exercises to train sphincteric control. Survival rates following this procedure are given in figure 353.

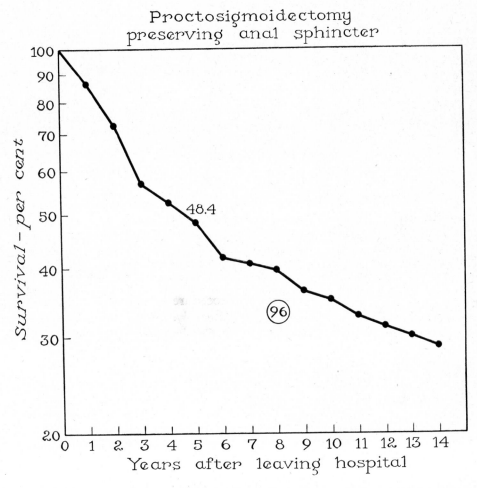

FIG. 353. Survival rates after proctosigmoidectomy in ninety-six cases.

Posterior Proctectomy and Local Excision.[16] These procedures are not radical resections for cancer but situations arise in which a compromise procedure may occasionally be performed. For example, blind or otherwise debilitated persons do not master a colonic stoma well. Furthermore these procedures are applicable to the removal of benign lesions or certain strictures. Some small lesions of low-grade malignancy situated on the posterior wall below the pelvic peritoneal field may be treated by fulguration.

It is frequently advantageous to precede the operation by temporary sigmoidal colostomy. This permits inspection of the liver, peritoneal cavity

and mesosigmoid. If the sigmoid is mobilized in this procedure it may provide more free sigmoid to anastomose to the rectum.

With the patient in the prone position, incision is made from the coccyx
to the posterior margin of the anus. The incision is carried through the
levator ani muscle, avoiding injury to the sphincter muscles. The coccyx is
excised and the fascia propria of the rectum is separated from the hollow
of the sacrum as far as the promontory. The middle hemorrhoidal stalks
are ligated if necessary. When the rectum is retracted to one side, the anterior attachments are divided. When the peritoneum of the pouch of
Douglas is reached it is incised and the incision is continued around the
rectum. The sigmoid is then mobilized sufficiently to allow an end-to-end
anastomosis after resection of the lesion. The superior hemorrhoidal
vessels above and the rectal stalks below the lesion are then ligated. Rubber
covered curved clamps are placed above and below the lesion. The upper
clamp should be placed so that when the anastomosis is made the upper end
is given a quarter turn. The sigmoid and rectum harboring the lesion are
resected. The opening in the peritoneum is closed and end-to-end anastomosis is performed, thus reestablishing continuity of the bowel (Fig. 354).
Five grams of sulfathiazole is scattered over the anastomosis, a Penrose
cigaret drain is inserted, the levator ani is sutured and the skin is closed,
the drain being brought out at the posterior angle. If there has not been
a temporary colostomy a large rectal tube should be inserted beyond the
anastomosis.

The recurrence rate following this procedure is high. Fistula along the
drain site is frequent but it heals spontaneously.

Local Operations for Squamous Cell Carcinoma of the Anus. Results
following radical excision of squamous cell carcinoma of the anus are
poor. The incidence of these carcinomas is less than 2 per cent of all malignant lesions of the sigmoid, rectum and anus. The patient usually is advanced in years and the lesion is of high grade. Such lesions are most often
seen after spread to the inguinal lymph nodes so that only local application
of radium with roentgen therapy to the regions of lymphatic drainage is
advisable. If the lesion is of low grade, some surgeons perform an excision
by means of cautery, removing part of the sphincter. This is followed by
radium and roentgen therapy. Radical dissection of the inguinal nodes may
be carried out mainly with the idea of preventing their "breaking down."

Surgical Treatment of Polypi of the Sigmoid and Rectum. While not
all adenomatous polypi become malignant, the incidence is so high that
they must be treated accordingly. It appears that a large number of the carcinomas of this region begin as polypi. While they are still polypi they can
be fulgurated through a proctoscope, but the region should be checked at
frequent intervals. If the polypus is above the pelvic peritoneal fold and
the pedicle is distinct it may be fulgurated. Otherwise transsigmoidal excision may be indicated so that the sigmoidal wall can be examined for
stippling, dimpling or induration. Low-grade sessile lesions are sometimes
resected locally as described in the previous section, or the sphincter may

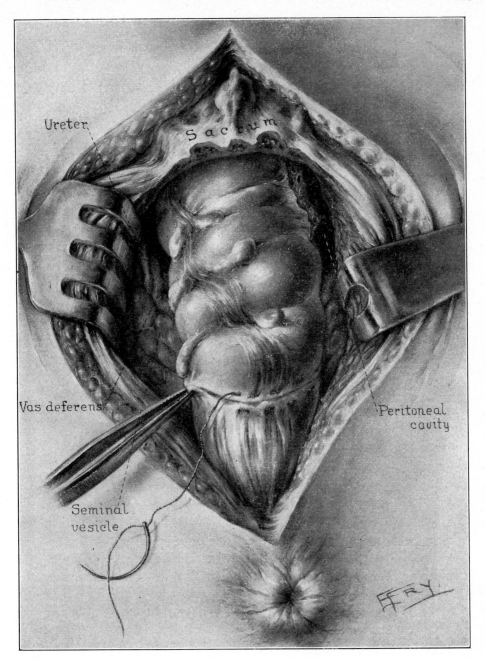

FIG. 354. End-to-end anastomosis after posterior proctectomy.

be split and the lesion and its surrounding tissue may be removed by cautery excision under direct vision. The incision is left open by some surgeons while others reconstruct the sphincters, inverting the rectal mucosa. Again the region of excision must be examined at frequent intervals.

In polyposis of the diffuse familial variety an attempt is made to prevent permanent ileostomy. If the polypi in the rectum have not undergone ulcerative malignant degeneration an exclusion type of ileosigmoidostomy is established through a low right or left rectus incision. The second stage consists of subtotal colectomy which the senior author carries out through a long diagonal abdominal incision extending from the right midcostal margin to the left superior iliac crest. The colon is divided immediately proximal to the ileosigmoidostomy. The remaining end is inverted. Finally, about three weeks after colectomy the polypi of the remaining bowel are fulgurated through a proctoscope. Frequent "check-ups" of the rectum and sigmoid should be made. Fulguration of polypi of the lower bowel seems unwise as an initial procedure because it has been observed in such cases that ileosigmoidostomy following fulguration produces a thickened and somewhat narrowed sigmoid which for many weeks is unsuitable for anastomosis.

SURGICAL TREATMENT OF BENIGN NEOPLASMS AND INFLAMMATORY LESIONS OF THE RECTUM, LOWER PART OF THE SIGMOID AND PRESACRAL SPACE

The relative infrequency of these lesions as compared to malignant lesions of the sigmoid and rectum makes it necessary for the surgeon to be vigilant so that the rectum is not unnecessarily sacrificed.

Adenomyoma or Endometrioma. Heterotopic endometrial tissue in the colon of women may be found incidentally at operation or may produce hemorrhage or partial obstruction. Frequently removal or inactivation of the ovarian tissue will cause regression of the lesion. Occasionally local excision or anterior resection is necessary.

Hemangioma. This rare lesion produces rectal hemorrhage. It may coexist with hemangiomas elsewhere. Low lesions may be treated by radium. It is occasionally necessary to remove them by local excision or transcolonically.

Myoma and Lipoma. These tumors are removed by local excision.

Presacral Tumors. Dermoid cysts, teratomas and chordomas occur in the presacral region. Roentgenograms of the pelvis must be taken to see if spina bifida is present, if the sacrum is involved or if teeth are present. If the lesion feels anything like a pelvic kidney, excretory urograms should be made.

The approach is the same as for local excision of the rectum with the patient in the prone position. Incision is made from the coccyx to the posterior margin of the anus and the coccyx is removed. Excision of the tumor occasionally requires introduction of a finger into the rectum to avoid injury to its wall. Excision of part of the sacrum is necessary sometimes. Five grams of sulfathiazole is inserted in the cavity. If bleeding is not controlled a pack or oxidized cellulose may be inserted; otherwise a Penrose cigaret drain is left in the wound. Levator ani muscle and the skin are approximated by suture. After three days the drain is removed and irrigation of the space is carried out. If there is evidence of malignancy in the tumor or invasion of adjacent structures roentgen therapy should be instituted. Perforation or invasion of the rectal wall necessitates segmental or local excision of the rectum either by anterior resection or by local excision via the posterior route, depending on the level of the involvement.

Lipomas of the ischiorectal space are excised through a perineal incision over the mass.

Benign Stricture of the Rectum and Sigmoid. Strictures present difficult problems in therapy and the cause of the stricture must be borne in mind. Gentle, gradual dilatation should always be tried. If dilatation is too vigorous, friable granulomatous tissue may split, causing perirectal sup-

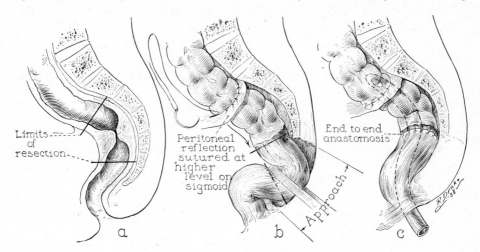

FIG. 355. Resection of region of stricture by posterior proctectomy. (From Pemberton and Stalker, *Surgery*, 4:81-83, [July], 1938.)

puration or even peritonitis. When an increase in lumen is obtained it must be maintained by continual dilatation for a long period. If these methods fail, low strictures or narrow diaphragms may be incised vertically and the increased lumen may be maintained by repeated passage of bougies. Granulomatous tubular strictures such as occur after venereal lymphogranuloma or injection of petroleum oils in the perirectal space may simulate carcinoma. It is occasionally necessary to perform operations similar to those for carcinoma, such as anterior resection, posterior proctectomy (Fig. 355) or colostomy to permit emptying of the colon. Every effort must be made to preserve sphincteral function. When stricture follows multiple anal operations, plastic procedures must be performed to reestablish normal mucocutaneous relationships. Rectal stricture caused by venereal lymphogranuloma rarely requires resection of the rectum. Posterior resection in such cases is usually extremely difficult because of lack of planes of cleavage.

Diverticulitis. Diverticulitis of the rectum is rare in the experience of the senior author but it does occur, causing severe pain, tenesmus and occasionally ischiorectal abscess. The treatment consists of temporary colostomy (loop type). As a rule the stoma should not be closed for one to two years. During the interim warm saline irrigations or diathermy causes a subsidence of the inflammatory process and eventually permits closure of the colonic stoma.

The surgical treatment of diverticulitis is quite similar to that of carcinoma of the same segment. While one may suppose that it is not necessary to remove as much mesentery as in surgical treatment of carcinoma, frequently induration and thickening in the mesentery are so severe that the mesenteric resection is almost as extensive as in removal of carcinoma. If there is acute inflammation proximal colostomy is about all that can be done.

Perforation of diverticulitis of the sigmoid into the bladder makes surgical intervention imperative. A loop transverse colostomy is performed through an upper midline incision to put the distal portion of the colon to rest for a month or two. Sulfasuxidine paste should be instilled into the distal loop of the colostomy daily to aid in treatment of the pyuria. The region of diverticulitis in the sigmoid must be resected because a sigmoidovesical fistula rarely if ever heals. The resection is performed according to the technic given under anterior resection. Small openings in the vesical wall can be closed by suture if they are not surrounded by brawny tissue, and one can depend on urethral catheter drainage. However, if a section of the vesical wall is removed the opening is closed by two rows of inverting sutures and a large suprapubic cystostomy tube is brought through the anterior wall of the bladder through the space of Retzius, emerging from the lower angle of the incision. The suprapubic tube may be removed in about eighteen days, and the drainage of urine will cease within a day or two. After the anastomosis in the sigmoid heals, the colonic stoma may be closed as described previously.

SURGICAL TREATMENT OF ABSCESS AND FISTULA OF THE ANORECTAL REGION

Postoperative care plays such an important role in obtaining successful results after proctologic operations that the reader is advised to consult a text devoted exclusively to that field of surgery.

Ischiorectal Abscess. In cases of early cellulitis sulfadiazine is administered by mouth and warm moist compresses are applied to the perineum. As soon as an abscess is defined, crescentic incision concentric with the anus is made over the fluctuant area. The external sphincter must be avoided. Pockets are opened by gentle digital exploration. In the presence of extension of the abscess above the levator ani muscle the finger is introduced into the rectum to guide a blunt curved forceps into the pelvirectal space. Five grams of sulfathiazole is inserted into the cavity and it is packed lightly with gauze. The pack is removed in twenty-four hours and another is inserted. Then sitz baths and irrigations are instituted.

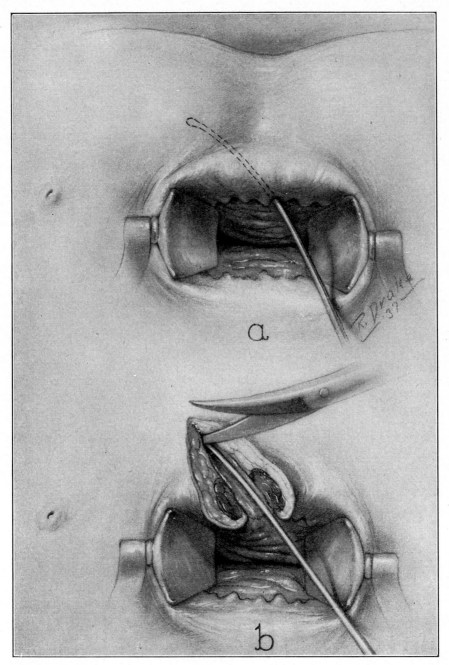

FIG. 356. Unroofing of a simple fistula in ano (Buie). (From Buie, L. A., *Practical Proctology,* Courtesy of W. B. Saunders Company, Philadelphia, 1937.)

Fistula in Ano.[2] If acute inflammation is present operation is deferred and warm moist compresses are applied. In the presence of complicated fistulas, advantage is gained by the preoperative oral administration of sulfa-suxidine. The presence of ulcerative colitis or regional enteritis must be ruled out, for any degree of activity of these diseases will prevent healing.

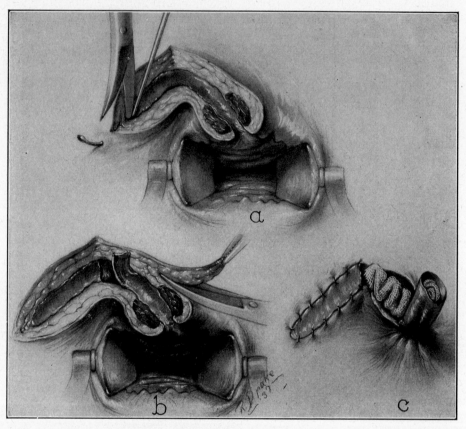

FIG. 357. The further reaches of the tract are unroofed. Part of the wall of the tract may be sutured to the skin as shown in c (Buie). (From Buie, L. A., *Practical Proctology*, Courtesy of W. B. Saunders, Philadelphia, 1937.)

Tuberculous fistulas of the anal region have become less common than formerly.

In the operative treatment the fistulous tracts are unroofed and allowed to granulate in from below. The operation is performed with the patient under spinal, sacral or caudal anesthesia and in the prone position. If anesthesia does not give sufficient relaxation the anus is gently dilated to permit location of primary anal openings, which are frequently found in infected crypts of the posterior quadrant (Fig. 356a). The tortuous secondary tracts are explored by probing and the skin roofing the tract is incised segment by segment (Fig. 356b). The external sphincter muscle is cut over a probe passing through the primary opening in the anal canal. Success is dependent on postoperative measures which insure granulation from below. When the lumen of the fistula is large Buie [17] advocates the use of the unroofed wall of the tract with suture of its lining to the skin (Fig. 357). It is unnecessary to dissect out and resect the entire wall of the tract.

Recto-urethral Fistula. Repair is difficult and success in initial operations is limited. Wide and free mobilization of the structures is essential. It is wise to prepare the patient with oral administration of sulfasuxidine. The operation is performed with the patient under low spinal or general anesthesia and the patient is placed in the prone position with an indwelling urethral catheter in place. Incision is made in the perineum, and the anterior wall of the rectum is dissected free from the urethra and the prostate. When a previous attempt at repair has been made the dissection is extremely difficult making preliminary suprapubic cystostomy advisable. The urethra must be partially mobilized and the opening must be closed transversely with fine sutures. The defect in the rectum is closed with two inverting rows of sutures. Such muscle fibers and connective tissue as are available laterally are sutured together in the midline to keep the structures apart. Hemostasis is secured and the skin is closed. If there is a large defect in the rectum it is wiser to dissect the rectal mucosa free, starting at the dentate line and mobilizing enough mucosa anteriorly so that the defect can be ignored, and normal mucosa can be sutured to the skin, forming a new dentate line.

Rectovesical Fistula. The treatment of fistulas due to diverticulitis has been discussed previously. When the fistula results from perforation of carcinoma of the rectosigmoid or trauma from previous operation or irradiation, anterior resection of the carcinoma with the attached portion of bladder, suprapubic cystostomy and transverse colostomy should be performed at the first operation, for defunctioning the distal portion of the colon does not reduce the difficulty of the resection. Experience has shown that after preliminary transverse colostomy there is little reduction of the inflammation in the bladder if the fistula is due to perforation of a carcinoma.

Rectovesical fistulas resulting from trauma, congenital defects or operative injury are often repaired by an abdominal approach to permit visualization of the ureters. The pouch of Douglas is incised, the bladder is separated from the rectum and all inflammatory tissue is removed. If the defects are small they may be closed by inverting the mucosal edges and reinforcing the closure by a second row of sutures. The blood supply to the rectum must be verified for it is occasionally impaired in the dissection and a segment of the intestine must be resected. The omentum should be interposed between the repaired surfaces. A large rectal tube should be inserted in the rectum and after the abdomen is closed a urethral catheter is inserted. In difficult procedures as previously mentioned suprapubic cystostomy is performed and gentle suction is applied for twelve to eighteen days after operation.

Fistulas Associated with Osteomyelitis. Fistulas following gunshot and shrapnel wounds, pelvic fractures and rupture of an abscess originating in bone are extremely indolent. Preliminary transverse colostomy should be

performed, followed by prolonged treatment with antibiotic and chemotherapeutic agents. Fistulous tracts passing through or along bone heal very
slowly. Even after six months of defunctioning of the distal portion of the
colon the tissues are the seat of brawny inflammation and the segment of
intestine involved must be resected to effect a cure.

SURGICAL TREATMENT OF OTHER ABNORMALITIES
OF THE RECTUM AND ANUS

Prolapse of the Rectum.[18,19] If the patient is an infant prolapse usually
responds to conservative treatment. The buttocks are kept strapped together
as much as possible.

Minor prolapse of the mucosa is occasionally treated by linear cauterization to produce retraction by scar tissue. More commonly the redundant
mucosa is amputated and the mucocutaneous juncture is reestablished.

With the patient in the lithotomy position, with the head of the table
depressed, the prolapsed portion of the rectum is drawn out as far as possible.
Transverse incision is made in the mucosa of the anterior portion of the
outer layer about 1 cm. from the dentate line, avoiding injury to the sphincter muscle. The incision is continued around the rectum, freeing the outer
tube so that the intussusception can be unfolded. If the peritoneum appears
on traction it should be incised all the way around to the vascular stalk.
It is resutured to the peritoneum covering the sigmoid as high as possible.
The inner tube is then amputated one quadrant at a time, its mucosa being
sutured to that at the dentate line before proceeding to the next quadrant.
At the posterior section the superior hemorrhoidal vessels must be ligated.
The mucosal suture line is then placed inside the sphincters and a rectal
tube is inserted.

When prolapse occurs in a patient whose prognosis is poor, and when the
surgeon can be sure that there is no small intestine in the prolapse, it is
occasionally possible to perform amputation by ligation over a grooved val-
canite cylinder. The cylinder is slipped inside the prolapse and a heavy silk
ligature is applied close to the dentate line. The ligature is made to lie in
the circular groove in the cylinder to prevent slipping. The bowel projecting
beyond the cylinder is cut off. The cylinder is usually expelled in four to
five days.

The great variety of procedures suggested for the treatment of prolapse
indicates that none has met with satisfaction in the hands of a majority of
surgeons. An abdominal procedure in which the rectum is mobilized extensively gives the best results. The trauma of dissection causes adhesion of
the rectum to the sacral hollow.

Pemberton and Stalker[19] have outlined this procedure in detail. The
lower part of the sigmoid and the rectum are mobilized (Figs. 358 and 359)
as described previously, freeing the rectum as low as the levator ani muscle.
The peritoneum of the pouch of Douglas is not incised. With the redundant
portion of the rectum drawn out of the pelvis, the peritoneum is resutured

behind it so that a peritoneal reflection is made on the posterior surface as low as possible (Fig. 360). The denuded posterior surface of the rectum is peritonized by suturing the lateral edges of the peritoneum to the new pos-

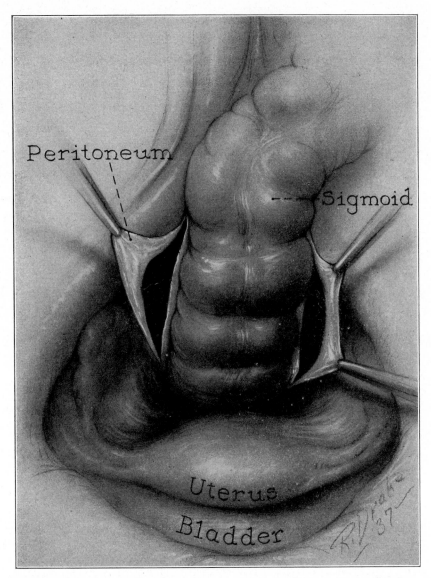

FIG. 358. Mobilization of the sigmoid and rectum. (From Pemberton and Stalker, *Ann. Surg.*, 109:799-808, [May], 1939.)

terior parietal peritoneum (Fig. 361). The pouch of Douglas may be obliterated by suturing the peritoneum of the posterior surface of the uterus or bladder to the peritoneum covering the rectosigmoid (Fig. 362).

Since relaxation of the sphincters frequently accompanies prolapse, plastic reefing of the external sphincter muscle is sometimes indicated.

Hemorrhoids.[17] The surgeon's work has only begun when the procedure in the operating room is finished, for good results are obtained only after

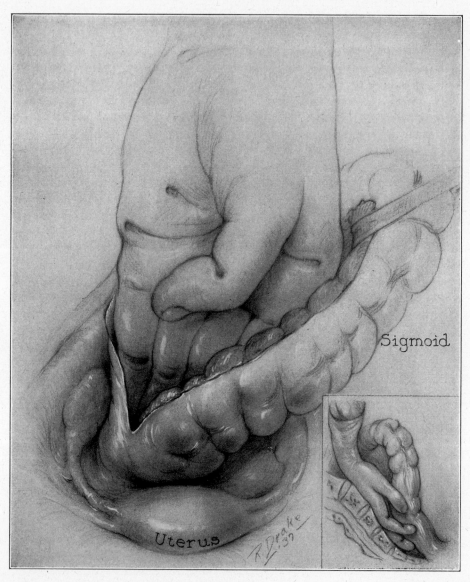

FIG. 359. The rectum is freed from the hollow of the sacrum. (From Pemberton and Stalker, *Ann. Surg.*, 109:799-808, [May], 1939.)

painstaking postoperative care. When edema or infection is present in or about the hemorrhoids, operation should be deferred until it has been reduced by witch hazel packs.

EXCISION OF EXTERNAL HEMORRHOIDS. The skin over the hemorrhoid is excised with the hemorrhoidal tissue attached to it. It is occasionally necessary to clamp and tie the pedicle. Thrombotic masses are enucleated. The skin is left open.

EXCISION OF INTERNAL HEMORRHOIDS (Buie). The operation is performed with the patient in the prone position with the hips elevated. The anesthesia usually gives enough relaxation of the sphincter to enable the surgeon to

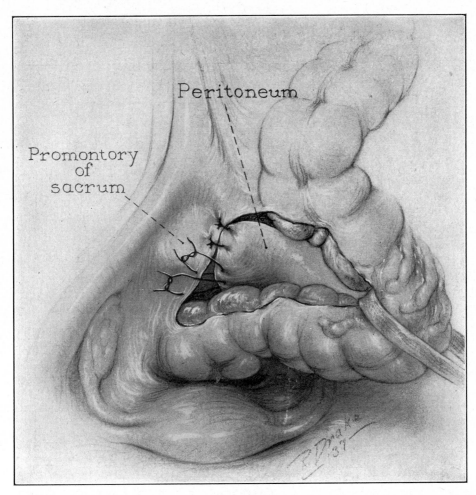

FIG. 360. A new posterior parietal peritoneum is created.

perform the procedure. A strip of gauze is packed into the rectum and it is pulled out slowly to prolapse the hemorrhoids. The most prominent mass is grasped with a clamp (Fig. 363a). If coexistent external hemorrhoids are present a V-shaped segment of skin is excised (Fig. 363b); otherwise incision is made at the dentate line and the varicosities are dissected free from the external sphincter (Fig. 363c). A clamp is then placed across the base of the hemorrhoid in the longitudinal axis of the rectum (Fig. 363d). The hemorrhoid is excised and the clamp is replaced by a transfixion ligature (Fig. 363e). The end of this ligature is used to suture the stump to the distal edge of the external sphincter (Fig. 363f). A few stitches are similarly placed attaching the mucosa to the external sphincter but the cutaneous edges are left open for drainage (Fig. 363g). A Penrose drain is inserted in the rectum and

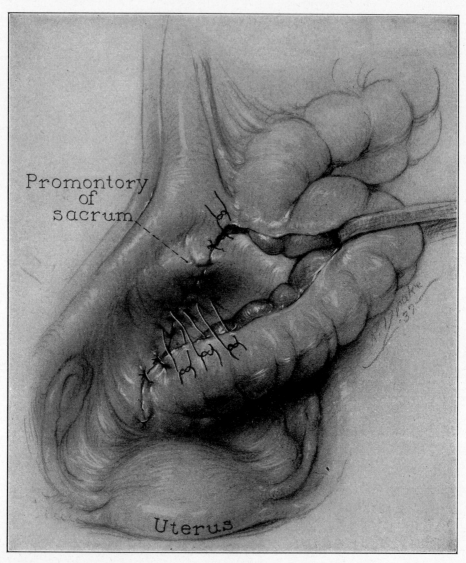

Fig. 361. The sigmoid is then sutured to the new peritoneal bed. (From Pemberton and Stalker, *Ann. Surg.*, 109:799-808, [May], 1939.)

petrolatum gauze is smoothed over the open areas. When the hemorrhoids have previously been treated by injection the dissection may be extremely difficult.

COMBINED INTERNAL AND EXTERNAL HEMORRHOIDS ASSOCIATED WITH PROLAPSE. In this situation Buie advocates an amputative and plastic procedure. Incision is made at the dentate line along one half the circumference together with excision of a wedge-shaped segment of skin which permits removal of the external hemorrhoids of that side. After hemorrhoidal tissue

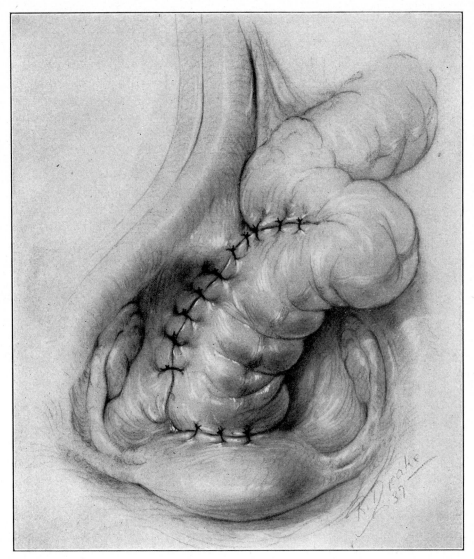

FIG. 362. The pouch of Douglas is obliterated. (From Pemberton and Stalker, *Ann. Surg.*, 109:799-808, [May], 1939.)

and mucosa have been dissected away from the external sphincter on that side, a crushing clamp is placed circumferentially above the bases of all the varicosities on that side. The hemorrhoidal tissue is then excised and the clamp is removed. Each bleeding point is clamped and ligated. The muco-cutaneous relations are reestablished by a Lembert suture which catches the

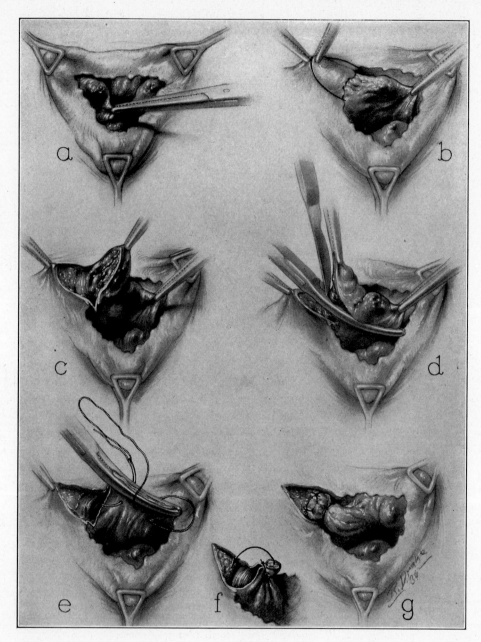

FIG. 363. Excision of internal hemorrhoids. For further explanation see text (Buie). (From Buie, L. A., *Practical Proctology*, Courtesy of W. B. Saunders Company, Philadelphia, 1937.)

mucosa, picks up a small bite of the inner surface of the external sphincter and causes the cutaneous edge to overlap the mucosa, thus preventing eversion of mucosa. Where the wedge-shaped region of skin was excised the mucosa is merely stitched to the external sphincter, leaving lateral sulci for drainage. The procedure is then repeated on the other side. A Penrose drain is inserted in the rectum and the external wound is covered with petrolatum gauze.

When the history suggests the presence of ulcerative colitis or regional enteritis, activity of these diseases should be ruled out before any operation on the rectum or anus not of pressing necessity is performed.

Fissure in Ano.[17] If the anesthesia does not relax the sphincter sufficiently it is gently dilated. Vertical incision is made through the center of the ulcer down to the external sphincter and out on the perianal skin (Fig. 364a). All ulcerated, indurated or fibrosed tissue is excised (Fig. 364b and c). This usually involves excision of a bit of the external sphincter muscle. Hypertrophied papillae or infected crypts are excised. Hemostasis is secured and the edge of the mucosa is sutured to the inner edge of the external sphincter (Fig. 364d).

Anal Incontinence. Gratifying results are obtained when third degree obstetric lacerations are repaired immediately after they occur. Delayed repair is attended with less success. Relative continence can be secured if all scar tissue between the muscle ends is excised and the muscular structures of the perineum are approximated anatomically. The colon should be prepared with sulfasuxidine as described previously.

The patient is placed in the lithotomy position. It will usually be found that dimples mark the point of retraction of the sphincter muscle. An H-shaped incision is made with the bar through the membrane separating the rectum and the vagina. The rectum and the vagina are separated until the plane between them is clearly demarcated. The retracted ends of the sphincter are grasped by forceps and all scar tissue is dissected away until good muscle tissue is obtained. The anterior rectal wall is then closed with two rows of interrupted sutures which invert the edge into the rectum. Successful repair of the sphincter is dependent on clear understanding of the normal anatomic relations of the anal musculature. The normal anal canal does not close like a purse string. In the resting state it is a vertical slit with the tone of the muscle pulling on the anococcygeal ligament and the perineal body. Closing the ends of the sphincter is not sufficient; a perineal body must be provided from which it can draw taut. The levator ani muscle and the transversi perinei muscles must be approximated in the midline to provide a point for the attachment of the united ends of the sphincter. Tension on the sutures must be applied exactly to prevent cutting or compromise of circulation. Perineorrhaphy is then performed in the usual manner, the vaginal mucosa and skin being sutured with a subcuticular suture. Intestinal movement should be delayed for a week. Painstaking perineal care is essential postoperatively.

In the treatment of anal incontinence following multiple operations for anal fistulas or abscesses, Buie stresses the importance of eradicating all residual fistulas, sinuses and abscesses. Prolapsed mucosa, hemorrhoids or hypertrophied papillae which impede anal closure must be removed. All scar tissue must be excised to permit approximation of the freshened ends of the muscle by a type of scar tissue that permits function. Attachments of the muscles of the perineal body must be reestablished. Just as in the treatment of fistula in ano, all sinus tracts must be unroofed and left open to permit granulation from below.

Pilonidal Cysts and Sinuses. If active inflammation is present excision must be deferred. Operation is performed with the patient under low spinal or caudal anesthesia and in the prone position.

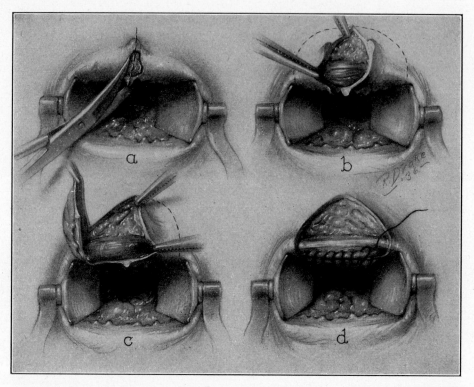

Fig. 364. The excision of the fissure in ano. For further explanation see text (Buie). (From Buie, L. A., *Practical Proctology*, Courtesy W. B. Saunders Company, Philadelphia, 1937.)

The sinus tracts are probed and an elliptic incision is made with a cautery around the widest ramifications. The incision is carried down to the fascia covering the sacrum and coccyx, and the bloc of tissue is removed en masse. Occasionally it is necessary to dissect out a tract under the coccyx.

There is wide divergence of opinion about the feasibility of primary closure. No doubt when the tract is short and narrow and it never was the site of inflammation, primary closure will be attended with reasonable success. Mobilization of flaps and undermining of the cutaneous edges to permit closure will invite persistent drainage. Open packing of the wound with gauze impregnated with sulfathiazole gives the most uniformly good results but the convalescence is prolonged. It is the procedure of choice when the sinuses have been the seat of recurrent abscesses. In a modified method of partial closure the cutaneous edges are sutured to the fascia over the sacrum by interrupted mattress sutures, bringing the cutaneous edges close together but not touching. Undercutting and tension must be avoided. Buie frequently employs a marsupialization method in which the sinuses are carefully unroofed and the wall of the tract is used in the closure. The cutaneous edges are trimmed back sufficiently to allow suture of the unrolled wall of the tract to the skin.

Imperforate Anus. The time of performance and the procedure are dictated by the distance between the blind end of the rectum and the perineum, and the presence of external openings into the urethra, bladder, vagina or perineum. In the absence of an external opening or in the presence of a rectovesical fistula, operation should be performed without delay. In the absence of an external opening gas appears in the rectum in twelve hours and distention develops in twenty-four hours. The distal extent of the rectum may be determined by a lateral roentgenogram of the pelvis taken with the infant suspended by the ankles after a lead marker has been placed in the anal dimple.

If the rectum is more than 3 cm. from the anal dimple or if there is a rectovesical fistula, sigmoidal colostomy should be performed with the infant under local anesthesia supplemented by administration of pentobarbital sodium, or under anesthesia produced by administration of ether by the open-drop method. A left McBurney incision is made and the finger is slipped along the left parietal wall until the sigmoid is located. A loop is brought out of the wound and supported by a rubber tube passed through the mesentery. The abdomen is closed in layers around the emerging loop. The meconium is relatively sterile for eighteen hours and during that interval the colonic stoma can be opened immediately. A subsequent reconstructive operation is deferred until the child is five to eight years of age. At that time the rectum can be brought down to a perineal incision and an attempt can be made to establish a mucocutaneous juncture. Rectovesical fistula requires a combined abdominoperineal approach in which the rectum is first mobilized abdominally and the defects in the rectum and the bladder are closed. The procedure is difficult because the opening in the bladder is usually in the region of the trigone and the ureters are in jeopardy. Then through a perineal incision the rectal blind pouch is brought down, opened and sutured to the skin. The colonic stoma is closed when irrigations reveal complete healing.

When the rectum is within 3 cm. of the perineum the blind end can be approached from the perineum. Incision is made from the anal dimple toward the coccyx. Dissection is carried down the midline toward the rectal blind pouch. For identification this can be made to bulge by pressure on the abdomen. One must beware of injuring the urethra if the infant is male. When the rectum is found it is grasped with an Allis clamp and mobilized enough to bring it out of the incision. If possible, opening into the rectum is deferred to the last, for the flow of meconium obscures the field. The mucosa is sutured to the skin at the site of the anal dimple and the remainder of the incision is closed. Despite the fact that the sphincter is not usually identified, continence after these operations usually is good. The opening must be kept dilated at intervals. Otherwise subsequent plastic procedures will be necessary to prevent acquired megacolon.

When there is a fistula into the vagina or perineum it can be dilated so that the repair can be deferred until the infant is older. Repair of recto-urethral and rectovaginal fistula has been described previously. The repair of a cloaca requires multiple operations which are best deferred until the patient is past the age of eleven years.

Injuries to the Rectum. When impalement or projectile wounds cause suspicion of injury to the rectum the surgeon cannot afford to wait for signs of peritonitis or suppuration. Laparotomy gives opportunity for inspection of neighboring viscera when the laceration is above the pelvic peritoneal fold and for the performance of colostomy. Extensive injury requires anterior resection if the lacerations cannot be closed. Proximal colostomy is essential.

When the surgeon is certain that the injury is below the pelvic peritoneal fold he may use the posterior approach to examine the rectum. The laceration is closed or the segment of rectum is resected as indicated. Drains are inserted before the incision is closed. The patient's interest is usually best served if a proximal colonic stoma is established in addition. This will also permit exclusion of additional damage.

There always is danger of secondary hemorrhage in wounds of this region. Sulfonamides, antibiotic agents and antiserums must be used to full advantage, guarding against gas bacillus, tetanus and coliform bacterial infections, which take hold easily in traumatized perirectal tissues.

REFERENCES

1. GILCHRIST, R. K. and DAVID, V. C.   Lymphatic Spread of Carcinoma of the Rectum, *Tr. Am. S. A.*, 56:141-157, [May], 1938.
2. MILES, W. E.   The Pathology of the Spread of Cancer of the Rectum, and Its Bearing upon the Surgery of the Cancerous Rectum, *Surg., Gynec. & Obst.*, 52:350-359, [Feb.], 1931.
3. BACON, H. E.   Evolution of Sphincter Muscle Preservation and Re-establishment of Continuity in the Operative Treatment of Rectal and Sigmoidal Cancer, *Surg., Gynec. & Obst.*, 81:113-127, [Aug.], 1945.
4. WANGENSTEEN, O. H.   Primary Resection (closed anastomosis) of Rectal Ampulla for Malignancy with Preservation of Sphincteric Function; Together with a Further Account of Primary Resection of the Colon and Rectosigmoid and a Note on Excision of Hepatic Metastases, *Surg., Gynec. & Obst.*, 81:1-24, [July], 1945.
5. WAUGH, J. M. and CUSTER, M. D., JR.   Segmental Resection of Lesions Occurring in the Left Half of the Colon with Primary End-to-end Aseptic Anastomosis; Report Based on Fifty Cases, *Surg., Gynec. & Obst.*, 81:593-598, [Dec.], 1945.
6. DIXON, C. F.   Anterior Resection for Carcinoma Low in the Sigmoid and the Rectosigmoid, *Surgery*, 15:367-377, [Mar.], 1944.
7. COFFEY, R. C.   Cancer of Rectum and Rectosigmoid, *Am. J. Surg.*, 14:161-214, [Oct.], 1931.
8. JONES, D. F.   A Two-stage Combined Abdomino-sacral Operation for Carcinoma of the Rectum, *J.A.M.A.*, 65:757-762, [Aug. 28], 1915.

9. LAHEY, F. H. and CATTELL, R. B. Two Stage Abdominoperineal Resection of Rectum and Rectosigmoid for Carcinoma, *Am. J. Surg.*, 27:201-213, [Feb.], 1935.

10. LOCKHART-MUMMERY, J. P. Perineal Excision for Cancer of Rectum, *Surg., Gynec. & Obst.*, 67:655-660, [Nov.], 1938.

11. MAYO, W. J. The Radical Operation for the Relief of Cancer of the Rectum and Rectosigmoid, *Ann. Surg.*, 56:240-255, [Aug.], 1912.

12. JONES, T. E. Technique of Abdominoperineal Resection for Carcinoma of Rectum, *Am. J. Surg.*, 27:194-200, [Feb.], 1935.

13. MAYO, C. W. One Stage Combined Abdominoperineal Resection for Malignant Tumors of the Rectum, Rectosigmoid, and Lower Part of Sigmoid, *Surg., Gynec. & Obst.*, 76:649-654, [June], 1943.

14. MILES, W. E. *Cancer of the Rectum*, Harrison and Sons, Ltd., London, 1926, 72 pp.

15. PAUL, F. T. Personal Experiences in the Surgery of the Large Bowel, *Brit. M. J.*, 2:172-181, [July 27], 1912.

16. MAYO, C. H. Cancer of the Sigmoid and Rectum, *Surg., Gynec. & Obst.*, 3:236-241, [Aug.], 1906.

17. BUIE, L. A. *Practical Proctology*, W. B. Saunders Company, Philadelphia, 1937, 512 pp.

18. MAYO, C. W. Complete Rectal Prolapse: a Fascial Repair, *Tr. West. S. A.*, 1:164-169, [Dec.], 1937.

19. PEMBERTON, J. DE J. and STALKER, L. K. Surgical Treatment of Complete Rectal Prolapse, *Ann. Surg.*, 109:799-808, [May], 1939.

16

LYMPHATIC SYSTEM, SPLEEN, AND PORTAL HYPERTENSION

R. K. Gilchrist, M.D., W. H. Cole, M.D. and N. A. Womack, M.D.

THE LYMPHATIC SYSTEM

R. K. Gilchrist, M.D.

Anatomy. Lymphatic capillaries are found in all tissues which are supplied by vascular capillaries. They are thin walled and elastic and communicate freely with other lymphatic capillaries in their immediate neighborhood. They drain into lymph channels which have valves. The channels are elastic and tend to accompany blood vessels. The lymph channels may be several feet in length. They empty their contents into lymph nodes. Several channels may drain into one node. In most parts of the body a number of nodes in close proximity to each other receive lymph from channels draining contiguous structures. The nodes are the source of lymphocytes and of some phagocytes. They also act as filters for bacteria and foreign particles and cells. After the lymph has passed through the node, it enters a larger efferent lymph channel. The efferent lymph channels may empty into more centrally placed nodes, or they may drain directly into the thoracic duct. All lymph passes through at least one node before entering the thoracic duct. The thoracic duct is thick walled. It collects lymph from all of the body, with the exception of the right arm and neck which pour their lymph into the right lymph duct. These two vessels empty into the veins of the neck (Fig. 365).

Pathology. *Injuries* to the lymph vessels occur with every wound. Tears of the capillaries heal rapidly and without sequelae. Repeated injury in the absence of infection will not result in any permanent interference with lymph drainage.

Infections involving the lymphatic capillaries of the skin produce one form of reticular lymphangitis (erysipelas). It causes stasis and lymphedema. Stagnation of lymph increases the concentration of fibrinogen and proteins in the lymph. This results in a fibrosis. If this process is repeated, chronic lymphangiectasis and fibrosis occurs.

Infections of the long lymph vessels which drain into the lymph nodes (tubular lymphangitis) produce a red streak which extends from the point of injury, up the arm or leg, to the node draining the area. There is fever, pain, malaise, and leukocytosis. Chills are common. The onset is acute; the pulse rises. The infecting organism is usually a streptococcus. The inflammation produces exudation and the vessel is blocked by coagulated lymph, leukocytes, and cellular debris. A single episode of this sort leaves no after effects.

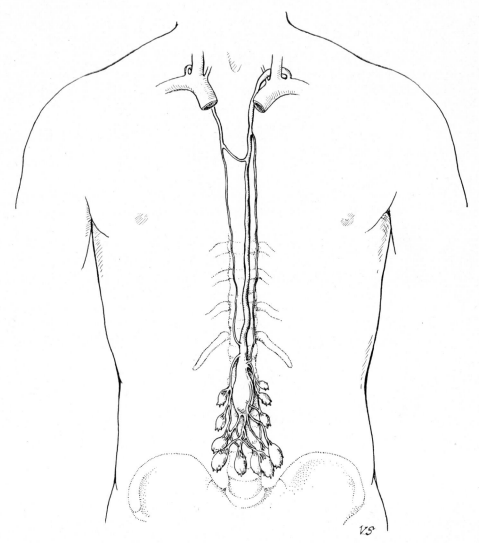

FIG. 365. Modified from Gray's Anatomy showing both the thoracic duct and the right lymphatic duct. The connection between the two is inconstant. (Redrawn from Gray's *Anatomy,* 33rd edition, Lea and Febiger, Philadelphia.)

Lymphadenitis causes pain, swelling and tenderness in the nodes draining an inflamed part. The swelling of the nodes is caused by edema and exudation as well as by the multiplication and infiltration of phagocytes and other leukocytes. If the part is put at rest and warm moist dressings are used, surgery is seldom indicated, the inflammation gradually subsiding leaving a somewhat enlarged firm node. When the infecting organism is more virulent, the defense of the node may be overwhelmed and suppuration may

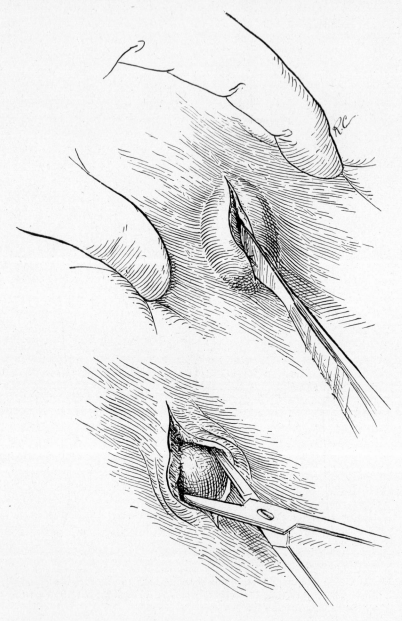

Fig. 366. Showing method of incision of the skin over suppurating lymph node and opening into the abscess in the node with a blunt forceps.

occur in the center of the node. In such cases, there is fever and much more pain and tenderness and edema of the soft parts surrounding the involved node. Redness of the skin over this area will appear and this usually indi-

cates that suppuration has developed. The more central area will be exquisitely tender. As soon as fluctuation can be demonstrated, such an area
should be incised along the flexion creases of the skin. The incision should
extend through the skin. Then a blunt forceps should be forced into the
abscess and the points spread. This will help prevent injury to adjacent
structures. A collapsible rubber drain should be inserted to keep the wound
open (Fig. 366).

Lymphangiectasis. If there is a chronic lymph stasis such as is seen following thrombophlebitis or following radical surgery for carcinoma, or after
infection with filaria, the limb is apt to be subject to repeated attacks of
reticular or tubular lymphangitis. This results in a marked fibrosis and
lymphangiectasis. The skin becomes thickened and soaked with lymph. The
protein content of the lymph increases to as much as 4 per cent (Drinker).
Fibrosis follows with increasing lymphatic blockade. Marked deformity follows producing elephantiasis. The same picture is seen in tropical elephantiasis where the original lymphatic obstruction is due to *Filaria bancrofti*
lodging in a lymph node. The first lymphangitic streak following invasion
by the filaria often progresses in a retrograde direction from the node harboring the worm. There is evidence to show that this early lymphangitis may
be due to an allergic reaction which follows the death of the worm (Hibbard).[1] This allergic reaction, when repeated, causes lymphatic obstruction,
with the same end result. The stage is set for infection to occur following
any trivial injury, and the massive deformity so often described eventually
results.

Treatment of Elephantiasis. In the earlier stages, elevation will allow
the lymph which collects in the tissue spaces to escape into normal areas
where it is removed. Dependency initiates the swelling again. Support will
correct many mild cases. Elevation and restricted activity will help. When
the enlargement and fibrosis progress, surgery is indicated. The Kondoleon [2] operation as modified by Sistrunk [3] and Ghormley [4] has given 50 to
80 per cent good results in various hands. In this operation wide areas of
subcutaneous tissue and fascia are excised in order to reduce the deformity
and to allow the lymph to be drained through the lymphatics of the muscles.
Pratt and Wright [5] have devised a modification of the Kondoleon operation
to augment lymphatic drainage into contiguous normal skin, thus short-
circuiting the obstructed lymphatics. The technic as utilized by them is
described as follows:

TABLE 6. *SURGICAL CLASSIFICATION OF LYMPHEDEMA* *

   I. Amenable to surgical treatment
      1. Modified Kondoleon procedure
         a. Idiopathic
            1. Praecox
            2. Congenital or familial (Milroys)

* Pratt and Wright, *Surg., Gynec. & Obst.*, 72(2):244, [Feb.], 1941. By permission of
Surgery, Gynecology and Obstetrics.

    b. Acquired
       1. Trauma (accidental or surgical)
       2. Filariasis bancrofti
       3. Occasionally the group secondary to venous pathology.
  2. Local surgical intervention
    a. Pressure—growth, etc.
    b. Traumatic or operative scars
    c. Most venous obstructions
    d. Local inflammation
    e. X-ray, radium and other burns
    f. Congenital lymph collections (Cystic hygroma, etc.)
II. Not Recommended for surgical treatment
  1. Mild idiopathic lymphedema
  2. Fungus infections
  3. Malignancies with invasion
  4. Allergic or systemic lymphedemas.

From the Surgical and Vascular Services of New York Post-Graduate Medical School and Hospital (Columbia University).

"This operation was performed on 12 patients and in a modified form on 6 others. They had surgical improvement in a high percentage of patients. Measurement of 6 extremities observed one and a half to three and a half years after the radical operation showed a maintained reduction in the circumference of the leg from a minimum of seven inches to a maximum of twenty-one inches.

"PREOPERATIVE PREPARATION. The leg is elevated a minimum of two weeks and diuretics, usually in the form of mercurials, are administered. The fungus infection, which as a rule accompanies this process, is controlled. Sulfonamides are prescribed prophylactically for several days prior to operation. If the pedicle graft is to be used, it is prepared during this time. Careful measurements of both limbs are recorded. For two days prior to operation a careful skin preparation, consisting of green soap and alcohol cleansing and the use of sterile drapes, is carried out.

"OPERATION. Under prolonged spinal anesthesia an elliptical incision is made in the lateral aspect of the thigh from the iliac crest to the femoral condyle. Below the knee this elliptical incision is continued posteriorly in the calf to its lower margin, when it again runs laterally to the external malleolus. This type of incision exposes the area of greatest lymph collection (Fig. 367). In selected instances the incision is modified to run entirely laterally. A sufficient ellipse is excised to allow the residual skin, when approximated, to equal the circumference of the normal limb. The skin alone then is undermined until three-fourths of the circumference of the leg has been exposed; this is done without transverse incisions, which would produce further scars. The incision is then carried through the superficial tissue and the deep fascia throughout three-fourths of the circumference of the leg; and a block of tissue, which includes the ellipse of skin and the three-fourths circumference of the superficial and deep fascia, is excised en masse (Fig. 368). Bleeding is controlled, the skin is then united with interrupted alloy steel wire, and directly approximated to the denuded muscle. The insert in figure 367 illustrates in cross section by the dotted lines, the tissue excised and remaining after the plastic closure. In one case they removed 100 per cent of the fascia, thus entirely encircling the leg. In the modified Kondoleon operation just described, the leg is covered without graft.

"In instances in which the skin becomes devitalized by constant over-stretching, it is necessary partially or completely to remove it. These areas are covered by broad based pedicle tube grafts as in Figs. 369, 370 and 371. The pedicle graft will drain the skin lymphatics and thus a shunt is made to by-pass the obstructed lymphatics. The tubes are made five inches in width. This would seem to be well worth doing routinely.

"*Postoperative Care.* The limb is maintained in an elevated position for about three weeks, after which time the patient is gradually allowed to lower the leg and bear weight, always with support. Support is needed for at least six months." *

Lymphedema of the Arm. This is one of the most trying complications following radical surgery for carcinoma of the breast. It is caused by recurrent tumor, by irradiation fibrosis, by infection or occasionally by partial occlusion of the axillary vein with superimposed infection. In the early stages, there is pitting edema which disappears on elevation. This edema may be controlled

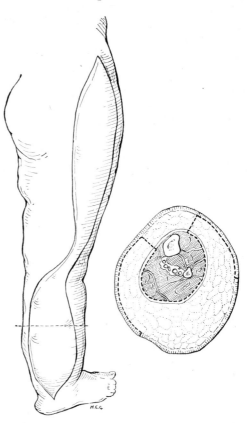

FIG. 367. Outline of skin incision. Dotted line on the cross section shows the amount of undermining. Excision of both the deep and superficial fascia and of the excess tissue lying between them. (Redrawn from Pratt and Wright.)

by support. Chemotherapy gives promise of lessening the incidence of infection. Treatment in the past has been unsatisfactory. In many cases the process follows much the same course seen in elephantiasis of the leg, the arm eventually becoming so heavy that amputation is welcomed. A Kondoleon type of operation has not given better than 50 per cent satisfactory results. The burial of long silk threads, the lymphangioplasty of Handley, has been abandoned. Standard has devised a short-circuiting operation which

* Pratt and Wright, *Surg., Gynec. & Obst.*, 72(2):244, [Feb.], 1941. By permission of Surgery, Gynecology & Obstetrics.

consists of the excision of an oval segment of skin and deep fascia exposing bare muscle on the medial aspect of the arm. The skin of the chest is then opened opposite the arm incision and the fascia of the chest wall is sutured to the arm, using silk. The arm is immobilized until healing has occurred. The incision need not be more than 5 inches long. This results in fixation of the arm to the chest wall. It will not remove fibrous tissue, but it does give relief.

It appears to the author that an operation such as the one described for elephantiasis of the leg would give equally satisfactory results in the arm.

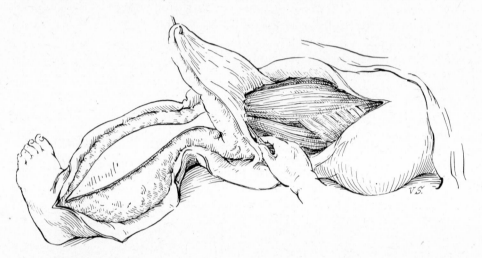

FIG. 368. This shows the manner in which the excision is carried out. (Redrawn from Pratt and Wright.)

The pedicle should be turned as in figure 372. Any tight scars or bands should be replaced by the pedicle. This would allow full motion of the arm. If there is marked deformity, the Kondoleon principle should be followed, removing enough of the excess skin and subcutaneous tissue to give freedom of motion.

Guthrie and Gagnon, reporting on an operation recommended by William C. Beck, report excellent results in elephantiasis of the arm when the following operation is performed:

"A small incision is made on the arm, about 2 cms. long, which is deepened into the edematous tissue. Into this incision a large eight inch forceps is introduced. The forceps is pushed subcutaneously as far as it will go and a second small incision is then made over the tip of the forceps. The tip of the forceps now grasps a celloidin strip 1 cm. wide by 16 cms. long and pulls it through. The ends of the celloidin strip are then pushed beyond the incision so that the entire strip lies in the subcutaneous tissue. Usually two strips are used in front and three behind pushed through the subcutaneous tissue from the arm to the chest. The small incisions are then closed with 1 or 2 sutures. The arm is placed in an aeroplane splint and the strips

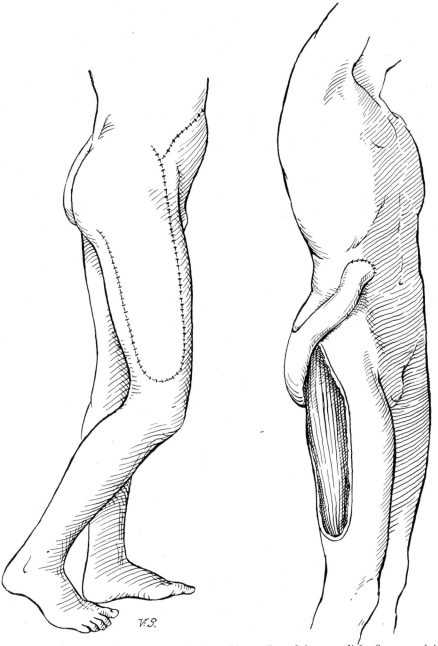

FIG. 369. Showing the method of making a broad base pedicle flap supplying new lymphatic drainage to the normal tissue. (Redrawn from Pratt and Wright.)

remain in place for three weeks. At this time, the incision in the normal tissue is reopened and the strips removed. This is done under local anesthesia." *

Radical Excision of Lymph Nodes for Carcinoma. Malignant growths spread by direct extension, by blood vessel embolism and through the lymphatics. The manner and incidence of metastasis varies with different types of tumors and with their location. In carcinoma, metastasis occurs

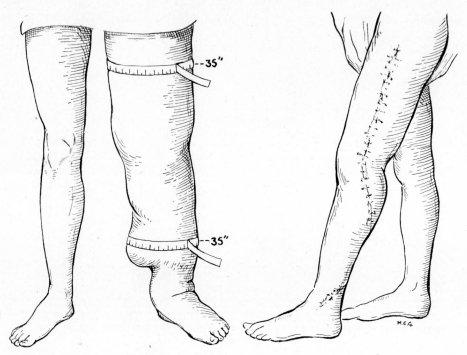

FIG. 370. This is a representation of the type of result obtained with this operation. (Redrawn from Pratt and Wright.)

predominantly through the lymphatic system. Surgical treatment of a neoplasm rests on the ability to remove all malignant cells. If all of the tumor can be removed locally, and if blood vessel embolism has not occurred, cure will be determined by the extent of lymphatic spread. The fate of cancer cells invading the lymphatic system can be predicted.

The lymph is collected into thin walled elastic channels which run for a variable distance from their origin in the structure to be drained to the lymph nodes. The nodes are made up of a capsule, thick or thin, or the small nodes may have no capsule, but there does seem to be a definite boundary between the lymphoid tissue and the surrounding fat. In those nodes having a capsule the collecting lymph channels pierce the capsule and discharge their contents into the subcapsular space which lies between the capsule and the lymphoid tissue. The center of the node has a connective tissue frame-

* Guthrie and Gagnon, *Ann. Surg.*, 123:925, 1946.

work, the reticular cells. The larger nodes are divided into gross compartments by connective tissue trabeculae leading from the capsule to the hilus of the node. The lymph cells are found between the reticular cells. There are many collecting lymph channels entering each node. It is possible to make injection directly into ten to fourteen different afferent channels entering one node in a dog's mesentery. These all empty into the subcapsular space. Many large afferent lymph channels break up into two, three or more short channels just outside of the node, and then these shorter channels pierce the capsule to empty into different parts of the subcapsular space, or

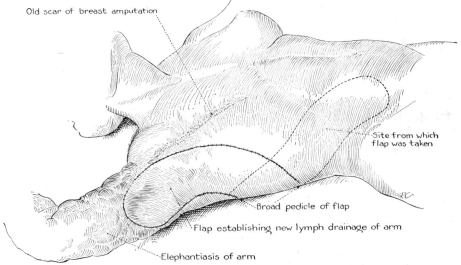

Old scar of breast amputation

Site from which flap was taken

Broad pedicle of flap

Flap establishing new lymph drainage of arm

Elephantiasis of arm

Fig. 371. Suggested operation using broad based pedicle flap to supply a new lymph drainage of the arm short circuiting the lymphatic obstruction in the axilla.

one of the short channels may empty into the lymph sinus of an adjoining node (Fig. 373). In addition, there are usually several different anastomosing channels between the large efferent channels draining a given region, and the channels draining into adjacent nodes on either side (Fig. 373).

When a colored solution is injected into an afferent lymph channel,[7] using very low pressure, the solution will penetrate through the node without coloring all of it if the node is large. The node seems to be divided grossly into separate anatomic units so that material from a given channel seems to drain to a limited part of the node. When pressure is used in the injection, the entire node will be colored before any dye appears in the efferent channel. If, instead of a colored solution, a suspension of carbon particles, or silica particles or carmine or barium particles, all less than 1 u in diameter, is used to inject into the afferent channel using very low pressure, a different picture is seen. The suspension of colored particles will partially fill its own compartment in the subcapsular space (Fig. 373A). If more pressure is used, the suspension will either overflow into the remainder of the node or it will enter the adjacent parts of the node through one of the short channels leading into a different part of the subcapsular space (Fig. 373B). If there is much pressure, the node is soon solid black in color, and the suspension may pass into one or even two or three of the adjoining nodes through the short channels (Fig. 373C). At the same time it may back up one of the tributary channels emptying into the original channel injected,

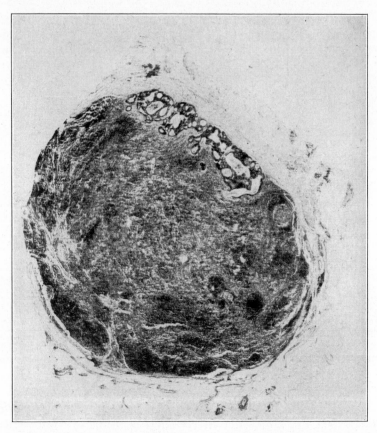

FIG. 373. Photomicrograph of a lymph node almost completely replaced by carcinoma metastasis showing thickened capsule over the area of metastasis. (From Gilchrist, *Ann. Surg.*, 111:631, 1940.)

and it is often possible to get it to go through a retrograde anastomosing channel and come through another afferent channel into an adjoining normal node (Fig. 373D). Even great pressure to the point of rupturing the walls of the afferent channel will not force any one of the fine suspensions through the node. If the animal is killed immediately, or is allowed to live for a week and then killed, no sign of passage through any node is seen, either in transparent preparations or in microscopic sections. Drinker [9] perfused a popliteal node with an undiluted serum broth culture of a strain of hemolytic streptococci. The culture contained 600,000,000 colonies per cc. The perfusion pressure was 34 mm. of mercury. In one hour and twenty

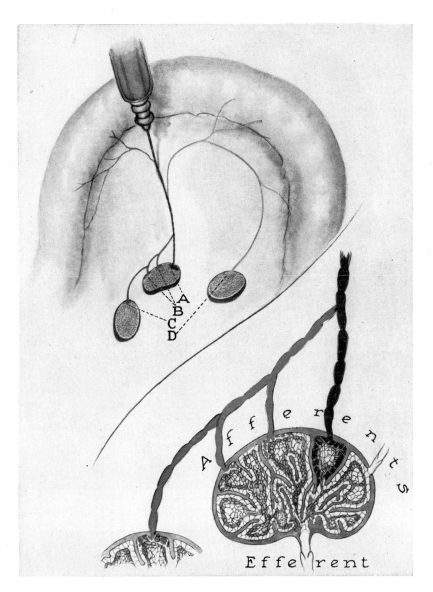

FIG. 372. Showing the manner of spread of a suspension of insoluble particles injected into a single afferent lymph channel. (From Gilchrist, *Ann. Surg.*, 111:631, 1940.)

minutes 5 cc. of the culture ran into the node and were collected from the efferent lymphatic. Cultures of the entire effluent showed 4,500,000 colonies per cc. Filtration, therefore, was 99 per cent complete. These experiments show how, when a node is destroyed or blocked, the lymph drainage is rerouted through collateral channels, or by retrograde means, into a channel draining into a normal node. Carcinoma cells are many u in diameter in contrast to the particles or bacteria, which were all less than 1 u in diameter. The normal system of collateral lymph channels, plus the demonstration of retrograde channels available when nodes are blocked, shows how much more likely spread of the large carcinoma cells is apt to be by collateral channels than by growth through lymph nodes. Even if the carcinoma cells do enter the efferent channel, the entire barrier system will again have to be overcome before the next node, central to the first one involved, is passed. Metastatic cells are arrested in the node; they do not grow through it.

Of 10,000 lymph nodes examined microscopically in resected specimens of the colon and rectum, metastases were found in 1100 different nodes. A study of this material from patients having operable lesions brought out the following facts.

Lymph channels packed with carcinoma were seen only when the lymph nodes central to the channel involved were already heavily involved with carcinoma.

Carcinoma metastases do not completely destroy the function of a node until all of the node is destroyed. This was shown in a surgical specimen of carcinoma of the breast. The lymph channels in the neighborhood of the tumor were injected with a suspension of carbon particles just before surgery. The specimen was cleared and some of the lymph channels, and several lymph nodes were seen to be outlined in black. The particles did not pass through the nodes. Figure 374 shows how the carbon particles could still flow into a node which was almost destroyed by carcinoma. Most of the carbon is found in the normal part of the node although some of it penetrates a short distance along spaces between the cancer cells.

Throughout the entire series of 10,000 lymph nodes studied a common pattern of lymph node metastasis was seen. The earliest metastasis is limited to the subcapsular space just beneath the capsule as illustrated in figure 373. When the metastasis has grown larger than the small subcapsular lesion, the spread is by expansion around the subcapsular space and into the depth of the node. This is usually accompanied by a thickening of the capsule over the area adjacent to the growth (Figs. 373 and 374). There may be a more or less heavy layer of fibrous tissue between the cancer cells and the lymph cells. In many cases there is so much interference with nutrition that we see a thick layer of fibrous tissue, a thin rim of live cancer cells within this, and necrosis in the center. Growth progresses until one or several large nodes, usually lying close to the main blood vessels, are completely replaced by carcinoma. Groups of lymph nodes which are completely replaced by metastases tend to be found in certain regions. The group of heavily involved nodes is along the main or primary line of lymph drainage.

Nodes involved central to or lateral to these nodes are apt to be subcapsular lesions or ones which are obviously late metastases.

In none of the 1100 different nodes containing metastases has there been any evidence of penetration of carcinoma outside of the capsule of any node, except where there was a collection of large involved nodes lying tightly

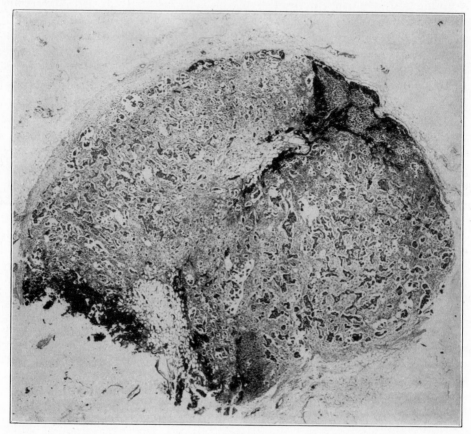

FIG. 374. Photomicrograph of a carcinoma metastasis confined to the subcapsular space. The thickened capsule over the region of the metastasis is clearly seen. (From Gilchrist, *Ann. Surg.*, 111: 631, 1940.)

packed together. Usually when this occurred, the main artery supplying the region was blocked by pressure of the nodes. Several such nodes contained necrotic material.

Postmortem studies of patients dying within two weeks of resection for carcinoma of the colon or rectum, repeatedly showed that resection had "just missed" removing all of the tumor bearing nodes, when resections were done in those having many nodes involved at the time of resection. A resection only 1 or 2 cm. wider would usually have removed all of the tumor bearing nodes. The liver, lungs, etc., were all free of metastases in these specimens.

All of these facts lead us to the conclusion that the lymphatic spread of carcinoma is primarily embolic. The nodes where the emboli lodge prevent further spread until the node is completely overwhelmed by carcinoma. Further embolic spread is through the collateral channels, each new node involved tending to make a longer and more difficult channel for a new embolus to travel. Spread from one node to another does not seem to be common, at least during the period when lesions are operable. The extreme importance of doing the widest possible resection of the lymph nodes which drain a carcinoma is evident. Any compromise with this principle, in order to avoid deforming scars or in order to preserve a more adequate blood supply as in the bowel when doing end-to-end suture, will lead to a greater incidence of recurrence.

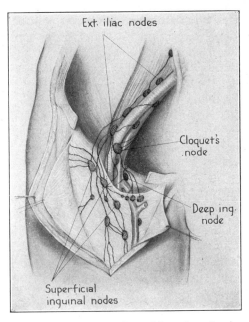

The inguinal lymph nodes are found in the anterior surface of the thigh, in the region bounded by the inguinal ligament above and by the point of intersection of the sartorius and adductor medius muscles below. These nodes are divided into superficial and deep groups.

The superficial inguinal nodes are placed in the subcutaneous tissue between the superficial and deep fascia. These nodes are divided according to their position in relation to the point of junction of the saphenous with the femoral veins. A line drawn almost horizontal through this point will divide the nodes into superior and in-

FIG. 375. Distribution of lymph nodes in the groin (after Rouviere). The superficial inguinal lymph nodes drain the major number of superficial lymphatics from the lower extremity. The deep inguinal and retrofemoral nodes receive the lymphatics accompanying the femoral vessels. Both groups communicate and may empty into the higher chain of deep iliac nodes. (From Pack and Rekers, *Am. J. Surg.*, 56:555, 1942.)

ferior; while another line which follows the saphenous vein and its prolongation downward will subdivide each of the superior and inferior groups. These four groups are the superolateral, superomedial, inferolateral and inferomedial. The nodes of the superolateral group are elongated in the direction of the inguinal ligament. They are also most nearly arranged in chain formation parallel and subjacent to the inguinal ligament. The superomedial nodes are rounded.

The superficial inguinal lymph nodes, according to Rouviere,[10] receive almost all of the superficial lymphatics of the inferior extremity, those of the scrotum, of the labia majora and minora, the cutaneous lymphatics of the penis, of the preputium clitoris, of the cutaneous zone of the anus, of the umbilicus and of the infraumbilical part of the abdominal wall. They also receive, though uncommonly, the lymphatics of the glans penis and the glans clitoris. The afferent vessels of the superficial inguinal nodes do not preside over any particular lymphatic region; indeed, the lymph vessels from a given region end most often in the nodes of several different inguinal groups.

The cutaneous lymphatics from the inferior extremity terminate in the inferolateral and inferomedial groups of nodes; those of the buttock reach the superolateral but also the inferolateral groups. The superficial lymphatics of the umbilicus and of the infraumbilical part of the abdominal wall flow into the superomedial and superolateral groups. The cutaneous lymphatics of the external genital organs run predominantly to the supero, but also to the inferomedial, groups. The lymphatics from the perineum and from the cutaneous anal zone end in the supero and inferomedial groups and sometimes in the inferolateral group. The medial nodes sometimes receive lymphatics from the glans penis and glans clitoris. There are lymphatic channels which unite the superficial lymph nodes to each other. In general, the vessels which run from node-to-node extend from the inferior to the superior nodes of the same side.

Of the efferent lymph trunks which leave the superficial lymph nodes, some proceed to the deep inguinal lymphatics and nodes; the majority, however, run directly to the external iliac nodes. Several superficial efferent trunks pass through the femoral canal and reach the medial retrofemoral nodes directly. Other superficial efferent trunks reach the external iliac nodes by passing in front of the femoral vessels in the femoral sheath; still others, the most laterally placed and generally the greater number, run from the inguinal region to the iliac fossa by passing through the interstices between the inguinal ligament and the fascia which covers the iliopsoas muscle, lateral to and often some distance from the femoral vessels. The trunks which ascend in front of the femoral vessels or lateral to the femoral canal end in the nodes found along the external iliac vessels.

The deep inguinal nodes are placed beneath the fascia lata and medial to the femoral vein. They are small nodes. They are usually found along the medial aspect of the femoral vein. The uppermost of these nodes is called the node of Cloquet and it is situated in the femoral canal between the femoral vein and the lacunar ligament. Inflammation in this node may simulate the symptoms of a strangulated hernia.

Indications for Groin Dissection. Resection of the inguinal lymph nodes should be done routinely in all melanomas of the extremities and genitalia, since 73 per cent of those having melanomas developed node metastases (Pack and Rekers).[11] Epitheliomas of the scrotum have a bad prognosis and require a bilateral inguinal node dissection. This should be done en bloc removing a large area of skin. Carcinoma of the vulva metastasizes to the superomedial group of nodes, often bilaterally. The superficial inguinal nodes should be removed; if any nodes are found to have metastases, the complete dissection should be done bilaterally. Epitheliomas and melanomas of the perianal and perineal region metastasize bilaterally in many cases. If either group of nodes contain metastases, both sides should be dissected. Patients with adenocarcinoma of the rectum which involves the skin should be examined for evidence of inguinal involvement. Dissection is indicated when nodes are enlarged. In carcinoma of the prepuce and skin of the penis, the superomedial group of nodes is involved. If the lesion is early, a super- ficial dissection may be adequate. However, if metastases are found, a com- plete dissection must be done bilaterally. In carcinoma of the glans penis or clitoris, metastases may not only involve the superficial inguinal nodes, but the external iliac nodes may be involved primarily. For this reason, a radical dissection must be seriously considered in every case. Sixty-three per cent of epidermoid carcinomas of the lower extremity develop inguinal node metastases. When nodes are enlarged, dissection is indicated. If an expectant program is adopted, a close watch must be maintained and a punch biopsy of any enlarged node must be made.

A successful groin dissection requires that the primary tumor should be controllable, and it should be removed first; that there be no evidence of blood stream metastasis; that the lymph stream must not show evidence of retrograde extension; that it must be technically possible to excise all of the lymph nodes involved; that there must be some possibility of the in- terruption of the lymphatic spread of the tumor by the excision of these nodes.

The groin dissection should either be done en bloc with the tumor, or ten to fourteen days may be allowed after removal of the primary, in order for all tumor emboli to lodge in the nodes draining the area. Never resect the nodes first and the tumor later. This invites further metastasis, as the natural filters are removed first and metastasis will occur into the interven- ing soft parts.

TECHNIC OF OPERATION (Pack and Rekers).[11] "Spinal anesthesia is desir- able. The scrotum is sutured to the opposite thigh for better exposure (Fig. 376). Because of the death of skin which so often follows extensive operations in this region, a wide ellipse of skin is excised. The incision extends from 2 inches above and 1 inch medial to the anterior-superior iliac spine, sweeping downward in a wide ellipse, and then in a medial direction over the inguinal region, then over the femoral trigone, to terminate in the mid-thigh over Hunters canal. Towels are clipped to the skin. The skin edges are then elevated and the subcutaneous fat is dissected widely until the entire upper one-third of the anterior thigh, the inguinal region and the lower abdominal wall over the iliac quadrant has been denuded of skin. The dissection now persists deeply to the underlying muscles, through the fascia which is dissected with the fat and lymphoid tissue en bloc in a medial direction. This dissection proceeds from above downward exposing the inguinal canal and femoral vessels. The adventitial layer of the artery and vein is stripped together with the fat and fascia intervening between these vessels. The external saphenous vein is severed and ligated near its junction with the femoral vein. The dissection proceeds downward, removing all of the fascia from the sartorius, pectineus, adductor brevis, and rectus femoris muscles (Fig. 377). The sartorius is retraced as Hunters canal is

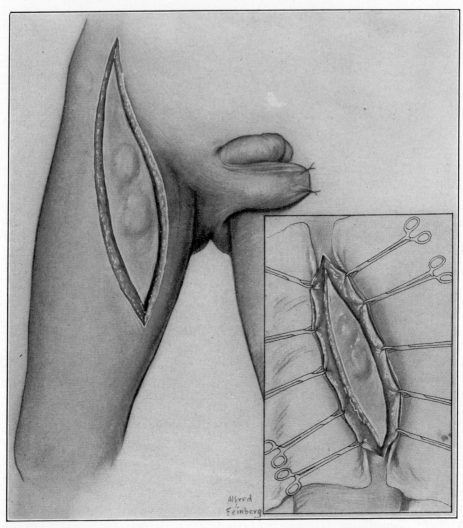

FIG. 376. Scope of incision for groin dissection. The ellipse permits necessary sacrifice of condemned skin. Note direction of incision and upper and lower limits. Scrotal skin is sutured temporarily to opposite thigh. Insert shows use of tenacula to facilitate subcutaneous and fascial dissection. (From Pack and Rekers, *Am. J. Surg.*, 56:549, 1942.)

entered. The external saphenous vein is again severed and ligated where it enters the field overlying the middle portion of the sartorius muscle. This bulk of tissue is removed.

"Now the inguinal canal is opened from the external ring to the point where the round ligament or spermatic cord dips downward into the pelvic cavity. The canal is further exposed laterally by incising the external oblique

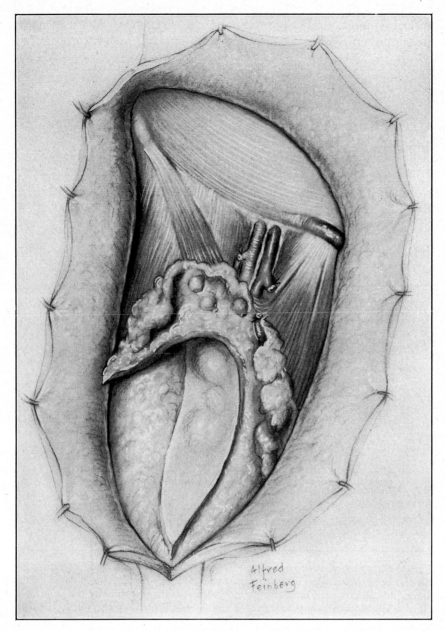

FIG. 377. Superficial stage of groin dissection partly completed. Skin flaps dissected widely back. Lower abdominal, inguinal and femoral regions freed of fat, fascia, lymphoid and areolar tissues from above downward. Observe medial and lateral extent of fascial dissection. (From Pack and Rekers, *Am. J. Surg.,* 56:549, 1942.)

fascia and the transversalis muscles down to the properitoneal fat. The occasional lymph node in the inguinal canal is removed. The external fascia and the inguinal ligament are then severed about 2 inches from the attach-

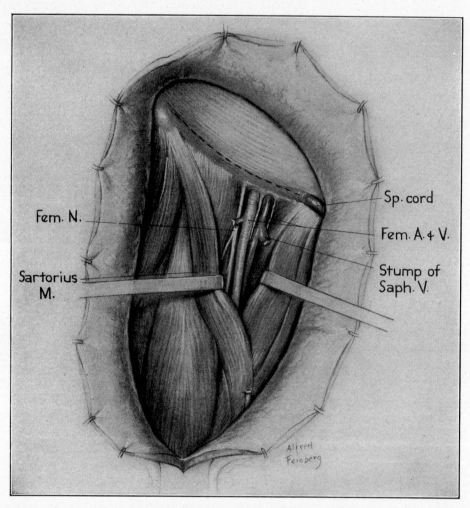

Fem. N.

Sartorius M.

Sp. cord

Fem. A. & V.

Stump of Saph. V.

Alfred Feinberg

Fig. 378. Completion of superficial stage of groin dissection. The neurovascular femoral bundle has been cleanly dissected down through Hunter's canal. The fascia overlying the pectineus, iliacus, sartorius, adductor brevis and rectus femoris muscles has been removed. Proposed incision to expose the inguinal canal is indicated by the dotted line. (From Pack and Rekers, *Am. J. Surg.*, 56:550, 1942.)

ment to the pubic spine (Fig. 378). This opens the femoral ring and improves the exposure of the vessels and lymphoid tissue situated retroperitoneally along the iliac vessels. Deep retractors now draw the peritoneum upward and medially outside of the operative field. The dissection is entirely retroperitoneal. The chain of lymph nodes, fat and areolar tissue found along the external iliac vessels are dissected from above downward, including those overlying the obturator foramen. Ligation of the deep epigastric vessels at the external artery and vein aids in the dissection.

"The inguinal ligament is resutured and the inguinal canal is closed. The edge of the sartorius is sometimes sutured medially in an attempt to obliterate the dead space of Scarpa's triangle. If the tumor was fungating through the skin or if an irradiation burn was present, closure is with catgut,

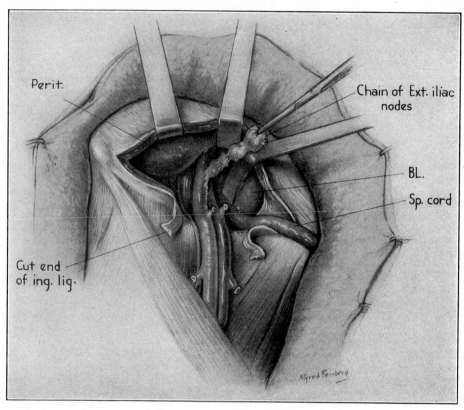

FIG. 379. Dissection of deep iliac lymph nodes. Displacement of peritoneum medially to afford adequate exposure. (From Pack and Rekers, *Am. J. Surg.*, 56:551, 1942.)

with drainage in the most dependent part of the wound. If there is little likelihood of an infection, silk is used throughout." *

The leg is kept in slight flexion and the skin and muscles must be kept in apposition by a sponge or voluminous mechanic's waste dressing held in place with a spica dressing. Pack had an operative mortality of 1.6 per cent in 122 cases.

Hemorrhage following sloughing of the skin, especially if preoperative radiation has been done, may be serious. Wound infection will occur in some. Twenty per cent required skin grafting because of necrosis of skin flaps. Lymphedema of the entire lower extremity invariably follows this radical operation. This edema is increased if infection is present or if the

* Pack and Rekers, *Am. J. Surg.*, 56:545, 1942.

scar is tight. This lymphedema may be temporary. If grafting is necessary, pedicle grafts should be used as described under the treatment of chronic lymphedema.

REFERENCES

1. HIBBARD, JAMES J.   *U. S. Nav. M. Bull.*, 44:27, [Jan.], 1945.
2. KONDOLEON, E.   *Zentralbl. f. Chir.*, 39:1022, 1912.
3. SISTRUNK, W. E.   *Minnesota Med.*, 6:173, 1923.
4. GHORMLEY, R. K.   *Ann. Int. Med.*, 9:516, 1935-1936.
5. PRATT, GERALD H. and WRIGHT, IRVING J.   *Surg., Gynec. & Obst.*, 72:244, [Feb.], 1941.
6. GUTHRIE, DONALD and GAGNON, GERALD.   Prevention and Treatment of Postoperative Lymphedema of the Arm, *Ann. Surg.*, 123:925, 1946.
7. GILCHRIST, R. K.   *Ann. Surg.*, 111:634, [April], 1940.
8. BATSON, O. V.   *Ann. Int. Med.*, 16:38, [Jan.], 1942.
9. DRINKER, CECIL K.   *Lymphatics, Lymph and Lymphoid Tissue*, Howard Press, 1941.
10. ROUVIERE, H.   *Anatomy of the Human Lymphatic System* (translated by Tobias), Edward's Press, Ann Arbor, 1938.
11. PACK, GEORGE T. and REKERS, PAUL.   *Am. J. Surg.*, 56:545, 1942.
12. STANDARD, SAMUEL.   *Ann. Surg.*, 116:816, [Dec.], 1942.

SPLENECTOMY

WARREN H. COLE, M.D.

INDICATIONS FOR SPLENECTOMY

During recent years, appreciation of the fact that inhibition of the bone marrow is one of the normal functions of the spleen has given rise to a better understanding of the indications for splenectomy. In addition to hemolytic jaundice and purpura, in which there is strong indication for splenectomy as discussed below, there are numerous other diseases for which splenectomy may be very beneficial; in general, most of these represent one or more of the manifestations of hypersplenism. Splenomegalia alone, regardless of cause, may give rise to hypersplenism.

Hemolytic Jaundice. In this disease the spleen is the primary cause of symptoms. Therefore, as would be expected, splenectomy is followed by good results in at least 90 per cent of patients. Although the disease was originally classified as being of the familial or acquired type, it is probable that all belong to the congenital group except, of course, patients having hemolytic jaundice produced by chemicals and poisons. Cardinal manifestations are splenomegalia, spherocytosis, and anemia. Crisis may develop, at which time fever, weakness, abdominal pain, extreme anemia and related symptoms may develop. Splenectomy in the presence of crisis is dangerous, and should be avoided if possible; however, on many occasions the danger of a fatality from the crisis alone is so great that splenectomy must be performed. If a large amount of blood is available and its transfusion started as soon as the splenic artery is ligated, the mortality rate will be quite low.

Thrombocytopenic Purpura. In this disease the spleen is likewise the primary cause of symptoms. For this reason, splenectomy is usually strongly indicated if the symptoms are very severe. Cardinal manifestations are anemia, low platelet count, lack of clot retraction, prolonged bleeding time (with normal coagulation time), and hemorrhage from mucous membranes or other sources. The disease occurs with varying degrees of severity. In the mild cases, symptoms sometimes disappear without treatment. The disease must be differentiated from the so-called symptomatic purpura (non-thrombocytopenic). Bone marrow studies are of great value in determining the advisability of operation, since in the primary disease responding so well to splenectomy, megakaryocytic hyperplasia in the bone marrow is present.

Banti's Disease or Splenic Anemia. In this disease splenomegalia is indicative of obstruction of the splenic or portal vein, with or without mild cirrhosis. Portal hypertension develops because of a peculiar but mild type of cirrhosis and possibly obstructive lesions in the veins. The author is convinced that in late cases splenectomy offers no favorable effect other than partial relief of portal hypertension afforded by ligation of the splenic artery. Splenectomy may be of some permanent value in early cases of Banti's disease. For the above reasons, the author is convinced that splenectomy should not be performed in the late stage of the disease because of the high mortality rate and the low incidence of relief. Cardinal manifestations of the disease are splenomegalia, anemia, mild jaundice and leukopenia. Ultimately, cirrhosis of the liver develops which usually leads to ascites in the late stages. Hematemesis because of dilated esophageal varices is common. Years ago, Smith and Farber[1] described a disease of childhood consisting of splenomegalia and mild changes in the liver, associated with hematemesis; the lesion described by them was probably similar to Banti's syndrome.

Felty's Syndrome. Cardinal manifestations of this disease are splenomegalia, chronic arthritis, leukopenia and anemia, for which splenectomy was first performed by Hanrahan and Miller[2] in 1932. The disease is relatively uncommon. The splenomegalia is probably a secondary manifestation, although the primary source of symptoms is not known.

Primary Splenic Neutropenia. The primary manifestations of this disease are splenomegalia and neutropenia; it probably represents a selective form of hypersplenism in which only one of the functions (viz. maturation of granulocytes) of the bone marrow is inhibited. Splenectomy is curative.

Splenic Panhematocytopenia. Though not common this condition may be primary, or secondary to many conditions such as Gaucher's disease, etc. The spleen exerts an excess inhibition on the bone marrow giving rise to decreased production or maturation of granulocytes, erythrocytes and platelets from the bone marrow. Splenectomy will relieve the defects just named, but if the disease is secondary, it will not influence the primary lesion.

Gaucher's Disease. This is a rare disease, encountered usually in young girls. Important manifestations are splenomegalia, pigmentation of the skin, anemia and the presence of Gaucher's cells in the spleen. On many occasions, splenectomy exerts a very favorable influence in this disease.

Traumatized Spleen. The normal spleen is a rather friable organ and is readily lacerated even though it is fairly well protected by the ribs. Bleeding from lacerations of the spleen is profuse and may lead to shock and death. The history of the injury will be helpful in determining the site of trauma although no local evidence may be found. If hemorrhage is significant, symptoms of shock including pallor, tachycardia, low blood pressure, cold sweat, etc., will be present. Transfusion is obviously indicated immediately. If the condition of the patient returns to normal after one or two transfusions it may be assumed that the hemorrhage has stopped and operation will be unnecessary if injury to other organs, particularly the intestine can be eliminated. However, if the symptoms are improved only slightly, or persist in spite of one or two transfusions, splenectomy should be undertaken at once.

Miscellaneous Diseases. Occasionally, splenomegalia produced by syphilis, cirrhosis of the liver, and malaria may be treated effectively by splenectomy. Years ago, splenectomy was performed somewhat on an experimental basis in patients with leukemia, polycythemia and aplastic anemia, but it is quite definite now that removal of the spleen in these diseases is contraindicated. Splenectomy is likewise contraindicated in agnogenic myeloid metaplasia of the spleen, but it is usually very difficult to diagnose this disease without microscopic examination of the spleen.[4]

PREOPERATIVE CARE

Preoperative preparation of the patient is extremely important in splenectomy, particularly because the patient is so commonly very anemic and suffering from nutritional disturbances. The amount of preoperative therapy is determined by the disease and its severity. For example, a patient who is bleeding profusely because of purpura hemorrhagica may require three or four transfusions before operation. Intravenous fluids will be necessary in some cases to combat dehydration when anorexia and nausea are pronounced.

In hemolytic jaundice severe reaction can be sustained following preoperative transfusions. In the majority of patients transfusion in hemolytic icterus will not be followed by reaction but Doan and associates[5] have called attention to the fact that a severe hemolytic reaction following a transfusion even though relatively uncommon may actually produce death. Therefore, it may be considered safer to prepare the patient for operation with other means available and start blood in the operating room immediately after the splenic artery and vein have been ligated.

Hepatic insufficiency is a common cause of death following splenectomy. Accordingly, the patient should be examined closely for primary or secondary hepatic disease, and measures including forced food, intravenous glucose and amino acids, transfusions, etc., utilized in an effort to combat it. Liver insufficiency will be most pronounced in Banti's disease.

Before the patient goes to the operating room, a tube should be inserted into the stomach to decompress it, thereby allowing optimum exposure of the spleen. The surgeon should make certain that several bottles of blood have been cross-matched and are available for transfusion immediately.

TECHNIC OF SPLENECTOMY

Incision. Numerous types of incision are used for splenectomy. The author prefers one which starts slightly to the left of the midline just below the ensiform, proceeding downward for 2 or 3 inches paramedially to the rectus muscle, and curving transversely to the left, parallel to the costal margin (see Fig. 380A). The external sheath of the upper portion of the rectus muscle is opened with a longitudinal incision and the muscle along with adjacent structures severed transversely after the incision is carried laterally to the left. This incision usually requires cutting the eleventh intercostal nerve. It is well known that section of only one of the intercostal nerves going to the abdominal wall results in no muscle weakness. However, section of two or more nerves will result in muscle weakness and encourage development of postoperative hernia. The twelfth nerve is located near the end of the incision, but can be avoided and retracted away from possible harm. This incision gives optimum exposure and is particularly valuable insofar as its extension up to the ensiform allows good exposure of the diaphragmatic attachments which may be quite vascular. Years ago, Singleton [6] advised use of an oblique transverse incision which is begun in the midepigastrium half way between the ensiform and umbilicus, and extended laterally and downward to a point just above the crest of the ileum. Anatomically this is a good incision, but it does not allow good exposure of the diaphragmatic attachment to the spleen and the upper group of vessels in the gastrosplenic ligament which always requires ligation.

Some surgeons utilize a left paramedian incision. However, the author is firmly of the opinion that exposure with this incision is entirely inadequate, insofar as exposure is confined largely to the midportion of the abdomen. It is true that in the majority of splenectomies the spleen may be rolled out safely into such a wound. However, in 10 to 20 per cent of cases blind mobilization of the spleen with the hand will result in such severe hemorrhage that the patient's life may be jeopardized.

Exploration. Before starting ligation of the vessels and isolation of the spleen, thorough exploration should be conducted to determine the extent of adhesions and particularly their vascularity. Inspection of the adhesions for vessels will be of great help insofar as the surgeon will be forewarned as to which adhesions can be severed without ligature and which ones must be ligated. Thorough exploration also will reveal the extent of adhesions of other organs to the spleen. Frequently the colon is densely adherent to the spleen and may be injured if the surgeon is not constantly aware of its presence. In hemolytic jaundice the gallbladder should be palpated for the presence of stones. As emphasized by Curtis and Movitz, [7] thorough exploration must be made for accessory spleens, particularly in hemolytic jaundice and purpura. On all occasions except when the spleen is being removed for secondary disease of the spleen, accessories should be removed.

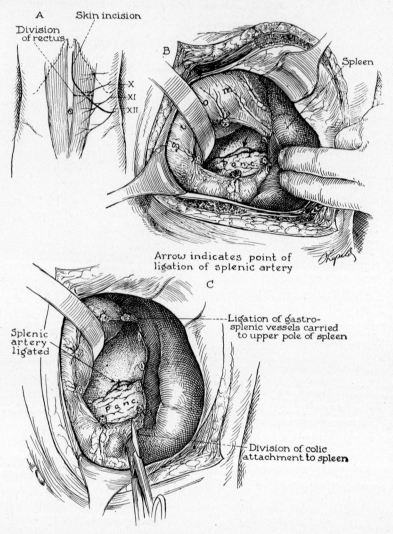

FIG. 380. (A) The incision preferred by the author starts high in the left upper quadrant, extending paramedially downward and laterally cutting the rectus muscle and enough of the muscles of the anterior abdominal wall to allow exposure. Only the eleventh nerve is sacrificed. (B) The gastrocolic and gastrosplenic attachments are cut to allow exposure of the splenic artery and its *ligation* just proximal to its bifurcation. (C) Ligation of the gastrosplenic vessels and division of the colic attachments to the spleen. (Modified from Cole, *Surg. Clin. N. Amer.*, 22:46, 1942.)

Ligation of the Splenic Artery. The author strongly advises preliminary ligation of the splenic artery before an attempt is made to mobilize the spleen. When the spleen is small, as in purpura hemorrhagica, traumatized spleen, etc., there will be little advantage in ligation of the splenic artery, insofar as vascularity is of little consequence. However, when the spleen is enlarged and surrounded by vascular adhesions, preliminary ligation will be of tremendous value. In general, the size of the artery is related to the size of the spleen. As the artery becomes enlarged, it becomes tortuous and more readily isolated for ligation.

After incision through the gastro-colic omentum the splenic artery, with few exceptions, is readily palpated along the superior border of the pancreas several centimeters from the hilus of the spleen (see Fig. 380B). Incision through the posterior layer of peritoneum allows isolation of the artery and application of a ligature without difficulty. Rarely will more than two or three minutes be required for isolation of the artery. However, it must be emphasized that dissection of the artery from adjacent structures must be carried out carefully, since the splenic vein lies near it and injury to this structure would result in troublesome bleeding which might be difficult to control. Ligation of the splenic artery preceding splenectomy reduces sharply the vascular pressure in the spleen which then contracts appreciably within three or four minutes after ligation of the vessel, providing the splenic vein is left intact during this interval. Ligation of the artery likewise allows the patient to have an autotransfusion. When the spleen is large, 500 to 700 cc. of blood may escape into the systemic circulation following ligation of the artery. The decreased vascularity of adhesions make the operation much easier. Miller [8] has described temporary ligation of the splenic artery, exposing the vessel near its origin from the celiac trunk, through an opening in the gastrohepatic omentum. He compresses the artery with a small rubber tube, and releases it after the spleen is removed. The author has found the artery more accessible in the floor of the lesser peritoneal cavity at the superior edge of the pancreas as mentioned previously.

Ligation of Ligamentous Attachments and Splenic Pedicle. The first attachments encountered are the gastrocolic and gastrosplenic ligaments; both of which are vascular but readily ligated because of their position in the wound (see Fig. 380C). The lienorenal ligament, which is located posteriorly fixing the spleen to structures adjacent to the kidney, is a constant and rather dense structure, but avascular except when portal hypertension is present. In the presence of portal hypertension this structure must be cut and ligated, particularly if it appears to be vascular. The diaphragmatic ligament is likewise avascular except in portal hypertension. It is cut with, or without ligation depending upon its vascularity. Before rolling the spleen medially into the wound (see Fig. 381A), the surgeon must make sure that the uppermost vessels in the gastrosplenic ligament are ligated, since the delivery of the spleen will tear these vessels unless they are previously ligated. These vessels are always of considerable size and if bleeding from them is not recognized and controlled, considerable blood may escape into the splenic fossa and jeopardize the condition of the patient. After all the ligamentous attachments have been severed (see Fig. 381B) and ligated as indicated, the splenic pedicle is ligated (see Fig. 381C). In general, it is

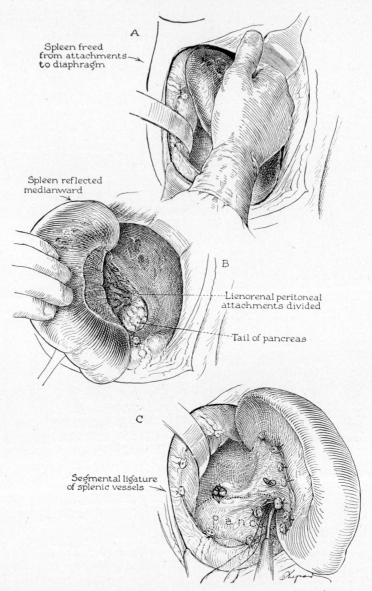

Spleen freed from attachments to diaphragm

Spleen reflected medianward

Lienorenal peritoneal attachments divided

Tail of pancreas

Segmental ligature of splenic vessels

FIG. 381. (A) After mobilization anteriorly the ligamentous attachment to diaphragm and kidney can usually be accomplished with the hand. In portal hypertension, these folds may be vascular, requiring ligation. (B) After separation of these folds the spleen can be rotated medially exposing the pedicle and tail of the pancreas. (C) The vessels are ligated individually allowing secure ligations. (Modified from Cole, *Surg. Clin. N. Amer.*, 22:47, 1942.)

much safer to ligate the pedicle in segments rather than include all of it in one ligature. With care, segmental resection is readily carried out. The artery should be ligated twice unless it was ligated preliminary to mobilization of the spleen.

If the patient is a poor risk, or bleeding is present and uncontrollable because of the presence of the spleen, it may be justifiable to place one large clamp on the pedicle and remove the spleen rapidly. If this procedure is adopted three curved clamps should be applied to the pedicle, as illustrated

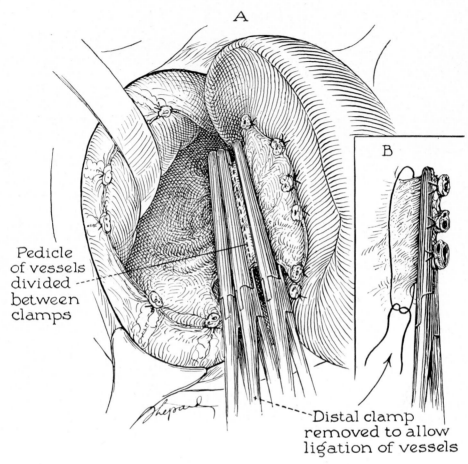

A

B

Pedicle
of vessels
divided
between
clamps

Distal clamp
removed to allow
ligation of vessels

FIG. 381a. (A) If the splenic artery is not ligated before section of the pedicle it is preferable to place three clamps cutting between, as shown. Removal of the middle clamp will allow individual ligation of the vessels as shown in (B) and a mass ligation later. Usually the clamps used for the pedicle must be curved or right-angled instead of straight, as shown. (From Cole in *Surg. Clin. N. Amer.*, 22:48, 1942.)

in figure 381a and the pedicle severed at the point indicated. Removal of the central clamp will allow the surgeon to ligate the vessels individually. A transfixing ligature may then be applied to the entire pedicle thereby supplying a double ligature to the pedicle. Such a procedure will rarely save time, but may be strongly indicated if bleeding is occurring in the depths of the wound and cannot be controlled because of the presence of a large spleen. During ligation of the gastrosplenic ligament and the splenic pedicle, care must be taken in dissection lest a bit of the stomach be included in the clamps, and damage inflicted upon that organ. These clamps should be applied under direct vision, thereby making it necessary to have an incision which affords good exposure. Injury to the stomach by one of the artery clamps, or inclusion of part of its wall in a ligature may result in perforation later if it is not detected at the time of injury.

After removal of the spleen, careful search is again made for accessory spleens, particularly in thrombocytopenic purpura and hemolytic anemia, Gaucher's Disease and Felty's Syndrome. Accessory spleens are usually found in the hilus, but Curtis and associates [7] have emphasized that they may be found almost anywhere in the peritoneal cavity. Before the wound is closed all the raw areas must be inspected closely for bleeding points (particularly in portal hypertension) and ligatures applied as indicated.

Closure of the Wound. A continuous zero or 1 chromic catgut is used to close the peritoneum. Drainage is not indicated. The rectus fascia as well as internal oblique and external oblique muscle and aponeurosis are approximated with interrupted silk or cotton. This makes an adequate closure and postoperative hernia will rarely be encountered. Likewise, rupture of the wound seldom develops.

POSTOPERATIVE CARE

Blood transfusions are given after operation as indicated. Gastrointestinal decompression is maintained for 24 hours, or longer if ileus develops. Maintenance of fluid balance by intravenous or subcutaneous fluids is important as in any other celiotomy.

Fever and tachycardia are common 24 to 36 hours following operation. An explanation of this complication is not available. There is no indication that it is explainable on the basis of infection, but if infection appears to be present, chemotherapy would obviously be indicated.

For several hours following splenectomy, the blood pressure and pulse must be watched closely for signs of hemorrhage from the splenic pedicle, particularly in patients with portal hypertension. In portal hypertension, hemorrhage from the splenic pedicle will be the most common cause of postoperative fatality. A sudden drop in blood pressure may indicate necessity for reopening the abdomen for control of a bleeding vessel. However, reopening the abdomen is not indicated in all patients having splenectomy, and showing a fall in blood pressure immediately after operation. The author has observed depression of the blood pressure in such instances 2 or 3 hours after operation, which responded rapidly and effectively to adequate transfusion.

PRECAUTIONS IN SPLENECTOMY

1. It is essential that ample blood be available to take care of the anemia, and unforseen demands brought about by the accidental loss of blood during operation.

2. Good exposure must be obtained by the proper incision. In a small percentage of patients good exposure will be life-saving.

3. Preliminary ligation of the splenic artery will give the patient an autotransfusion and make the ligamentous attachments much less vascular, thereby making the operation much easier.

4. The vascular ligaments and fibrous adhesions should be cut and ligated before the spleen is delivered into the wound.

5. The tail of the pancreas must be dissected free from the spleen before the pedicle is ligated.

6. Care must be taken not to injure the stomach during ligation of the gastrohepatic omentum or the splenic pedicle.

7. Ligate the splenic pedicle in segments except when necessary to ligate it en masse to obtain good exposure for the control of bleeding.

8. Search carefully for accessory spleens in all diseases in which the spleen may be the primary cause of symptoms.

9. Perfect hemostasis must be obtained before the abdomen is closed, particularly in all patients with portal hypertension.

TABLE 7. *ANALYSIS OF SPLENECTOMIES*

(Illinois Research and Educational Hospitals, 1936-1948)

SPLENECTOMIES	NO. OF CASES	OPER. DEATHS
Hemolytic anemia	28	1
Thrombocytopenic purpura	26	0
Thrombosis of the splenic vein	5	0
Banti's disease	13	5
Felty's disease (Secondary panhematocytopenia)	5	0
Atypical hemolytic anemia	1	0
Sickle cell anemia	1	0
Congenital cyst	1	0
Gaucher's disease	1	0
Aneurysm of splenic artery	1	0
Agnogenic myeloid metaplasia	1	0
Atypical aplastic anemia	1	1
Hodgkins disease	1	0
Myeloid leukemia	1	0
Unclassified splenomegalia	1	0
Total	87	7
Mortality 8.0%		

RESULTS

The mortality rate will vary somewhat depending upon the type of patients chosen for splenectomy, but in a large series of patients should be under 10 per cent. All surgeons note a higher mortality rate in Banti's disease and other lesions accompanied by portal hypertension. Although patients may enter the hospital seriously ill because of anemia with hemolytic jaundice and purpura hemorrhagica, operation is tolerated relatively well in these patients because hepatic insufficiency is uncommon in such patients and portal hypertension absent.

In 87 splenectomies performed at Illinois Research Hospital during the past 10 years, 7 patients died postoperatively, constituting a mortality rate of 8.0 per cent. In this series, 28 splenectomies were performed for hemolytic anemia, and 26 for thrombocytopenic purpura, with but 1 death. In 13 patients with Banti's disease, upon whom splenectomy was performed, 5 postoperative deaths were encountered, thus constituting a mortality rate of 38 per cent. This high mortality rate in Banti's disease is added reason why the patient should be studied thoroughly before splenectomy is advised. The seventh fatality in our series was encountered in a patient with atypical aplastic anemia resembling purpura hemorrhagica.

REFERENCES

1. SMITH, R. M. and FARBER, SIDNEY.   Splenomegaly in Children with Early Hematemesis, *J. Ped.*, 7:585, 1935.
2. HANRAHAN, E. M., JR. and MILLER, S. R.   Effect of Splenectomy in Felty's Syndromes, *J.A.M.A.*, 99:1247, [Oct. 8], 1932.
3. de J. PEMBERTON, J.   Splenectomy, *South. Med. & Surg.*, 102:46, 1940.
4. LEVINSON, SAMUEL A. and LIMARZI, L. R.   Agnogenic Myeloid Metaplasia of the Spleen, *Amer. J. Clin. Path.*, 17:449, [June], 1947.
5. DOAN, C. A., CURTIS, G. M. and WISEMAN, B. K.   Hemolytopoietic Equilibrium and Emergency Splenectomy, *J.A.M.A.*, 105:1567, [Nov. 16], 1935.
6. SINGLETON, A. O.   Splenectomy, *Surg., Gynec. & Obst.*, 70:1051, 1940.
7. CURTIS, G. M. and MOVITZ, D.   The Surgical Significance of the Accessory Spleen, *Ann. Surg.*, 123:276, 1946.
8. MILLER, E. M.   Temporary Complete Control of Main Blood Supply as Preliminary Step in Difficult Splenectomies, *J.A.M.A.*, 112:229 [Jan. 21], 1939.

THE SURGERY OF PORTAL HYPERTENSION

NATHAN A. WOMACK, M.D.

Portal hypertension may be produced by obstruction of the portal vein or some of its branches, before it reaches the liver, within the liver, or in the hepatic vein or vena cava. The last site is so unusual and lends itself so rarely to surgical attack that it might well be ignored in this discussion.

Physiologic Considerations of Portal Hypertension. Ordinarily in the portal vein the pressure generally is low, ranging from 6 to 12 mm. of mercury (8 to 16 cms. of water) in the normal human, although in disease this often is elevated four or five times as high. Since the pressure in the hepatic vein is close to that of atmospheric level, liver capillary pressure is extremely low and blood flow in the portal system is slow. However, this pressure in the portal vein within the liver probably is modified considerably by the influence of the hepatic artery. Hepatic artery blood probably merges with portal vein blood before these vessels reach the sinusoids of the liver. The volume of blood entering the liver through the hepatic artery under normal conditions has been variously estimated but probably is approximately 25 per cent. This in itself would serve as one factor modifying the pressure level in the portal system, and this effect would vary with systemic arterial pressure. In cirrhosis this effect is markedly exaggerated. Many other factors come into play to make the regulation of portal pressures extremely complicated. Among these are the action of the splanchnics, the presence of sphincters at the junction of the hepatic vein and the vena cava, probably sphincters near the central veins within the liver, the sinusoids of the liver, and the intrahepatic tension as affected by parenchymal metabolism such as lipid infiltration or edema.

The effects of intrahepatic obstruction are variable. Obstructions outside of the liver are much more consistent. Most dramatic of these is occlusion of the splenic vein. This is most often seen in that portion of the vein adjacent the pancreas and usually is secondary to trauma. This results in increased intrasplenic tension with gradual hypertrophy and hyperplasia of the reticulum as a result of congestive effects. Apparently the spleen takes on increased function insofar as its destructive capacity is concerned and the patient seen presents a picture of so-called hypersplenism. There usually is moderate to severe secondary anemia, decrease in blood platelets, and leukopenia. The spleen is enlarged and firm. Often due to the collateral circulation through the vasa brevia and the left gastro-epiploic, there is a marked gastric congestion and the patient may have episodes of hematemesis. The clinical picture is a classical one, and the condition responds adequately to splenectomy.

Another type of extrahepatic portal obstruction is generally seen near the entrance of the vein into the liver and generally occurs in infants or early childhood. This may consist of either a fibrous replacement of an obliterative type or in a cavernomatous transformation. Both of these types have been recently stressed by Whipple.[1]

When the obstruction is within the liver and the pressure within the portal system is elevated, an increasing amount of blood must enter the liver through the hepatic artery; and this generally is accomplished by the formation of so-called collateral circulation. There are two groups of veins which play an important part in this collateral circulation. In one group fall the so-called accessory veins of Sappey, which are the veins which enter the liver directly without passing through the portal vein. While these are small structures, in disease they may become quite large. They are the veins seen in the supporting ligaments of the liver, namely, the suspensory ligament, the gastrohepatic omentum, the veins between the gallbladder and the liver, and the hepatocolic and hepatorenal veins. The other groups of veins involved in the collateral circulation are numerous, but the chief groups are those anastomosing with the coronary vein, the middle hemorrhoidal, and the para-umbilical veins.

The importance of this collateral circulation to the surgeon lies in the fact that the collaterals of the coronary especially may become huge, sometimes 1 centimeter or more in diameter. As they extend up the lesser curvature of the stomach and invade the wall of the stomach and esophagus, erosions are frequent and massive hemorrhage occurs. These hemorrhages may be exsanguinating in amount and often are fatal. Therefore, the patient who has had a single such hemorrhage and survived, lives in constant terror of others.

Besides the clinical picture of congestive splenomegaly and recurrent attacks of hemorrhage, the patient with portal hypertension frequently is embarrassed by a third finding, namely, the appearance of ascites. At the present time there is some question as to whether or not ascites as seen in portal hypertension is due entirely to increased intrahepatic resistance. Other factors seem to be involved, perhaps related to protein synthesis and hormonal influence. The effect of lowering portal hypertension on ascites, however, is at times dramatic; and it, therefore, should be considered along with congestive splenomegaly and hematemesis as one of the indications for surgery.

The surgical approach to the relief of portal hypertension historically has followed one of two general principles. The first is the establishment of a fistulous connection between the portal and general circulation, and the latter has to do with lowering the portal tension by excision of viscera or portions of viscera within the portal system, thus reducing the amount of blood necessary in the portal vein. The shunt between the portal and venous systems is the method used by the body in overcoming intrahepatic occlusion of the portal vein. As this collateral circulation increases, the relative amount of blood supplied the liver by the hepatic artery increases; and it has been estimated that in some advanced states of cirrhosis approximately 85 per cent of the hepatic circulation is arterial. This effective arterial supply probably explains why some patients with a huge amount of scarring in the liver present no clinical evidence of hepatic dysfunction and suggests that probably functional decompensation occurs in advanced cirrhosis chiefly when the arterial branches become occluded. In the light of such a functional consideration, the surgical performance of a shunt between the two circulations would seem to be less formidable physiologically; and this concept would seem to be verified experimentally.[2] At the same time one must bear in mind the possible ill effects of the sudden removal of a large amount of portal circulation from the liver with possible episodes of intoxication. This will be particularly hazardous to proper protein metabolism.

The most classical of the older operations for the establishment of such a shunt is the Talma-Morrison procedure of omentopexy. Although this procedure has had its enthusiastic supporters in times past, the over-all picture has not been too satisfactory. While many patients have had a probable decrease in the amount of ascites for a variable period of time, the shunt has never been very effective in lowering portal hypertension. Modifications of this procedure such as excision of the parietal peritoneum along with omentopexy have had their supporters but this, too, has been effective chiefly in the partial relief of ascites but not in the other effects of portal hypertension.

While a direct approach in the performance of such a shunt has been known for many years following the work of Eck, it is due to the more recent aggressive attack through this method by Whipple, Blakemore,[3] and others that the performance has been applied clinically.

The first procedure tried by them in a considerable number of cases was an anastomosis between the splenic and renal veins after removal of the spleen and the left kidney. Several technics have been developed by them and others for the performance of this anastomosis which are described in detail in several reports. In the few years which have elapsed since the utilization of this type of shunt, there have been a considerable number of dramatic results described in the literature. However, as results have been evaluated with the passage of time, at the present writing it is becoming more and more evident that this procedure is unsatisfactory in many instances. The hazard of the operation is great. Its technical performance is most difficult and even impossible in those patients who have had previous splenectomy. Leaks, thrombosis and stenosis of the anastomotic site probably have made this a less desired procedure to that of the direct portacaval shunt.

Numerous technics have been described for the direct portacaval anastomosis. Perhaps the most effective is a side-to-side anastomosis between the vena cava and portal vein just beneath the liver, and the one which we shall describe here is that established by Blakemore (see Fig. 382a).

Technic of Portacaval Shunt. The portal vein and vena cava are best approached with a posterolateral incision by subperiosteal excision of the right ninth rib, although a lower incision may be utilized. The anterior approach is much more difficult technically. The duodenum, common bile duct, and gallbladder are pushed forward by gentle dissection, the portal vein and vena cava isolated at that site where they run parallel and in juxtaposition. Because of the danger of long occlusion of the vena cava, continuity of circulation in this vein is maintained by the use of a modified clamp after the type used by Potts in operations upon the thoracic aorta. The circulation in the portal vein is occluded by bull dog clamps above and below the site of anastomosis (see Fig. 382a). A single row of continuous mattress sutures of fine silk is used producing an intima-to-intima contact after the method of Blalock in his operation for pulmonic stenosis. As soon as the anastomosis is established, the clamps are removed from the portal vein, and then from the vena cava. Thrombosis is rare, due to the fairly rapid circulation of the vena cava. There is an immediate adjustment of pressures so that the pressure in the portal vein becomes almost identical to that in the vena cava, as can be measured by manometers placed in radicals of the portal vein before closure of the abdomen.

Although this procedure has, at the present writing, been performed in a relatively small number of patients, and the time during which they have

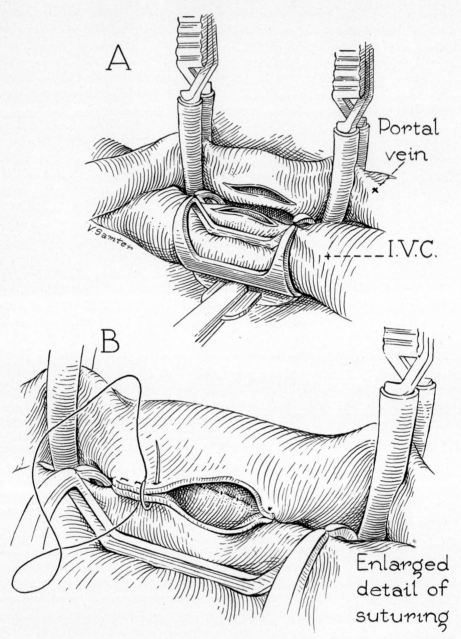

Fig. 382a. Side-to-side portacaval anastomosis utilizing the principles advocated by Blakemore.

been observed is relatively short, it probably represents the best direct approach to the problem in the performance of a portacaval shunt.

Splenectomy for Portal Hypertension. The second general approach toward the lowering of portal tension, as mentioned above, has had to do with

the excision of viscera which drain into the portal vein. The most classical of
these is that of splenectomy. It has been estimated by some that approximately 40 per cent of the blood going to the portal vein has its origin from
the spleen; and it, therefore, would seem that excision of the spleen would
offer considerable relief in the symptoms resulting from portal hypertension

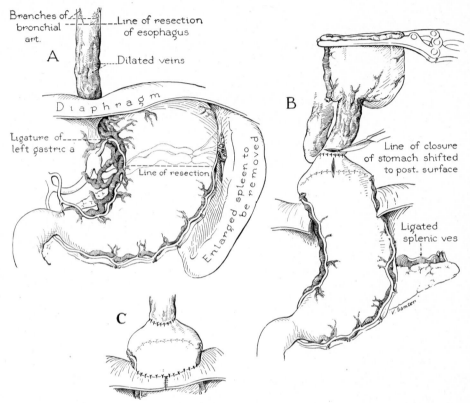

FIG. 382b. Resection of upper half of stomach and distal end of esophagus for hemorrhage from esophageal varices. A. After exposure through a combined thoraco-abdominal
incision the left gastric artery and vein are ligated and the stomach transected at its midportion; B. After removal of the spleen the esophagus is anastomosed to the stomach;
C. After completion of the anastomosis the diaphragm is anchored to the stump of
stomach to prevent herniation.

as well as those from congestive splenomegaly. For a number of years now
splenectomy has been performed particularly in those patients in whom the
symptoms of congestive splenomegaly have been dominant and in whom
functional liver damage has been minimal. By and large, the results have
been good for only a relatively short length of time. The effect of splenectomy on esophageal varices and ascites has been most disappointing. While
the use of this procedure is dramatic when the hypertension is limited to
the splenic vein, used elsewhere its limitations are so great as to raise some
question as to the advisability of its use as a sole procedure.

Gastrectomy and Resection of Distal End of Esophagus for Portal Hypertension. Recently Phemister and Humphreys [4] reported two instances of a more aggressive approach in such visceral excision. One consisted of a total gastric resection and the other of resection of the lower esophagus and upper stomach. The immediate results in both of these patients were good. Both operations were performed for massive hemorrhage from esophageal varices, and subsequent hemorrhage was completely alleviated in both instances.

Recently, we have modified the procedure of Phemister and Humphreys slightly to include the lower portion of the esophagus, the upper half of the stomach, and the spleen. The technic which we have used is illustrated in figure 382b.

The left eighth rib is removed subperiosteally with an incision carried from the angle to the costal cartilage. The suspensory ligament of the lower lobe of the left lung is sectioned and the lung reflected upward. The abdomen is opened by a radial incision through the diaphragm with or without previous paralysis of the left phrenic nerve. Because of the large number of fragile veins, it is wise first to approach the spleen from behind. The splenic artery is ligated proximal to the origin of the vasa brevia and the left gastroepiploic. This artery often is as much as twice its normal diameter, and double ligation is advisable. The left gastro-epiploic artery and vein are ligated at a point about opposite the level of the origin of the left gastric artery. If there is evidence of varicosities involving the entire stomach wall, more stomach may be removed. The splenic vein is doubly ligated and the spleen removed. By gentle dissection the left gastric artery is brought into view just beyond its origin from the celiac and doubly ligated. The mediastinal pleura is now reflected off from the esophagus about 10 centimeters above the diaphragm at the level of rich blood supply to the esophagus from branches of the bronchial artery. The large veins which exist behind and to the right of the esophagus are then doubly ligated. The coronary vein is then ligated just before it enters the portal. It then is possible to excise huge masses of dilated veins along the course of the coronary without a considerable loss of blood. The stomach then is sectioned at the mid-portion of the body and the mucosa closed with a running suture of very fine catgut. This is best done without clamps on the lower segment in order to visualize properly the presence of intragastric varicosities which might be left behind. If such varicosities are seen, the stomach necessarily will have to be resected at a lower site. Serosa is brought to serosa on the stomach by interrupted mattress sutures of fine silk. The upper portion of the stomach and the lower esophagus are gently lifted from their beds and a row of interrupted sutures of fine silk placed transversely between the esophagus and stomach well in front of the previous gastric suture line. A longitudinal incision then is made in the stomach and an inner row of sutures placed between the esophagus and stomach with fine mattress silk. The esophagus then is transected and the outer row of fine silk sutures continued. The stomach is brought well up into the mediastinum in order that there be no tension and the diaphragm closed. The stomach wall is sutured to the diaphragm in order to prevent subsequent

herniation. The lung is expanded, the thoracic incision closed with interrupted silk, and a Foley catheter inserted through a small (air tight) intercostal incision and the catheter connected to a small flask of water and all
pneumothorax relieved. This tube generally is withdrawn within 24 to 48
hours.

Because it is necessary to sacrifice both vagus nerves, Urecholine generally is administered hypodermically and later given by mouth. The patient
is started on liquid diet usually in 48 hours.

We have not been able, as yet, to observe a considerable group of patients
in which this procedure has been performed for a long enough time to express
a final opinion. Where the operation is performed properly and all varicosities removed, subsequent gastric hemorrhage is alleviated. Obviously, the
effects of congestive splenomegaly also are done away with. We have been
pleased to observe the disappearance of ascites in every instance in which
it has been present. All of the patients have been able to resume their work
and have gained weight. Because of the importance of nutrition in cirrhosis
of the liver, this has been most satisfying.

Discussion of Relative Values of Various Operative Procedures. Less
drastic approaches to the relief of gastric and esophageal hemorrhage from
varicose veins by ligation of the veins or injection with sclerosing substances,
in our experience, have been futile. Attempts to relieve ascites by the insertion of glass buttons have been at the best of only temporary value in
establishing such relief, and we doubt seriously their indication.

The underlying pathologic disease producing intrahepatic origin of
portal hypertension always is of a serious nature. The most common cause
is that of fibrosis of a progressive sort which may have its origin from several
underlying causes. This picture of cirrhosis of the liver is, at the present
writing, a most confused one. As new light is being shed upon the subject,
the historical classifications of the disease seem no longer to hold. Because
a detailed discussion of the disease would be most involved, it cannot be
considered here. Suffice it to say, in every instance where the condition has
progressed to the extent that there is a marked increase in portal pressures,
liver function is considerably altered. Oftentimes the intensity of liver
damage cannot be ascertained by the common laboratory tests of liver function. The liver function may be compensated adequately in the face of
severe disease and yet decompensate within a very short interval. We have on
numerous occasions encountered situations in which extensive cirrhosis of
the liver was present but all functional tests within normal limits. It is
assumed that in these instances the hepatic arterial circulation has been the
compensating mechanism. As yet, one has no way of knowing when this
compensating circulation, however, will become embarrassed. We have
come to feel more and more insecure by relying on so many of the present
functional tests. There are two such estimations, however, which seem to be
of considerable value. The most important of these is the ability of the liver
to synthesize albumin. When the level of albumin in the blood is markedly
diminished, surgery of any sort becomes exceedingly hazardous. Another

test that has proven to be of clinical value has been the ability of the liver to excrete bromsulfalein from the blood stream. Where the liver damage is great enough to have a level of bromsulfalein of as much as 40 per cent left in the blood stream thirty minutes after injection, we are loath to advocate extensive surgery of any sort.

It must be understood that both the portacaval shunt and the massive resection of esophageal and gastric tissue and the spleen are at the present time hazardous procedures. They should never be undertaken lightly. Perhaps the best indication for either of them is impending death from massive hemorrhage from esophageal varices. Where this situation co-exists in a patient with compensated liver function, the indication for such surgery is greatest. Which of the particular procedures is preferable, it is impossible to state at the present writing. It is well to consider the habitus of the patient, the technical skill of the surgeon, and many other individual factors.

It also is well to remember that the surgery of portal hypertension, as described above, may influence the preservation of liver function but little. Progressive decompensation of liver function, therefore, often continues; and the main function of the surgical procedure is that of maintaining comfortable existence for a longer period of time. At its best then, it is surgery of desperation. Eventually the best treatment of portal hypertension will be its prevention.

REFERENCES

1. WHIPPLE, ALLEN O. The Problem of Portal Hypertension in Relation to the Hepatosplenapothies, *Ann. Surg.*, 122:449-473, 1945.
2. WHIPPLE, G. H., ROBSCHPIT-ROBBINS, F. S. and HAWKINS, W. B. Eck Fistula Liver Subnormal in Producing Hemoglobin and Plasma Proteins on Diets Rich in Liver and Iron, *J. Exp. Med.*, 81:171-191, 1945.
3. BLAKEMORE, ARTHUR H. and LORD, JERE W. The Technic of Using Vitallium Tubes in Establishing Portacaval Shunts in Portal Hypertension, *Ann. Surg.*, 122:476, 1945.
   WHIPPLE, ALLEN O. The Rationale of Portacaval Anastomosis, *Bull. New York Acad. Med.*, 251, 1946.
   BLAKEMORE, ARTHUR H. Portacaval Anastomosis for the Relief of Portal Hypertension, *Gastroenterology*, 11:488, 1948.
   BLAKEMORE, ARTHUR H. The Portacaval Shunt in the Surgical Treatment of Portal Hypertension, *Ann. Surg.*, 128:825, 1948.
4. PHEMISTER, DALLAS B. and HUMPHREYS, ELEANOR M. Gastroesophageal Resection and Total Gastrectomy in the Treatment of Bleeding Varicose Veins in Banti's Syndrome, *Ann. Surg.*, 126:397, 1947.

17

ABDOMINAL HERNIA

Edwin P. Lehman, B.A., M.D. and Charles E. Davis, Jr., M.D.

INTRODUCTION

Operation for hernia has two phases, the treatment (usually the excision) of the sac and the repair of the defect through which the hernia has passed. These may be of varying importance in different types of hernia. In principle it can be said that in hernia of congenital origin the treatment of the sac is of the first importance, whereas in acquired hernia it is the treatment of the defect. Since an acquired hernia may occur following operation for congenital hernia, the repair of the defect must be a part of treatment in both types.

A sound surgical technic is the *sine qua non* of successful hernia surgery. The maintenance of asepsis, the division of tissues with sharp instruments, the minimum of dissection for the accomplishment of a specific purpose, complete hemostasis, the strangulation of the smallest possible amount of tissue by ligatures and sutures, the minimal tension of sutures, and the use of interrupted sutures of the finest nonabsorbable material adapted to the purpose at hand are all essential elements in this technic which need not be further described here. In many illustrations and descriptions of hernia operations, whether diagrammatic or not, there is presented a complete anatomical dissection of all layers for a considerable distance around the central point of operation. For instance, certain authors advise that the external oblique aponeurosis be cleaned of all fat and areolar tissue from the inguinal ligament to the edge of the rectus muscle. This offers a demonstration which is more fitted to the anatomical laboratory than to the operating room. The limitation of dissection to the minimal needs of orientation and repair means in the above example that only that portion of the external oblique aponeurosis be cleaned of fat that is to be imbricated as the deep layer. In the illustrations accompanying the following descriptions of operations an attempt to maintain this principle has been made.

Descriptions of operations for hernia are necessarily somewhat standardized on the basis of the normal anatomy of the structures concerned. Since the presence of a hernia, particularly one of long standing or large size, distorts normal relationships, the operator must vary standardized procedures to fit the pathological state encountered. Such variations are often an index of the experience and ingenuity of the surgeon. A number of the commoner variations from the standardized operations are so frequently useful that they are included in this chapter.

The custom of applying to certain operations the names of the surgeons who first described them is fixed in the literature of hernia. The terms "Bassini operation," "Ferguson operation," etc. have become established. The development of surgery, however, and the application of many minds to the problems of hernia have resulted in variations in practice from the original descriptions. In fact, almost every surgeon varies the technical minutiae of standard operative principles on the basis of his own training and experience. In this text, therefore, the authors have been careful to use terms such as "Bassini principle," "Halsted principle," etc. in order not to imply that the operations described follow faithfully the originals. After all, the principles involved are the most important contributions of the pioneer surgeons whose names it is proper thus to honor.

Preoperative preparation and postoperative care in hernia surgery have no individual deviations from standard practice. In the experience of others, as well as ourselves, early postoperative ambulation seems not only adaptable to but also a great advantage in the surgery of hernia. It is too early to attempt a final appraisal of its value since its effect on the late recurrence rate is not as yet known. For non-strangulated hernia in good-risk cases the choice of anesthetic is immaterial; the surgeon may be guided by his individual choice.

The descriptions in this chapter are limited to operations for the common hernias of the abdominal wall. Diaphragmatic hernia is included in the chapter on surgery of the chest; and strangulated hernia and internal concealed hernia are included in the chapter on surgery of the intestine. The rare hernias of the abdominal wall, such as the obturator, lumbar, sciatic, etc., have been omitted because of the limitations of space and the necessity for describing in greater detail the more common types. Excellent descriptions of these uncommon hernias may be found in Watson's monograph.[21] The operations to follow have with few exceptions been employed by the authors as described and represent in their opinion a repertory of technical devices adequate to permit the repair of any individual hernia.

INDICATIONS AND CONTRAINDICATIONS

In general, the diagnosis of hernia is an indication for operation. There are, however, conditions that modify this general principle and serve as contraindications of varying importance. These, in turn, are nullified by a single absolute indication for operation, namely, strangulation. The history or the observation of incarceration or the complaint of incapacitating pain may also serve as strong reasons to override otherwise compelling contraindications.

To assert that the diagnosis of hernia makes operation justifiable in the absence of complications is not always helpful, since the diagnosis, particularly in the case of inguinal hernia, is often uncertain. A surgeon is well advised not to perform operation for hernia unless he can be sure that a sac is present. The problem has not been simplified by the unfortunately popular terms "potential hernia" and "dilated external ring" applied to large rings. No ring, of course, has been dilated except by the repeated passage through it of the content of an easily diagnosed hernia. A large ring without definite hernia is of congenital origin. It may be an index of poor development of other structures and hence may often be associated with a persistent processus vaginalis. But, of itself, a large external ring does not mean hernia and is not an indication for operation.

A further complicating factor is the attitude of industry. Since in most courts hernia is compensable if it appears initially during work, industrial employers rarely take the chance of hiring men who in their opinions might develop hernia. As a result applicants for employment, who have been denied urgently necessary jobs because of large external rings, may come to the surgeon demanding repair. The decision is a difficult one if examination reveals only a large ring with no evidence of a hernia sac. The sound surgical principle is to avoid even the slight risk of operation under such circumstances. The desperate economic plight of the patient may move the surgeon in rare instances to violate his surgical conscience. In these instances the least he can do is to make the reasons for operation unmistakably clear to the patient. The young surgeon must be warned that this type of compromise with surgical principles is in general a dangerous practice.

In the presence of a single proven inguinal hernia for which operation is being carried out, the decision as to whether to operate also on the opposite side presents its own problems. Since the danger from the anesthetic is not usually appreciably affected by the duration of the operation within ordinary limits, this decision is less difficult than when one must decide for or against any operation. Bilaterally persistent processus vaginalis is common as are bilaterally deficient fascial and muscular structures. Operation limited to one side is, therefore, occasionally followed at some later time by the appearance of a hernia on the opposite side. These considerations justify an attack on the clinically uninvolved side on the slightest indication of poor structures. Of these, the large external ring is the commonest and most obvious. As their experience has increased, the authors have tended to perform bilateral operations more and more frequently when a single hernia is diagnosed.

The age of the patient, particularly at the extremes of life, must be considered in planning operation. Contrary to a certain body of surgical thought, operation for hernia in earliest infancy is not contraindicated by the danger of postoperative wound soiling or by the small size of the structures. The former can be prevented by an adequately occlusive dressing of silver foil attached with collodion, liquid adhesive or one of the newer plastic glues. If one should not operate on hernia in infancy because of the size of the structures concerned, then most ophthalmic surgery is unjustified. There is, however, a sound reason for delaying the repair of uncomplicated inguinal and umbilical hernias in infancy. Both result from a failure of prenatal development. This failure may be only a delay, and the further steps of development, particularly the obliteration of the sac, may take place after birth. The latter can occur only if the sac is kept empty. A processus vaginalis or an umbilical sac filled with omentum or bowel will not become obliterated spontaneously in the normal manner. If one is to delay operation, therefore, it is essential that the hernia be kept reduced constantly by a proper apparatus. In umbilical hernia, the commonly employed adhesive strapping to approximate the rectus abdominis muscles is effective. In inguinal hernia, a well-fitted truss of the usual type or the simpler yarn truss may be employed. In both cases, the surgeon must be convinced that the mother is intelligent and conscientious enough to use the appliance correctly. The danger of strangulation under a truss is real. There are several indications for the abandonment of such conservative treatment no matter how young the child. These include strangulation, irreducibility, a large musculo-fascial defect, ineffectiveness of the retaining apparatus and psychological deficiencies of the responsible parent. In such instances, operation should be promptly performed.

At the other extreme of life, ordinary surgical judgment governs. The risk of operation in old age has often been exaggerated; the risk lies in the concomitant degenerations and diseases of senility rather than in operation itself. The life-expectancy curve of individuals undergoing elective operation in the older age-groups does not greatly differ from the curve without operation. It is, therefore, proper to operate electively for hernia at advanced ages, provided only that careful appraisal be first made by hospital study of the functional capacity of the heart, lungs, peripheral vessels and kidneys. The comfort that can be given to aged men by the repair of hernia is often worth the risk involved. If there is strangulation, any risk must be taken. If there is incapacitating discomfort, only severe functional deficiencies in vital systems should serve to contraindicate surgical attack.

At any age, the preoperative study of the patient to determine operability must be complete. Nothing need be said here of the common physical defects that affect decision for or against any elective operation. The surgical treatment of hernia, except when strangulated, is clearly an elective procedure and therefore should be carried out only when conditions are as favorable as possible. A specific problem in choosing the time for operation is chronic cough, not only because of the risk of dehiscence of a suture line but also on account of increased postoperative discomfort and the danger of postoperative pulmonary complications. It is well to make a determined effort, in association with the internist and possibly even with the thoracic surgeon and otolaryngologist, to abolish or diminish cough before operation, even if weeks of delay ensue.

An additional contraindication to elective operation is one which is less and less commonly encountered in inguinal hernia but still occasionally encountered in umbilical and postoperative ventral hernia, namely, large size combined with irreducibility. In huge hernias which cannot be reduced by manipulation before operation, the surgeon must keep in mind the possibility that reduction will be impossible at operation. When much of the abdominal content has escaped and has not been replaced for months or years, the fasciae and muscles of the abdominal wall shorten and the capacity of the cavity is permanently decreased. An attempt to crowd intestine into the narrowed space, if not physically impossible, often results in severe postoperative reactions and may terminate in a fatality. It is occasionally necessary to refuse relief of any sort except external support to these neglected cases.

Finally, occupation may have a modifying effect on indications for elective operation. The sedentary individual without discomfort may be refused operation because of complicating diseases of less importance than the workman whose livelihood depends on muscular effort.

INDIRECT AND DIRECT INGUINAL HERNIA

The Approach. The approach to inguinal hernia, as well as often to femoral hernia, opens the inguinal canal through the external ring and the external oblique aponeurosis. The first structure to be identified is the pubic spine. The external ring lies in the adult about 1 inch cephalad and 1 inch lateral to this point. The inguinal ligament, from the pubic spine to the anterior-superior spine of the ilium, parallels the direction of the fibers of the external oblique aponeurosis. The incision is made about 1 inch mesial to and parallel to the inguinal ligament from the pubic spine to a point slightly more than halfway the distance from the latter to the anterior-superior spine (Fig. 383).

The incision is carried down through the superficial fascial layers to the external oblique aponeurosis which, at this stage of the operation, is cleaned only sufficiently to permit identification of the external ring. The exposed skin is then walled out of the operative field by the attachment of towels (Fig. 384). The edge of the external ring is defined by thrusting a blunt object, such as the handle of the knife or the finger, into the ring and lifting upward. The external oblique aponeurosis is opened along the line of its fibers upward to the limit of the incision and downward to divide the intercolumnar fibers, including the free border of the external ring. In this maneuver great care must be exercised to avoid injury to the ilio-inguinal nerve (Fig. 385). The canal may then be spread open either by the application of fine hemostats or fine silk or cotton traction sutures (Fig. 402) to the divided borders of the external oblique aponeurosis. The ilio-inguinal nerve is carefully dissected from its bed and held out of harm's way by placing it behind one of the hemostats or traction sutures on the mesial leaf of the external oblique aponeurosis (Fig. 386). In conforming to the principle of minimal dissection, the iliohypogastric nerve, which emerges from the internal oblique muscle at a higher level, is rarely seen. If it becomes necessary to dissect more widely, the location of this nerve must be remembered. At this stage further procedure depends on the type of hernia under attack.

Indirect Inguinal Hernia. THE SAC. After opening the inguinal canal as described above, a search for an indirect sac is always indicated irrespective of the preoperative diagnosis, since the clinical differentiation between direct and indirect hernia is often inaccurate. The cremaster muscle surrounding the cord presents in the exposed portion of the inguinal canal, appearing at the edge of the internal oblique muscle and disappearing at the

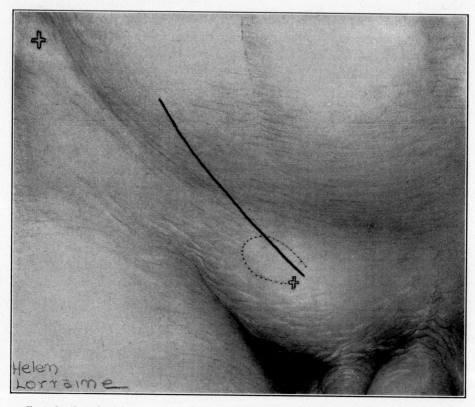

FIG. 383. Inguinal hernia. Skin incision for opening the inguinal canal. The approximate position of the external ring is indicated by the dotted line.

lower limit of the incision beneath the fat. This structure is picked up and incised in the direction of its fibers. Beneath it there may immediately be found a glistening white structure which is recognized as the peritoneal sac, the usual position of which is on the anteromesial aspect of the cord (Fig. 386). On other occasions the surgeon may have to search almost to the internal ring before the sac is found. In such instances it is sometimes possible that an artificial sac may be created by traction on the cord which pulls down the adherent parietal peritoneum into a small knuckle. During this dissection great care must be exercised to avoid damage to the spermatic artery, pampiniform plexus, and vas deferens. If a vein is wounded, it must immediately be seized with a fine hemostat and ligated. If the sac is found early, the cord structures are more completely protected by opening it and dissecting close to the outer surface of the peritoneal layer. Fingers or a gauze sponge are employed to define the extent of the sac from within. The sac will usually separate easily from the areolar tissue of the cord except at two points. At the lower pole in the position of the obliterated processus vaginalis there are usually adhesions. At the upper pole near the neck the relationship of the vas to the sac becomes increasingly intimate, and sepa-

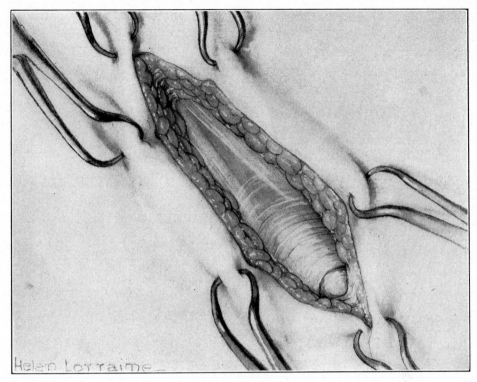

Helen Lorraine

Fig. 384. Inguinal hernia. The skin and subcutaneous tissue have been divided. Note limited exposure of the external oblique aponeurosis and protection of the wound from skin contact with drapes. The external ring with intercolumnar fibers is exposed. A partial split often seen in the external oblique aponeurosis is indicated. (For the sake of simplicity the covering of the skin has been omitted in subsequent illustrations but it is understood to be always applied.)

ration must be carried out with increasing care. All properitoneal fat, which may be so localized as to suggest a lipoma, must be removed during this dissection.

If after careful search of the cord no indirect sac is found and there is no bulging in Hesselbach's triangle, the fibers of the internal oblique and transversalis muscles should be split above the level of the internal ring and the peritoneum opened as in a McBurney abdominal incision. Examination of the hernia area with the finger inside the peritoneum will reveal the opening of a sac, as well as the strength of the floor of the inguinal canal. If no sac is found by this maneuver, the symptoms and signs of hernia were probably caused by the prolapse of properitoneal fat through the external ring. It should be noted that LaRoque [14] and others proposed the above approach as the best means of handling the sac neck in many cases. In such operations the sac opening is closed from the peritoneal side.

After the sac has been completely isolated and the structures at its neck freed from the peritoneum, the internal ring is recognized, usually marked by a slight thickening of the neck of the sac and a glistening white band on

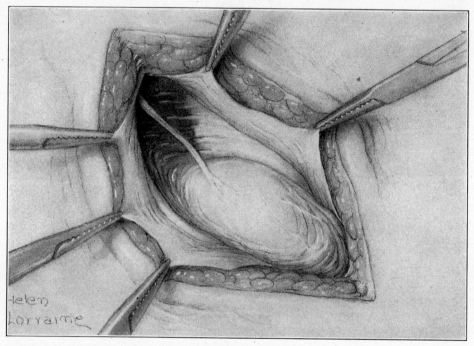

Fig. 385. Inguinal hernia. The external oblique aponeurosis has been divided in the direction of its fibers from the upper end of the incision through the external ring and the edges are spread apart by fine hemostats using small bites, attached to the divided borders. The position of the ilio-inguinal nerve is indicated, as well as a general bulging below the border of the internal oblique muscle which indicates the presence of a hernia.

the peritoneal surface. With traction on the sac the dissection should be carried so high that the final position of the internal ring is actually 1 to 2 centimeters superficial to its normal level, with the resulting production of an artificial neck, consisting of the nearby parietal peritoneum (Fig. 387). This maneuver insures high ligation of the neck and absence of a post-operative pouch on the inside of the peritoneal cavity. To accomplish this high dissection the internal oblique muscle must be sharply retracted.

The open end of the sac is now widely spread so that a complete inspection of its interior is possible. Adhesions of omentum or bowel or a sliding hernia of bladder or bowel are sought. Adhesions are carefully freed with ligation of all bleeding points, and the liberated sac content is dropped back into the abdomen. Excess omentum may be amputated distal to ligatures. If a sliding hernia of the bowel is found, a special procedure to be described later is indicated.

When the sac is empty, a fine needle carrying fine silk or cotton is introduced through the neck of the sac proximal to the original level of the internal ring under direct vision within the sac so as to avoid injury to intra-

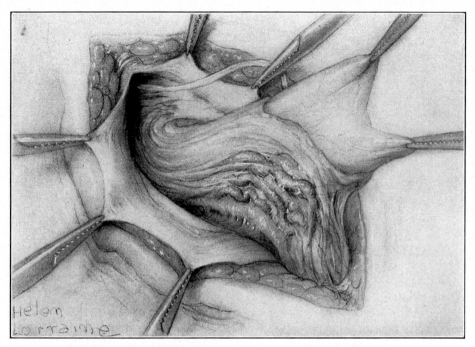

FIG. 386. Indirect inguinal hernia. Dissection of the sac. The ilio-inguinal nerve has been dissected free and has been displaced behind a clamp placed on the mesial border of the external oblique aponeurosis. The cremaster muscle has been incised, and the external surface of the sac has been identified. The sac is being drawn out of the incision in the cremaster muscle preparatory to opening it and completing its dissection. The position of the vas deferens is indicated.

abdominal structures (Fig. 387). This suture is tied with care not to include omentum or bowel within it. At this point one may twist the sac by rotation about its long axis so as to prevent escape of abdominal content while the ligation of the rest of the neck is carried out. The latter consists in passing the already anchored suture completely around the neck of the sac and tightening it again proximal to the level of the internal ring. It is well not to tie the second loop of the knot until after amputation of the sac. The neck of the sac should next be divided about 0.5 centimeter distal to the ligature with care to avoid accidental division of the latter. If tension is kept on the first loop of the knot while the sac neck is being cut, there is usually a little extra give which can be taken up before throwing the second loop. With the completion of this maneuver and the removal of the retractor from the edge of the internal oblique muscle, the ligated neck of the sac retracts out of sight beneath the muscle, leaving the two ends of the ligature projecting (Fig. 388).

Since the prevention of recurrence of hernia probably depends on conditions which prevent its beginning rather than on the strength of the

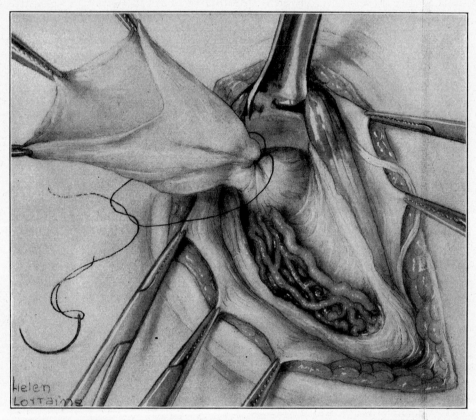

FIG. 387. Indirect inguinal hernia. The cremaster muscle has been widely split, and the structures of the cord, including the vas, are lying at the bottom of the canal. The internal oblique muscle has been sharply retracted upward. The former position of the internal ring in relation to the sac neck is indicated by a slight constriction. A transfixion suture has been passed and tied once above the neck, and the final tie is about to be made below. After the first loop of the knot, the sac will be amputated about 1/2 centimeter distal to the ligature. After taking up any additional slack, the knot will be completed.

structures which might hinder its progress later, it is a general principle that the most proximal weak spots should be most completely protected. The proximal weak spot after the removal of an indirect inguinal hernia sac is at the peritoneal position of the former neck, where there remains a small dimple the direction of which is down the canal. An attempt to direct any potential thrust against a stronger area of the abdominal wall may be made by anchoring the stump of the neck of the sac high beneath the internal oblique muscle [13] (Fig. 388). To accomplish this purpose each end of the ligature projecting from the divided sac neck is threaded on a half-round medium curved needle which is then insinuated carefully between the fibers of the internal oblique muscle, with special care to avoid the ilio-inguinal nerve. The needle is passed eye-first in order to avoid the danger of dividing any small vessel within the substance of the muscle. After the

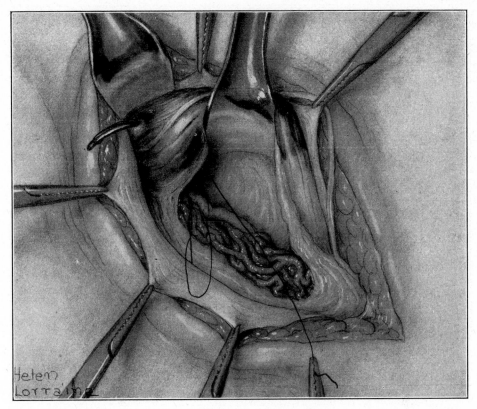

FIG. 388. Indirect inguinal hernia. Transplantation of the stump of the sac. The sac has been amputated, and the stump has retracted beneath the internal oblique muscle. One end of the transfixion ligature is held in a clamp, and the other end has been partially passed through the fibers of the internal oblique muscle on a needle directed eye-first. The remaining end will be carried through at a short distance from the first, and the two ends will be tied together, anchoring the residual dimple on the peritoneal surface firmly under the muscle.

two ends have thus been placed through the internal oblique a short distance apart, they are tied together and cut short. This has the effect of placing strong muscle over any residual pouch of the peritoneum remaining after the ligation of the sac neck.

The treatment of the sac described above is, of course, limited to sacs which are not of congenital type, i.e., which are not continuous with the tunica vaginalis. The general principle of the treatment of the congenital sac is to divide it in the middle, dissect the upper end as though one were dealing with the ordinary indirect inguinal sac, as described above, and treat the lower end either by ignoring it completely (Fig. 389) or by everting it over the testis (bottle operation). Elevation and freeing of the testis, procedures which are needed to make possible the bottle operation, are rarely justified, since the distal open sac does not usually give trouble. When the lower end

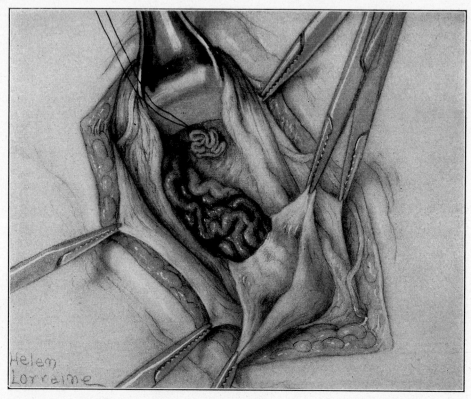

Fig. 389. Indirect inguinal hernia. Congenital sac. The sac has been separated from the structures of the cord and transected. Dissection of the proximal portion with ligation and division of the neck has been carried out, as already described, and the stump of the neck can now be transplanted beneath the internal oblique muscle. The distal portion of the sac is wide open. The clamps are to be removed, and the sac allowed to retract towards the scrotum without further treatment. This is preferable to the extensive dissection and mobilization of the testis which must precede the "bottle operation."

of the sac has been dropped back into the wound, it disappears into the scrotum.

Since the peritoneum is always closely applied to the elements of the cord, separation of the congenital sac from the cord may be difficult, especially in a small child where the wall of the sac is excessively thin. In dividing such a sac across the middle there is, therefore, grave danger of wounding the cord. A useful maneuver to protect the structures of the cord is to infiltrate beneath the peritoneum with normal salt solution, using a hypodermic needle. The wheal so created actually dissects the peritoneum from the cord structures so that the former may be divided without risk to the vas or vessels (Fig. 390).

THE REPAIR. An operation for indirect inguinal hernia which includes high extirpation of the sac and transplantation of its stump is rarely followed by a recurrence of the hernia as an indirect hernia. If recurrence takes place it is apt to occur through the floor of the canal as a direct hernia.

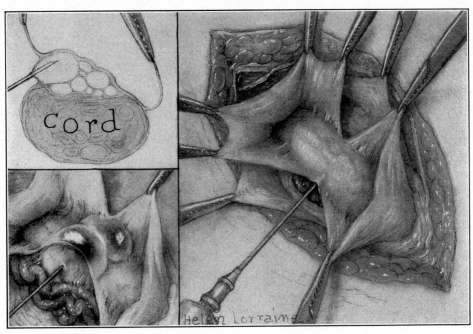

FIG. 390. Indirect inguinal hernia. Congenital sac. Method of facilitating separation of the posterior third of the sac from the structures of the cord preliminary to transection of the sac. A hypodermic needle is introduced just beneath the peritoneum, and wheals of normal saline are formed in this plane. Note cross-section diagram and insert demonstrating wheal formation. After this procedure it becomes possible to divide the peritoneum with less threat to the structures of the cord. The needle shown is of much greater caliber than the hypodermic needle actually employed.

Any operative procedure adopted must, therefore, be chosen with the need in mind to prevent a future direct hernia. There are three main methods of strengthening the inguinal region. In the first, as typified by the Ferguson principle,[8] the cord bears its normal relationship to the floor of the canal, and the weak area is buttressed by bringing the internal oblique and conjoined tendon to the inguinal ligament superficial to the cord. In the second type, typified by the Bassini principle,[3] the floor of the canal is reconstituted by bringing the internal oblique muscle and the conjoined tendon to the inguinal ligament beneath the cord which then leaves the canal through an opening left just below the normal origin of the internal oblique muscle from the inguinal ligament. The result is an increased obliquity of the course of the cord through the parietes. This maneuver and the following are called "transplantation of the cord." In the third method, as typified by the Halsted principle,[12] the cord is brought directly out to the subcutaneous tissue beneath the edge of the internal oblique muscle so that there lies beneath it the internal oblique muscle and conjoined tendon and the external oblique aponeurosis as well. Although Halsted himself later abandoned this principle as a routine procedure, it is still employed occasionally. Whether one is to use the Ferguson type or the Bassini type of repair will depend on the quality of the structures encountered. In a great many instances the internal oblique muscle is weak and the conjoined tendon malformed to the point, even, of absence. In such cases neither type of operation may be possible, and other variations to be described below may have to be employed.

As soon as the sac has been dealt with and hemostasis is complete, the surgeon should appraise the quality of tissues available. The most important fact to determine is the strength and tension of the transversalis fascia making up the posterior wall of Hesselbach's triangle, since, as already stated, the most important part of the repair is the prophylaxis of direct hernia. In those cases of indirect inguinal hernia with a loose, weak or defective transversalis fascia, the Bassini type of operation should always be employed in order to interpose a firm buttress to the first thrust through the weak area. In young individuals with strong musculature and particularly with a strong floor to the canal, the Ferguson type of repair is permissible. The authors are accustomed in all instances in which the Bassini principle of repair is indicated to add a maneuver described by Edmund Andrews [1] which will be referred to below.

FERGUSON PRINCIPLE. The fundamental maneuver of the Ferguson operation consists of approximation of the internal oblique muscle and conjoined tendon to the inguinal ligament superficial to the cord. Interrupted nonabsorbable sutures of fine caliber are passed through the free border of the internal oblique muscle and conjoined tendon and then beneath the inguinal ligament. These sutures begin just below the lowest point of origin of the internal oblique muscle and end at a point sufficiently far above the pubic spine to leave a comfortable exit for the spermatic cord after they are tied. This exit should permit introduction of the tip of the index finger. The sutures take a wide bite of muscle and fascia and a correspondingly wide bite of the inguinal ligament, including perhaps even a little of the origin of the external oblique aponeurosis (Fig. 391). Healing of muscle to fascia takes place only between the fine connective tissue fasciculi of the muscle and the connective tissue of the fascia. For early strong union, therefore, a considerable surface of muscle must be held in contact with the fascia. Such broad approximation is afforded by the use of the large bites illustrated. The sutures should be passed under the inguinal ligament from within outward with traction on the lateral leaf of the aponeurosis so that the immediately underlying external iliac artery and vein are protected from damage. It is highly important that the structures are sufficiently mobile to permit tying the sutures without strangulation

of the embraced tissue. In the event that the conjoined tendon cannot be
brought over without tension, other additional procedures may be employed
as described below.

FIG.
391

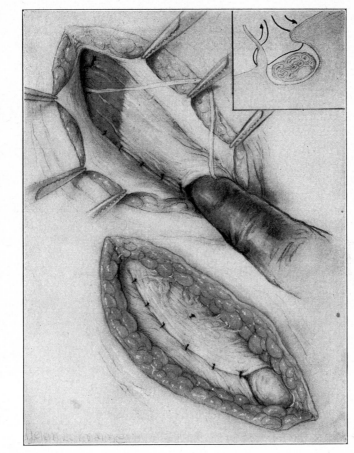

FIG.
392

FIG. 391. Indirect inguinal hernia. Ferguson principle. Sutures uniting the internal
oblique muscle and conjoined tendon to the inguinal ligament have been placed and tied.
There is no tension, and the exposed portion of the sutures is small. The exit for the
cord is tested for capacity with the tip of the finger, which hides the cord beneath it. The
opening shown is larger than that usually made. Insert shows in cross-section diagram
the size of the bites taken and the direction of passing the sutures. It will be seen that
broad approximation between the sutured structures is attempted.

FIG. 392. Indirect inguinal hernia. Ferguson principle. The lateral leaf of the external
oblique aponeurosis has been cleaned and imbricated beneath the mesial leaf with a
mattress suture. The free edge of the mesial leaf has been tacked down to the superficial
surface of the lateral leaf, creating a new external inguinal ring.

The next step is the treatment of the external oblique aponeurosis, the
lateral leaf of which is cleaned of fat so that, on imbrication beneath the
mesial leaf, clean fascial surfaces will be approximated. Following the release
of the ilio-inguinal nerve, the lateral leaf is anchored beneath the mesial leaf

with a single mattress suture. The free edge of the mesial leaf is then attached to the superficial surface of the lateral leaf with multiple interrupted fine sutures creating a new external ring at the lower margin (Fig. 392). Many surgeons close the external oblique aponeurosis by simple approximation sutures without imbrication.

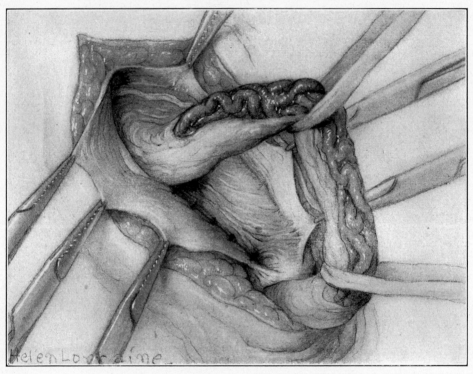

FIG. 393. Indirect inguinal hernia. Bassini principle. The spermatic cord has been freed and elevated. The internal oblique muscle and the conjoined tendon have been united beneath it to the inguinal ligament. Interrupted sutures, passed as illustrated in figure 391, (insert) beginning just above the pubic spine and ending cephalad at a point which leaves an exit for the cord from beneath the internal oblique muscle, have been tied. The most caudad suture grasps also a few fibers of Cooper's ligament. The cord will be dropped down upon this layer and the external oblique aponeurosis imbricated superficially to it. The floor of Hesselbach's triangle has been completely closed.

The subcutaneous tissue is closed with interrupted sutures and the skin with either interrupted or continuous sutures. Closure of the subcutaneous tissue and the skin need not be further mentioned in this chapter, since it is uniform in all hernias.

BASSINI PRINCIPLE. The Bassini operation is carried out in the same way as the Ferguson operation except that the internal oblique muscle and the conjoined tendon are united to the inguinal ligament beneath the spermatic cord. This entails the careful separation of the cremaster muscle from the inguinal ligament in order to permit elevation of the spermatic cord. The latter passes to its position beneath the external oblique aponeurosis through an opening at the upper end of the canal where an arch of the free edge of the internal oblique muscle is constructed by the most cephalad of the sutures that unite the muscle to the ligament. This opening should permit comfortable introduction of the tip of the finger. Caudad, the lowermost suture should be just proximal to the pubic spine and should pick up the upper end of Cooper's ligament so that there is complete closure at the inferior point of Hesselbach's triangle (Fig. 393). The manner of passing the individual sutures is the same as in the Ferguson procedure (Fig. 391, insert).

After release of the ilio-inguinal nerve, the external oblique aponeurosis is imbricated over the cord exactly as it is imbricated over the deep suture line in the Ferguson procedure.

HALSTED PRINCIPLE. In this operation the Bassini principle is employed up to the point of imbrication of the external oblique aponeurosis. Here an exit through that aponeurosis is provided for the cord opposite its exit from beneath the internal oblique muscle, and the external oblique aponeurosis is imbricated beneath the cord, leaving it in a subcutaneous position. A modification, of historic interest only, is the Wyllys Andrews procedure [2] of uniting the edge of the mesial leaf of the external oblique aponeurosis to the under surface of the lateral leaf beneath the cord and bringing the lateral leaf above the cord so that the latter lies between two layers of the aponeurosis.

EDMUND ANDREWS PRINCIPLE. In order to make more effective the strengthening of the posterior wall of the canal as attempted in the Bassini type of operation, a maneuver, originally described by Edmund Andrews [1] as a part of an operation including other features, has been found useful. It consists fundamentally in the pleating or tightening of the transversalis fascia or the closure of a defect therein. Whenever the floor of the canal is so weak that the Bassini principle is to be employed, the authors supplement it by this procedure. The transversalis fascia is identified and cleaned. Its surface is then picked up by interrupted sutures placed not far from the position of the conjoined tendon, which are then passed beneath the inguinal ligament as though a Bassini repair were being done (Fig. 394). When these are tied, there results commonly a strong, tight fascial layer constituting the floor of Hesselbach's triangle. The most caudad of these sutures picks up Cooper's ligament as well as the inguinal ligament. Following this maneuver it is necessary to unite the internal oblique muscle and conjoined tendon to the under surface of the lower leaf of the external oblique aponeurosis slightly mesial to the inguinal ligament which has been preempted by the deeper layer of sutures (Fig. 395).

SPECIAL TECHNICS. In those hernias in which the conjoined tendon is defective either in position, width or substance, closure of the canal may be difficult without too great tension, or even impossible. In all such instances the Bassini principle of transplantation of the cord is to be employed, since the conjoined tendon moves a shorter distance in reaching the inguinal ligament beneath the cord than when placed superficial to it. Even with

this advantage it may not be possible to close the floor of the canal completely. A number of special operative procedures have been devised to
circumvent this difficulty. With the use of one or more of the following it
will usually be possible to close any defect in the inguinal region.

FIG.
394

FIG.
395

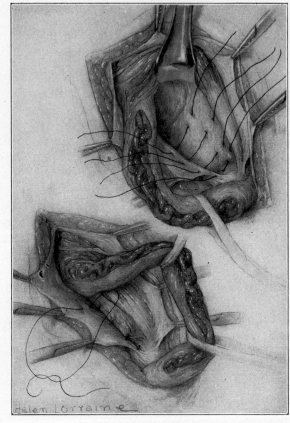

FIG. 394. Indirect inguinal hernia. Edmund Andrews principle. Before making use of
the internal oblique muscle and the conjoined tendon, the transversalis fascia which has
been cleaned of areolar tissue is picked up near the border of the conjoined tendon and
brought over to the inguinal ligament. The lowest suture picks up the origin of Cooper's
ligament.

FIG. 395. Indirect inguinal hernia. Edmund Andrews principle. The transversalis
fascia has been united to the inguinal ligament. The first suture uniting the internal
oblique muscle to the under surface of the lateral leaf of the external oblique aponeurosis
just mesial to the inguinal ligament is shown. Similar sutures are placed down to the
lower limit of the dissection.

Incision of Rectus Fascia. The external oblique fascia is dissected from
the anterior rectus sheath for a distance of about 2 centimeters. An incision
is then made through the rectus sheath parallel to the fibers of the muscle
(Fig. 396). This allows lateral displacement of the border of the rectus
muscle together with the defective conjoined tendon. It will sometimes
permit complete closure of Hesselbach's triangle without tension.

Pedicled Rectus Sheath Flap.[6] After exposing the rectus fascia as above, a quadrilateral flap of rectus sheath is cut on three sides, leaving the outer border of the rectus sheath as a hinge. This is turned over any remaining defect in Hesselbach's triangle and sutured to the inguinal ligament (Figs. 397 and 398).

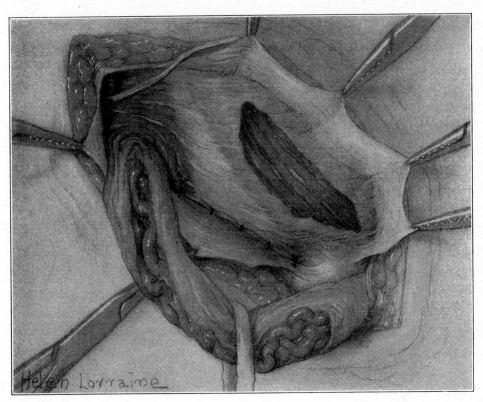

FIG. 396. Indirect inguinal hernia. Incision of the rectus sheath. The anterior sheath of the rectus muscle has been exposed by dissecting away the external oblique aponeurosis mesially. An incision has been made in the sheath parallel to the fibers of the rectus muscle permitting dislocation of the conjoined tendon outward and suture to the inguinal ligament beneath the cord without tension.

Free Fascia or Cutis Graft. If the defect is so large that the pedicled rectus sheath flap will not completely close it, a free graft either of fascia lata or of cutis [7] may be employed. A sheet of fascia or cutis cut to the proper size is sutured to the inguinal ligament, the internal oblique muscle, the conjoined tendon and Cooper's ligament to close the defect completely (Fig. 399). In doubtful cases such a transplant may be used to supplement a pedicled rectus sheath graft.

McArthur Method.[17] In this operation the canal is closed by a pedicled fascial suture or sutures derived from the free edges of the external oblique aponeurosis (Fig. 400). The authors have had no experience with this method.

Gallie and LeMesurier Method.[9] This is similar to the McArthur method except that the fascia is not pedicled and is obtained from the fascia lata. It has the advantage of a more generous supply of suture material. Free fascia may be obtained by either one of two methods. A longitudinal

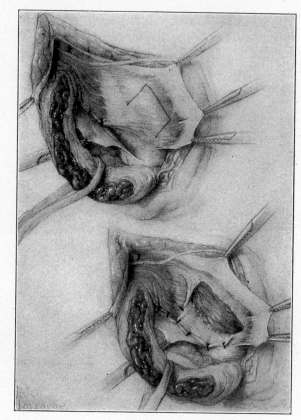

FIG. 397

FIG. 398

FIG. 397. Indirect inguinal hernia. Pedicled rectus sheath flap. The conjoined tendon cannot be brought down to the inguinal ligament without undue tension. The anterior rectus sheath has, therefore, been exposed, and an incision has been made outlining three sides of a rectangular flap.

FIG. 398. Indirect inguinal hernia. Pedicled rectus sheath flap. The rectus sheath flap has been reflected, revealing the fibers of the rectus muscle, and its free edge has been sutured to the inguinal ligament, to complete the closure of the floor of Hesselbach's triangle.

incision exposes the fascia lata from which a large square is excised to be split into suture width before use.[9] In the second method two transverse incisions are made, one just below the greater trochanter and one just above the lateral femoral condyle. These are carried through the fascia lata. The cut edge of the fascia is then ribboned and each ribbon separated from the next by an instrument resembling a vein stripper which is passed from one incision subcutaneously to the other.[15] The authors have not employed the

Gallie principle in the inguinal region but have employed it in ventral hernia (Fig. 401).

Other Methods. Many other methods have been employed for closure of the defect in difficult cases, such as the use of a pedicled fascia lata flap [19]

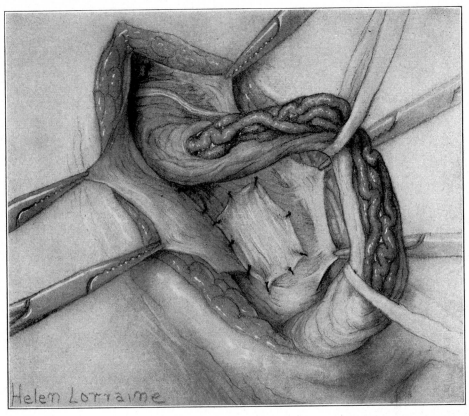

FIG. 399. Indirect inguinal hernia. Free fascia or cutis graft. A free graft has been cut and sutured to the inguinal ligament, the surface of the internal oblique muscle and conjoined tendon, and the beginning of Cooper's ligament. Fascia lata is illustrated, but cutis may also be used.

or of a tantalum mesh. The authors have also had no experience with these methods. As a general surgical principle it is felt that the problem of inguinal hernia should be solved without the necessity of employing a foreign material such as a metal obturator.

Direct Inguinal Hernia. THE SAC. After the canal has been opened, the protrusion caused by a direct inguinal hernia is found projecting from the floor of Hesselbach's triangle mesial to the deep epigastric vessels and beneath the spermatic cord on its mesial aspect. The cremaster is carefully dissected from the inguinal ligament and the cord retracted with a tape. The transversalis fascia is frequently defective in direct inguinal hernia. If it is present, it must be first incised before a search is made for the sac. Since the area of Hesselbach's triangle is one in which a considerable amount of properitoneal fat exists, the sac is usually found deeply buried in adipose tissue (Fig. 402). The treatment of the sac in direct hernia depends somewhat on how well-developed it is. In some instances it may be dissected free and opened and the neck transfixed and ligated, in exactly the same manner as the indirect sac. In other instances where a definite neck is not found the

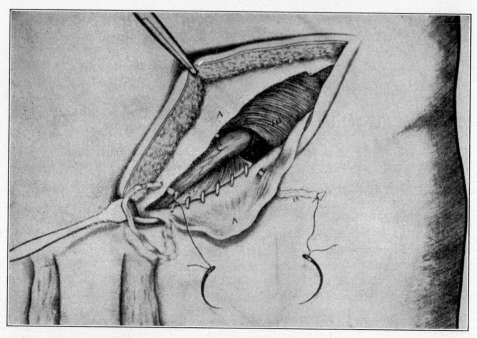

Fig. 400. Indirect inguinal hernia. McArthur method, showing the use of a fascial suture cut from the mesial leaf of the external oblique aponeurosis to unite the conjoined tendon to the inguinal ligament beneath the cord and a suture from the lateral leaf to unite the free borders of the external oblique aponeurosis over the cord. (From McArthur, *J.A.M.A.*, 43:1039, 1904.)

peritoneum may have to be closed as following laparotomy with or without imbrication. In the treatment of the sac one must keep in mind the fact that not infrequently the peritoneal reflection over the bladder is a part of the sac wall and that there is, therefore, a partial sliding hernia of the bladder (Fig. 403). For this reason when the sac is to be opened it should be incised on the lateral side after the fat has been thoroughly cleaned away. In general, to open the sac is the preferable method of treatment when it is well developed. Some surgeons pass purse-string sutures about the bulging portion and suppress the sac by plication without opening it. This method should be reserved for instances of diffuse bulging. In many cases this plication is in fact plication of the transversalis fascia.

THE REPAIR. In direct hernia the strengthening of Hesselbach's triangle is of primary importance and, therefore, the Bassini principle[3] is to be employed. The first step is the closure of the defect in the transversalis fascia. If the fascia is well formed, this may be carried out by imbrication of the borders of the defect. If the lateral border cannot be identified, then the mesial portion of the fascia may be brought over to the inguinal ligament in accordance with the Edmund Andrews principle [1] (Figs. 394 and 395). Following this maneuver the internal oblique muscle and conjoined tendon are brought over to the inguinal ligament as already described (Figs. 393 and

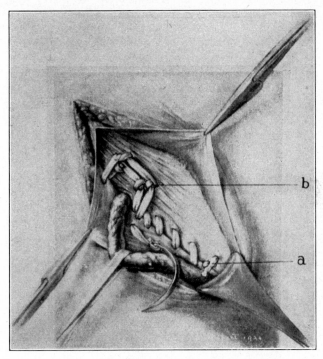

FIG. 401. Indirect inguinal hernia. Gallie and LeMesurier method, showing approximation of the internal oblique muscle and conjoined tendon to the inguinal ligament beneath the cord employing a free fascial suture taken from the fascia lata. (From Gallie and LeMesurier, *Brit. J. Surg.,* 12:289, 1924.)

395). The superficial tissues are closed in the usual way (Fig. 392). Any of the modifications previously illustrated may be employed to close the defect in cases presenting deficient structures.

Combined Direct and Indirect Hernia ("Saddlebag" — "Pantaloon"). THE SAC. In combined direct and indirect hernia two sacs are present, one of the indirect type and one of the direct type, separated by the deep epigastric vessels. This combination may be present in all degrees. It is, therefore, important when either a direct or an indirect sac is opened to search from within the peritoneum for a sac of the other variety (Fig. 404). This is particularly important in the operation for indirect inguinal hernia when the transversalis fascia is found to be weak or defective. In the combined type of hernia the most satisfactory method of treating the sacs is to separate the peritoneum from the deep epigastric vessels and dislocate the neck of the direct sac cephalad so that it presents near the position of the internal

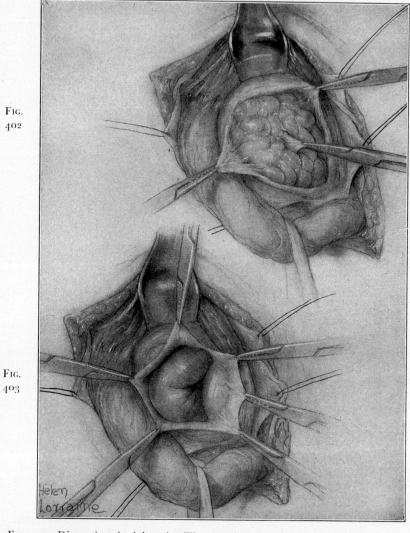

FIG. 402

FIG. 403

FIG. 402. Direct inguinal hernia. The canal has been opened. Note use of traction sutures rather than hemostats in exposing the contents of the canal. The cord has been dissected free and retracted laterally, and the transversalis fascia has been incised. After dissecting through the properitoneal fat, the tip of the sac has been identified and is being drawn outward for further dissection.

FIG. 403. Direct inguinal hernia. The sac has been opened, and an early sliding hernia of the bladder is demonstrated together with a free loop of bowel. This type of sac must be closed as in a laparotomy.

ring (Fig. 405). The double sac neck is then treated as a single indirect sac by transfixion, ligation, excision and transplantation.

THE REPAIR. Repair is made as in direct inguinal hernia.

Inguinal Hernia in the Female. The problem of inguinal hernia in the female is much simplified by the presence of the round ligament instead of

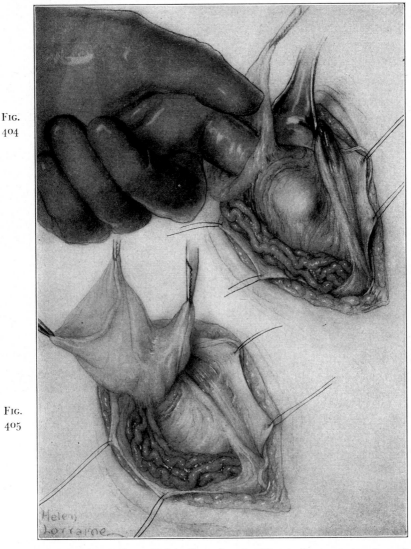

FIG.
404

FIG.
405

FIG. 404. Combined direct and indirect hernia. The indirect sac has been freed and opened, and a finger, thrust beneath the deep epigastric vessels, demonstrates a direct sac.

FIG. 405. Combined direct and indirect hernia. The peritoneum has been separated from the deep epigastric vessels, and the direct sac, unopened, has been dislocated lateral to them. The combined sacs will now be treated as a single sac with transfixion, ligation, amputation and transplantation. Repair will follow the principles of repair of direct inguinal hernia.

the spermatic cord, since no serious results will follow constriction of the former. This means that complete closure of the canal can be made simply by the Ferguson principle without the necessity of leaving a weak spot for exit of the cord. The most caudad suture can be tied snugly down on the round ligament which at that level begins to lose its identity (Fig. 406).

Sliding Hernia. The mechanism of sliding hernia is difficult to visualize. The clearest description of the peritoneal relationships of this type of hernia has been furnished by Graham (Fig. 407) and his article should be read.[11] On opening a sac containing a sliding hernia one finds that a part of the wall

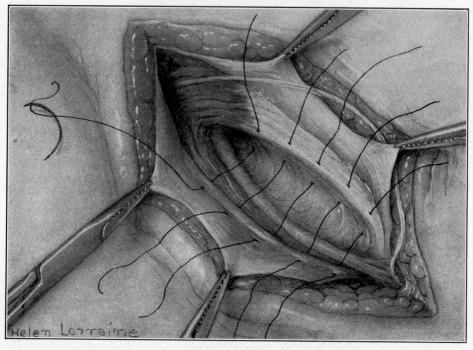

Fig. 406. Inguinal hernia in the female. The sac has been treated as in hernia in the male. Sutures are placed to unite the internal oblique muscle and conjoined tendon to the inguinal ligament snugly from the pubis to the origin of the internal oblique muscle without concern for the round ligament. If the conjoined tendon is not mobile, other maneuvers described earlier can be employed.

consists of bowel with its mesenteric attachment. If one were to open the abdominal cavity without dissection of the inguinal region and deliver the sliding hernia sac into the abdominal cavity by traction on the bowel, the only peritoneal evidence of hernia would be the detachment of a portion of the peritoneum from the vascular layer of the mesentery. In the case of the sigmoid the sac is formed primarily from the outer leaf of its mesentery, and it is here that detachment would be found. Since the diagnosis of sliding hernia is usually not obvious until the sac is opened at operation, delivery of the sac into the abdomen will reveal also a wound in the outer leaf of the mesentery of the sigmoid where the sac was opened in the inguinal canal (Fig. 408). The reduction of the sac by traction on the bowel from within the abdomen is the principle of Graham's operation which the authors have employed. Since the blood supply of the herniated bowel lies in the wall of the sac itself (Fig. 407), the separation of the bowel from the remaining sac is both difficult and unsafe. An operation of the latter nature was described by Bevan [5] and has been used by many surgeons.

GRAHAM PRINCIPLE. The inguinal canal is exposed and the sac identified and opened in the usual way. When a sliding hernia has been diagnosed, a paramedian laparotomy incision is made, and the cecum or sigmoid is

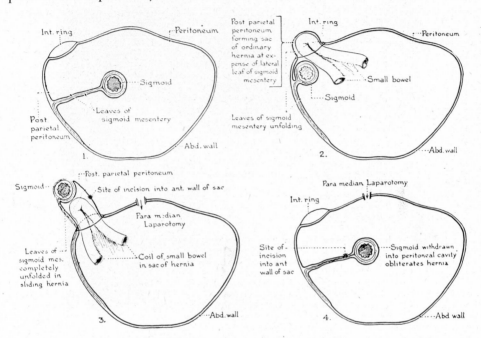

FIG. 407. Sliding hernia. Genesis and anatomy as illustrated by Graham.[11] Note the relationship of the mesenteric vessels to the peritoneal lining of the sac, and the part played by the outer leaf of the mesentery in forming the sac. Note also the final position of the exploratory opening in the sac after the sigmoid has been withdrawn from the inguinal canal. (See Fig. 408). (From Graham, *Ann. Surg.*, 102:784, 1935.)

identified and drawn through the abdominal wound. The delivery of the bowel reveals the situation previously described, namely a rent in the outer leaf of its mesentery representing the incision made in the peritoneum of the sac while it was in the inguinal canal. The neighboring peritoneum of the outer leaf of the mesentery, together with the bowel itself and often a part of the inner leaf, has constituted the wall of the sac before delivery. Treatment consists in suturing the rent in the mesentery and repairing the inguinal canal in the usual way, together with closure of the laparotomy wound.

Graham's method is particularly adapted to large sliding hernias. In small sliding hernias in which the bowel is just entering the sac, treatment of the sac may be effected through the inguinal exposure alone by pushing the bowel as high as possible and imbricating the rest of the sac distal to its attachment.

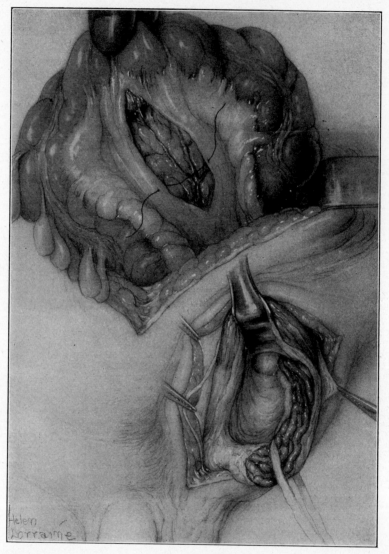

FIG. 408. Sliding hernia. Graham principle. The hernia sac has been identified, the cremaster muscle and sac have been opened, and the latter has been found to contain a sliding hernia. A left paramedian laparotomy incision has been made and the sigmoid withdrawn from the inguinal region, carrying the sac with it. (See Fig. 407). When this has been done, the opening in the sac is revealed as a slit in the lateral peritoneal leaf of the mesentery of the sigmoid, exposing the blood vessels immediately beneath. This rent will be sutured, the inguinal wound will be treated as in any inguinal hernia and the laparotomy wound will be closed.

FEMORAL HERNIA

Femoral hernia passes first through the internal femoral ring and then through the femoral canal which lies between the lacunar ligament and the femoral vein. The neck of the sac is found about 2 centimeters lateral to the corresponding pubic spine. The hernia, after descending through the canal, reaches the subcutaneous tissue through the fossa ovalis and Scarpa's triangle where the bulging is recognized.

The Approach. Femoral hernia may be approached either from above the inguinal ligament or from below. From above, the approach is that already described to approach inguinal hernia until after the inguinal canal has been opened. The approach from below[4] is made through an incision usually longitudinally placed over the position of the hernia (Fig. 409). The

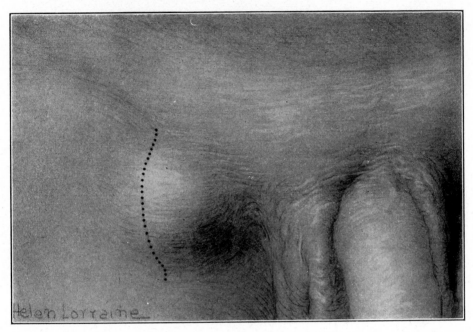

FIG. 409. Femoral hernia. Inferior approach. The skin incision. The inguinal incision shown in figure 383 is employed for the superior approach.

femoral canal is funnel-shaped with the large end above. The approach from below, as will be seen, permits closure of only the lower small end of the funnel as compared with the approach from above which permits closure of the upper large end. Failure to close the upper portion of the funnel is the probable reason for recurrence of femoral hernia when the inferior approach is employed. Protection from recurrence is, therefore, more satisfactorily obtained when femoral hernia is approached from above. Unfortunately, in many cases of incarcerated femoral hernia or in hernia of long standing, the sac and its content cannot be safely delivered from above alone. In such instances the superior approach is supplemented by an inferior incision.

THE SAC. (*Superior Approach*). After opening the inguinal canal and retracting the cord, as described above, the transversalis fascia is incised and the peritoneum is separated from the lateral and inferior walls of the pelvis. In carrying out this dissection the neck of the sac will be discovered mesial to the external iliac vessels and passing beneath the inguinal ligament (Fig. 410). Gentle traction on the neck of the sac combined with blunt dissection and pressure on the hernia sac in the thigh may serve to deliver the entire sac without difficulty. If the sac is not easily delivered and obviously contains

Fig. 410

Fig. 411

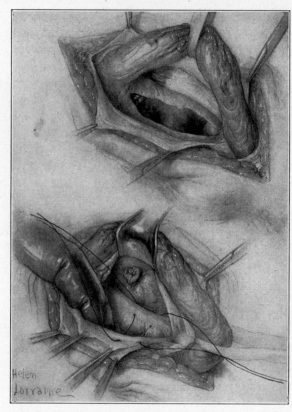

FIG. 410. Femoral hernia. Superior approach. The inguinal canal has been opened, the cord retracted and the transversalis fascia incised. The separation of the peritoneum from the lateral and inferior walls of the pelvis reveals the neck of the sac passing out of sight beneath the inguinal ligament.

FIG. 411. Femoral hernia. Superior approach. The sac has been delivered from the femoral canal, opened, transfixed, ligated, amputated and allowed to retract mesially. This reveals the defect in the femoral canal. Sutures are being placed, uniting the inguinal ligament to Cooper's ligament, which will completely close the weak point. The femoral vein has been retracted with the finger to prevent its being wounded. Closure of the inguinal canal will be carried out as previously described.

intraperitoneal structures, one may open the peritoneum above the neck and attempt to withdraw the contents before delivering the sac itself. If, without exerting undue force, these maneuvers fail, it may be necessary to open the sac through a separate incision in the thigh, as described later, and make a combined attack. After the sac has been delivered, it is opened (if not already opened by a supplementary inferior approach), the contents reduced, and the neck transfixed, ligated and divided as in indirect inguinal hernia. Occasionally it may be necessary to divide the inguinal ligament to effect safe reduction of the sac content.

THE REPAIR. (*Superior Approach*). After the sac has been delivered, the internal femoral ring beneath the inguinal ligament and superficial to Cooper's ligament is revealed. This opening can be satisfactorily occluded by suturing the former to the latter. Interrupted sutures are passed through Cooper's ligament and beneath the inguinal ligament and tied snugly (Fig.

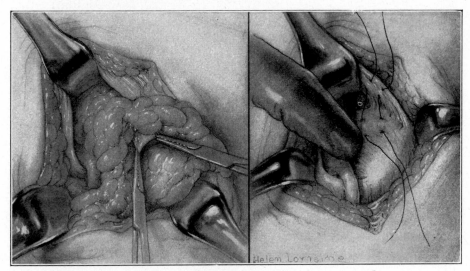

FIG. 412   FIG. 413

FIG. 412. Femoral hernia. Inferior approach. The subcutaneous tissue has been incised, and the long saphenous vein is seen disappearing beneath it. The properitoneal fat has been isolated and incised. The sac has been identified and will be opened.

FIG. 413. Femoral hernia. Inferior approach. The properitoneal fat has been excised. After reduction of the content of the sac, the neck has been transfixed, ligated, amputated and allowed to retract. Interrupted sutures are being placed between the under surface of the inguinal ligament and the pectineus fascia. The finger is guarding the femoral vein. The drawing illustrates the fact that this closure represents the occlusion of only the lower end of the funnel-like femoral canal.

411), with care to protect the external iliac vein. The inguinal canal is then closed as in inguinal hernia with due respect to the strength of its floor as a prophylaxis against the possible development of later direct inguinal hernia.

THE SAC. (*Inferior Approach*). After incision of the subcutaneous tissue and superficial fascia, the hernia is first encountered as a bulging mass of properitoneal fat, the actual sac being buried deep within it (Fig. 412). The fat must be carefully separated until the peritoneum is identified. Since a sliding hernia of the bladder is sometimes encountered, the possibility of this type of content must be remembered if the sac wall seems unusually thick. After the sac has been identified and opened, the properitoneal fat is cleaned away and the sac neck freed beneath the inguinal ligament. The neck is drawn down as far as possible, transfixed, ligated, divided and allowed to retract. During the clearing of the properitoneal fat proximity of the femoral vein must be kept in mind.

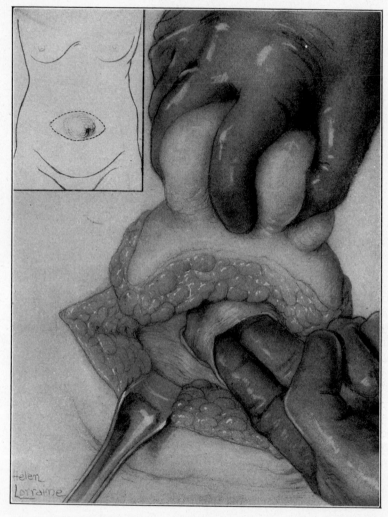

FIG. 414. Umbilical hernia. The incision has been carried down to the level of the rectus sheath which has been cleaned of subcutaneous tissue to the neck of the sac. The border of the fascial defect has been cleaned, and an incision has been made into the neck of the sac. The fingers are separating any adhesions which may lie in this plane and protecting the contents of the sac. Insert shows the size and position of the elliptical incision in relation to the size of the hernia. In small hernias the umbilicus may be preserved by omitting the upper limb of the elliptical incision and dissecting the umbilical scar from the sac.

THE REPAIR. (*Inferior Approach*). After removal of the sac and properitoneal fat, the borders of the defect can be seen to consist of the common femoral vein laterally, the lacunar ligament mesially, the inguinal ligament superficially, and the pectineus fascia deeply. Closure consists of approximation of the under surface of the inguinal ligament to the pectineus fascia by interrupted sutures with careful protection of the common femoral vein

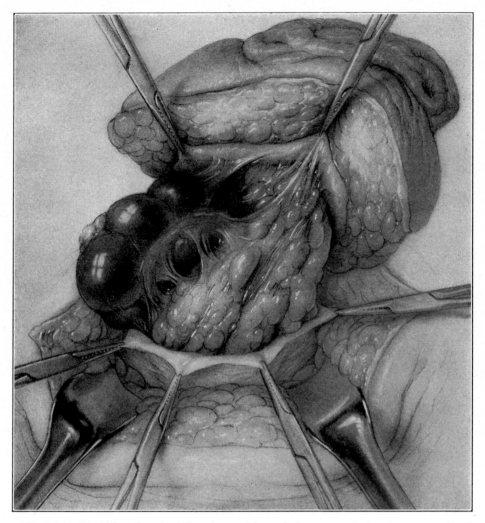

FIG. 415. Umbilical hernia. The circumcision of the sac neck has been completed, amputating the distal portion of the sac. The adherent content is being drawn out of the sac as indicated by the dimpling of the redundant skin. Separation of adhesions will now proceed, including amputation of the adherent omentum where no bowel is involved. The remaining sac content can then be reduced into the abdominal cavity and the redundant tissue discarded.

(Fig. 413). When these sutures are drawn snugly, one must be careful to see that the femoral vein is not compressed. In closing the femoral ring an occasional anomalous branch of the obturator artery winding about the mesial surface of the neck may be wounded if not identified.

UMBILICAL HERNIA

The Approach. The treatment of hernia at the umbilicus is identical whether the lesion is a true umbilical hernia, *i.e.*, eversion of the umbilicus, or the more common para-umbilical hernia. In large hernias a transverse elliptical incision including the umbilicus is made, varying in size with the extent of the palpable sac and the amount of redundant skin (Insert, Fig.

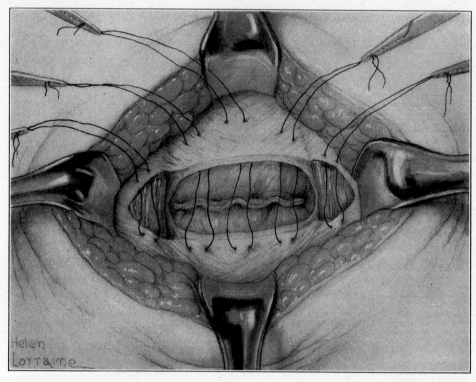

Fig. 416. Umbilical hernia. Mayo principle. The peritoneal defect has been closed with a running horizontal mattress suture everting its edges. The anterior rectus sheath has been incised at both ends of the defect to expose the muscle fibers. Multiple mattress sutures have been placed so as to approximate the superficial surface of the inferior flap to the under surface of the superior flap. When these are snugly tied, the two flaps will be imbricated for a distance of from 1 to 3 centimeters.

414). The incision is carried down perpendicularly until the sheath of the rectus muscle is encountered. Ramifications of the sac may project beyond the limits of the skin incision, and it is, therefore, important to watch for the sac during the incision. When the plane of the deep fascia has been identified, the subcutaneous tissue and any adherent sac are dissected centripetally until the border of the fascial defect is encountered.

In small hernias it may be possible to limit the incision to the lower element of the ellipse. The scarred skin of the umbilicus is dissected from the sac which is then further defined. By this maneuver a flattened umbilicus is preserved.

THE SAC. The edge of the fascial defect is carefully cleaned entirely around the neck of the sac, and the peritoneum is separated from the fascial ring. The neck is opened with care to avoid damaging possible adherent content. When the peritoneal plane of cleavage is identified within the neck, fingers can be introduced and further freeing of adhesions carried out (Fig.

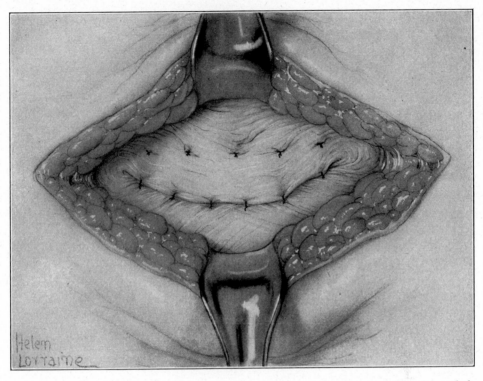

FIG. 417. Umbilical hernia. Mayo principle. Sutures of the deep row have been tied, and approximation sutures have been placed, tacking the free edge of the superior flap to the superficial surface of the inferior flap.

414). The incision in the neck of the sac is then continued completely around its circumference, with cautious liberation of adhesions as the amputation advances. Fine hemostats are applied to the divided margin. At the close of this manipulation the content of the sac projects from a ring of free peritoneum. If there are additional adhesions within the distal portion of the sac, the ellipse of skin and subcutaneous tissue will remain attached to the content (Fig. 415). In this case, the adhesions between the interior of the sac and its content must be carefully freed everywhere. If these adhesions involve only omentum, it may be ligated in segments and amputated, both to save time and to diminish the bulk of the material that must be replaced within the abdominal cavity. Following the discarding of the redundant tissue, the sac contents are reduced within the abdomen. The opening in the peritoneum is closed transversely with a horizontal running mattress suture as in a laparotomy (Fig. 416).

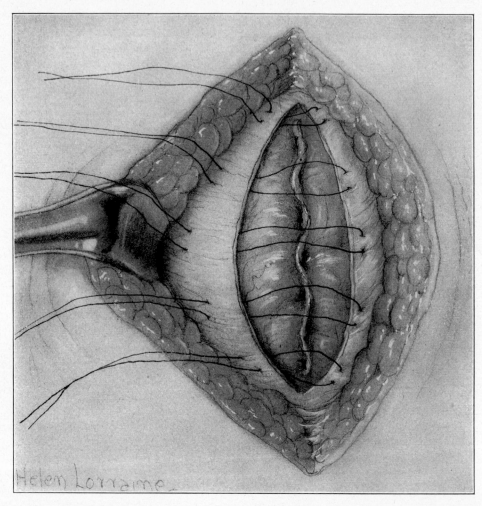

Fig. 418. Ventral hernia. An incision has been made excising the scar of a previous operation and exposing the deep fascia which has been cleaned to the border of the defect. The sac has been opened and amputated. The contents have been freed from adhesions and dropped back into the abdominal cavity, and the peritoneal opening has been sutured just as in umbilical hernia. Mattress sutures have been placed to effect a horizontal imbrication of the edges of the defect, resembling the vertical imbrication of the Mayo operation for umbilical hernia.

THE REPAIR. After closure of the peritoneum there remains a cleaned fascial border, usually of oval shape. The principle of repair is the overlapping of the upper and lower fascial layers in a vertical direction across the defect, a procedure first proposed by W. J. Mayo and now bearing his name.[16] In order to insure overlapping at the lateral corners, the anterior rectus sheath is divided for about 2 centimeters laterally from the angles of the defect. The typical Mayo procedure consists of drawing the inferior flap beneath the superior flap, but the reverse procedure is also successful. Su-

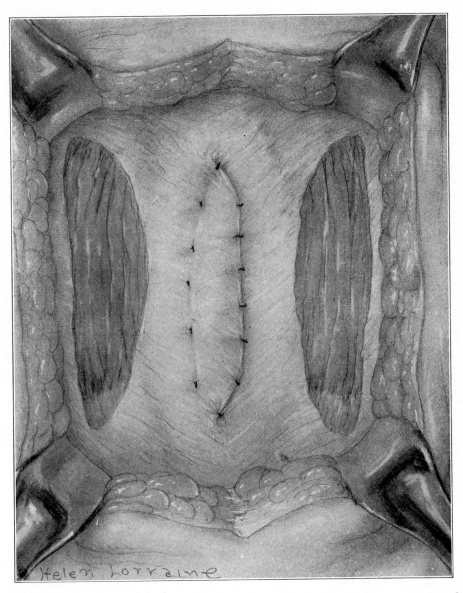

Fig. 419. Ventral hernia. To permit imbrication, relaxation incisions have been made in the anterior rectus sheath, exposing the fibers of the muscle and permitting mesial dislocation of both edges of the defect. The drawing shows the completed overlap as begun in figure 418.

tures are passed through the superior flap from without inward at a distance of from 1 to 3 centimeters from its free border. Bites are taken of the inferior flap, and the sutures pass outward through the superior flap at points close to their origin. These sutures are placed at intervals of about 1 centimeter (Fig. 416). After they are tied, the free edge of the superior flap is then anchored by a row of approximation sutures to the superficial surface of the inferior flap, completing the imbrication (Fig. 417). The subcutaneous tissue and the skin are closed in the usual manner. If there is a large pocket in the fat once occupied by the sac that cannot be obliterated by suturing and pressure, a small rubber drain may be left in place for from twenty-four to forty-eight hours.

VENTRAL HERNIA

The Approach. The problem presented by a postoperative ventral hernia may be one of the most difficult in hernia surgery, being complicated often by intraperitoneal adhesions and sometimes by an enormous defect. The ap-

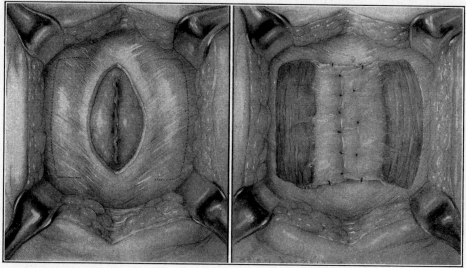

FIG. 420   FIG. 421

FIG. 420. Ventral hernia. Rectangular flaps of the anterior rectus sheath have been outlined on three sides in the case of a defect the edges of which cannot be overlapped by simpler methods.

FIG. 421. Ventral hernia. The flaps indicated in figure 420 have been imbricated over the defect.

proach depends on the position and size of the hernia and the direction of the long axis of the defect. Any variety of skin incision, with or without the sacrifice of skin and subcutaneous tissue, is permissible. Almost universally the scar of the wound through which the hernia has passed is excised. As in umbilical hernia, the primary incision is carried down to the deep fascia with care to avoid projecting arms of the sac. The surface of the deep fascia is then cleaned by sharp dissection up to the edge of the defect.

THE SAC. The handling of the sac is the same as in umbilical hernia. Occasionally it may be necessary to open the sac near the apex, if a free peritoneal space is not easily encountered at the neck. The sac neck is closed as in a laparotomy (Fig. 418).

THE REPAIR. On account of the great variation in the size of the fascial defect, a number of different procedures have been devised, one or more of

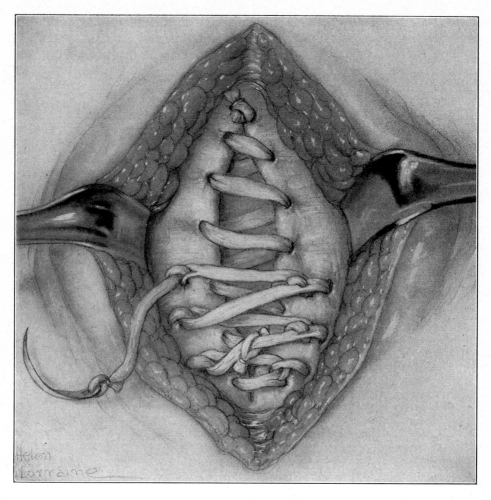

FIG. 422. Ventral hernia. Gallie and LeMesurier method. A continuous suture of fascia lata has been placed in the edges of the defect. This should approximate the edges, if possible. If not, a latticework of fascial sutures will be constructed until the interstices between the strips are exceedingly small.

which may have to be called upon by the surgeon in any individual case. If the hernia is in such a position that two fascial layers can be developed on each side of the defect—for example, through the upper portion of the rectus muscle where one layer may consist of the posterior sheath and one layer of the anterior sheath—these layers should be defined by splitting the single layer presenting at the free edge of the defect. If the combined layers are thin, one can do more harm than good by this maneuver. If two good layers can be developed, particularly in small ventral hernias, closure of the defect can often be made exactly as the surgeon would close the original laparotomy.

In defects which cannot be closed by suture of normal layers, it is a general principle that at least two thicknesses of tissue must be placed across the defect. If there is not too large an opening, this may be effected by overlapping the two flaps horizontally just as they are overlapped vertically in umbilical hernia (Fig. 418). If there is not sufficient tissue to permit overlapping without tension, additional material may be made available by vertical relaxation incisions in the anterior rectus sheaths as proposed by Gibson [10] (Fig. 419).

Additional devices employed are types of fascia or cutis transplant similar to those already described in inguinal hernia. If an incision in the rectus sheath does not permit imbrication of the edges of the defect, rectangular flaps of rectus sheath cut on three sides and hinged at the mesial border may be thrown across the defect and there imbricated [18] (Figs. 420 and 421). One may also employ the principle of the free sheet-graft of fascia or cutis from the thigh or Gallie's living suture [9] (Fig. 422). The last has proved particularly valuable in huge postoperative defects in the upper abdomen in obese patients. The fascia is obtained in the manner already described. Wangensteen reports the use of a lower abdominal flap of fascia and muscle to close the upper abdominal defect and a pedicled flap of fascia lata to close the resulting deficiency in the lower abdominal wall.[20] In all these fascia transplants the details of technic are those already described. Koontz [13a] reports the use of tantalum mesh.

REFERENCES

1. ANDREWS, E.   A Method of Herniotomy Utilizing only White Fascia, *Ann. Surg.*, 80:225-237, 1924.

2. ANDREWS, E. W.   Technique of the Andrews Operation for Hernia, *Surg., Gynec. & Obst.*, 11:89-92, 1906.

3. BASSINI, E.   Ueber die Behandlung des Leistenbruches, *Arch. f. klin. Chir.*, 40:429-476, 1890.

4. BASSINI, E.   Neue Operatione—Methode zur Radical Behandlung der Schenkel—Hernie, *Arch. f. klin. Chir.*, 47:1-25, 1894.

5. BEVAN, A. D.   Sliding Hernias of the Ascending Colon and Caecum, the Descending Colon and Sigmoid, and of the Bladder, *Ann. Surg.*, 754-760, [Oct.], 1930.

6. BLOODGOOD, J. C.   The Transplantation of the Rectus Muscle or its Sheath for the Cure of Inguinal Hernia When the Conjoined Tendon is Obliterated, *Ann. Surg.*, 70:81-88, 1919.

7. CANNADAY, J. E.   The Use of the Cutis Graft in the Repair of Certain Types of Incisional Herniae and Other Conditions, *Ann. Surg.*, 115:775-781, 1942.

8. FERGUSON, A. H.   Oblique Inguinal Hernia, *J.A.M.A.*, 33:6-14, 1899.

9. GALLIE, W. E. and LE MESURIER, A. B.   The Transplantation of the Fibrous Tissues in the Repair of Anatomical Defects, *Brit. J. Surg.*, 12:289-320, 1924.

10. GIBSON, C. L.   Post-Operative Intestinal Obstructions, *Ann. Surg.*, 63:442-451, 1916.

11. GRAHAM, R. R.   The Operative Repair of Sliding Hernia of the Sigmoid, *Ann. Surg.*, 102:784-792, 1935.

12. HALSTED, W. S.   The Radical Cure of Hernia, *Bull. Johns Hopkins Hosp.*, 1:12-13, 1889.

13. HALSTED, W. S. The Cure of the More Difficult As Well As the Simpler Inguinal Ruptures, *Bull. Johns Hopkins Hosp.*, 14:208-214, 1903.

13A. KOONTZ, A. R. Preliminary Report on the Use of Tantalum Mesh in the Repair of Ventral Hernias, *Ann. Surg.*, 127:1079, 1948.

14. LaROQUE, G. P. The Permanent Cure of Inguinal and Femoral Hernia, *Surg., Gynec. & Obst.*, 29:507-510, 1919.

15. MASSON, J. C. Strips of Fascia Lata as Suture Material in the Repair of the More Difficult Abdominal Hernias, *Virginia M. Monthly*, 62:148-150, 1935-36.

16. MAYO, W. J. An Operation for the Radical Cure of Umbilical Hernia, *Ann. Surg.*, 34:276-280, 1901.

17. McARTHUR, L. L. Autoplastic Sutures in Hernia and Other Diastases, *J.A.M.A.*, 43:1039-1048, 1904.

18. ROTHSCHILD, N. S. Treatment of Recurrent Incisional Hernia by Flap of the Anterior Sheath of the Rectus, *Ann. Surg.*, 101:754-758, 1935.

19. WANGENSTEEN, O. H. Repair of Recurrent and Difficult Hernias and Other Large Defects of the Abdominal Wall Employing the Iliotibial Tract of Fascia Lata as a Pedicled Flap, *Surg., Gynec. & Obst.*, 59:766-780, 1934.

20. WANGENSTEEN, O. H. Repair of Large Abdominal Defects by Pedicled Fascial Grafts, *Surg., Gynec. & Obst.*, 82:144-150, 1946.

21. WATSON, L. F. *Hernia*, The C. V. Mosby Company, St. Louis, 1938.

18

THE BREAST

Thomas G. Orr, M.D.

INFECTIONS OF THE BREAST

Infection in the breast producing suppuration requires drainage. Tuberculosis of the breast is rare, but when it exists partial or complete mastectomy may be indicated. Persistent sinuses may result from multiple abscesses of the breast and complete removal of the breast or mastectomy with preservation of the nipple may be the operation of choice in such cases.

Technic of Incision and Drainage of Infections of the Breast. A superficial abscess should be drained through a linear incision radiating from the nipple. A deep abscess in the breast tissue should also be drained through an incision radiating from the nipple to avoid cutting across ducts. The abscess cavity is explored with a finger and all communicating abscess pockets are connected into a single abscess. When extensive counter drainage is advisable, the counter incision may be made over the tip of a hemostat introduced through the original incision and pointing toward the periphery of the breast. When multiple incisions are made, through-and-through drainage is established by using Penrose or cigarette types of drains. Bleeding vessels may require ligation. Sutures are seldom necessary (see Fig. 423). Drains should usually be removed in three to five days.

A deep submammary abscess may be drained through a curved incision of the Gilliard-Thomas type at the lower margin of the breast (Fig. 423). Through this type of incision the breast may be partially dissected from the chest wall. Single or multiple abscesses are incised and are drained with cigarette or rubber tissue drains. The skin incision is partially closed about the drains with interrupted silk or cotton sutures. Warm moist dressing will promote drainage.

As an adjunct to surgical treatment the proper sulphonamide drugs and penicillin should be used.

BENIGN TUMORS AND CYSTS OF THE BREAST

It is frequently impossible to make an accurate clinical diagnosis of a small mass in the breast. When in doubt about the nature of any growth in the breast the growth should be excised. If a biopsy is done the entire local tumor should be removed when possible.

Simple mastectomy may be indicated for multiple cystic disease of the

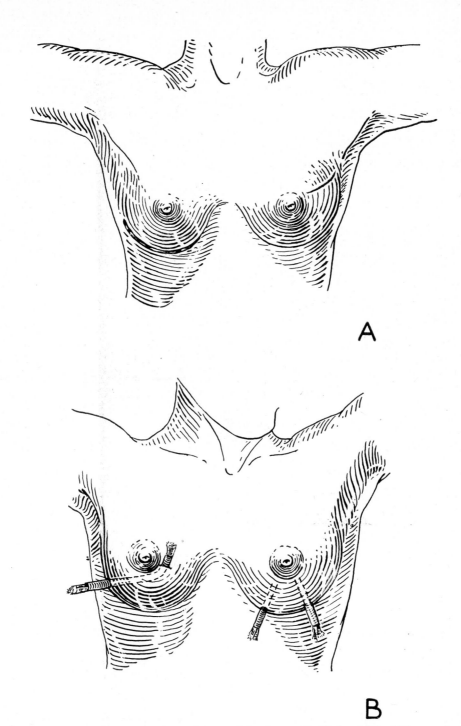

FIG. 423. Incisions for drainage of breast infections. (A) *Right:* Gilliard-Thomas incision. (B) *Left:* Incision radiating from nipple. (B) Drainage for breast abscesses.

breast, for large benign tumors, and occasionally as a palliative operation for incurable carcinoma with ulceration.

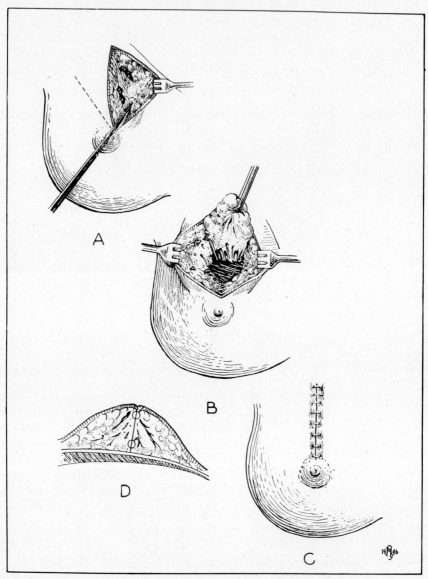

FIG. 424. Technic of excision of benign tumor or cyst. (A) Incision radiating from nipple with partial exposure of tumor. (B) Involved breast tissue partially excised. (C) Wound in skin closed with interrupted sutures of fine silk or cotton. (D) Section through breast showing closure of breast tissue with fine sutures.

A bleeding nipple may be due to a benign intraductal papilloma or to an early malignancy. Local excision is indicated for the benign lesions. If evidence of malignancy is found either by gross or microscopic examination, removal of the breast is indicated.

Technic of Excision of Benign Lesions of the Breast. An incision is made over the tumor radiating outward from the nipple. The tumor or cyst is excised with a thin covering of breast tissue. All bleeding vessels are carefully ligated. The breast tissue is sutured with fine silk or catgut. Unless an accurate closure of the wound is made a hematoma will often form and delay healing (see Fig. 424).

Lesions deep in the breast tissue in the lower half of the breast may be removed through a curved incision made in the skin fold below the breast

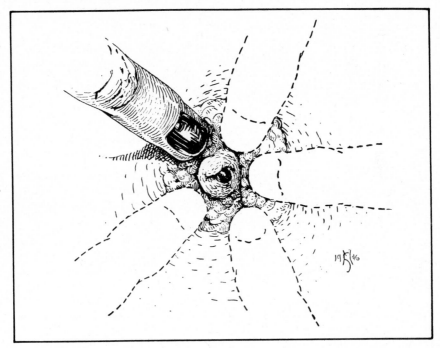

FIG. 425. Method of systematic digital palpation to locate bleeding duct.

(Gilliard-Thomas). After dissecting the breast from the chest wall the tumor or cyst is removed through an incision radiating from the center of the breast. The breast tissue is carefully closed with two or more rows of interrupted sutures. The skin is closed with silk or cotton. A small drain placed beneath the breast, to be removed in 48 hours, is usually advisable. A firm dressing is applied to prevent the collection of exudate in the wound.

Technic of Excision of Intraductal Papilloma. A bleeding nipple is very frequently caused by a papillomatous growth in a duct. Such a growth should be explored to determine its type and extent. If a malignant growth is found, a radical or sub-radical removal of the breast is indicated.

The duct containing the papilloma can usually be located by palpation around the nipple (Fig. 425). When the involved duct is compressed a drop of serous or bloody fluid will appear at the duct opening. The diseased duct in some cases may be identified by the method of Babcock (Fig. 426).

An incision is made radiating from the nipple. The duct containing the papilloma and a thin portion of surrounding tissue should be excised. The wound is closed as in excision of any benign tumor or cyst.

Technic of Simple Mastectomy (Fig. 427). Incisions are made about the breast so that sufficient skin is preserved to close without tension. The skin margins are dissected up to points well beyond the breast tissue. The breast with its surrounding fat is then removed. Complete removal exposes the muscles of the chest wall. All vessels are carefully ligated with fine catgut,

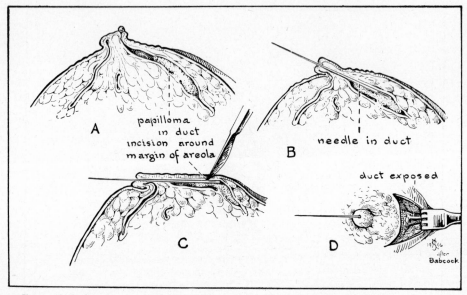

Fig. 426. Babcock's method of locating and excising papilloma of duct. (A) Section through breast showing location of papilloma in duct. (B) Small round needle inserted through nipple into duct containing papilloma. (C) Needle in duct used as a guide for skin incision. (D) Type of incision at margin of areola with exposure of duct. (Redrawn from Babcock, Wayne W., *Surgery*, 4:914, 1938.)

silk, or cotton. The wound is closed with silk or cotton. If the breast is large and the patient is obese, drainage may be indicated for 48 hours to remove serum from beneath the skin flaps. A pressure dressing is applied.

Simple mastectomy with preservation of the nipple may also be performed by a method described by Dean Lewis. The Lewis operation is best suited for the small breast in a thin individual. A curved incision is made at the margin of the areola. The nipple and areola are dissected up by cutting across the ducts beneath the nipple. The breast is grasped with a tenaculum and gradually withdrawn through the incision as it is dissected free from the subcutaneous fat. After ligating all bleeding vessels, the subcutaneous tissues are closed with a series of purse-string sutures. The skin is closed with silk and a pressure dressing is applied.

Simple mastectomy is occasionally indicated for chronic mastitis of the male breast. In such a case the breast may be removed without the nipple

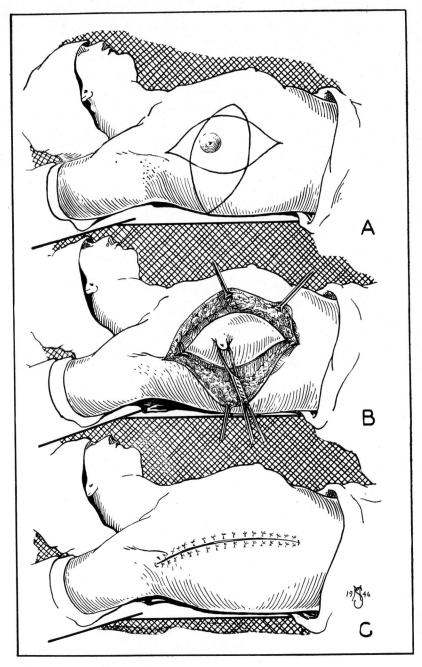

FIG. 427. Technic of simple mastectomy. (A) Types of incisions. (B) Skin flaps undercut and retracted to expose entire breast. (C) Wound closed with fine silk or cotton.

and areola. A curved incision is made below the nipple at the margin of the areola. The skin and nipple area is undercut and the entire breast is excised. The skin is closed with silk and a pressure dressing is applied to prevent collection of serum beneath the skin.

Operations for gynecomastia may be advisable for cosmetic reasons. Enlarged breasts in the male may be removed by simple mastectomy or by a plastic operation to preserve the nipple and areola. The breast may be excised through a curved incision made at its lower margin, by undercutting the skin over the breast and beneath the nipple. In order to properly locate the nipple, after removal of the breast, it may be necessary to excise sections of skin above and below the nipple. If too much skin is removed there is some danger of necrosis of the nipple area of skin. Careful hematosis, suturing of the wounds and pressure dressings are necessary for smooth healing and a good cosmetic result.

CARCINOMA OF THE BREAST

General Considerations. The breast is a multiglandular organ having an abundant blood and lymph supply. The blood supply is received from branches of the internal mammary, intercostals, and axillary artery. Since cancer cells spread along lymphatic channels, it is very important that the lymphatic drainage of the breast be understood. The major portion of the lymphatic vessels from the breast extend to the axilla (Fig. 428). Some of the lymphatics from the upper and lower medial quadrants of the breast pass directly into the chest along the perforating mammary vessels. Other paths of dissemination of cancer cells through lymphatic vessels are to the supraclavicular nodes, the opposite axilla, the intercostal vessels, along the skin vessels, downward through the rectus fascia and along the round ligament into the liver. Late metastases from the breast are most frequently found in the lungs, pleura, bones, and liver.

It is generally believed that malignant tumors of the breast grow more rapidly in young individuals. Malignant tumors also grow more rapidly during pregnancy. To prevent the rapid growth and spread of cancer in women before the menopause, radiation castration has been recommended. Oophorectomy is preferred by some surgeons.

There is not a unanimity of opinion concerning the treatment of carcinoma of the breast. Radiation alone has been recommended by some authors, and surgery alone has been advised by others. Most surgeons believe that radical mastectomy is the treatment of choice in operable cases. Either preoperative or postoperative radiation therapy is advised by many. In selected cases, which are obviously incurable, a simple palliative mastectomy may be done to remove a large or ulcerating mass of cancer tissue.

When the diagnosis of cancer is in doubt, a biopsy or local removal of the tumor for study is indicated. Although the possible dissemination of cancer cells by biopsy is still a disputed point, it is wise to proceed immediately with the surgical or radiation therapy as soon as the diagnosis is made.

Technic of Radical Mastectomy. The general plan of the operation should follow that described by Halsted. Halsted's operation included the complete removal of the breast with a wide area of skin, the pectoralis major and minor muscles, and the contents of the axilla. The dissection should extend from the latissimus dorsi muscle to the midsternum and below to costal margin. Handley believed that most cancer cells spread

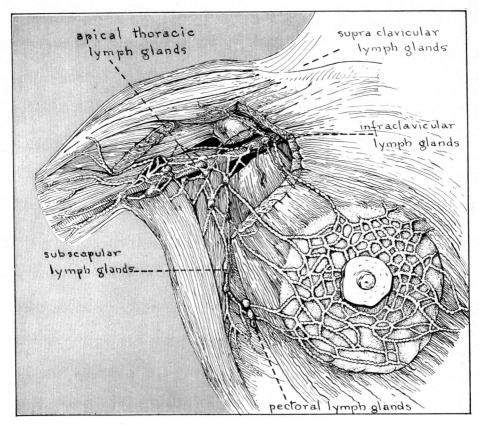

FIG. 428. Approximate distribution of lymph nodes in the axillary region. (Redrawn from Babcock, *Principles and Practice of Surgery*, Lea and Febiger, 1944.)

through the lymphatics along fascial planes and recommended a wide excision of subcutaneous tissue and fascia extending laterally beyond the anterior border of the latissimus dorsi muscle, medially beyond the sternum and inferiorly to a point about midway between the ensiform process and umbilicus, including excision of the anterior rectus sheath on the side of the tumor and a portion of the opposite rectus sheath. With the Handley technic the wound can usually be closed without skin grafting. White has recently stated that: "There is no sufficient proof that the Halsted skin removal with Thiersch graft gives a reduced incidence of local recurrence over the plastic skin closure of Handley."

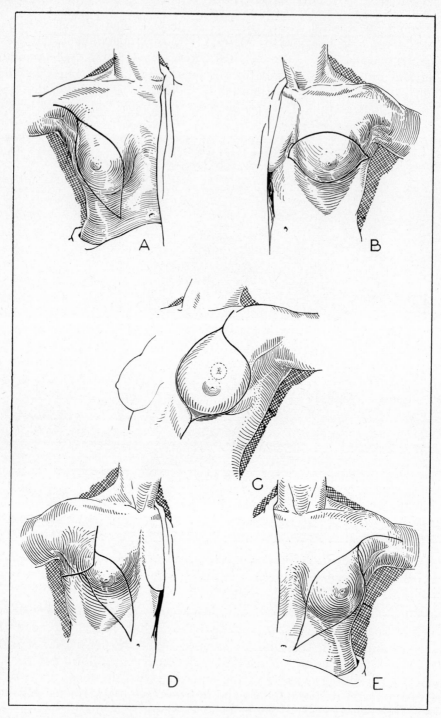

FIG. 429. Examples of skin incisions. (A) Willy Meyer's incision. (B) Stewart incision. (C) Haagensen's incision. (D) Orr's incision. (E) Deaver's incision.

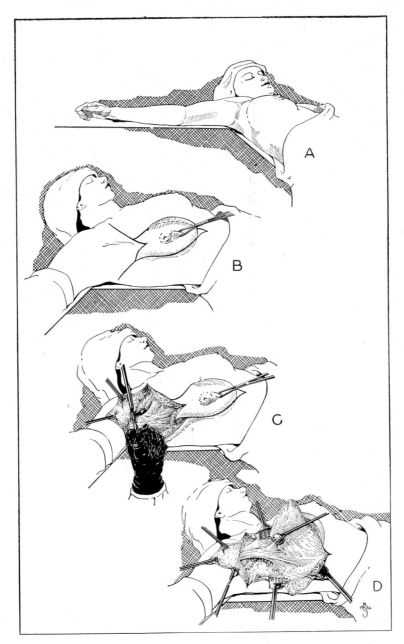

Fig. 430. Technic of radical mastectomy. (A) Position of patient on the operating table. (B) Lines of incisions forming triangular axillary skin flap. (C) Pectoralis major muscle exposed ready for division near insertion. (D) Pectoralis major muscle divided and retracted exposing pectoralis minor muscle.

All tissue should be removed down to the serratus anterior muscle and the fascia should be removed from that portion of the rectus muscle attached to the chest wall. All fat, areolar tissue and lymphatics should be removed from between the chest wall and the latissimus dorsi and subscapularis muscles. Meticulous dissection is necessary to entirely denude the vessels and nerves in the axilla of all fat and areolar tissue which may contain lymphatic vessels and lymph nodes.

One of the gas anesthetics is suitable for breast operations. The patient is placed on the operating table with the arm on a support at right angles to the body. The draped area should expose the entire half of the anterior surface of the chest, the lateral chest wall, the upper abdominal wall, the supraclavicular area, and the upper arm and shoulder.

If a preliminary diagnostic incision is made into the tumor, the wound should be closed with sutures, the instruments and surgeon's gloves discarded and the operative field again prepared for radical operation.

The type of incision used will depend upon the choice of the surgeon, the size and location of the tumor, and the size and shape of the breast. A single type of incision is not suitable for all cases. Types of satisfactory incisions are shown in figure 429. The Stewart and triangular axillary flap incisions prevent the formation of scar tissue across the axilla from the chest wall to the arm and minimize disturbing contractures. The incision described by Haagensen places the scar medial to the axilla and gives adequate exposure.

The triangular axillary type of incision is here described and shown in the illustrated technic of operation (Figs. 430, 431 and 432). The incision is begun about 6 cm. below the middle of the clavicle and extended downward and outward to meet an incision extended downward and inward beginning over the latissimus dorsi muscle about 6 cm. below the posterior axillary fold. These two incisions outline a triangular flap of skin which covers most of the axillary area. Curved incisions are made around the breast branching off from the oblique incisions. These incisions join at the costal margin in the midclavicular line.

The triangular skin flap is dissected up and retracted over the shoulder. This dissection exposes the axillary area, and the margins of the pectoralis major and latissimus dorsi muscles. The medial and lateral skin flaps are freed and retracted to give adequate exposure for the axillary dissection. The pectoralis major muscle is severed near its attachment to the humerus. This muscle is to be removed with the exception of its clavicular portion. The pectoralis minor muscle is next severed at its attachment. Retraction of the pectoral muscles exposes the axilla ready for dissection.

Beginning at the apex of the axilla the fat and fascia, which contain lymphatic vessels and nodes, are completely removed from the nerves and vessels. This dissection exposes the chest wall and the medial surfaces of the latissimus dorsi and subscapular muscles.

As the dissection proceeds all branches of the great vessels are clamped and ligated as soon as exposed. Fine cotton, silk, or catgut may be used for

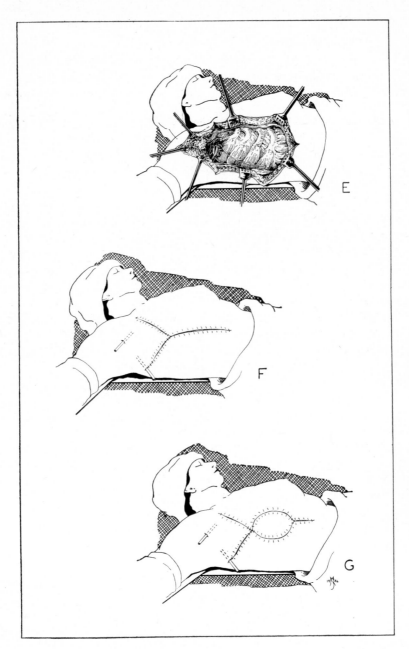

FIG. 431. Technic of radical mastectomy, continued. (E) The breast has been completely removed with pectoral muscles and axillary contents. Long thoracic and thoracodorsal nerves have been preserved. (F) Skin closed and axillary drains in place. (G) Skin graft sutured in position to fill defect after removal of large area of skin.

ligatures. The nerves supplying the pectoral muscles are severed and removed with the muscles. The intercostobrachialis nerve is usually removed but may be preserved in selected cases. The subscapular nerve to the subscapular muscle, the thoracodorsal nerve to the latissimus dorsi muscle, and the long thoracic nerve to the serratus anterior muscle, must be carefully preserved.

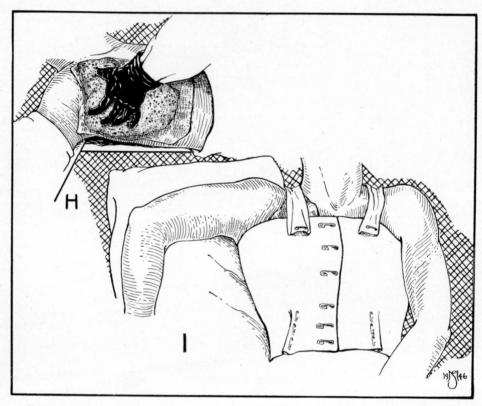

Fig. 432. Technic of radical mastectomy, continued. (H) Application of marine sponge to axillary area. (I) Type of breast binder which may be used to hold dressings securely in place.

When the axillary dissection has been completed the skin incisions are extended around the breast and reflected medially to the sternal midline and laterally to the latissimus dorsi muscle. The upper end of the rectus muscle is exposed and denuded of its fascia. The entire breast and axillary contents are removed in one mass. As the breast is dissected from the chest wall each bleeding vessel is clamped and later ligated. Careful hemostasis may be very tedious but is very necessary for proper wound healing. It is advisable to thoroughly wash the wound with warm physiologic sodium chloride solution before closure.

The skin flaps can usually be closed completely. If the area of skin removed is too large for closure, a skin graft should be immediately prepared and sutured into the defect. A suitable split graft may be taken from the thigh or abdominal wall with the Padgett dermatome. Such a graft may be cut to fit a measured defect. An axillary drain of the Penrose or cigarette type is inserted into the axilla through the end of the lateral incision. It is wise to add an additional axillary drain passed through a stab wound in the axillary flap. These drains should usually be removed in 48 hours. The axillary flap may be sutured to the intercostal muscle and the stumps of the pectoralis muscles with mattress sutures to aid in the obliteration of the axillary space.

The entire wound is covered with a thin layer of gauze dressing and over this is placed a moist marine sponge to hold the skin snugly in the axilla and against the chest wall. A chest binder is used to hold the dressings firmly in position. A pressure dressing prevents the accumulation of serum beneath the skin and aids in early attachment of the skin flaps.

Complications. The danger of hemorrhage and shock are not great if an infusion of 5 per cent dextrose solution is given during the operation and blood for transfusion is immediately available when needed. Blood loss during radical mastectomy was found by Coller and his associates to average 821 cc. or 17.7 per cent of the total volume of blood. This estimate of blood loss would indicate the need of transfusions during the operation.

Collection of blood and serum beneath the skin flaps not only delays healing but predisposes to infection and increases scar tissue. Careful hemostasis and pressure dressings will reduce this complication to a minimum.

To prevent contractures and restore early function, motion of the shoulder should be started gradually within three to five days after operation. Motion should be increased as the skin flaps become more firmly adherent.

Swelling of the arm is a frequent complication when the axillary dissection has been complete. By avoiding accumulations of blood and serum in the axilla immediately following operation, swelling of the arm will be minimized. Late swelling of the arm may mean a recurrence of the carcinoma about the vessels of the axilla.

The death rate following radical breast operation should not exceed 1 or 2 per cent.

UMBILICATED OR DEPRESSED NIPPLE

Operation is indicated for congenital umbilication or depression of the nipple when the deformity is sufficient to prevent nursing. Operations are designed to constrict the tissues about the nipple to hold it in normal position. Such operations should not injure the ducts leading to the nipple.

Technic of Mammilliplasty for Umbilicated Nipple. For deep umbilication the method of Ashford is advised (Fig. 433a). The nipple is grasped with forceps and withdrawn as far as possible to stretch the surrounding skin. Traction on the skin makes it possible to accurately place the small incisions around the nipple. Three spindle-shaped areas of skin about the nipple are removed with the ends of the areas almost in contact. The

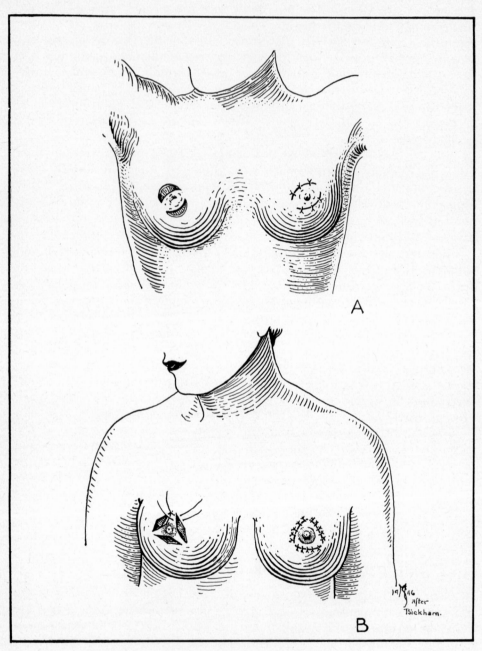

Fig. 433. (A) Incisions and wound closure in Kehrer's method of mammilliplasty. (B) Ashford's technic of mammilliplasty. (After Bickham.)

incisions should be placed about 1.5 cm. from the nipple. After the spindle-shaped areas are carefully denuded of skin, a purse-string suture of chromic catgut is passed around the nipple through the denuded areas and tied. This purse-string suture puckers the tissues about the nipple and forces it

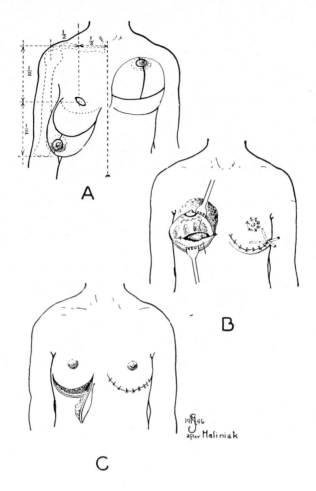

FIG. 434. A two-stage plastic operation for hypertrophy of the breasts. *First Stage:* (A) The site of the relocated nipple is outlined at a point midway between clavicle and elbow joint directly below the midpoint of the clavicle. Incisions outlining the areola and areas of skin to be removed. (B) Nipple sutured into its new position. The skin is closed and the wound is drained. *Second Stage:* (C) Excess of skin beneath the breast is removed and the wound is sutured without drainage. (Redrawn from Maliniak.)

outward. Strangulation of the nipple must be avoided. The wounds are closed with interrupted sutures of fine silk or cotton.

When the nipple is slightly umbilicated the technic described by Kehrer is satisfactory (Fig. 433b). Kehrer makes a double crescentric incision on each side of the nipple. An area of skin about 2.5 x 5 cm. in size is denuded down to the fascia. When the incisions are closed with interrupted sutures, the nipple is projected outward.

Hypertrophy of the Breast. Four types of hypertrophy of the breast have been described. They are true hypertrophy, congenital hypertrophy with a difference in size of the breasts, fatty hypertrophy, and hypertrophy due to mastitis.

The indications for operation to be considered are, the general attitude of the patient toward the deformity and the degree of deformity. A plastic operation is designed to reduce the size of the breast and to relocate the breast in its normal position. In true hypertrophy amputation may be the operation of choice.

The large pendulous breast rarely retains its normal lactating function. Lactation is lost after plastic operations upon the breasts.

Technic of Operation for Pendulous Hypertrophic Breast. Much difficulty may be experienced by any surgeon who attempts to correct breast deformities by plastic operations. To make smooth symmetrical breasts after plastic procedures requires the greatest care in making measurements and estimates of size and shape before the operation is done. The blood supply to the skin must be carefully preserved to prevent necrosis and excessive scarring. Clean-cut incisions, careful and painstaking dissection, and accurate suturing are necessary for good results.

The operation of Maliniak is here described and illustrated (Fig. 434). There are many other procedures described which may be found in more elaborate treatises on the subject.

FIRST STAGE. After careful measurements are made and the site for relocation of the nipple is selected and outlined, a circular incision is made around the nipple at the outer margin of the areola. A concave incision is made across the breast above the nipple from the median to lateral mammary fold. The flap thus outlined is separated upward from the breast as high as the second rib interspace. An opening is cut in this flap at a predetermined site for relocation of the nipple. A second curved incision is made below the nipple from one submammary fold to the other. The skin between the two curved incisions is dissected away from the breast. Meticulous care must be used in controlling bleeding.

The upper pole of the breast is sutured to the pectoral fascia beneath the upper flap to fix it in position. The areola is next sutured into the prepared opening in the upper skin flap. Closure of the skin flaps completes the first stage of the operation. Drainage at each end of the incision for 48 hours is advisable to prevent accumulation of serum beneath the flaps. A firm dressing is applied and held in place by a breast binder.

SECOND STAGE. The second stage may usually be done in from four to six weeks. The scar, excess skin, and fat, and a portion of breast tissue are removed through a crescent-shaped incision in the submammary fold. Minor operations may later be necessary to properly shape the breast.

REFERENCES

1. COLLER, F. A., CROOK, C. E. and IOB, V.   *J.A.M.A.*, 126:1, [Sept. 2], 1944.
2. HAAGENSEN, C. D.   *Surgery,* 19:100, [Jan.], 1946.
3. HALSTED, W. S.   *Ann. Surg.*, 20:497, [Jan.], 1894.
4. HANDLEY, W. S.   *Cancer of the Breast and Its Operative Treatment,* John Murray, London, 1922.
5. LEWIS, D.   *Surg. Clin. of Chicago,* 1:117, [Feb.], 1917.
6. MALINIAK, J. W.   *Arch. Surg.*, 31:587, [Oct.], 1935.
7. ORR, T. G.   *Ann. Surg.*, 106:454, [Sept.], 1937.
8. WHITE, W. C.   *Surgery,* 19:149, [Jan.], 1946.

19

THE THYROID AND PARATHYROID GLANDS

John deJ. Pemberton, M.D. and B. Marden Black, M.D.

THE THYROID GLAND

Introduction. Technical difficulties, principally in securing hemostasis and in the avoidance of sepsis, were so great prior to the development of efficient artery forceps and aseptic surgery that practical operations on the thyroid gland were not possible. By the 1880's the major technical problems inherent in thyroid surgery had been defined and largely solved by Central European surgeons. Kocher in 1883, on reexamination of eighteen patients on whom he had performed total thyroidectomy, found that sixteen were suffering from a condition which he described as cretinoid and which he termed "cachexia thyreopriva." The spontaneous development of the condition, later known as myxedema, had been described previously by Gull and by Ord. In 1884 Horsley produced myxedema experimentally in monkeys by the removal of the thyroid gland. It was thus amply evident that some thyroid tissue must be preserved to avoid myxedema and Kocher, after 1883, largely limited his operations on the thyroid to single lobectomy. Single lobectomy had obvious disadvantages and Mikulicz proposed in 1886 that both lobes should be resected, but that a portion of the gland on either side near the inferior thyroid arteries should be preserved. Postoperative tetany and postoperative myxedema were observed, frequently together and often singly, following total thyroidectomy and the two conditions were originally thought to be different phases of the same disease. Vassale and Generali were able to demonstrate in 1896 that the two conditions were quite different and that postoperative tetany was due to the removal of the parathyroid glands. It is not surprising that injury to the recurrent laryngeal nerves was encountered frequently during these earlier years. In a series of Billroth's cases, reported in 1882, the inferior laryngeal nerves were uninjured in thirty-one cases but were paralyzed on one side in eleven cases and on both sides in two cases. Because of the rather fortunate anatomic relationship between the usual sites of the parathyroids and the inferior laryngeal nerve, it was soon evident that nerve injuries and tetany could be avoided, as could postoperative myxedema, by preserving thyroid tissue on both sides, as had been suggested by Mikulicz.

In spite of the demonstration in the 1880's that hyperthyroidism could be effectively controlled by subtotal thyroidectomy, and in spite of the fact that the operation could be safely done in cases of nontoxic goiter, the surgical treatment of hyperthyroidism lagged behind that of nontoxic goiter, principally because of the high surgical risk associated with operations on hyperthyroid patients. In an effort to reduce this risk the principle of carrying out the operation in stages was evolved. While Kocher employed the principle of graduated operations to some extent in the treatment of hyperthyroidism, credit for the development of the method is due chiefly to surgeons in this country, notably to C. H. Mayo. In 1908 C. H. Mayo reported a mortality rate of 6 per cent in a series of operations on 234 patients who had exophthalmic goiter. By the adoption of multiple-stage operations it was possible to reduce this figure to about 3 per cent. H. S. Plummer in 1922 proposed the use of iodides to prepare for operation patients who had hyperthyroidism and it was possible, after preparation with iodine, to carry out one-stage operations on all but 2 to 3 per cent of patients who had exophthalmic goiter. This was in sharp contrast to the years just preceding the iodine era when multiple-stage operations were carried out in the treatment of approximately two out of every three patients with exophthalmic goiter who were operated on at the Mayo Clinic. Under modern conditions, with satisfactory preoperative preparation with iodides, the risk of subtotal thyroidectomy on patients with exophthalmic goiter has been reduced to less than 1 per cent and is largely dependent on the amount of visceral damage the patient has sustained as a result of hyperthyroidism.

Anatomy. The thyroid gland lies in the lower third of the neck deep to the infrahyoid and sternocleidomastoid muscles and closely applied to the larynx and the upper part of the trachea. It has two lobes, one on either side of the trachea, connected by the isthmus, and, in about 50 per cent of the cases, there is a cephalad prolongation of thyroid tissue, the pyramidal lobe, extending upward from the anteromedial surface of either lobe or from the isthmus. The two lobes are roughly symmetrical, although often one lobe, usually the right, is somewhat larger than the other. The size and weight of the gland vary greatly depending on age, sex, physiologic status, geographic location and the presence or absence of pathologic enlargement (goiter). On an average, and within wide limits, the diameters are as follows: vertical 3 to 6 cm., transverse, whole gland, 6 to 7 cm., and anteroposterior 2 to 3 cm. The weight varies between 20 and 60 gm. The lobes are roughly conical in form and are applied to the trachea so that the medial surface is concave. The anterolateral surface is rounded and the posterior surface is usually molded by surrounding parts. The lobe narrows to an apex superiorly, the superior pole. The inferior extremity of the lobe, the inferior pole, is broad and rounded. The isthmus varies in size and may be absent altogether; on the average it is about 0.5 cm. thick and 2 cm. wide and connects the two lobes at the junction of the lower and middle thirds. The pyramidal lobe, when present, varies in size and it may extend as high as the hyoid bone, to which it is sometimes attached.

Each lobe is more or less densely attached to the sides of the trachea. The attached zone extends from the anterolateral surface of the cricoid cartilage superiorly to the second or third cartilaginous ring of the trachea inferiorly. In addition to the attachments between the trachea and the medial surface of each lobe, fibrous or muscular bands are present, which connect the isthmus, pyramidal lobe or medial surfaces of the superior poles to the hyoid bone. When muscular, these are known as the levator glandulae thyroideae. Other bands, one on either side, which run medially, the suspensory ligaments, connect the lobes with the thyroid and cricoid cartilages. The thyroid gland is so intimately connected to the larynx and trachea that the gland follows the upward movement of the trachea on swallowing.

The thyroid lies in the visceral compartment of the deep cervical fascia, which also contains the larynx and trachea, the esophagus, the recurrent laryngeal nerves, the parathyroid glands and the great vessels. The compartment is bounded anteriorly by the middle layer of the deep cervical fascia, which ensheathes the subhyoid muscles, and posteriorly by the deep, or prevertebral, layer of the deep cervical fascia. The gland is loosely surrounded by areolar tissue. The true capsule of the thyroid gland is inseparably connected with the parenchymatous tissue and is continued into the lobe in the form of numerous septa which subdivide the lobe. Studies by Rienhoff of wax model reconstructions of the gland demonstrated that the thyroid is not subdivided into lobules, as was previously thought, but that the septa ramify irregularly, dividing the gland into masses of parenchyma of irregular shapes and sizes, which are always connected by bars or strips of thyroid tissue. The blood vessels, lymphatics and nerves course through the septa.

The functioning unit of the thyroid gland is the follicle or vesicle, a closed sac of irregular shape and size, lined by a single layer of cuboidal or low columnar epithelium, and containing a viscid, usually acid-staining, homogeneous fluid called "colloid." The parenchymal cells rest directly on the connective tissue. The follicles and contained colloid vary with the functional activity of the thyroid. In very active glands the follicles are reduced in size, the epithelium is taller and may be thrown into papillary infoldings and the colloid is reduced. The converse is true for the resting or sluggish gland; the follicles are larger and may be very large so that it appears that they are actually distended with colloid, the epithelium is cuboidal or even flattened and the colloid stains more deeply.

ARTERIES. The chief arteries supplying the thyroid gland are the two superior thyroid arteries, the two inferior thyroid arteries and the inconstant thyroidea ima. Constant collateral branches anastomose with the arteries that supply the larynx, trachea and esophagus. The superior thyroid artery, the first branch of the external carotid artery, leaves the carotid slightly above the bifurcation, usually arches upward in a so-called shepherd's crook form and descends to the tip of the superior pole or to its medial aspect. The branches are distributed to the superior and anterior surfaces of the lobe. One branch usually runs in the suspensory ligament and another anastomoses with a corresponding branch from the opposite superior thyroid artery across the isthmus. The inferior thyroid artery is a branch of the subclavian, arising from the thyrocervical trunk. The artery passes behind the common carotid and, after ascending a variable distance in the neck, descends to reach the lobe near the junction of the lower and middle thirds. The branches are distributed along the posterior surface of the lobe and constant branches pass anteriorly beside the trachea. The artery anastomoses freely with the superior thyroid artery and through the isthmus with the contralateral arteries. The thyroidea ima artery arises from the aorta or the innominate artery and runs upward anterior to the trachea to reach the lower poles or isthmus. It is inconstant, and, when present, varies in size. The collateral blood supply is extremely well developed. Colored injections through any one thyroid artery color not only the entire thyroid gland but the larynx, upper part of the trachea, esophagus and neighboring muscles. All four thyroid arteries may be ligated, during the course of subtotal thyroidectomy, without fear of depriving the remnants of thyroid tissue or the parathyroids of adequate blood supply, provided that the remnants of thyroid tissue are not detached from the trachea.

VEINS. The veins arise within the lobes and form an extensive plexus beneath the true capsule. More or less constant channels, the superior, the middle and the inferior thyroid veins, connect the plexus with the systemic circulation. The superior thyroid veins, usually paired and constant, follow the course of the superior thyroid artery and empty into the internal jugular vein. The middle thyroid vein, frequently multiple but inconstant, runs from the posterolateral surface of the lobe to the internal jugular vein. The inferior thyroid veins, usually two on each side, descend from the lower pole or isthmus to enter the innominate vein. A fairly constant vein connects the pyramidal lobe with the anterior jugular system. The thyroid veins lack valves.

LYMPHATICS. From an abundant lymph capillary system which surrounds the vesicles, the lymph passes into a lymphatic plexus beneath the true capsule. Lymph channels pass outward chiefly in the regions of the three sets of veins to enter the thoracic duct and right lymph trunk. The lymph drains through nodes in the deep jugular group and those situated anterior and lateral to the trachea. Some lymphatics are thought to enter the subclavian vein directly without passing through nodes.

NERVES. The thyroid receives the major portion of its nerve supply from the sympathetic system. Fibers pass outward from the cord through the first two thoracic roots to reach the superior, middle and inferior cervical sympathetic ganglia. Nonmedullated fibers run from these ganglia, particularly from the middle and inferior, to the thyroid, intimately associated with the superior and inferior thyroid arteries. Fibers from both the superior and inferior laryngeal nerves are thought to be distributed to the thyroid gland.

The Recurrent (Inferior) Laryngeal Nerves. The recurrent laryngeal nerves, one on either side, are the chief motor nerves of the intrinsic muscles of the larynx. The nerve on the left side, after arching around the aorta, passes upward deep in the tracheo-esophageal groove. On the right side the nerve arches around the subclavian artery and does not reach the tracheo-esophageal groove until it has passed above the level of the lower pole of the right lobe. The nerve on the right is almost 1 cm. from the trachea at the level of the clavicle. Rarely, once in 200 to 300 cases, the nerve on the right side leaves the vagus in the neck and passes medially to reach the adherent zone directly. On both sides the nerves continue upward in varying relationship to the adherent zones and inferior thyroid arteries, to enter the larynx just posteriorly to the inferior cricothyroid articulations. Berlin, from a study of seventy dissections of 140 recurrent laryngeal nerves of cadavers, found that the right nerve arched up to pass through thyroid gland tissue in 13 per cent, passed through the adherent zone in 27 per cent and continued in the tracheo-esophageal groove in 60 per cent of cases. The left nerve arched up into the lobe in 7 per cent, passed through the adherent zone in 23 per cent and ran in the tracheo-esophageal groove in 70 per cent of cases. On the right side, the nerve passed posterior to the artery in 44 per cent, anterior to the artery in 40 per cent and between its branches in 16 per cent. On the left side the nerve ran posterior to the artery in 63 per cent of cases, anterior to the artery in 24 per cent and between the terminal branches in 13 per cent. Before reaching the adherent zone or larynx, the nerve divides frequently into two trunks, which may not follow the same course upward.

Indications for Operation on the Thyroid Gland. The varieties of goiter of particular concern to the surgeon are as follows (classification of H. S. Plummer):

1. Diffuse colloid goiter
2. Adenomatous goiter without hyperthyroidism
3. Adenomatous goiter with hyperthyroidism
4. Exophthalmic goiter
5. Thyroiditis, acute and chronic
6. Malignant lesions.

The indications for surgical intervention in the several diseases of the thyroid gland are generally well known. With colloid goiters, as a rule, resection is not indicated since medical management with desiccated thyroid by mouth and iodine will reduce the size of the gland satisfactorily. It occasionally happens, after the size of the colloid goiter has been thus reduced, that persisting adenomas can be palpated, and in such cases surgical removal of the adenomas or resection of the involved lobe or lobes may well be indicated. With patients who have adenomatous or nodular goiters without hyperthyroidism, surgical treatment is indicated when the goiter has produced pressure effects on the trachea or esophagus, or when there is evidence of obstructed venous return. Similarly, substernal adenomas should be resected. More frequently no pressure effects are present and in such cases the indications for operation are less well defined. In general, when there is definite nodular or adenomatous enlargement of the thyroid, and particularly when the nodules are 2.5 cm. or more in size, operation for removal of the adenoma should be advised.

The potential risks of neglected adenomatous goiters are very real. Approximately 60 per cent of the malignant lesions of the thyroid gland encountered at the Mayo Clinic could not be diagnosed clinically, and the malignant lesions were found only on microscopic examination of resected nodular goiters. Three or 4 per cent of patients with adenomatous goiters have an established malignant lesion at the time of the removal of the goiter. In addition, in an unknown, but material, percentage of cases of adenomatous goiter malignant lesions will subsequently develop if the adenomatous goiter is not removed. The proportion of patients with adenomatous goiter without hyperthyroidism who will ultimately become hyperthyroid, similarly, is not known with certainty. It has been estimated that in from 35 to 50 per cent of such cases signs of toxicity will develop, usually many years after the appearance of the goiter. The onset of hyperthyroidism is often so insidious in such cases that serious cardiac damage may be produced before the patient seeks medical care. The advanced age of the patient and the visceral damage, particularly cardiac, increase the risk of operation from approximately 0.2 per cent for patients who have adenomatous goiter without hyperthyroidism to 2 to 3 per cent for patients who have adenomatous goiter with hyperthyroidism.

With patients suffering from hyperthyroidism, either adenomatous goiter with hyperthyroidism or exophthalmic goiter, surgical treatment is strongly indicated after adequate preparation. A small proportion of patients who have exophthalmic goiter may be treated adequately with iodides, but the control of the disease is uncertain and the disease is prone to recur. Certain goitrogenic drugs, notably propylthiouracil, will control the symptoms of exophthalmic goiter and those of adenomatous goiter with hyperthyroidism, though they control the latter less readily than the former. However, the treatment with such agents must be continued for many months, if not indefinitely, and during the treatment the patients must be observed regularly for the possible development of toxic effects and for the effect of the drug on the basal metabolic rate. Such drugs have found less place in the definitive treatment of hyperthyroidism than was originally hoped. Because of the small but definite incidence of malignancy (about 4 to 6 per cent) associated with adenomatous goiter, no medical treatment should be employed without taking into consideration this potential risk. In recent years radioiodine has proved to be an effective means of controlling hyperthyroidism in many cases. The permanence of the results has not been determined. Until greater accuracy in gauging the dose is established and until the potential radiation hazard in the treatment of hyperthyroidism with radioiodine is known, caution demands that its employment be limited to those patients on whom thyroidectomy is regarded as unduly hazardous.

In acute thyroiditis surgical treatment is limited largely to the prompt drainage of abscesses should the disease progress to this point. In chronic thyroiditis the thyroid should be explored surgically, in most cases, to verify the diagnosis and to relieve or prevent tracheal compression. The operation, in such cases, is limited usually to the removal of the isthmus and to the resection of the anterior third of each lobe. The trachea, in this way, is freed from the semicircle of thyroid tissue and the remaining thyroid tissue is separated completely into two masses.

The most satisfactory treatment of carcinoma of the thyroid gland is surgical removal combined with irradiation.

In children there is some difference of opinion as to whether hyperthyroidism, that is, exophthalmic goiter, since adenomatous goiter with hyperthyroidism has not been observed, should be treated by subtotal thyroidectomy. The operation is somewhat more difficult technically, preparation for operation takes a longer time, and hyperthyroid reactions following operation are more pronounced than in adults. Furthermore, there is greater chance for the development of both myxedema and recurrent hyperthyroidism than in adults. In spite of such disadvantages, subtotal thyroidectomy remains the treatment of choice, since the hyperthyroidism in most cases can be efficiently controlled without excessive risk. In the series of children operated on for hyperthyroidism at the Mayo Clinic, the mortality rate was less than 3 per cent. In children with nodular goiters, surgical exploration is more imperative than in adults because of the likelihood of the nodules being malignant. Thus, eighteen in a series of fifty-one children less than fifteen years of age who had nodular goiters were found on surgical exploration to have carcinoma of the thyroid gland.

Preoperative Preparation. No particular preparation is necessary for patients without hyperthyroidism, and there is some evidence to indicate that prolonged medication with iodide may incite the development of hyperthyroidism in patients with adenomatous goiter who are not hyperthyroid.

Patients who have exophthalmic goiter should receive 10 drops of strong solution of iodine (Lugol's solution) three times a day for seven to fourteen days before operation, and occasionally for much longer periods, provided that improvement is continuing. During the time of preparation the patient need not be confined to the hospital, and the patient should not be confined to bed because of the muscular weakness that continued rest in bed promotes. An ample diet (3,000 calories or more) and ample intake of fluids should be provided. When congestive heart failure is present, digitalis is, as a rule, not indicated since the congestive heart failure is treated more rationally by treating the hyperthyroidism. However, if the patient does not readily respond to the foregoing regimen, the mercurial diuretics may be indicated to rid the patient of excessive fluid. Most patients may be prepared satisfactorily so that subtotal thyroidectomy may be carried out in one stage. In about 3 per cent of cases, however, the patient cannot be got into satisfactory condition for a one-stage operation and for this group of patients operations divided into stages may be considered. Goitrogenic drugs, such as propylthiouracil, are finding their greatest usefulness in the preoperative preparation of this relatively small group of patients, since with such drugs it is usually possible to control the hyperthyroidism until the patient has had an opportunity to recover from its effects and so withstand operation more satisfactorily. Lugol's solution (strong solution of iodine) should be administered during the three weeks preceding the operation in place of the goitrogen.

Patients who have adenomatous goiter with hyperthyroidism respond less dramatically to iodides than do patients who have exophthalmic goiter. However, such patients should receive the same dose of strong solution of iodine preoperatively as is given to patients who have exophthalmic goiter.

Anesthesia. The method of anesthesia of choice in thyroid surgery, with rare exceptions, is the combination of local, superficial, cervical field block, using 0.5 per cent procaine hydrochloride, with light general anesthesia, employing nitrous oxide and oxygen. The general anesthesia is needed usually only while the first lobe is being elevated and resected. This method of anesthesia allows the patient to be awakened after the first lobe has been resected and before the second lobe has been disturbed, so that the integrity of the recurrent laryngeal nerve on the first side may be determined. If there is evidence of injury to the recurrent laryngeal nerve, it is obvious that the injured nerve is on the side of the resected lobe, and it can be dissected out without danger of producing bilateral paralysis of the vocal cords.

If there is impairment of the airway prior to operation, as evidenced by stridor, or if definite narrowing, flattening or distortion of the trachea exists, the operation is more safely conducted using local anesthesia only. This is particularly true in the presence of large substernal or retrotracheal masses of thyroid tissue, since the airway may be even further diminished during the mobilization of such tissue. After the misplaced tissue has been elevated and the trachea exposed, the general anesthetic agent may be more safely added. Very rarely the airway is so seriously decreased, usually by large adenomas wedged in the superior strait of the thorax, that any mobilization of the lobe may produce tracheal obstruction. In such cases, after complete cocainization of the pharynx and hypopharynx, a Magill intratracheal tube may be introduced past the obstruction and general anesthesia induced. The tube acts as an internal splint and insures an airway during mobilization and resection of the offending tissue. After the lobe has been resected and with the trachea still exposed, the intratracheal tube should be removed, so that tracheotomy may be carried out if the trachea should collapse.

With children, the plan of anesthesia is essentially the same as that for adults. As a rule, it is necessary to induce general anesthesia before the local block can be done. General anesthesia usually is necessary during the resection of the second lobe.

Subtotal Thyroidectomy. The prototypic operation on the thyroid gland is subtotal thyroidectomy, the basic principles of which are as follows: 1. The removal of sufficient tissue. In cases of exophthalmic goiter this ordinarily implies the removal of 65 to 85 per cent of each lobe. In cases of adenomatous goiter it implies that no whole adenomas are left behind and that a symmetrical neck is achieved. 2. The preservation of adequate tissue to secure normal function. In cases of exophthalmic goiter it is necessary to preserve tissue equal to one-fourth to one-sixth of a lobe of normal size on either side. 3. The control of bleeding, both immediate and late. 4. The avoidance of sepsis. 5. The avoidance of injury to surrounding structures. 6. The securing of a satisfactory cosmetic result. Under modern conditions, the technical complications are largely limited to injuries of the recurrent laryngeal nerves and to bleeding.

POSITION OF PATIENT. By the use of small pillows and the head rest on the operating table, the neck is moderately extended. Since the patient is to be awake during most of the operation, a position not too trying for him should be found. The arms are pulled firmly toward the foot of the table to depress the shoulders and the operating table is so tilted that the head is well elevated above the feet. Venous blood is thus kept from pooling in the great veins of the neck. A suitable foot rest and a strong strap across the legs just above the knees are essential to prevent the patient from sliding downward. The draping is arranged so that the face of the patient is excluded from the field of operation. Sufficient room must be provided for the anesthetist and for the application of the anesthetic mask to the patient's face.

INCISION. The incision has become well standardized. Because of its importance from the cosmetic standpoint, it should be carefully made. It is placed about 2 cm. above the sternal end of the clavicle, the actual position depending on the length and contour of the neck (Fig. 435, inset). The length varies somewhat with the size of the goiter but is usually from 7 to 12 cm. An incision made through a natural crease in the skin of the neck, or parallel to such a crease, leaves the least noticeable scar. The incision should be almost horizontal when the patient's neck is extended and must be symmetrical. A horizontal incision made with the neck extended will have approximately the proper curve when the neck is in the more normal position or flexed, because of the tenting effect of the chin on the skin of the neck. A necklace or a piece of string may be used to mark the position of the incision. Unsightly scars result from incisions which are asymmetrical or too curved, and from those which slant. If the incision is too low and lies at the level of the sternoclavicular articulations, the resulting scar is unsightly. If the incision is placed too high it cannot be concealed by a collar or beads.

ELEVATION OF FLAPS. The incision is deepened through the subcutaneous layer and the platysma. The proper cleavage plane is found readily if the upper flap is firmly retracted anteriorly and upward. The plane lies just anterior to the first layer of the deep cervical fascia, which covers the sternohyoid muscles and in which the anterior jugular system of veins passes (Fig. 435). None of the anterior jugular veins need be divided if the dissection is carried upward in the proper plane. If an anterior jugular vein should be opened inadvertently, transfixion ligatures should be used to occlude the vein above and below the opening, since ordinary ligatures are prone to slip. The upper flap is elevated by combined blunt and sharp dissection to well above the level of the laryngeal prominence. The lower flap need be elevated only sufficiently to afford engagement to a self-retaining retractor, such as the Beckman. All bleeding points are secured by fine ligatures before going deeper, and skin towels are applied to the edges of the incision.

An alternative cleavage plane may be found just deep to the superficial layer of the deep cervical fascia. In this plane, the subhyoid muscles must be separated from the fascia by sharp dissection and the anterior jugular veins divided and secured. This plane is more vascular than the more

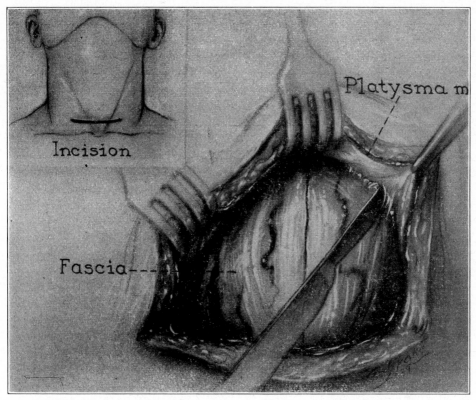

FIG. 435. The inset illustrates the position, length and curve of the incision. In the main part of the figure the upper flap is being raised in a cleavage plane just superficial to the first layer of the deep cervical fascia. (From Pemberton and Black, *Surg. Clin. N. Amer.*, [Aug.], 1946.)

superficial one but its advocates believe that more ample exposure is secured.

EXPOSURE OF THE GLAND. A vertical incision is made in the midline between the two sternohyoid muscles and carried through the fused layers of the superficial and middle layers of the deep cervical fascia. The loose areolar tissue which surrounds the thyroid gland is encountered as soon as the denser fascial layer is incised. The vertical incision should extend from the sternum to above the level of the thyroid cartilage. The sternohyoid muscles are loosely connected to the underlying thyroid and, more laterally, to the sternothyroid muscles and this space may be readily opened into by blunt dissection to provide more adequate exposure (Fig. 436). The sternothyroid muscles are closely applied to the lobes of the thyroid gland.

DIVISION OF STERNOHYOID MUSCLE. In many cases, particularly with large goiters (and some surgeons prefer in all cases), the sternohyoid muscle

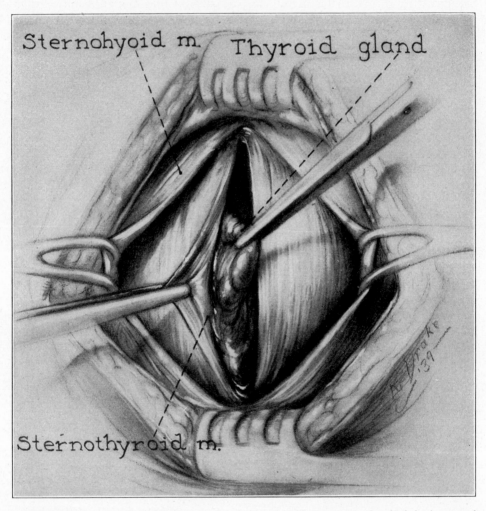

FIG. 436. The deep fascia has been incised in the midline from the level of the laryngeal prominence to the sternum. The space between the sternohyoid and the sternothyroid muscles on either side has been opened up. (From Pemberton and Black, *Surg. Clin. N. Amer.*, [Aug.], 1946.)

may be divided transversely on one or both sides to provide more ample exposure. The muscle, contained in a compartment of the deep cervical fascia, is sectioned between clamps to prevent retraction of the cut ends of the muscle and to control bleeding. The incision may be continued laterally into the sternocleidomastoid muscle, although this usually is not necessary. Annoying bleeding may be avoided if the lateral border of the

sternohyoid muscle is separated from the sternocleidomastoid muscle before
the former muscle is sectioned, and the small vessels which run between the
two muscles are ligated separately. The sternohyoid should be divided in
its upper third to minimize injury to its motor nerves. In the closure of the

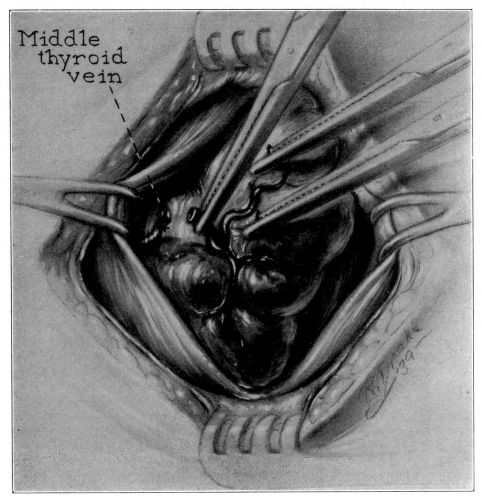

FIG. 437. The thyroid gland is being mobilized, the Ochsner hemostat being used to
grasp the capsule. The middle thyroid vein has been ligated. (From Pemberton and Black,
Surg. Clin. N. Amer., [Aug.], 1946.)

incision the cut ends of the muscle are approximated by suture and the
cut anterior jugular veins carefully secured. No deformity in the contour
of the neck results from sectioning the muscles.

ELEVATION AND ROTATION OF THE LOBE. Usually, the right lobe of the
thyroid gland is resected first. With large goiters, and particularly when
tracheal compression is present, it is often desirable to expose the trachea
before proceeding with the elevation of the first lobe because of the possi-

bility that tracheotomy may become necessary. Should the airway become obstructed during the elevation of the lobe, tracheotomy can be carried out promptly if the trachea has been well exposed and all hemostats have been removed after securing the bleeding vessels. If this emergency is not

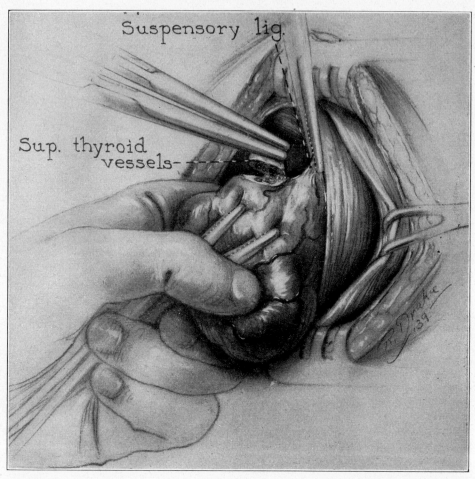

FIG. 438. The superior pole of the thyroid gland has been exposed and the superior thyroid vessels have been doubly clamped. The suspensory ligament has been clamped. (From Pemberton and Black, *Surg. Clin. N. Amer.,* [Aug.], 1946.)

foreseen, there may not be sufficient time to expose and open the trachea before the patient is beyond aid.

In the usual case the more medial fibers of the sternothyroid muscles are pushed laterally and the lobe is grasped with forceps (Fig. 437). Many types of grasping forceps have been devised for this but the ordinary toothed Ochsner hemostat is entirely satisfactory. With friable glands several hemostats may be thrust into the lobe side-by-side, each grasping a different segment of capsule to secure a firm hold on the lobe. The lobe is lifted anteriorly and rotated medially as the overlying sternothyroid muscle is separated from the lobe by combined blunt and sharp dissection. The proper cleavage plane, just outside of the true capsule, is readily followed in the usual case. The plane may be largely obliterated, however, when the thyroid has been resected previously or has been involved by thyroiditis. In such cases sharp dissection may be necessary throughout.

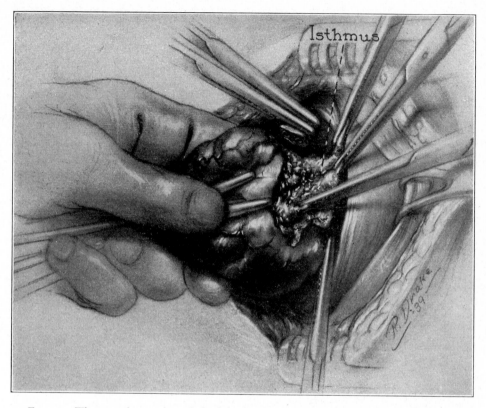

FIG. 439. The actual resection of the lobe has been started from the medial or tracheal side. The surgeon's left hand keeps the lobe elevated and controls bleeding. (From Pemberton and Black, *Surg. Clin. N. Amer.*, [Aug.], 1946.)

As the elevation and rotation of the lobe progress, the middle thyroid vein is encountered near the lateral border of the sternothyroid muscle. This is a major collecting trunk from the subcapsular plexus of veins and empties directly into the internal jugular vein. There may be several such veins. The vein should be carefully isolated, clamped and tied immediately, so that the clamps cannot be pulled off inadvertently (Fig. 437). If the vein should be torn across or avulsed from the jugular, frequently all that remains is a hole in the jugular vein. The wound fills promptly with a gush of venous blood which is difficult to control at this stage of the operation. There is also some danger of air embolism. It usually is safer and far easier to pack the area with gauze until the lobe has been removed, when, with the more adequate exposure attained by removal of the lobe, the opening in the jugular vein may be found and closed. After the division and ligation of the middle thyroid vein, the lobe is exposed completely by blunt dissection and elevated well out of the incision.

RESECTION OF THE LOBE. Exposure of the superior pole of the thyroid gland and the superior thyroid vessels is secured by downward traction on

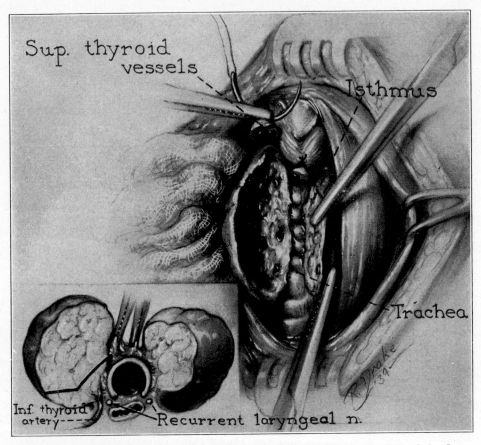

FIG. 440. The insert shows the proper line of resection. In the main part of the figure the lobe has been resected and the superior thyroid vessels are being ligated. (From Pemberton and Black, *Surg. Clin. N. Amer.*, [Aug.], 1946.)

the lobe and by upward and outward retraction of the strap muscles (Fig. 438). The exposure must be ample so that no thyroid tissue will be left above the clamps. The superior thyroid vessels are doubly clamped and divided. Because of the troublesome and possibly dangerous bleeding that may result if the superior thyroid artery should escape, two clamps with subsequent double ligatures would seem a reasonable precaution. After the superior thyroid vessels have been divided, the suspensory ligament, the base of the pyramidal lobe, if present, and the isthmus are clamped and divided in this order. It is easier to continue with the dissection than to stop to remove the pyramidal lobe at this time. The lobe, by this stage, is connected to the trachea only in the adherent zone and care should be taken not to encroach on the adherent zone during the resection.

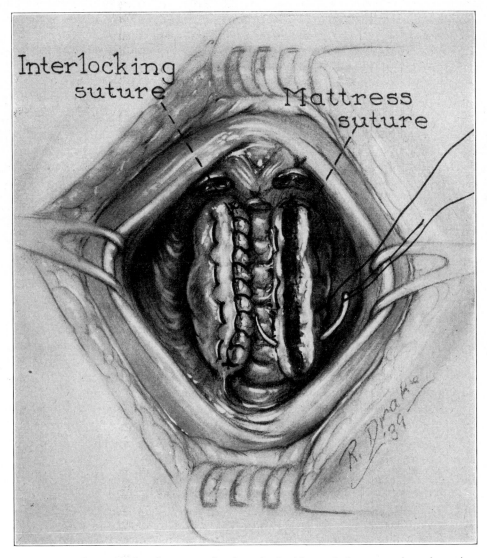

FIG. 441. Resection has been completed on both sides and the posterolateral portion of the capsule is being sutured to the tissue which was preserved alongside the trachea. (From Pemberton and Black, *Surg. Clin. N. Amer.*, [Aug.], 1946.)

The actual resection of the lobe proceeds from the tracheal side outward, even in cases in which the isthmus is unusually thick (Fig. 439). With the lobe under tension, secured by the surgeon's left hand lifting upward on hemostats caught in the lobe or its capsule, the medial surface of the lobe is caught in several places by hemostats placed in a frontal plane which passes through the anterior wall of the trachea. The gland caught in the hemostat is sectioned. This first row of hemostats serves several useful functions: they secure branches of the inferior thyroid artery, they mark the anterior limit of the thyroid tissue to be saved, they prevent the dissection entering the adherent zone of the lobe, and finally the tissue in their grasp will afford anchorage for subsequent hemostatic sutures. Other hemostats are successively placed and the gland tissue is sectioned above them. The lobe is sectioned horizontally for about 5 mm. and then posterolaterally, carefully preserving the gland tissue beside the trachea and along the posterior portion of the capsule (Fig. 440). As the capsule is approached, the line of resection through the capsule is delineated by the application of two to four hemostats to the lateral surface of the capsule, and the capsule is sectioned above them. These hemostats are placed in the capsule 1.5 to 2 cm. anterior to the posterolateral line of resection through the lobe so that the sectioned surface of the lobe is V-shaped. Thus, far more parenchymatous tissue is resected than capsule. All clamps are removed after the vessels have been ligated. Transfixion ligatures are used generously, particularly in the capsule and along the anterior border of the adherent zone beside the trachea. The preserved remnant of thyroid tissue is sutured to the trachea for the double purpose of controlling any remaining oozing and of anchoring the remnant firmly to the fascia covering the trachea (Fig. 441). In suturing, the needle is always passed anteriorly to a plane passing through the anterior wall of the trachea. The suture is started at the superior pole and, using a continuous mattress suture, the capsule is tightly approximated to the tissue adherent to the trachea. The suture is reversed at the inferior pole and, using an interlocking suture, laid just posteriorly to the mattress suture, is returned to the superior pole.

Testing for Integrity of Recurrent Laryngeal Nerve. Following the resection of the right (first) lobe and before any dissection has been started on the second side, the patient is awakened and allowed to talk, cough and strain in an effort to determine if the recurrent laryngeal nerve has been injured. With nerve injury, the voice changes, as a rule, quite unmistakably, although at times the voice changes so little that uncertainty exists as to whether the changes are due to preoperative medication, removal of false teeth, collection of mucus in the larynx and trachea, or other causes. The uncertainty may be dispelled easily by having the patient cough. The character of the cough of the patient who has had a recurrent nerve recently injured is pathognomonic. Instead of the normal single explosive sound, a high pitched squeaky note precedes an enfeebled explosive effort. Some patience may be necessary on the part of the surgeon and the anesthetist to secure satisfactory co-operation of the patient, but unless the preoperative sedation has been too great or the general anesthesia too deep, satisfactory tests may usually be carried out.

The status of the nerve on the first side must be determined satisfactorily before resection of the second lobe is begun in order that the side of the injured nerve, if one of the nerves has been injured, may be known with certainty. If such an injury has occurred, the nerve should be dissected out, in its course through the operative field, and the cause of the injury found. If a ligature has been placed around the nerve the paralysis will be permanent unless the ligature is removed. If the ligature is removed, or if the nerve has been injured by pressure or tension, recovery of function is to be expected and can be detected on laryngeal examination in from two to twelve weeks. The operation should be terminated usually after the nerve has been dissected out, the cause of the injury found and corrected, and the remnant resutured to the trachea. The removal of the remaining lobe can be carried out after a period of three months when function of the nerve has returned. In this way the possibility of bilateral paralysis of the vocal cords is minimized. If the injury to the nerve occurs during the removal of the second lobe, time should be taken to dissect out the nerve and repair the damage, in order to correct a potentially permanent injury into a temporary one.

As a rule, permanent paralysis of one vocal cord causes little disability, usually no obstruction of the airway and relatively minor impairment of the speaking voice, although singers, public speakers and persons who use the voice vigorously or for prolonged periods may find that their use of the voice has been impaired. In decided contrast, bilateral permanent paralysis of the vocal cords is a catastrophe which may lead to death and which, at best, will be followed by serious consequences. In many cases, immediate tracheotomy is necessary; in other cases the airway, ample soon after the injuries, becomes progressively impaired so that tracheotomy is ultimately necessary or the activities of the patient must be greatly limited. The development of pneumonia is common because of anoxia, impaired cough, and the aspiration of mucus, liquids and food. Formerly, the most satisfactory method of treatment was permanent valve tracheotomy. More recently King has proposed an operation which provides an adequate airway by the lateral dislocation of one of the arytenoid cartilages, to which the vocal cord is attached posteriorly. When this operation is skillfully done, an ample airway can be provided without impairing the speaking voice too markedly. The operation has proved most satisfactory but requires skill, experience and a thorough knowledge of laryngeal and cervical anatomy.

RESECTION OF PYRAMIDAL LOBE. A search should be made in all cases for the pyramidal lobe, which is removed completely if present. If such thyroid tissue is not removed it may hypertrophy or adenomas may develop in it. Such so-called recurrent tissue is very disfiguring because of the superficial location of the pyramidal lobe.

RESECTION OF THE SECOND LOBE. The resection of the second lobe is carried out in the same manner as that of the first lobe. The second lobe can be mobilized more easily than the first lobe, because the removal of the first lobe allows the larynx and trachea to be rotated more readily and further than when the opposite lobe is present. Because of this, caution should be exercised to avoid carrying the dissection into the adherent zone and to avoid exposure of the lateral tracheal wall. Furthermore, the resection of the left lobe may be needlessly radical because of the fact that the right-handed surgeon stands on the patient's right and therefore his view of the posterior and lateral parts of the lobe on the left is less satisfactory than on the right. The left recurrent laryngeal nerve, in spite of its more protected position, is injured more often than the right, probably because of these two factors.

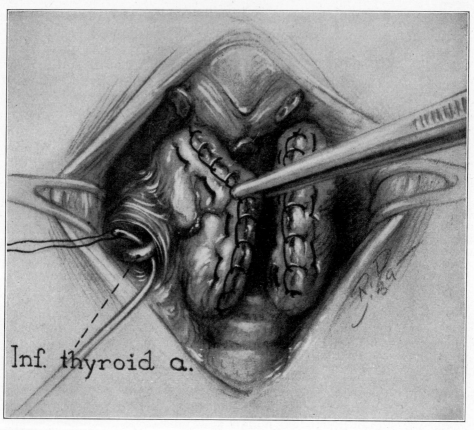

Inf. thyroid a.

FIG. 442. The inferior thyroid artery has been ligated well laterally. (From Pemberton and Black, *Surg. Clin. N. Amer.*, [Aug.], 1946.)

The patient is urged to cough and strain, or the anesthetist may cause the patient to gag or retch by intermittent pressure on the oropharynx before closure of the incision is started. Unsecured veins are thus caused to bleed so that they can be caught and ligated.

LIGATION OF INFERIOR THYROID ARTERY. It is common practice, as a further measure to prevent bleeding, to ligate one or both of the inferior thyroid arteries separately before they have entered the corresponding lobe (Fig. 442). The position of the artery can usually be found by palpation and the artery can be quickly exposed by blunt dissection. The main trunk is ligated in continuity far laterally to avoid the inferior laryngeal nerve. The dissection is facilitated by retracting the common carotid laterally. In some cases, to minimize bleeding during the resection, the inferior thyroid artery can be ligated before the lobe is resected. As previously mentioned, the collateral circulation to the thyroid is very rich, and extensive experience has proved that the ligation of the inferior thyroid artery does not seriously impair the blood supply to the remnant of the resected lobe or to the parathyroid glands, provided the remnant of the gland is not detached from

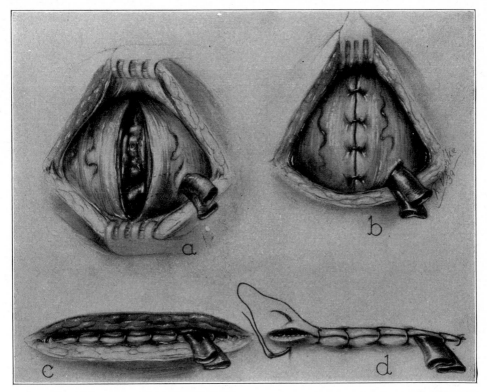

Fig. 443. Steps in the closure of the incision. The fascial layer has been closed in the midline and the drains have been brought out through the incision well laterally. (From Pemberton and Black, *Surg. Clin. N. Amer.*, [Aug.], 1946.)

the lateral wall of the trachea, thus destroying the principal collateral blood supply.

DRAINAGE. Drains, if used, should be of soft rubber to prevent erosion of neighboring structures. Penrose drains are entirely satisfactory and two are used as a rule. One drain is left on either side down to the remnant of the thyroid tissue, and the two drains are brought out together through an opening in the deep cervical fascia between the sternohyoid and sterno-cleidomastoid muscles (Fig. 443). The drains are not brought out through the original vertical incision in the midline because of the possibility that adhesions may form between the skin and the trachea, but the drains are led out near one extremity of the skin incision. Stab wounds through the skin are needless and leave an added scar in the neck. Whether drainage is necessary following thyroidectomy has been long debated. Soft rubber drains, removed after forty-eight hours, produce no permanent increase in scarring, no impairment in wound healing and, in addition to providing for the escape of serum, their presence permits of earlier diagnosis of postoperative bleeding.

CLOSURE. The vertical incision through the deep cervical fascia in the midline is closed by means of interrupted sutures (Fig. 443). The skin flaps are carefully checked for bleeding and closed with skin clips or by dermal sutures after first approximating the cut edges of the platysma with interrupted fine catgut sutures. The skin sutures, or clips, should be removed in seventy-two hours; otherwise permanent scars from the stitch holes will remain.

Recurrent and Persistent Goiter. Secondary operations on the thyroid gland are more difficult technically than primary operations. Secondary operations are fairly frequently necessary because of recurrence and occasionally because of inadequate removal of thyroid tissue at the time of the first operation. It would appear from the frequency with which substernal and retrotracheal masses of thyroid tissue are encountered at secondary operations that such masses of tissue are fairly often overlooked at the time of the original operation. However, the frequency with which the retrotracheal and substernal projections are encountered in secondary operations for recurrent goiter can be explained in part by the fact that the tissues anterior and lateral to the remnant of the gland are unyielding because of the presence of scar tissue, and therefore the extension of the growth is downward or behind the trachea, in the line of least resistance. It is evident that both remnants of thyroid tissue should be well exposed in any secondary operation, and that the dissection should be complete enough to expose any possible retrotracheal or substernal masses of thyroid tissue.

In secondary operations, particularly when there has been a true recurrence following a reasonably radical primary operation, two situations are encountered which have resulted from the scarring after the first operation. First, the recurrent tissue on either side of the trachea is solidly fused with the trachea so that there is little or no play between the gland tissue and the trachea. Serious distortion and rotation of the trachea occurs as the remnant is elevated unless it is dissected free from the trachea. The thyroid tissue along the lateral wall of the trachea must be preserved as in any subtotal lobectomy. Secondly, the internal jugular vein is commonly adherent to the lobe and tends to be pulled upward with the lobe as the lobe is elevated. Consequently, the vein is likely to be injured unless it is carefully dissected from the lobe.

The vocal cords should be checked before any operation on the thyroid gland, and particularly before secondary operations, because of the possibility of previous nerve injury. Injuries of the recurrent laryngeal nerves are more frequent during secondary operations because of anatomic distortion which has resulted from scarring and the regeneration of thyroid tissue.

Postoperative tetany develops after secondary operations rather commonly, and planned effort should be made to preserve a reasonable amount of the posterolateral capsule to avoid removing the remaining parathyroids.

OPERATION. Secondary operations on the thyroid gland are carried out in essentially the same manner as primary operations. The incision is almost invariably made through the scar of the original incision, even if the original incision is improperly placed or shaped, since two incisions would produce a most unsatisfactory cosmetic effect. More sharp dissection is necessary to raise the flaps and more small bleeding vessels are encountered than in primary operations. After the lobes have been well exposed, the recurrent tissue is freed, in part at least, from the trachea before the lobe is elevated, and laterally the internal jugular vein is dissected away from the lobe as the lobe is elevated. Masses of recurrent tissue are sought in the regions of the superior poles and any remaining portion of the pyramidal lobe is carefully removed. The posterior and inferior portions of the lobes are well exposed in a search for substernal or retrotracheal projections of thyroid tissue. Bleeding is controlled meticulously, but far more oozing of blood is to be expected than after primary resections. Drainage is usually indicated after secondary operations and frequently small gauze packs are employed to aid in the control of the oozing. The gauze is removed in from seventy-two to ninety-six hours.

Substernal and Intrathoracic Goiter. Substernal and intrathoracic goiters may be removed almost invariably through a cervical approach. This approach is made possible by, and the safety of the operation depends on, the fact that the displaced thyroid tissue in the thorax has carried the major portion of its blood supply from the cervical region. Hence the intrathoracic masses of thyroid tissue may be dislocated out of the thorax without opening large and inaccessible vessels. The operation is essentially the same as the prototypic thyroidectomy although the steps are carried out in a different order; that is, the lobe is partially freed from its cervical attachments before it is elevated. Too early elevation of the lobe results in torn blood vessels, particularly the lateral and inferior thyroid veins, or even the inferior thyroid artery. If there is serious distortion of the trachea, the operation should be carried out using local anesthesia alone.

OPERATION. The usual incision is made and the sternohyoid muscles are divided on one or both sides, if more ample exposure is thought necessary. The superior pole is exposed, clamped and ligated, as is the suspensory ligament. The isthmus is divided. In some cases it is desirable to expose the trachea as the first step in the operation. The cervical portion of the lobe is elevated and rotated as it is being resected and the resection, as in the usual lobectomy, is started at the tracheal side. The resection is continued laterally, the thyroid tissue beside the trachea and along the adherent zone being carefully preserved. As much as possible of the blood supply of the lobe is secured before the substernal mass is mobilized. It is possible usually to secure the middle thyroid veins and to ligate the inferior thyroid artery at this stage of the operation. Hemostats are removed after ligation of the vessels to prevent too many clamps accumulating in the field of operation. After the cervical portion of the lobe has been largely freed from its attachments, and almost completely resected, mobilization of the substernal mass is started. Delivery of the mass is accomplished gradually by traction, as it is being cautiously separated by finger dissection from the mediastinal tissues. The inferior thyroid veins are clamped and tied as they appear during the elevation of the mass.

If the intrathoracic mass of thyroid tissue is too large to be delivered intact from the thorax, it is safer and easier to remove the contents of the mass piecemeal, after finger morcellation, than to perform anterior mediastinotomy. The substernal mass is mobilized as much as possible and held by forceps which grasp the capsule. The contents of the mass are broken up by thrusting a finger into its center, and thoroughly morcellating the thyroid tissue. The resulting pieces of thyroid tissue are removed by placenta forceps. The capsule is allowed to collapse and as a rule can be delivered readily into the neck with the help of the forceps applied to the capsule. The removal of the capsule and loose thyroid tissue can be facilitated by having the patient strain or cough. The procedure is less bloody if the inferior thyroid artery is ligated before the morcellation than if ligation of this artery is deferred. The intrathoracic cavity may be packed loosely with gauze, which can be removed in from forty-eight to ninety-six hours.

Stage Operations. As previously discussed, multiple-stage operations are indicated far less frequently than they were before the use of iodine to prepare patients for operation. Recently, the use of goitrogenic drugs, such as propylthiouracil, has further decreased the number of patients who cannot tolerate the single-stage operation. Ligations are still rarely indicated and are considered somewhat of a test of surgery. Single lobectomy, as the first stage of a double lobectomy, has a definite place in the treatment of severe hyperthyroidism, while injections, using sclerosing solutions or hot water, are largely obsolete.

LIGATION OF THE SUPERIOR POLE. One superior pole is ligated at a time and the second pole is not ligated until the reaction following the first ligation has subsided, usually seven to fourteen days. The operation is relatively simple and can be carried out in the patient's hospital room. However, it is more easily and safely done in the operating room. Local anesthesia is used. A short (4 to 5 cm.), lateral transverse incision is made in a natural crease in the skin over the superior pole, which can be readily found by palpation. Skin flaps including the platysma muscle are raised superiorly and inferiorly and the cervical fascia is incised longitudinally. The anterior belly of the omohyoid muscle is located and with a small right angle blunt retractor, this muscle is retracted anteriorly and medially, exposing the superior pole of the gland. The superior thyroid artery and vein are exposed, divided between clamps and ligated, or simply ligated with silk suture by passing an aneurysm needle beneath the vessels.

LOBECTOMY. Technically, lobectomy is done exactly as the first side of the prototypic operation. The decision to terminate the operation as a lobectomy may be made at the operating table. Marked increase of pulse rate, restlessness, extreme lack of co-operation, or similar symptoms, may lead to this decision. As previously discussed, the operation is usually terminated as a lobectomy if the recurrent laryngeal nerve has been injured during the removal of the first lobe. If lobectomy was done as a stage procedure, either because of the severity of the disease or because of nerve injury, resection of the remaining lobe can be considered after the lapse of about three months. The exact time will depend on the individual patient, the status of the hyperthyroidism, and whether function has returned to the paralyzed vocal cord.

It is evident that lobectomy is indicated only when the disease is limited to one lobe. It follows that single lobectomy alone is virtually never indicated in cases of exophthalmic goiter except as the first stage of a bilateral resection, since the disease involves the entire thyroid gland. Whenever single lobectomy alone is carried out on patients who have adenomatous goiter, the second lobe should be fully exposed since adenomas may be present which have not been palpable clinically. Such adenomas are frequently concealed in either retrotracheal or substernal positions and if not removed may necessitate a subsequent operation for so-called recurrent adenomatous goiter.

Carcinoma of the Thyroid Gland. Carcinomas of the thyroid gland are generally considered to be of three types: (1) papillary adenocarcinoma (30 per cent of cases); (2) adenocarcinoma in an adenoma or malignant adenoma (40 per cent of cases); and (3) diffuse adenocarcinoma (30 per cent of cases). Epitheliomas and sarcomas develop rarely in the thyroid and do not merit consideration here.

PAPILLARY ADENOCARCINOMA. Papillary adenocarcinomas are of a low grade of malignancy, spread slowly and, apart from metastasis to the cervical lymph nodes, metastasize late. They have a marked tendency to spread to the cervical lymph nodes and often the cervical metastatic growths overshadow the primary lesion. The metastatic lesions in cervical lymph nodes have been called lateral aberrant thyroids. It should be emphasized that in all cases of so-called lateral aberrant thyroid, there is a primary adenocarcinoma in the thyroid gland. Total lobectomy, or subtotal lobectomy getting well around the primary lesion, along with the removal of the grossly involved lymph nodes, should be carried out in such cases. In the average case, the usual thyroid incision is made and extended upward along the posterior border of the sternocleidomastoid muscle on the side of the involved lymph nodes. After the skin flaps are elevated the exposure is usually ample to remove the lobe of the thyroid and the involved lymph nodes. In most cases, the internal jugular vein and the sternocleidomastoid muscle are preserved, as are the strap muscles. In more advanced cases, block neck dissections sacrificing the strap muscles, the sternocleidomastoid and the internal jugular vein may be carried out as described in Chapter 6. Postoperative irradiation is advisable. The five year survival rate of treated patients is excellent (90 per cent or more).

Adenocarcinoma in an Adenoma or Malignant Adenoma. Lesions of this type are somewhat more malignant than papillary adenocarcinomas. The tendency to metastasize to the regional lymph nodes is less marked, but there is a marked tendency toward dissemination through the blood stream. Subtotal lobectomy with complete removal of the capsule or total lobectomy is the treatment of choice. Some authors prefer a radical block dissection of the involved lobe of the thyroid, together with the strap muscles and the thyroid veins including the segment of the internal jugular vein from the level of the superior thyroid vein to the junction of the jugular with the innominate vein. If extensive regional metastatic lesions have occurred the operation probably will be palliative. Postoperative irradiation should always be employed. The prognosis is excellent for those cases in which the malignant lesion has not extended beyond the capsule of the adenoma. The five year survival rate of treated patients for the group as a whole is approximately 70 per cent.

Diffuse Adenocarcinoma. The diffuse adenocarcinomas of the thyroid are of high-grade malignancy. They have marked infiltrative tendencies and metastasize at an early stage through both the lymphatics and the blood stream. If the primary lesion is still movable an attempt at resection should be made. If infiltration into the esophagus or the trachea has occurred, radon seeds may be left in the unremoved malignant tissue or large rubber tube drains may be left in the incision, through which radium may be applied subsequently to the remaining tissue. In many cases resection is impossible because of local fixation. In such cases, surgical exploration is often advisable, not only to establish the diagnosis, but also to free the trachea from the surrounding malignant mass. Tracheotomy may be indicated because of existing or potential tracheal obstruction. Irradiation often increases temporarily the degree of tracheal obstruction. Virtually all patients who have diffuse adenocarcinoma of the thyroid should have the benefit of irradiation. Diffuse adenocarcinomas are somewhat less predictable than other high-grade malignant lesions and with irradiation alone occasional patients will survive for many years. The five year survival rate of treated patients for the group as a whole is approximately 37 per cent.

Complications. The postoperative complications peculiar to subtotal thyroidectomy are crisis, bleeding, inadequate airway and tetany. The late complications have to do with the function of the remaining thyroid tissue; that is, myxedema or recurrence, and the two conditions are not mutually exclusive. The usual complications, common to any operation, such as pulmonary and cardiac complications, are observed perhaps more frequently after subtotal thyroidectomy than after other major operations. Bronchopneumonia is common, and its development has to do with increased tracheal secretions and difficult, painful cough, as well as the debilitated condition of the patient. Pulmonary embolism is virtually unknown following operations on the thyroid gland. If it should occur, it is usually attributable to associated congestive heart failure. Arterial embolism is occasionally observed, particularly if the patient has had atrial fibrillation for some time.

It should be remembered that coronary occlusion and congestive heart failure are fairly common after subtotal thyroidectomy because of the large numbers of patients with damaged coronary arteries and myocardium who undergo thyroidectomy.

CRISIS. The development of postoperative crisis or thyroid storm is rare if the patient has been prepared adequately for operation with iodides. The symptoms are sufficiently well known not to demand further discussion. Treatment, when the condition has developed, is none too successful. Iodides are given in large doses, the patient is placed in an oxygen tent, fluids are given in ample amounts, and morphine and other sedatives are freely used in an effort to control the extreme restlessness. Expert nursing and even restraints are frequently necessary. Since treatment is of so little avail, emphasis should be placed on prevention. All patients who have hyperthyroidism, suspected or evident, either with nodular goiter or with exophthalmic goiter, should be given iodides (10 drops of strong solution of iodine three times a day) for from eight to fourteen days before thyroidectomy. The administration of iodides may be continued for prolonged periods without inducing so-called iodine fastness and, in some cases, preparation with iodides for operation may continue for some weeks before the operation is undertaken. As previously mentioned, goitrogenic drugs such as propylthiouracil may be used advantageously in the relatively small group of severe cases to control the hyperthyroidism until the patient can recover sufficiently to tolerate operation. In this group of patients iodides should always be given during the three weeks prior to operation to counterbalance the excessive vascularity of the gland induced by the goitrogens.

HEMORRHAGE. Because of the marked vascularity of the thyroid gland, postoperative bleeding is fairly common. The danger of such bleeding lies not as much in the loss of blood as in the effects of pressure produced by bleeding into the confined spaces in the neck. The prevention of postoperative bleeding is an inherent part of the operation and consists of four measures: 1. Individual vessels are ligated separately. 2. The remnant of thyroid tissue is sutured and the entire remnant is anchored to the trachea so that it will not be avulsed by swallowing movements. 3. One or both inferior thyroid arteries are ligated separately before the vessels reach the lobe. 4. The patient is made to strain and cough before the incision is closed in order that any open veins may be found and secured.

Following subtotal thyroidectomy patients should be observed meticulously for bleeding. The use of drainage has the advantage that bleeding may be diagnosed somewhat more readily by observing blood dripping from the drains than by waiting for the effects of pressure to become manifest. The pressure effects include tenseness of the skin of the neck, certain rather characteristic changes of the voice, and most important, impairment of the airway. When it is evident that the patient is bleeding, or even with serious suspicion of bleeding, the patient is returned to the operating room and the wound is reopened. Anesthesia is usually not necessary and *general anesthesia should never be used*. All clots are evacuated and the bleeding point is secured. Tracheotomy may be necessary if the stridor is not relieved by removing the blood.

INADEQUATE AIRWAY; STRIDOR. The development of stridor following subtotal thyroidectomy is a complication of the utmost gravity, which demands prompt and energetic treatment. If the patient is cyanotic or is using accessory muscles of respiration, emergency tracheotomy is strongly indicated. The tracheotomy should not be postponed until the patient is in serious difficulty. With close observation, it is usually possible to perform the tracheotomy before the patient's last desperate attempts at securing air have arrived. The tracheotomy is carried out readily through the thyroidectomy incision without anesthesia. A tracheotomy tube of ample size (No. 6 or 7) is inserted into the trachea after removal of a short segment of one of the cartilaginous rings well below the ring of the cricoid cartilage. A small gauze pack is left in the space about the trachea to localize any infection and to prevent mediastinitis. Sulfonamides, penicillin, or both should be administered systemically.

The most common cause of postoperative impairment of the airway is paralysis of the vocal cords. The vocal cords should always be observed before operation to determine whether an unsuspected paralysis of one vocal cord exists. A second check of the vocal cords is made soon after operation to determine whether any injury to the recurrent laryngeal nerves, with consequent paralysis of the corresponding vocal cord, has occurred. (See previous discussion of cord paralysis.) The narrowing of the laryngeal airway consequent on the injury of one recurrent nerve is, per se, usually not sufficient to impair respiration, but when the condition exists in association with marked laryngeal edema, which sometimes complicates the operation of partial thyroidectomy, serious respiratory difficulty may develop, which may require tracheotomy for its relief. Thus, caution demands that, during the immediate convalescence of all patients who have paralysis of the vocal cords, a tray containing the necessary equipment for emergency tracheotomy should be placed in the room. Occasionally one or both vocal cords which functioned normally immediately after operation may become fixed within twenty-four to forty-eight hours. At times this development is associated with marked respiratory stridor, for relief of which tracheotomy may be indicated. This secondary paresis is caused by edema of the laryngeal nerve and hence is temporary, persisting commonly for five to eight days. Other causes of postoperative impairment of the airway are edema, serious distortion of the trachea and possibly tracheal collapse. Such situations may demand tracheotomy but, as a rule, the impairment of the airway is temporary and the tracheotomy tube may be removed in five to fourteen days. Before the tube is removed, it should be occluded for a day or so to determine whether the airway is adequate.

The great value of the examination of the vocal cords immediately after the operation is that if movement of the cord can be detected at this time, it is safe to assume that a nerve injury has not occurred and that, if the cord subsequently becomes fixed, function will return. It is evident that collection of mucus in the larynx, or edema, may produce slight impairment of the airway which may not require tracheotomy. While such conditions demand meticulous observation, the use of oxygen, or of oxygen and helium, may be all that is required from the standpoint of treatment.

TETANY. Postoperative tetany is decidedly unusual (0.2 to 0.3 per cent of patients) following primary partial thyroidectomy on any patient, provided that a reasonable remnant of thyroid tissue and the posteromedial portion of the capsule have been preserved on either side. Unfortunately, tetany is fairly common following operations for recurrent goiter. The symptoms manifest themselves within a day or so following operation. The patient complains of numbness and tingling of the hands and feet and Chvostek's and Trousseau's signs may be elicited. Frank carpopedal spasms may be present. Blood calcium determination gives values lower than normal (10 mg. ± 1 mg. per 100 cc. of serum) and values as low as 5 to 6 mg. per 100 cc. of serum have been observed. As a rule, the symptoms respond satisfactorily to massive orally administered doses of calcium lactate (20 to 28 gm. per day). The relatively insoluble calcium lactate should be dissolved in boiling water and the solution allowed to cool. The administration of the drug is spaced over the twenty-four hours of the day. In most cases the symptoms disappear with time, and if sufficient parathyroid tissue remains, the blood calcium values return to normal and no further treatment is necessary. Occasionally, low blood calcium values persist and in such cases continued treatment is necessary to maintain a normal calcium level in the blood. Dihydrotachysterol (A.T.10) has proved of great value in the management of such chronic tetany.

MYXEDEMA. The development of the disease myxedema requires a period of time, so that postoperative myxedema is not observed until two to three months after subtotal thyroidectomy. The development of the condition depends not so much on the amount as on the type of tissue left behind at thyroidectomy. In cases of adenomatous goiter, when the only tissue that can be preserved is abnormal, myxedema occasionally develops and more than a minimal amount of thyroid tissue should be preserved in such cases. More commonly, myxedema develops following thyroidectomy which was done because of exophthalmic goiter, particularly in those cases in which the thyroid tissue was infiltrated with lymphocytes or involved in fibrosis (thyroiditis). In cases in which the lymphocytosis or fibrosis is more marked than usual, myxedema is quite likely to develop. The metabolic status of such patients should be evaluated about three months after the thyroidectomy so that treatment may be instituted if myxedema has developed. It has been our experience that the disease is more easily managed with desiccated thyroid given orally, if administration of strong solution of iodine is continued.

RECURRENCE. Recurrence of the disease exophthalmic goiter takes place in a small percentage of patients who have had adequate operations. Recurrences are more common in children and adolescents than in older patients. The recurrence may develop at any time from a few months to years after the thyroidectomy. Recurrences are not preventable by the surgeon and they cannot always be attributed to the leaving behind of excessive amounts of thyroid tissue. It is understood that a careful distinction is made between persistent exophthalmic goiter, which is due to inadequate resection, and recurrent exophthalmic goiter, which is presumably caused by the recurrence of the forces which caused the original disease. In about 25 per cent of cases of recurrent exophthalmic goiter, the symptoms may be controlled and the basal metabolic rate held within normal limits by the use of strong solution of iodine. In the remaining cases, and particularly in those cases in which the remnant has increased in size so that it is readily palpable clinically, another partial thyroidectomy is usually necessary. There is an understandable tendency to attempt a more radical resection of the thyroid gland for recurrent exophthalmic goiter than for the usual primary case, partly in an effort to prevent future recurrences, and partly because the recurrent remnant is smaller than the usual lobe. Frequently at operations for recurrent goiter, less than 10 gm. of tissue can be removed and cases have been reported of the removal of less than 1 gm. of tissue. Excessive radicalism is not warranted and leads only to greater incidence of nerve injuries and of tetany.

Recurrent adenomatous goiter with hyperthyroidism is decidedly unusual and many such so-called recurrences result from the inadequate removal of the original goiter. It is common at operation for so-called recurrent adenomatous goiter to find that the thyroid tissue in the neck had been well removed but that large adenomatous masses projecting retrotracheally from the posterior capsule or substernally from the region of the inferior pole had been left behind.

Postoperative Care. The care of the patient following the usual partial thyroidectomy is not onerous. The patient should, however, be observed meticulously for the usual complications and particularly for airway difficulties, evidence of bleeding, and pneumonia. A febrile reaction with temperatures as high as 103° F. is not unusual following operations done for exophthalmic goiter and may not indicate any complication. Vomiting is usual during the first day after operation. Parenteral administration of fluids usually is not necessary and a simple proctoclysis of tap water maintained for the first twenty-four to thirty-six hours will provide an ample fluid intake. Some degree of tracheitis and laryngitis is common and inhalations of steam give considerable relief. Adequate sedation in the form of morphine sulfate given in doses of from ⅙ to ¼ grain (0.01 to 0.016 gm.) every three to four hours for the first twenty-four to forty-eight hours may be advisable. Patients need not be urged to eat since the appetite returns when the nausea and vomiting have passed. The patient may be allowed out of bed after forty-eight hours and usually leaves the hospital after ninety-six hours. During the first twenty-four to forty-eight hours after operation patients are more comfortable propped well up in bed. The wound is dressed daily, drains are removed in forty-eight hours, and sutures or skin clips in seventy-two hours. Sutures removed at this time do not leave permanent scars.

In cases of hyperthyroidism, particularly exophthalmic goiter, a prolonged period of rest of two to three months seems advisable to allow the patient to recover from effects of the hyperthyroidism. The patient without hyperthyroidism needs only three to four weeks before full recovery takes place. Strong solution of iodine is prescribed following all operations for exophthalmic goiter for a period of one year. The first three months the patient is given 10 drops a day and the last nine months 5 drops a day. Some strong solution of iodine will do no harm when used indefinitely and usually 5 drops of strong solution of iodine is advised once every week for an indefinite period. The basal metabolic rate of hyperthyroid patients should fall to normal (+10 to −10 per cent) in three to four weeks following adequate subtotal thyroidectomy. When no hyperthyroidism existed before operation, the basal metabolic rate is not materially affected by the operation, unless the operation was unnecessarily radical.

THE PARATHYROID GLANDS

Collected experience in surgery of the parathyroid glands, in decided contrast to that of surgery of the thyroid gland, is still relatively meager and many problems associated with operations on the parathyroid glands are still unsettled. The parathyroid glands were described as anatomic structures by Sandstrom in 1880 but it was not until 1925 that Mandl demonstrated by removing a parathyroid adenoma in a case of von Recklinghausen's disease that the disease, hyperparathyroidism, existed. Unfortunately it was assumed early that hyperparathyroidism manifested itself as a disease of bone but by 1934, largely due to the efforts of Albright and his associates, it became evident that hyperparathyroidism could exist without disease of bone and that involvement in the urinary tract was a more common and a far more important manifestation of hyperparathyroidism than were changes in bone. Estimates of the percentage of cases of renal calculi which result from hyperparathyroidism vary from 2 to 10 per cent and it is of interest that the higher figures have been reported from institutions with the greatest experience with the disease.

Broadly speaking, two major problems are associated with surgery of the parathyroid glands: (1) recognition of the disease; and (2) the recognition and removal of the parathyroid adenoma or subtotal resection of hyperplastic parathyroid tissue. Consideration of the details of diagnosis of hyperparathyroidism is beyond the scope of this presentation but several diagnostic points will be included.

Hyperparathyroidism, in the absence of serious renal damage, is associated with an increase in calcium and a decrease in phosphorus in the blood. Such chemical changes may cause no distinctive symptoms per se. The symptoms of hyperparathyroidism result from secondary changes in the urinary tract (nephrocalcinosis, urinary calculi) or from involvement of bone (osteoporosis, osteitis fibrosa cystica generalisata). Changes in bone occur less commonly than changes in the urinary tract and the frequency with which the diagnosis of hyperparathyroidism is made depends largely on how frequently the disease is considered in cases of calculi of the urinary tract.

Anatomy. There are usually four, sometimes more than four and occasionally less than four parathyroid glands. The glands vary greatly in size but the average is about 6 by 3 by 2 mm. They weigh from about 0.030 to 0.040 gm. Usually they are oval but are molded by the surrounding structures. The color varies from reddish brown to yellow, depending on the amount of fat in the gland.

The two parathyroids on each side have a fairly constant position relative to each other and some symmetry is exhibited in the position of the glands on the two sides. The superior parathyroids are more constant in position than the inferior glands. They are situated on the anterior wall of the esophagus or lower part of the pharynx at the level of the lower margin of the cricoid cartilage and just medial to the posteromedial border of the corresponding thyroid lobes. They are connected to the thyroid gland only by loose areolar tissue. The glands lie anterior to the prevertebral layer of the deep cervical fascia. They receive their blood supply by means of slender vascular pedicles from the corresponding inferior thyroid artery. The glands may be situated as high as the upper border of the larynx or as low as the inferior pole of the thyroid gland, and they have been found anterior to the superior thyroid vessels. It is possible, theoretically, for a superior parathyroid gland to be within the thyroid lobe since it arises from the fourth branchial cleft contiguous to the lateral anlage of the thyroid.

The inferior parathyroid glands arise from anlagen contiguous to those of the thymus gland from the third branchial cleft and descend, on the two sides, lateral to the thyroid. The descent of the inferior parathyroid glands is arrested usually near the inferior pole of the thyroid gland while the thymus continues into the mediastinum. The inferior parathyroids are more anterior than the superior glands and usually lie anterior to the inferior thyroid artery and to the recurrent laryngeal nerve. The final position of the glands varies from the immediate vicinity of the thyroid gland, usually near the lower poles, to well within the superior mediastinum. Normal glands have been found within the thymus gland and one case has been reported in which an adenoma was found within the middle mediastinum between the pericardium and arch of the aorta. The arterial supply of the inferior glands usually comes from the inferior thyroid arteries but may come from other vessels, particularly when the gland is displaced. Apart from anomalous position resulting from arrested or faulty embryologic descent, enlarged parathyroid glands or parathyroid adenomas may be displaced into the superior mediastinum by swallowing movements and negative intrathoracic pressure, much as low-lying adenomas of the thyroid are drawn substernally. In such cases a vascular pedicle leading downward into the mediastinum from the inferior thyroid artery may indicate the position of the displaced gland.

Pathology. Hyperparathyroidism results from either an adenoma (or an adenocarcinoma) which develops in one or more of the parathyroid glands or from generalized primary hyperplasia which involves all of the parathyroid tissue. Considerable controversy exists as to the possible malignancy of the usual so-called parathyroid adenoma, although recurrence and metastasis are most unusual and radical removal of the tumor is not practiced. Multiple adenomas occur in from 5 to 10 per cent of cases. The adenomas vary in size from a few millimeters in diameter to relatively large tumors which

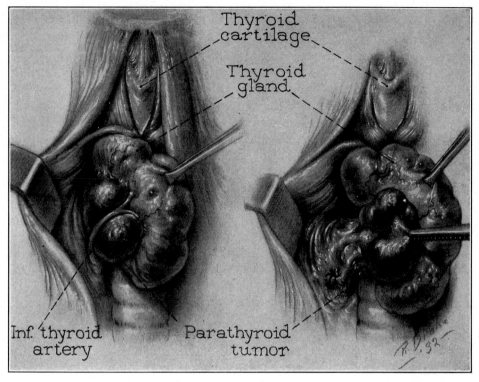

FIG. 444. Typical parathyroid adenoma, probably originating in right superior parathyroid gland. Patient had osteitis fibrosa cystica generalisata. The tumor weighed 5.0 gm.

may weigh as much as 100 gm. (Fig. 444). The adenomas are reddish brown and are composed of closely packed cells of the same types as those of the normal parathyroid gland. Mitotic figures may be present. The adenomas are not infiltrated by fat cells as is the normal adult parathyroid gland. When an adenoma is present in one parathyroid gland the other parathyroid glands may appear atrophic and contain more fat than usual.

In cases of hyperparathyroidism due to primary hyperplasia all parathyroid tissue is involved. On microscopic examination the glands are deep brownish red and have uneven surfaces with many projections. The cells are markedly enlarged and uniform. The cytoplasm is unusually clear and the nuclei are oriented toward the stroma (wasserhelle cells). As much as 52 gm. of such tissue has been reported in a single case.

Surgical Technic. It is evident from the foregoing that surgery for hyperparathyroidism consists in the location and removal of the offending adenoma or subtotal resection of the hyperplastic tissue. Experience is still so limited that specific steps of the procedure have not become standardized. The technic must be meticulous and the surgical field should be kept as bloodless as possible because hemorrhage may well obscure the color of the parathyroid glands and so make the search for the adenoma more difficult. The usual incision used for thyroidectomy is adequate for the cervical part of the operation. The sternohyoid muscles may be sectioned. One lobe of the thyroid, usually whichever is more prominent, is rotated and elevated completely. Unless the adenoma is quite evident, it may be safer to expose the inferior laryngeal nerve at the level of the inferior pole of the thyroid since the search for the parathyroid glands will be carried out in the immediate vicinity of the nerve. Because the superior parathyroid is more constant in position, it is searched for and found first. If it appears to be normal or is smaller and more yellow than usual, the search is continued until the inferior parathyroid on the same side is found. It is to be remembered that the inferior parathyroid may be embryologically displaced into the superior mediastinum or may have become displaced later by negative intrathoracic pressure and the movements of swallowing. In the latter case, a vascular pedicle leading into the mediastinum from a branch of the inferior thyroid artery may furnish a clue to the location of the gland. Presumably normal parathyroid glands should never be sacrificed but removal of a small amount of tissue for biopsy to verify the diagnosis is permissible.

After a thorough search of one side of the neck and posterior part of the superior mediastinum, the same procedure is carried out on the opposite side. Because of the rude symmetry of corresponding glands on the two sides, the finding of the parathyroids in the second part of the procedure may be somewhat facilitated. The search should extend well medially to the lobe of the thyroid gland, posteriorly to the esophagus and pharynx, between the trachea and the esophagus and within the sulci of the thyroid. The finding of four parathyroids does not exclude the presence of an adenoma in aberrant parathyroid tissue. Because of the possibility that parathyroid tissue may exist within the thyroid lobe, any suspicious appearing nodules of thyroid tissue should be removed, and even subtotal thyroidectomy may be considered if suspicious appearing nodules are found deep within the lobe.

Because of the intimate anatomic association of the parathyroids and the recurrent laryngeal nerve, the procedure should be carried out, as in the case of thyroidectomy, under combined local and light, general anesthesia, so that the functional status of the nerve on one side may be evaluated before the dissection on the other side is carried out. The search of the neck should be exhaustive and all parathyroids found should be identified by means of biopsy and frozen section if necessary.

If meticulous, complete cervical dissection fails to reveal a parathyroid tumor, a search of the anterior part of the superior mediastinum, upper middle and upper part of the anterior mediastinum must be carried out at a second stage. The dissection of the neck should have revealed which parathyroid gland or glands were missing from their usual location and that vascular pedicles leading down into the mediastinum were absent. The dissection of the mediastinum must be as meticulous as that of the cervical region. It is best carried out through a medial sternotomy incision. The search of the neck and mediastinum is best done in two stages, and the second stage should be postponed until the cervical incision is well healed.

When the adenoma has been found, it probably should be removed completely. In certain cases, notably those in which extensive changes in bone have occurred and the level of phosphatase in the blood is high, postoperative tetany of varying severity is to be expected and the proposal that subtotal resection be carried out has been made. Because of the question of malignancy, subtotal resection of adenomas should be avoided.

In primary hyperplasia of the parathyroid glands, subtotal resection of one gland with preservation of about 200 to 300 mg. of parathyroid tissue and total removal of the remaining parathyroid glands are carried out. Caution should be exercised to preserve the blood supply of the remnant of parathyroid tissue. Microscopic examination of a frozen section should be carried out immediately to establish the diagnosis in order that the surgeon may avoid removal of normal parathyroids. The uniform cellular pattern and the characteristic large clear cells make the microscopic diagnosis relatively easy.

Multiple adenomas situated in more than one parathyroid gland may be present and the removal of one parathyroid gland containing one adenoma will not cure the patient in such a case. Hence, bilateral complete cervical dissection probably should be carried out even if a tumor is found on the side first explored. The dissection should be extensive and meticulous enough to exclude other adenomas in the neck, since re-exploration presents serious technical difficulties. The mediastinum is never explored in cases in which cervical parathyroid adenomas have been removed until it has been demonstrated clinically and by determinations of blood calcium and phosphorus that this operation has not cured the patient.

REFERENCES

1. Astwood, E. B. Treatment of Hyperthyroidism with Thiourea and Thiouracil, *J.A.M.A.*, 122:78-81, [May 8], 1943.
2. Berlin, D. D. The Recurrent Laryngeal Nerves in Total Ablation of the Normal Thyroid Gland; an Anatomical and Surgical Study, *Surg., Gynec. & Obst.*, 60:19-26, [Jan.], 1935.
3. Halsted, W. S. Surgical Papers, 2:257-423, 1924, The Johns Hopkins Press, Baltimore.
4. King, B. T. A New and Function-restoring Operation for Bilateral Abductor Cord Paralysis; Preliminary Report, *J.A.M.A.*, 112:814-823, [Mar. 4], 1939.
5. Pemberton, J. deJ. Surgery of Substernal and Intrathoracic Goiters, *Arch. Surg.*, 2:1-20, [Jan.], 1921.
6. Pemberton, J. deJ. Malignant Lesions of the Thyroid Gland; a Review of 774 Cases, *Surg., Gynec. & Obst.*, 69:417-430, [Oct.], 1939.

7. PEMBERTON, J. DE J., STALKER, L. K. and BLACK, B. M.   Surgery of the Thyroid Gland. In PIERSOL, G. M.   *The Cyclopedia of Medicine*, F. A. Davis Company, Philadelphia. (In press.)

8. ALBRIGHT, FULLER, AUB, J. C. and BAUER, WALTER.   Hyperparathyroidism; a Common and Polymorphic Condition as Illustrated by Seventeen Proved Cases from One Clinic, *J.A.M.A.*, 102:1276-1287, [Apr. 21], 1934.

9. CASTLEMAN, B. and MALLORY, T. B.   Pathology of Parathyroid Gland in Hyperparathyroidism; Study of 25 Cases, *Am. J. Path.*, 11:1-72, [Jan.], 1935.

10. COPE, OLIVER.   Surgery of Hyperparathyroidism: the Occurrence of Parathyroids in the Anterior Mediastinum and the Division of the Operation Into Two Stages, *Ann. Surg.*, 114:706-731, [Oct.], 1941.

20

THE MUSCLES, FASCIAE, TENDONS AND BURSAE

Harrison L. McLaughlin, M.D.

THE MUSCLES

Myositis. Most conditions of myositis are secondary manifestations of some primary source of irritation which may be mechanical or toxic in origin. Therapy should be accompanied by investigation designed to identify the primary condition. The symptoms of myositis often may be relieved by certain surgical procedures.

Local Anesthesia by the Injection of Procaine Hydrochloride. Areas of myositis, especially those characterized by circumscribed "trigger points" of tenderness and pain, or by palpable indurated tender nodules, warrant infiltration with local anesthesia. Five to thirty cubic centimeters of a 1 per cent solution of procaine hydrochloride are injected into the painful and tender areas until the symptoms disappear. Deep massage and vigorous active motion of the previously painful structures are then instituted in an attempt to stimulate the local minute circulation. Repeated injections may be required, but if the first treatment has no beneficial effect subsequent injections are unlikely to be successful. A solution of local anesthetic in oil may be used for a more prolonged effect but must be injected with caution lest the accumulation of more than a few cubic centimeters of such a heavy solution produce an undue inflammatory reaction extending even to local necrosis in the tissues.

Surface Anesthesia by Ethyl Chloride Spray. Surface anesthesia may produce relief from pain originating in the muscles. Ethyl chloride is the most simple and convenient of the available surface anesthetics. Prior to spraying, a protective layer of vaseline or camphorated oil is applied to the area of skin to be treated in order to minimize the risk of blistering. Each subjective center of pain and tenderness is sprayed to the point at which the skin begins to blanche, but the procedure should be stopped short of actual freezing. Constant gentle massage, verbal reassurance and encouragement in relaxation and resumption of active motion of the part are essential adjuncts to the actual anesthetic effect which, per se, is of little benefit. The relief obtained probably results from a reduction in muscular and neurovascular spasm. For permanent relief a return of spasm must be prevented. Consequently, following a successful procedure it is essential that relaxed active function be maintained by the patient. His full cooperation is necessary to success, and the importance of voluntary maintenance of function should be explained fully. The use of splints or other restrictive dressings is obviously contraindicated by the necessity for continued function.

MUSCLE INJURIES

Hematoma. Overuse, strain or contusion of a muscle may result in a temporarily painful syndrome due to multiple minute hemorrhages into and between the muscle fibers. The resultant symptoms usually disappear quickly except when the lesion is followed by the formation of a hematoma. Small hematomata usually subside spontaneously within a short time. A large hematoma may require aspiration. This should be done early, while the contents of the lesion are still fluid in consistency. The skin is thoroughly prepared. A large bore needle is inserted through an 0.5 cm. incision in the skin, made through the site of a procaine hydrochloride weal. The skin nick should be large enough to allow free passage of the aspirating needle, so that a minimum of surface contamination is carried into the deeper tissues, since the introduction of organisms into a blood-filled cavity carries a considerable risk of infection. The needle is inserted into the depths of the hematoma and the enclosed fluid withdrawn.

The use of a small bore needle frequently results in a failure to aspirate the thick and viscid contents of the hematoma. Attempts to aspirate an old hematoma, even though a large needle is used, may be unsuccessful due to clot formation. At a still later date the clot may liquefy. Aspiration again becomes possible, but at this stage the walls of the cavity will have become thickened, organized and unable to collapse so that an early reaccumulation of fluid is to be expected. The treatment of choice for a long-standing hematoma is incision into the cavity, evacuation of its contents and obliteration of the residual tissue cavity by suture. The skin incision should be closed and the region compressed by a snug dressing for several days following the operation.

Rupture and Laceration of Muscle. Rupture through a muscle belly may result from direct or indirect violence. The presence of a large hematoma should arouse a suspicion of rupture. Spontaneous rupture due to violent contraction of the muscle belly often takes place at the musculotendinous junction.

Repair is made difficult by the friability of the lacerated muscle fibers at the site of rupture, by retraction of the proximal fragment and by the impossibility of maintaining apposition of the fragments against the tone of the muscle by ordinary suture methods. Repair should be preceded by a revision of the fragment ends (Fig. 445). All lacerated strands of muscle are excised until two flat vascular surfaces are available for approximation. These are held together while mattress sutures are placed around the entire circumference of their juncture. Each suture should penetrate sheath as well as muscle tissue. Such a circumferential suture line, per se, usually is inadequate. Reinforcement by additional deep sutures of fascia or tendon strip (Fig. 445) is advisable. The repair should be protected against strain for two to four weeks, following which gradually progressive resumption of function is indicated.

The Management of Muscles in Operative Approaches. Almost all operative approaches involve muscles. A good operative technic requires not only a knowledge of the anatomy and physiology of the muscles but also a utilization of this knowledge in muscle retraction and division so that their functional integrity is not jeopardized.

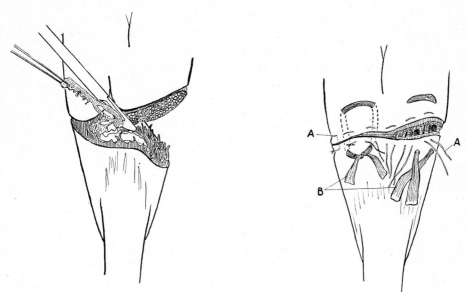

Fig. 445. Repair of ruptured muscle. *Left:* Lacerated muscle strands are débrided from each fragment to produce flat and viable surfaces for approximation. *Right:* A. Circumferential suture line. Mattress sutures are used and must penetrate both sheath and muscle tissue. B. Reinforcement of circumferential suture line by heavy autogenous sutures of fascia or tendon tissue.

The neurovascular supply usually enters and traverses a muscle at an angle, or parallel to the direction of its fibers. The point of entrance and the intramuscular distribution of this supply should govern the operative management of each muscle. Retraction should always be toward, never away from, the side at which nerves and vessels enter a muscle. Nerve and blood supply entering at one end of a muscle and running parallel to its fibers permits of retraction in either direction, but contraindicates transverse division of the structure except at its distal extremity. If an operative approach must go through such a muscle the fibers should be separated longitudinally. Nerve and blood supply passing through a muscle at right angles to the direction of the fibers makes transverse division permissible, providing the muscle sheath is stout enough to insure a strong repair. Longitudinal splitting apart of such a muscle never should be done except at the side opposite to the point of entrance of the neurovascular supply. Certain muscles have numerous and abundant sources of blood supply, or a double enervation, and may be handled with less risk of damage than those in which the neurovascular supply enters along a single pathway. In general, however, the result of ignoring the anatomical considerations outlined above is to incur the potential penalties of permanent paralysis or prolonged palsy and partial necrosis of the muscles encountered in the exposure of deep seated pathology.

The Use of Muscle Flaps. A pedicle flap of muscle tissue may be used to fashion an insulating cushion between a nerve and some adjacent point of irritation. The nerve is dissected free from its point of compression and a flap of adjacent muscle tissue is mobilized and sutured into place between the two. Such a flap need not be more than 1 centimeter in thickness and should be large enough to cover the extent of nerve insulation required. The procedure is especially useful in a compression lesion of the radial nerve due to fracture of the contiguous humeral shaft. In certain open reductions of humeral shaft fractures it may be advisable to transpose a flap of triceps muscle between nerve and bone if it appears that the production of callus subsequently may compress the nerve.

Pedicle flaps of muscle may be utilized to obliterate a dead space. A flap large enough to fill the defect in question is mobilized from the adjacent muscles, turned into the cavity without twisting, and stabilized by sutures placed in a manner to maintain its transposed position. Maintenance of position is aided by immobilization of the part and the use of a snug compression dressing for the first week following the operation. Such a flap should not be implanted into a cavity having avascular walls. It will not stay there. Whenever the walls of the defect to be obliterated are avascular, saucerization or scar tissue excision down to healthy bleeding tissues is an essential preliminary to transposition of the muscle flap, regardless of whether or not the recipient defect is in bone or soft tissue.

Free muscle transplants may be used as hemostatic agents. Small and otherwise uncontrollable hemorrhages from viscera or bone may be stopped at times by the application of a small free muscle graft to the bleeding point. The advent of oxidized gauze and fibrin foam, both of which accomplish the same purpose more efficiently than muscle, has minimized the use of this procedure.

THE FASCIAE

Certain affections of the fasciae may produce symptoms and disability necessitating operative intervention. The more common procedures carried out for relief of these derangements are discussed later in relation to the specific regions involved.

Removal of Fascia for Free Graft or Suture. Autogenous free grafts from the fascia lata of the lateral thigh region are used in many operative procedures. The use to which a graft is to be put must govern the size and shape of the piece of fascia removed. The operative approach to the donor area is made through an incision a little longer than the graft to be removed, on the anterolateral aspect of the thigh. The fascia lata is encountered

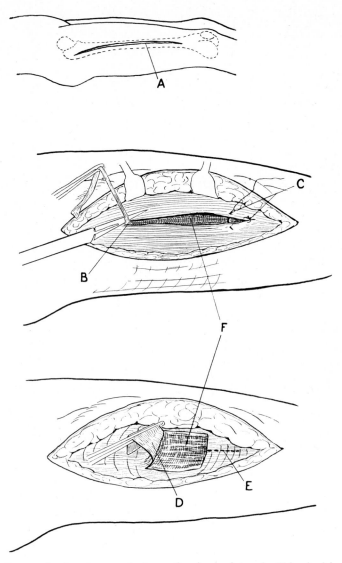

Fig. 446. Removal of a free graft from the fascia lata. A. Skin incision over the anterolateral aspect of the thigh should be a little longer than the estimated length of the graft to be removed. B. Removal of a long strip of fascia should be followed by, C. repair of the residual defect. D. Removal of a wide flap of fascia should be done in the distal portion of the thigh where the fascia is thickest and the risk of muscle hernia least. If removed from the proximal or middle thirds of the thigh the residual defect should be elongated by incision, E. to eliminate the risk of a sharply circumscribed hernia of, F. the vastus lateralis.

directly under the subcutaneous fat. Removal of a long narrow strip for use as an autogenous suture should be followed by repair of the resultant defect to prevent subsequent herniation of the vastus lateralis muscle (Fig. 446). Long narrow strips also may be removed by means of a fascial stripper. This technic requires only two small incisions, one at either end of the strip to be removed, but no hemostasis or repair of the fascial defect is possible and the risk of hematoma and muscle herniation is always present.

Removal of a rectangular flap of fascia leaves a defect that cannot be closed by suture. Because of this wide grafts should be taken from the distal portion of the thigh where the fascia is thickest and the risk of muscle herniation minimal. If a rectangular graft is taken from the proximal thigh region the residual defect should be elongated by incision so that any subsequent muscle herniation taking place (Fig. 446), will be diffuse and non-circumscribed.

THE TENDONS

Removal of Tendon for Use as Autogenous Graft or Suture. Tendon tissue is stronger than fascia and will not stretch under strain. When a strong strip of autogenous material is required, the peroneus longus tendon is a suitable donor. Heavy strips also may be obtained from the quadriceps or Achilles tendons. Free grafts for the bridging of tendon defects should be obtained from a tendon of equal or similar caliber to that requiring repair, whenever possible.

Removal of a Free Graft from Peroneus Longus Tendon. A skin incision is made 1 inch behind and parallel to the lower one-third of the fibula, its lower end curving slightly forward under the tip of the lateral malleolus. The peroneal tendons are easily located behind the fibula. The peroneus longus has much the longer tendon and is the better donor of the two. A partial thickness segment of the tendon is removed by sharp dissection. At both ends of the removed segment the plane of incision should be bevelled gently (Fig. 447) in order to minimize gross irregularities and localized weak points in the remaining tendon.

Removal of a full thickness segment from the peroneus longus is seldom necessary and is to be avoided when possible. If the peroneal tendons are so small that a partial thickness segment appears insufficient for the grafting procedure contemplated, it is advisable to expose the tendo achillis through the same skin incision and obtain a strip of the desired caliber from this structure. The operative wound is closed in layers and early motion and use of the extremity may be allowed.

Removal of the Palmaris Longus Tendon. This tendon is easy to remove, well suited for use as a free graft for repair of the small tendons and the functional defect following its removal is insignificant. When multiple small free tendon grafts are required the long extensor tendons of the toes may be removed. Removal of the palmaris longus tendon requires only two short transverse skin incisions, one over the tendon at the flexion crease of the wrist, and the other over its musculotendinous junction on the volar surface of the forearm. Through the latter incision the musculotendinous junction is identified, delivered into the wound and divided. Through the distal incision the insertion of the tendon is identified and a smooth instrument passed under it. The tendon then is avulsed from the forearm by traction

(Fig. 447). After avulsion has been accomplished the insertion of the tendon into the palmar fascia is divided and both skin incisions are sutured. Early motion of the extremity may be allowed.

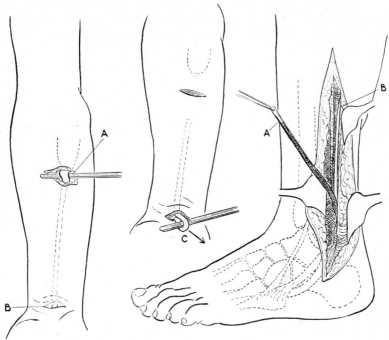

FIG. 447. Removal of palmaris and peroneus longus tendons. *Left:* Two short transverse incisions are made, one over the palmaris tendon at the flexion crease of the wrist and one over the musculo-tendinous junction of the muscle. A. Musculo-tendinous junction identified and delivered into the proximal wound prior to division. B. Terminal portion of the tendon identified through the distal wound. C. Musculo-tendinous junction has been divided and tendon is avulsed from the forearm by traction exerted upon a smooth instrument which has been passed under the exposed terminal portion. *Right:* Peroneal tendons are exposed by an incision 1 inch behind and parallel to the distal one-third of the fibula. The peroneus longus is the longer and larger of the two tendons lying posterior to the fibula. A. A partial thickness segment of the desired length is removed from the peroneus longus. B. At either end of the removed segment the tendon incision should be bevelled gently to eliminate the formation of a localized weak spot and to minimize the irregularity in contour of the remaining tendon.

TENDON REPAIR

Repair of a divided tendon should be carried out as an emergency procedure. The dangers and penalties of infection and the indications for emergency care are similar to those for a compound fracture. Repair of a ruptured tendon, however, even though it is not associated with a compound wound, should be done as soon as possible, but the absence of contamination and the almost inevitable intrinsic degeneration present in the tendon fibers at the site of a spontaneous rupture removes this lesion from the category of those demanding emergency care. Careful débridement and lavage of every compound wound is indicated as a preliminary to the repair of a divided tendon or tendons. The ultimate in atraumatic and aseptic operative technic is required since traumatization of the tissue or infection, no matter how trivial, may result in fibrosis sufficient to vitiate the results of the repair. Regardless of the actual technic by which a tendon repair is carried out, to obtain the optimum result the following prereq-

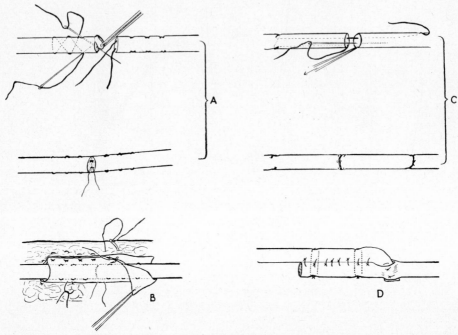

Fig. 448. Tendon repair. (A) End-to-end technic of Bunnell. The devitalized tendon ends are excised. Placement of sutures distributes strain along the intact tendon proximal and distal to the actual repair site. The only foreign material remaining in the repair consists of two knots where the sutures are tied. (B) Technic for fashioning a fascial sleeve around a repair site to minimize involvement of the repair by adhesions. (C) A method of end-to-end tendon repair which eliminates suture knots in the healing site. (D) Side-to-side tendon repair, with and without perforation of the tendons.

uisites are necessary: (1) a snug and accurate apposition of healthy to healthy tendon tissue; (2) a minimum of tension on the site of repair; (3) a minimum of foreign material in the site of repair; and (4) a maximum maintenance of function, compatible with integrity of the repair, during the healing period.

End-to-end Repair. This method is indicated in most tendon lesions resulting from division or rupture. The technic of Bunnell (Fig. 448) is widely used and is well suited to the repair of small round tendons. Properly carried out this method removes a large portion of the strain from the repair and distributes it along a considerable extent of intact tendon proximal and distal to the repair. A minimum of suture material remains at the site of healing. Occasionally additional protection against involvement of the healing site by adhesions is required. This may be provided by insulating the tendon from the neighboring tissues with a free graft of fascia fashioned as a sleeve around the repair (Fig. 448).

End-to-end Repair by Removable Suture. Repair by removable suture according to the technic described by Bunnell makes possible a maximum

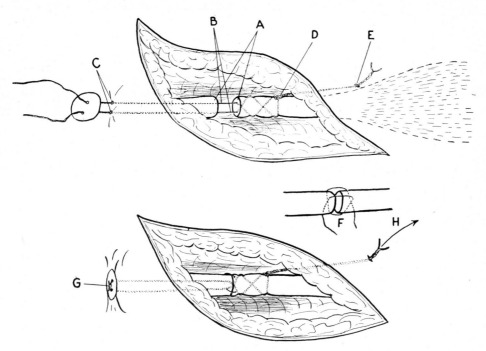

FIG. 449. Repair by removable suture (Bunnell). A. Devitalized tendon ends are excised to produce healthy tissues for approximation. B. Placement of traction suture, the free ends of which are threaded through both tendon fragments and brought out through the skin at C. The overall alignment of the traction suture should be as straight as possible. D. Removing wire is passed around the most proximal loop of the traction suture, twisted snugly and brought through a separate stab wound in the skin at E. F. Fine suture at healing site to insure accurate apposition of the tendon fragments. G. Traction suture pulled tight enough to neutralize all strain on the repair and tied over a button on the skin. H. Following union of the repair the ends of the traction suture are cut flush with the skin at G and the whole suture removed by traction on the removing wire.

attainment of the essential prerequisites for ideal tendon repair. The snug apposition of healthy-to-healthy tissues is obtained by a few very fine sutures. Tension on the repair site is neutralized by the placement of a proximal traction suture which is tied distal to the repair over a button on the skin (Fig. 449), or a bolt through the bone (Figs. 476 and 477). The introduction of a removing wire which makes possible complete removal of the main traction suture after healing has occurred, reduces to a minimum the amount of foreign material permanently left in the healing site.

Side-to-side Repair. This method may be carried out with or without perforation of the tendons involved (Fig. 448). Side-to-side repair should not be contemplated in any situation where it is necessary for the repair to pass through a narrow channel. Although it provides a strong repair especially well adapted to early function, the irregularity and bulk of apposed tendon tissues predisposes to a certain amount of scarring and adhesion formation. It is a useful technic for tendon transference procedures in the forearm or lower leg where the importance of adhesion formation is minimal, but

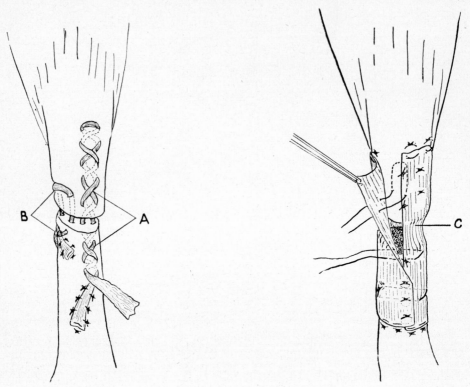

FIG. 450. Repair of ruptures through the large tendons often is made difficult by inability to obtain accurate approximation of the fragments and often requires autogenous sutures of fascia or tendon woven through the tendon tissue and across the rupture as in A. The use of two or three such sutures results in a bridging of the defect by a strong mass of fibrous tissue. Additional mattress sutures, B, of fascia or heavy silk may be used. C. Reinforcement of a repair or bridgment of a defect may be carried out by the use of a fascial sleeve firmly sutured into place.

should not be used in the hand where fibrosis and adhesion formation may be of great importance.

Reinforcement of Tendon Repair by Autogenous Free Grafts. Ruptures through the large tendons uniformly are characterized by intrinsic degeneration at the site of rupture, retraction of the proximal fragment by a strong muscular force and, when the lesion is of long duration, by a fixed contracture of the muscle belly in the retracted position. Apposition of the tendon ends frequently is difficult, and may be impossible, especially following excision of the degenerated and devitalized tendon fibers at the site of

rupture. Because of the poor quality of the tissues and the strength of the
retracting force ordinary sutures are very apt to pull out. Utilization of the
removable suture principle greatly facilitates the solution of these difficulties
in ruptures of the tendo achillis, quadriceps and infrapatellar tendons (Figs.
476, 478). When a removable traction suture is impractical, ordinary end-
to-end repair should be reinforced by heavy autogenous sutures of fascia or

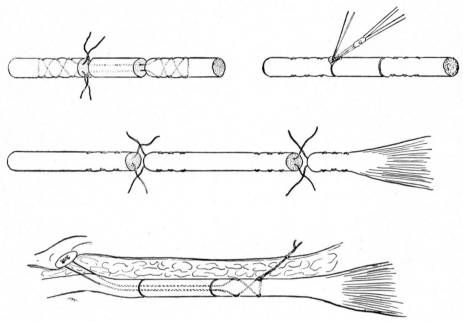

Fig. 451. Technic for implantation of a free tendon graft. *Top:* Method for placement and tying of suture with a short graft. *Middle:* Placement of sutures for implantation of a long graft. *Below:* Technic for implantation and stabilization of a free graft
by Bunnell removable suture.

free tendon graft (Fig. 450). A fascial sleeve also may be utilized to reinforce
such a repair, or to bridge an irreducible defect in the tendon (Fig. 450).

Tendon Grafting. Destruction by disease, injury, or long-established contracture may result in a tendon defect that must be bridged. The best material for bridging such a defect is a free tendon graft of a caliber equal to
the tendon to be grafted. The graft is inserted between the separated tendon
ends after freshening the end of each fragment by excision of a small terminal portion. The technic for attachment of short and long free grafts is
illustrated in figure 451. Irreducible defects in the large tendons seldom
are amenable to obliteration by the implantation of free grafts. They may
be bridged by fascial or tendon strip sutures with or without the added support of a fascial sleeve (Fig. 450).

Tendon Lengthening and Shortening. Tendon lengthening or shortening may be accomplished by many methods, some of the more useful of
which are illustrated in figure 452. The technic of choice depends upon

the shape and size of the tendon involved and the shape and size of the
channel through which the reconstructed segment of tendon must pass.
Following reconstruction the tendon must remain under physiological tension. Too loose or too tight a reconstruction of any tendon is disadvantageous
and the end result is likely to be vitiated by disruption of the suture line,

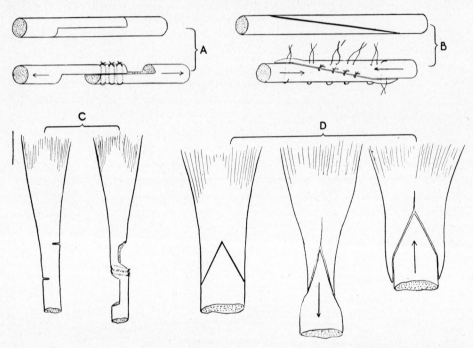

FIG. 452. Methods for lengthening or shortening a tendon. (A) Step-cut incision
through the tendon with side-to-side repair. End-to-end repair makes a little more length
available but is less stable. Excision of equal segments from each fragment followed by
side-to-side repair is a good method for shortening the tendon. (B) Oblique incision
through the tendon followed by side-to-side repair may be used to lengthen or shorten
a tendon. (C) Bayer's method of tendon lengthening. Traction following contralateral
incisions not quite half-way through the tendon makes the tendon fibers slip in opposite
directions. Firm through-and-through suture of the residual connection is necessary to
prevent complete separation of the two fragments. (D) V-incision well suited for use in
the larger tendons. May be used for both lengthening or shortening procedures.

atrophy of the muscle belly or loss of mechanical advantage to the structure
as a whole.

Tendon Transference and Reimplantation. The insertion of one tendon
into another for purposes of functional substitution may be done by side-to-
side suture, with or without perforation (Fig. 448), as the circumstances
may indicate. The long axis of the transferred tendon cannot under any
circumstances be allowed to twist or kink in following its new course and
must remain under physiological tension following the reconstruction. Transference of one tendon into the insertion of another by Mayer's technic is
similar to the method illustrated in figure 468. The transposed tendon is

passed through the sheath of that into which it is to be implanted when one is available.

Transposition of a tendon to a new body point of insertion must satisfy all prerequisites for tendon repair. In order to insure apposition of vascular to vascular tissues, it is necessary that the tendon end be sutured under a flap of periosteum or, better still, into a cavity or trench which has been fashioned in the bony cortex. The most secure fixation for such a reimplantation is obtained by anchoring the tendon with sutures passed through drill holes in the bones.

THE BURSAE

Normal bursae are to be encountered at the friction points along the course of certain tendons. In histological composition and function a bursa is identical to and should be considered as a form of tendon sheath. Its intimate association with a tendon is such that any affection of one must eventually involve the other. Bursitis seldom is encountered as a primary pathological entity and usually occurs as a secondary result of some irritative focus on the outside, in the associated tendon or in the neighboring bony structures. In either case removal of the irritation produces a spontaneous remission of the symptoms resulting from the bursitis. At times the primary source of irritation cannot be identified and in long-standing lesions the bursal wall may become irreversibly thickened. In both situations bursectomy is indicated as a therapeutic measure. Under ordinary circumstances bursectomy, unaccompanied by eradication of the primary source of irritation, is followed by a recurrence of symptoms.

Pyogenic infections of the bursae may be encountered and warrant early and wide incision and drainage. Unless the drainage is both early and adequate, the associated tendon and even the underlying bone rapidly may become involved by the infectious process. Specific infections of the bursae may complicate the systemic manifestations of tuberculosis, meningitis, syphilis or gonorrhea. When this occurs drainage usually is contraindicated and the therapy for the local condition is that required for the systemic disease.

THE SHOULDER REGION

Affections of the Subdeltoid Bursa. Approximately two-thirds of all painful shoulders, exclusive of those resulting from bony pathology, result from inflammation at the site of a calcific deposit situated in the tendon cuff formed by the short rotators. Such deposits remain quiescent so long as they are buried within the avascular tendon fibers. Eventually most quiescent lesions produce symptoms in some degree. These occur when the material enclosed within the tendon tissue works its way through the fibers, or is allowed to escape from the tendon by rupture of the fibers overlying the deposit due to mild trauma or overuse, and comes into contact with the vascular and well enervated floor of the bursa. Pain results from the ensuing foreign body inflammatory reaction.

Irrigation of the Subdeltoid Bursa. The rationale of irrigation origi-
nated in the misconception that the deposit formed in the bursa. The deposit
actually forms within tendon tissue and never enters the bursal cavity until
after the need for all but palliative measures has passed. Deposits characterized by chronic pain are dry and sandy in consistency, cannot be withdrawn
through a needle unless first diluted by saline and therefore respond favorably to any type of needling procedure in only a small percentage of cases.
Those accompanied by acute symptoms have been diluted by inflammatory
exudate until they become semi-fluid in consistency and enclosed within a
well-circumscribed cavity under considerable tension. Rupture of the tense
cavity, either spontaneously or as the result of therapy, is followed rapidly
by relief from pain and absorption of the irritant material.

Irrigation, in common with certain other needling procedures, may be
followed by relief from pain due to the chance rupture of the deposit by
one of the probing needles. The effect of the local anesthesia necessitated
by any needling procedure may make possible enough temporary pain-free
motion so that the tense deposit is ruptured spontaneously by forcible im-
pingement against the acromion, even though the actual procedure fails to
affect the lesion directly.

The technic for irrigation requires that two needles be inserted into
the bursal cavity at least 1 inch apart (Fig. 453). The needles may be inserted
at any point within the area limited by the coracoid and the lateral tip of
acromion in the horizontal plane, and the anterior edge of acromion and
a parallel line 1 inch distalwards in the vertical plane. If a needle is inserted
to humeral head and then withdrawn slightly, its point should be within
the bursal cavity. A 1 per cent solution of procaine hydrochloride is forced
into one needle, through the bursal cavity and out the other needle. After
comfort has been obtained copious quantities of normal saline are washed
through the bursal cavity until a thorough lavage has been accomplished.

Aspiration of the Calcific Material. Bursitis due to an inflamed deposit
is a self-limiting condition and nature eventually effects a spontaneous cure.
This is accomplished by the mobilization of an inflammatory reaction,
rupture of the deposit and disgorgement of the material into the bursal
cavity where rapid absorption takes place. Therapy by needling procedure,
if it is to be uniformly successful, must also rupture the tense deposit. In
lesions where the deposit material is semi-fluid in consistency (acute lesions),
this may be accomplished by aspiration. The patient is postured in the
position of least discomfort. The exact center of tenderness, which corresponds to the location of the deposit, is located by gentle palpation and
confirmed by comparison with the location of the lesion as disclosed by
preoperative roentgenograms. A small nick is then made through the skin
at this point using local procaine hydrochloride anesthesia. A large bore
needle is inserted through skin, subcutaneous tissues, deltoid muscle and
bursal roof to penetrate the substance of the intrinsic tendon cuff forming
the bursal floor. A minimum of local anesthesia should be used during
this stage of the procedure since the complete elimination of pain removes

all subjective guides to the center of tenderness. The deposit then can be entered only by chance. The needle is inserted to bone and then withdrawn a few millimeters before aspiration is attempted. If preoperative localization of the lesion has been accurate the needle point should be within the deposit and the semi-fluid contents may be aspirated (Fig. 453). Although rupture of the deposit is enough to produce a cure in the acute case, recovery of some of the calcific material should be aimed for since the appearance of calcific material in the aspirating syringe constitutes the only definite evi-

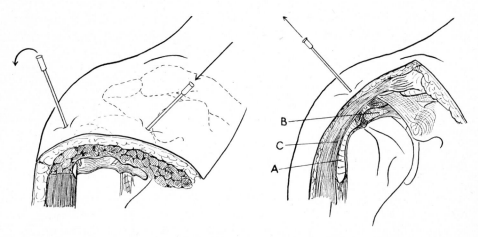

FIG. 453. *Left:* Irrigation of the subdeltoid bursa. The points of the inserted needles should be at least 1 inch apart to insure that lavage takes place through the bursal cavity and not through a false cavity in the tissues. *Right:* Aspiration of a calcific deposit from the short rotator tendons. The needle is inserted to bone at the exact center of tenderness which corresponds to the location of the deposit. It is then withdrawn a few millimeters and the aspiration carried out. A. Bursal cavity. B. The deposit situated in short rotator tendon cuff which forms the floor of the bursa. C. Deltoid.

dence available that the purpose of the procedure (puncture and deflation of the deposit) has been accomplished. This procedure will produce uniformly rapid and satisfactory results in acute lesions. Selected chronic lesions also may be aspirated after first infiltrating the dry chalky deposit with saline so that it becomes fluid enough to be withdrawn through a needle.

Excision of Calcific Deposit. Excision of the deposit is indicated when other therapies have failed or seem doomed to failure, and the symptoms, either by reason of severity or duration, warrant the minor operative procedure required. The presence of multiple deposits, even though only one of them may be responsible for the current symptoms, often makes excision of all deposits the procedure of choice in order to prevent future attacks of pain due to the others. Under any circumstances excision offers the most certain, uniform, rapid and permanent results. However, it is indicated in only about 5 per cent of all cases.

Accurate preoperative localization of the deposit is advisable but not essential. A 3 cm. skin incision in line with the skin creases is made just below the acromion about 5 cm. lateral to the coracoid process. The under-lying deltoid fibers are spread apart and the bursal roof is incised along the same line. With the bursal aperture retracted open, manipulation of the humerus serves to deliver the affected portion of tendon cuff into the field of vision (Fig. 454). The inflamed deposit is identified, the overlying tendon incised in line with the tendon fibers and the enclosed material evacuated. Neither the tendon cavity nor the bursal incision should be sutured. Deltoid, superficial fascia and skin are closed in layers with fine silk.

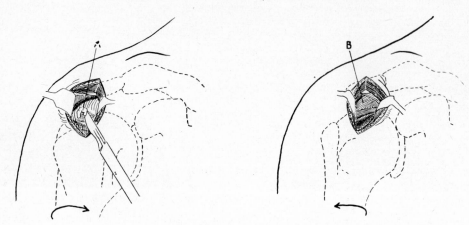

FIG. 454. Excision of a calcific deposit from the musculotendinous cuff of the right shoulder, viewed from in front. A 3-cm. incision is made distalward from the acromion at a point 5 cm. lateral to the coracoid. The deltoid fibers are separated and the bursal roof incised in the same line. By manipulation of the humerus the calcific deposit may be delivered into the incision. A. Infraspinatus lesion delivered into the operative incision by internal rotation. B. Exposure of the supraspinatus through the same incision by external rotation. Extension of the arm brings the proximal, and flexion, the distal portion of the tendon cuff into the operative field.

Early motion and use of the extremity is both beneficial and possible. The results are uniformly certain, rapid and permanent.

A more posterior or more extensive wound through the deltoid than that described carries a potential risk of damage to the axillary nerve fibers. Therefore, it is advisable to make a small anterior wound into which the lesion may be delivered by manipulation of the humerus. In order to do this the extremity must be draped in such a manner that free mobility is available without jeopardizing aseptic technic.

Occasionally visual identification of the calcific lesion is uncertain, especially in chronic cases characterized by a minimal inflammatory reaction. Exploration of the tendon cuff for such a deposit should not be done by incision. Incisions, no matter how small, are apt to bleed freely and obscure visibility. Suspicious areas of tendon should be perforated with a small hemostat which is then opened to spread apart the tendon fibers and expose the underlying tissue. Multiple small perforations of this type may be made without causing enough bleeding to obscure the field.

Excision of the Subdeltoid Bursa. Long-continued mechanical irritation commonly results in an irreversible proliferative inflammatory thickening of the bursal walls. The thickened bursa, no longer able to slide under the edge of the acromion and coraco-acromial ligament with ease, causes an

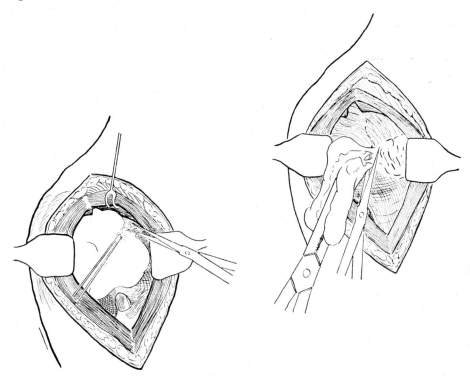

Fig. 455. Excision of the subdeltoid bursa. A 3-inch incision is made downward from the clavicle midway between the coracoid and the acromioclavicular joint. The deltoid fascia is incised in the same line and the anterior fibers of the deltoid spread apart to expose the roof of the bursa. *Left,* removal is commenced at the medial extremity of the bursa with the arm held in full external rotation. The dissection is carried lateralward and removal completed, *right,* with the arm held in full internal rotation. Only the roof of the bursa should be removed. Division of the anterior falciform edge of the coraco-acromial ligament as illustrated in the upper extremity of the wound should accompany removal of the bursa.

internal derangement of the subacromial mechanism in much the same way that a thickened synovial capsule affects a knee joint. Excision of the bursa produces relief from the symptoms. Elimination of the primary source of bursal irritation should accompany bursectomy whenever possible.

A 3-inch incision is made from the clavicle downward, midway between the coracoid and the acromioclavicular joint (Fig. 455). The deltoid fibers are separated at a point not more than 2 cm. lateral to the deltopectoral interval. Extensive spreading apart of the deltoid is safe only if done in the most anterior portion of the muscle. Retraction of the separated muscle fibers brings the bursal roof into view. Only the roof should be removed.

This is done by sharp dissection commencing at the medial extremity of the structure with the arm in external rotation. As the dissection progresses laterally the extremity is internally rotated in order to keep the field of dissection in full view. Bleeders are numerous but small, and many are amenable to control by temporary pressure with a moist sponge. The anterior edge of the coraco-acromial ligament is divided to reduce the pressure this structure normally exerts upon the subacromial structures. The deltoid fascia, subcutaneous tissues and skin are closed with fine silk. Gradually

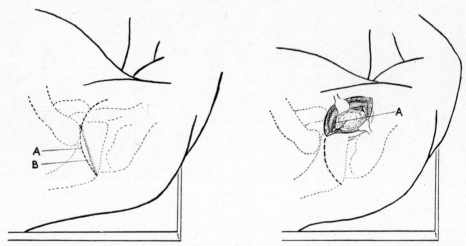

FIG. 456. Transacromial approach to the shoulder. Right shoulder viewed from above. *Left:* A. Skin incision. B. Average line of division of acromion. *Right:* Exploratory incision anterior to acromion is carried through deltoid and bursal roof to expose the underlying tendon cuff. Manipulation of the humerus delivers the various areas of tendon cuff into the operative wound for examination. A. The coraco-acromial ligament should be divided to facilitate exposure.

progressive resumption of motion and use of the arm should be commenced within 48 hours following operation. Postoperative management by balanced suspension of the extremity facilitates early return of function.

Incision and Drainage of the Subdeltoid Bursa. Pyogenic affections of the subdeltoid bursa seldom occur as an isolated lesion and usually are secondary to an infectious process in the adjacent humerus or shoulder joint. Drainage of the main infection should be so fashioned that the extension of suppuration into the bursal cavity is also controlled. Isolated pyogenic infections of the bursa may be incised and drained through the same route as described for bursal excision (Fig. 455). More adequate drainage may be obtained, if necessary, by utilization of a transacromial incision (Figs. 456, 457 and 458).

Acromioplasty. The pain in most derangements of the subacromial mechanism results from tissue tension due to the existing pathological process and from pressure exerted upon the involved structures by the overlying acromion and the anterior falciform edge of the coraco-acromial ligament.

The operation of acromioplasty minimizes the effect of the latter as a contributing cause of symptoms in many conditions. It is a particularly useful palliative measure in painful subacromial affections due to rheumatoid arthritis and is a useful adjunct to certain reparative and reconstructive procedures carried out on the shoulder mechanism, notably repair of ruptured rotator tendons and arthroplasty of the shoulder involving excision of the humeral head. The technic of acromioplasty is described coincidentally with the transacromial approach to the shoulder (Figs. 456, 457 and 458).

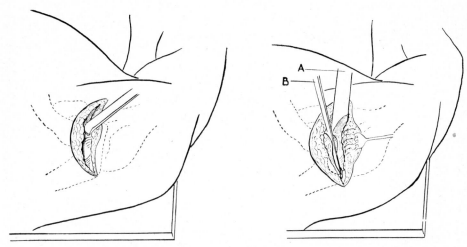

FIG. 457. *Left:* The skin incision is deepened to the acromion, the surface of which is exposed subperiosteally. *Right:* A. A flat instrument is passed between tendon cuff and acromion to act as a guard. B. The acromion is divided by osteotome. The line of division is governed by the amount of exposure required. The integrity of the acromioclavicular joint should be maintained whenever possible.

Affections of the Short Rotator Tendons. REPAIR OF COMPLETE RUPTURE. Complete rupture is a term used to designate a tear through the full thickness of the tendon cuff substance. The type and degree of both symptoms and disability depend upon the location and extent of the tear. Establishment of the diagnosis, per se, does not constitute an adequate indication for operation since both clinical experience and anatomical studies have demonstrated that such lesions are present and well compensated for in a considerable percentage of people past middle age. The only tenable indication for operation consists of symptoms or disability sufficient to make it worth while from the patient's viewpoint.

Exposure of the lesion is best accomplished through a superior transacromial approach. A gently curved skin incision is made over the top of the shoulder parallel to the strap or suspender line and extending from the posterolateral corner of the acromion, passing just lateral to the acromioclavicular joint to end at a point 3 cm. anterior to the acromion (Fig. 456). The anterior 3 cm. of the incision is deepened to the underlying deltoid, the fibers of which are spread apart to expose the roof of the bursa and the coraco-acromial ligament. Both are incised. A small and safe exploratory opening thus is made available through which, by manipulation of the humerus, almost all portions of the cuff may be brought into view (Fig. 456). Examination of the existing pathology will determine the amount of addi-

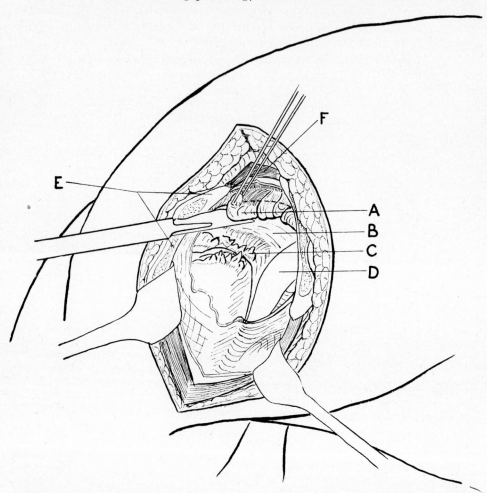

Fig. 458. The right shoulder, viewed from in front. The outer fragment of acromion along with attached deltoid is retracted laterally. A. The avascular edges of the tendon defect are excised back to healthy tissue. B. Head of humerus. C. Residual tendon tabs on greater tuberosity at point of avulsion. D. Biceps tendon. E. Retracted outer fragment of acromion. F. The posterior deltoid fibers may be split when necessary for increased exposure.

tional exposure necessary for repair. The remainder of the skin incision is deepened to acromion from which the periosteum is elevated with a sharp elevator (Fig. 457). A flat instrument is placed as a guard between the acromion and the tendon cuff and the acromion is divided with an osteotome. Division of the acromion is done at whatever point is necessary to provide adequate exposure and working room for the reparative problem encountered. Small lesions may require that only the anterolateral corner of the bone be separated, but the repair of large retracted ruptures or operative procedures in the region of the glenoid fossa are facilitated by removal of most of the bone lying lateral to the acromioclavicular joint. The latter

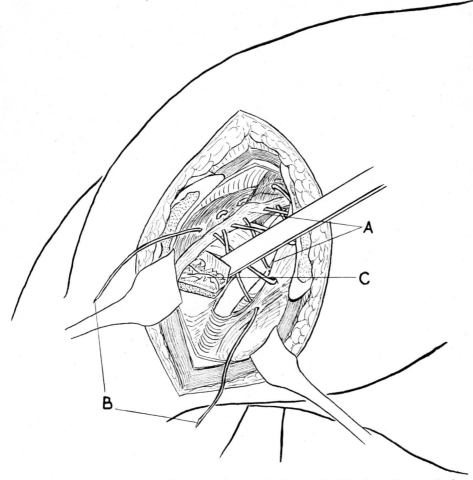

Fig. 459. The right shoulder viewed from in front. (A) Tendon edges excised and the residual defect fashioned in the shape of a wedge with apex pointing medially. (B) Continuous shoe-lace suture placed in such a way that traction upon its ends apposes the two sides of the wedge. (C) Raw bony bed for reinsertion of the residual sides of the tendon defect formed by removal of a portion of tuberosity and articular cartilage from the humerus.

structure should be left intact in order to preserve the integrity of the bony shoulder girdle, but unintentional involvement of this joint in the process of dividing the acromion has been followed by no appreciable functional or symptomatic defect.

The outer fragment of the acromion along with its attached deltoid origin is retracted laterally (Fig. 458). When needed, additional exposure may be gained by splitting the posterior deltoid fibers. On completion of the tendon repair or in carrying out the procedure of acromioplasty the outer fragment of divided acromion is separated from all soft part attachments by sharp dissection and removed. The remaining stump may be

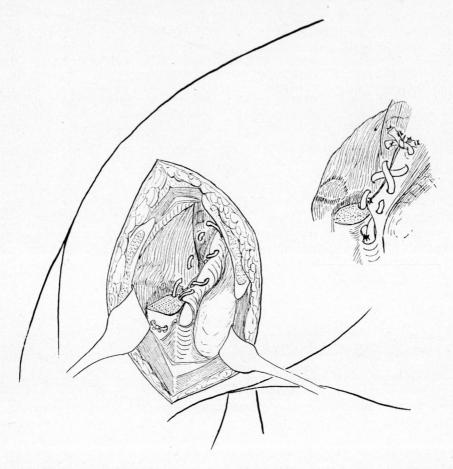

FIG. 460. Right shoulder viewed from in front. Repair is completed by passing the ends of the continuous suture through drill holes in the bone and tying them lateral to the tuberosity. Any increased tension on the suture resulting from motion of the arm makes more snug the apposition of tendon edges. The residual unapposed edges of the tendon defect are held in apposition to the raw bony bed which has been formed (Fig. 459). Additional sutures passed through drill holes in the bone may be required for this purpose. Inset shows alternate method for repair of selected cases. Long head of biceps is separated from the glenoid, split, and used as an autogenous suture.

reshaped by rongeur in order to obtain the optimum cosmetic result. The central tendon of deltoid origin then is sutured firmly to the terminal fibers of the trapezius muscle and the adjacent fascia and periosteum on the superior surface of the acromion. The remainder of the wound is closed in layers with interrupted sutures of fine silk.

The rupture almost invariably is an avulsion of tendon cuff insertion from the bone rather than a tear across tendon fibers. Retraction of the proximal fragment varies directly as the extent of the tear. It is always difficult and often impossible to secure and maintain anatomical reposition of the retracted fragment. Fortunately, anatomical integrity is not necessary to normal cuff function. The primary object of repair, therefore, is to restore continuity between the short rotator muscles and the humerus rather than accurate reposition of the avulsed tendon insertions.

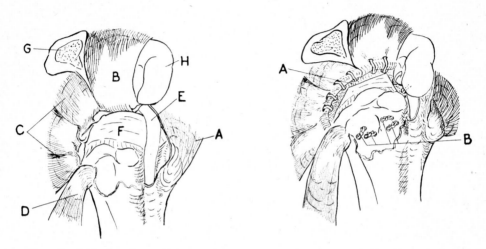

FIG. 461. *Left:* Massive avulsion of short rotator cuff from right humerus, viewed from the side, with acromion and deltoid removed. Retraction is marked and the detached tendon cuff lies between humerus and glenoid. A. Subscapularis, B. Supraspinatus, C. Infraspinatus, D. Teres minor, E. Biceps tendon, F. Humeral head, G. Scapular spine, divided, H. Coracoid. *Right:* Technic for reinsertion into the humeral head at whatever point the tendon cuff will reach without tension while the arm is at the side. Fixation is by mattress sutures passed through drill holes in the bone and tied lateral to the tuberosity.

The edges of the tendon defect always are degenerated and scarred. They are excised back to healthy tissue (Fig. 458) and the defect produced by the excision is fashioned in the shape of a wedge pointing medially (Fig. 459). A continuous, shoe-lace type of heavy silk suture is placed in such a way that it will produce side-to-side apposition of the healthy edges of this defect. The suture is then tightened to the point of maximum side-to-side apposition of the tendon edges without tension, while the arm is at the side. More apposition is possible in the abducted position, but a suture tightened in this position is apt to pull out when the arm is returned to the side. The tuberosity and humeral head are then denuded of cortex and cartilage over an area sufficient to accommodate the remaining unapposed tendon edges. Two drill holes are made into this denuded area, emerging lateral to the tuberosity and through these the ends of the continuous suture are passed and tied lateral to the bone (Fig. 460). Small tears in the supraspinatus insertion may be similarly repaired by an autogenous suture obtained by dividing the long biceps tendon at its glenoid attachment and using the split intra-articular portion as a continuous suture (inset, Fig. 460).

REPAIR OF MASSIVE AVULSION. A massive avulsion of all or almost all of the tendon cuff from its humeral attachment occasionally is encountered. Retraction is marked and the avulsed tendon flap may lie between humerus and glenoid. No attempt should be made to return the retracted tendon cuff to its normal point of insertion. Restoration of continuity between the muscles and the humerus should be accomplished by reinsertion of the retracted tendon cuff into the head of the humerus at whatever point it will reach without tension while the arm is at the side (Fig. 461).

No two ruptures will be encountered that are identical in size or shape or which are amenable to exactly the same reparative technic. Figure 460 represents side-to-side, and figure 461, an end-to-bone repair. Almost always, some combination of the two technics is called for. The size and shape of the original tendon defect must decide the exact number and type of sutures required for its repair. Regardless of the technic the repair must demonstrate the following characteristics in their order of importance. (1) There must be snug apposition of healthy to healthy tissues. (2) There should be no tension with the arm at the side. (3) There should be continuity between the intrinsic muscles and the humerus. (4) The apposition of repaired tissues should be snug enough to prevent the leakage of joint fluid through the site where healing is to take place. Restoration of anatomy is unimportant and never should be attempted at the expense of any of these four primary requirements.

REPAIR OF INCOMPLETE RUPTURE. Ruptures through a partial thickness of the tendon cuff fibers fall into three categories. The area of laceration may involve the superficial surface or the deep surface of the cuff or may be restricted to the internal fibers so that neither surface is affected. Regardless of its location an incomplete tear produces symptoms and disability by two mechanisms. Localized irregularity of the tendon cuff results in mechanical irritation of the subdeltoid bursa and the syndrome of bursitis. When the lacerated tendon fragments are large enough, there also results a mechanical internal derangement of the subacromial mechanism, the hypermobile tab of tendon becoming caught between humerus and acromion or ligament on motion of the arm in much the same way that a torn meniscus becomes caught between the bones of the knee.

Ruptures involving the superficial surface of the cuff, or restricted to the central tendon fibers, are visible in the floor of the bursa. The shoulder is explored in the manner described for complete tears so that adequate exposure of the pathology will be available. Many small ruptures may be repaired through the anterior, deltoid-splitting portion of the approach and do not require division of the acromion, but this circumstance cannot be foretold prior to visualization of the lesion, and the ability to enlarge the exposure as much as is necessary is of considerable importance.

Once identified the lesion must be eradicated in such a way that mechanical irritation of the surrounding structures is eliminated. When possible the lacerated area of tendon is excised by an elliptical excision paralleling the direction of the tendon fibers. The residual defect is then repaired by interrupted or vertical mattress sutures of fine silk while the arm is at the side (Fig. 462). The anterior horn of the coraco-acromial ligament is divided to lessen pressure upon the repaired cuff. The bursa need be excised only if it appears irreversibly thickened. The wound is closed in layers and early motion and use should be commenced within a few days.

The most commonly encountered incomplete rupture is the so-called "rim rent," characterized by an avulsion of the deep tendon fibers from their insertion into the tuberosity (Fig. 463). The hypermobile tab of

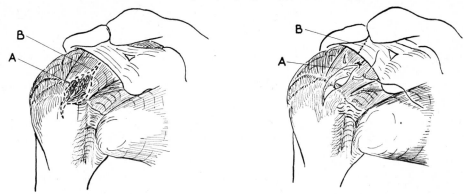

Fig. 462. The right shoulder with deltoid removed. Repair of incomplete rupture involving the superficial surface of the supraspinatus tendon, viewed from in front. *Left:* A. Area of lacerated tendon fibers. B. Line of incision for removing a full thickness block of tendon containing the lacerated area. *Right:* A. Repair of residual defect by side-to-side suture. B. Line of division of the anterior edge of the coraco-acromial ligament to lessen the friction normally occurring between it and the superficial surface of the cuff.

avulsed tendon causes an internal derangement of the subacromial mechanism as it becomes caught between humerus and acromion on appropriate motions of the shoulder. Even with the bursa open, identification of the lesion may be difficult since the surface of the cuff remains intact. A heaping up of the bursal floor into folds on motion of the arm is one abnormal visual characteristic of the condition. These blister-like folds may be reproduced by stroking the superficial surface of the tendon laterally with a flat instrument (Fig. 463). Similar folds cannot be reproduced in a normal cuff. Normally the cuff insertion is immovably fixed to humerus. The apparently intact tendon overlying a deep tear may be picked up with forceps and freely elevated from the bone (Fig. 463). By some combination of these signs one may arrive at the definite suspicion of a deep tear. A longitudinal incision through the tendon fibers then should be made for visualization of the suspected area. All such exploratory incisions should be firmly repaired with interrupted sutures of fine silk.

Repair of a deep surface tear requires elevation of a flap of tendon cuff for purposes of exposure (Fig. 463). This flap is best fashioned by separating the already damaged tendon insertion from the humerus and may be mobilized by incising the tendon fibers medially at each end of the separated area. The flap should be as extensive as the tear. A full thickness segment of the lateral extremity of the flap, including the avulsed tendon tab, is removed. The end of the flap is then inserted into a bony trench in the

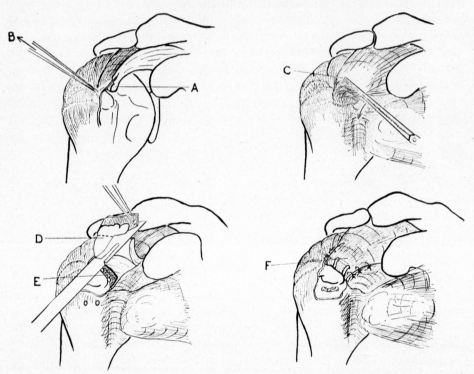

FIG. 463. The right shoulder viewed from in front with deltoid removed. Identification and repair of rim rent. A. Cross-section diagram showing deep surface avulsion of supraspinatus tendon. B. Intact surface of tendon may be lifted from the underlying tuberosity. C. Stroking the intact surface toward the tuberosity produces an abnormal blister-like elevation of the tendon substance from the bone. D. Elevation of a flap of tendon from the bone as wide as the tear is long and excision of the torn tab of tendon. E. Bony trench cut into an anatomical neck for reinsertion of tendon flap. Drill holes pass from the depths of the trench to lateral surface of tuberosity. F. Full thickness tendon flap inserted into bony trench and held in place by mattress suture, placed to invert the end of the flap into the depths of the trench, and tied lateral to the tuberosity. Additional fine sutures complete repair of mobilizing incisions made at either end of the tendon flap.

anatomical neck of the humerus and fastened by means of sutures passed through drill holes in the bone and tied lateral to the tuberosity. The mobilizing incisions at either end of the flap are firmly sutured with fine silk (Fig. 463). Division of the anterior edge of the coraco-acromial ligament removes a considerable amount of compression force from the repaired area and appreciably hastens rehabilitation of the extremity.

Repair of any incomplete tendon cuff tear is better not done unless it is accomplished in such a way as to satisfy the basic objectives of the procedure; *i.e.,* restoration of continuity between the short rotator muscles and humerus, elimination of hypermobile fragments of tendon which produce internal derangement of the subacromial mechanism and eradication of irregularities productive of mechanical irritation of the bursa on motion of the glenohumeral joint. Adequate repair is impossible without adequate exposure. One should never hesitate to divide the acromion or coraco-acromial ligament as far as is necessary to provide exposure and working room. Neither procedure is followed by any functional defect and the post-operative reduction of pressure upon the tendon repair following division of these structures definitely facilitates early recovery of motion.

Repair of Rupture of Long Biceps Tendon. Rupture of the long tendon of the biceps, per se, is not a particularly disabling condition. Commonly it occurs in the presence of a cuff rupture, and while the biceps lesion produces obvious objective signs, the cuff tear often accounts for most of the subjective complaints. For this reason the tendon cuff warrants a thorough inspection in any operation done for repair of the biceps tendon. An operative approach through the deltopectoral interval or anterior deltoid fibers (Fig. 455) provides adequate exposure. Retraction takes place in the distal rather than the proximal fragment of the ruptured structure. Frequently the tear is situated near the proximal end of the bicipital groove so that a portion of the tendon is pulled distalward by contraction of the muscle belly. The proximal tendon fragment requires no attention and may be excised if easily available. The distal fragment should be identified, pulled as far proximally as it will come without undue tension and firmly sutured to the nearest inelastic structure having sufficient strength to provide anchorage against contraction of the muscle belly; *i.e.,* the insertions of pectoralis major or subscapularis or the short head of the biceps. Attempts at end-to-end repair of the ruptured tendon usually are ill-advised, and predestined to failure.

Stabilization of Slipping Long Biceps Tendon. The long biceps tendon does not become unstable in its groove unless the transverse ligament which blends with the inserting supraspinatus and subscapularis fibers is torn. Biceps tendon instability, therefore, is rarely encountered except in the presence of a cuff tear. Repair of the cuff lesion should be designed to stabilize the slipping biceps tendon (Figs. 458 and 460). An unstable biceps tendon produces internal derangement of the subacromial mechanism in much the same way as a hypermobile tab of torn tendon cuff, and division of the coraco-acromial ligament, acromion, or both may be indicated. Further stabilization may be obtained by suturing the biceps tendon to the fibrous roof of the bicipital groove, the lesser tuberosity or the adjacent humeral cortex. Such a procedure eliminates the normal gliding of the tendon up and down the bicipital groove, may result in some defect in external rotation and abduction and is to be avoided when any other method of stabilization is available. Removal of the tendon from the glenoid and transposition to a new origin as in ruptures of the long biceps is a more satisfactory procedure than one which results in immobility of the tendon in its groove.

THE ELBOW REGION

Affections of the Olecranon Bursa. CHRONIC NONSUPPURATIVE BURSITIS. The most common lesion of the olecranon bursa results from mechanical irritation due to frequently repeated minor traumata of occupational origin. A proliferative inflammatory thickening of the bursal wall occurs and the bursal cavity becomes filled with excess fluid. Aspiration rarely is of any therapeutic benefit. Elimination of the mechanical cause of irritation eventually results in a subsidence of both signs and symptoms. Incision alone is of no therapeutic value and is strongly contraindicated by the risk of subsequent infection. Complete excision of the bursa followed by tight closure of the operative wound is the treatment of choice for any noninfected condition of the bursa in which surgical intervention is warranted by the subjective complaints on the cosmetic defects.

ACUTE BURSITIS DUE TO TRAUMA. A single trauma to the point of the elbow may produce an acute olecranon bursitis due to hemorrhage and the diffusion of inflammatory exudate into the bursal cavity. Aspiration, carried out under aseptic technic in the early stages of the condition, is indicated. A large bore needle is inserted into the bursal cavity through the most prominent portion of the fluctuant area and its fluid contents aspirated. A compression dressing by elastic bandage should be worn for several days following the procedure and, above all, the olecranon must be protected from undue pressure or minor traumata for a period of ten to fourteen days. Repeated traumata or undue pressure predisposes to transformation of the acute lesion into a chronic bursitis.

BURSITIS DUE TO GOUT. Repeated episodes of olecranon bursitis frequently prove to be local manifestations of gout. Colchicine therapy and dietary regulation should precede consideration of surgical intervention and may relieve the local condition completely. Large collections of urate crystals in the region of a gouty olecranon bursa may warrant excision. Usually the urate crystals are situated in the triceps tendon forming the floor of the bursa. The operative wound should be closed despite the fact that unremoved urate crystals may continue to be discharged through the healing site for some time.

ACUTE SUPPURATIVE BURSITIS. Incision and drainage without wound closure is indicated as soon as suppuration becomes localized. Unless the intrabursal tension resulting from an active infectious process is released at an early stage, rapid secondary necrosis of the triceps tendon in the bursal floor, and osteomyelitis of the olecranon, is likely to become superimposed upon the original condition. The bursal cavity is opened completely through a transverse or cruciate incision (Fig. 464). Care must be taken that the medial aspect of the incision does not damage the ulnar nerve lying between the olecranon and the medial humeral epicondyle. The bursal cavity should be packed open loosely and allowed to close by granulation tissue. The application of small deep skin grafts to the granulating wound may accelerate wound closure and rehabilitation of the extremity.

CHRONIC SUPPURATIVE BURSITIS. Chronic suppuration in the olecranon bursa usually is accompanied by some degree of infection in the triceps tendon and osteomyelitis of the olecranon. The most common cause consists of a previous ill-advised and improperly executed attempt to drain the excess fluid from an uninfected bursitis by a small incision into the bursal cavity. The proper operative management of a chronic suppurative lesion requires excision of all infected tissues. A transverse skin incision over the most prominent portion of the swollen bursa designed to include and excise

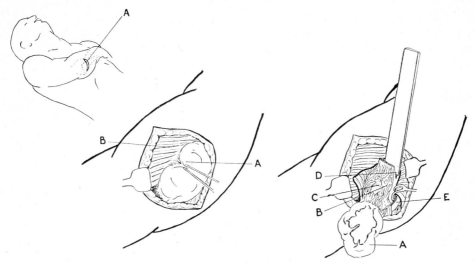

FIG. 464. *Left:* Excision of the olecranon bursa. A. The patient is postured with the arm lying across the chest. A transverse incision over the prominence of the bursa produces adequate exposure. *Middle:* A. The enlarged bursa, lying deep to subcutaneous tissue may be removed by a combination of sharp and blunt dissection. B. The triceps tendon and its expansions which form the floor of the bursa. *Right:* A. Bursa. B. Infected tendon in the bursal floor. C. Infected bone removed down to healthy tissue by osteotome, D. E. Ulnar nerve and recurrent ulnar artery which must be protected from injury.

the sinus opening in the skin when one exists, will produce an optimum cosmetic result. The ulnar nerve must not be molested in the medial extremity of the wound. The bursa is encountered directly under the skin and completely excised by sharp dissection. The triceps tendon forming the floor of the bursa should not be removed unless signs of necrosis and infection are present. In the latter circumstance all diseased tissue requires removal. The same holds true for any infected areas of olecranon lying deep to the tendon (Fig. 464). The operative wound should be packed open loosely and allowed to close by granulation tissue, aided, when necessary, by small deep skin grafts.

Aspiration of a Calcific Deposit from Lateral Epicondylar Region. Acute pain, tenderness, redness and swelling with local increased heat of the part may occur in the region of the lateral epicondyle. Almost always this is due to irritation centered around a calcific deposit situated in the tendinous origins of the extensor muscles of the forearm. The local condition may be very acute and simulate abscess formation sufficiently to suggest incision and drainage. X-ray identification of the presence and exact location of the inflamed deposit should precede any decision as to therapy.

Such deposits are superficial and may be localized accurately. A skin weal is made over the site of the lesion with procaine hydrochloride and a Wassermann needle inserted into the very center of tenderness. Aspiration of the creamy contents of the deposit is simple and relatively certain in acute cases once the site of the lesion is localized. Chronic lesions of this type are

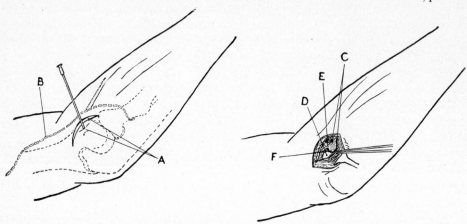

FIG. 465. A. Sites for incision and needling of tendon lesions at the origin of the forearm extensor muscles. B. The radial nerve the deep branch of which winds around the neck of the radius and may require protection from damage in the distal extremity of the approach. C. Edges of longitudinal exploratory incision through the tendon origin. D. Lateral epicondyle. E. The usual location of the local pathology, close to the epicondyle. F. Level for transverse division of the tendon origin.

encountered rarely. Early, complete and permanent relief from pain is to be expected following deflation of the tense deposit.

Needling of Lateral Epicondylar Region for "Tennis Elbow," Epicondylitis, etc. Pain in the lateral side of the elbow, aggravated by tension of the forearm extensor muscles, and tenderness localized to the lateral epicondyle, in the absence of a calcific deposit by x-ray, denotes a lesion of the tendinous origin of the forearm extensor muscles which has been given many names. Such symptoms seldom result from pathology in the radiohumeral bursa although this is commonly considered to be the offending lesion. The actual pathology usually is characterized by degenerative and inflammatory changes in the tendon tissue adjacent to the lateral epicondyle. Multiple needle perforations of the diseased tendon, either by reason of deflation of intratendinous tension or revascularization and fibrous tissue replacement of diseased tendon fibers, results in relief from symptoms in a large percentage of cases. Perforations may be carried out with a small needle inserted through the skin at the lateral epicondyle (Fig. 465). Through a single skin perforation the origin of the forearm extensors should be penetrated in all directions until the region of the epicondyle has been perforated ten or twenty times. Each perforation should be carried down to bone. The use of local anesthesia makes the procedure relatively free from pain. Following multiple perforation of the tendon origin deep massage over the affected area should be done. Restrictive dressings and splintage of the wrist in extension are purely palliative measures and seldom result in permanent relief of symptoms.

When conservative measures fail to produce relief operative intervention is warranted. A 2 centimeter incision is made over the lateral epicondyle (Fig. 465). Retraction of the skin exposes the superficial surface of the diseased tendon. If the operation is done under local anesthesia the patient's subjective reactions are an excellent guide to the location of the tendon lesion. The tendon is incised longitudinally (Fig. 465). Identification of an area of diseased tendon is followed by removal of all visibly abnormal tissue. When the diseased area cannot be found (frequently it may involve no more than 2 to 3 millimeters of tendon tissue) a transverse division of the tendon fibers just distal to the epicondyle should be done. Such a procedure produces relief by removing tension from that portion of the tendon immediately adjacent to the bone. The length of the transverse incision through tendon should not exceed 0.5 cm. No functional defect is produced by dividing the tendon origin and the prospects for relief from pain are reasonably certain.

Excision of Myositis Ossificans Traumatica from Brachialis Muscle. Abnormal bone formation may take place within the substance of the brachialis muscle following certain elbow injuries. The lesion may restrict elbow motion sufficiently to warrant operative intervention. The choice of time for operation is of the utmost importance. The activity of the abnormal bone forming mechanism progresses for nine to twelve months, and even complete removal of the lesion during this period is followed by prompt recurrence and an accelerated activity of the original condition. Cessation of activity is measurable by serial x-rays taken over a period of months. The abnormal bone may be removed with minimal risk of recurrence after it can be demonstrated that a stationary level has been reached. However, a further delay of several months prior to operation is usually advisable because many of these lesions tend to regress and may disappear spontaneously.

The lesion should be exposed through an anterior approach. A longitudinal incision crossing the flexion crease of the elbow never should be made. The skin incision providing optimum exposure and cosmetic result is illustrated in figure 466. Following reflection of the skin flaps the antebrachial fascia is incised longitudinally over the interval between the biceps and the brachioradialis. Excision of a segment of the cephalic vein at this stage facilitates exposure of the deeper regions and removes the danger of venous complications resulting from operative trauma to the vein. The radial nerve is next identified as it lies in the interval between the two muscles. Both nerve and brachioradialis are retracted laterally, en bloc, and the biceps medially. Excellent exposure of the underlying brachialis muscle may be obtained. The bony tumor is located by palpation and the overlying brachialis fibers spread apart (Fig. 467). Removal should be done by slow and careful sharp dissection accompanied by complete hemostasis. The best insurance against reformation of bone is a dry field, loosely closed,

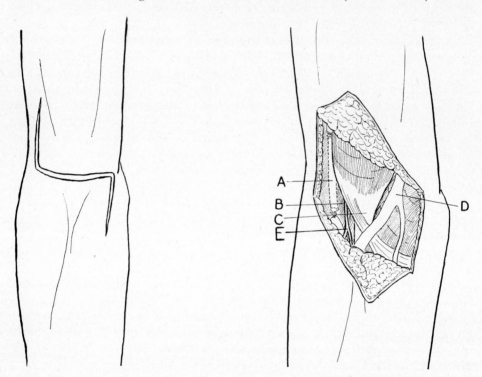

FIG. 466. Anterior approach to the elbow region for exposure and removal of a myositis ossificans in the brachialis muscle. A vertical incision across the flexion crease leads to subsequent contracture of the scar and is to be avoided. *Left:* A step-cut skin incision produces optimum exposure and cosmetic result. *Right:* The skin flaps are reflected and the antebrachial fascia incised longitudinally. A. The cephalic vein should be ligated and divided or a segment removed as it is encountered over the interval between B., the brachioradialis and C., the biceps. D. The remaining antecubital veins do not embarrass the approach and may be retracted. E. Lateral antebrachial cutaneous nerve.

following the operation. The fascia is left unclosed or, at most, closed very loosely. The skin is closed loosely with interrupted fine sutures.

Repair of Ruptured or Avulsed Biceps Insertion. This lesion is not common. Gross retraction of the tendon usually is prevented by remaining intact attachments to the lacertus fibrosus and deep fascia of the forearm. The end of the tendon usually is found lying free just under the antebrachial fascia (Fig. 468). Exposure is obtained through a transverse skin incision (Fig. 468). The biceps tendon is mobilized except for its lacertus attachments and the scarred and fibrotic terminal end excised. No attempt to return the tendon to its radial insertion is warranted. Some surgeons simply suture the tendon to the deep fascia of the forearm. Incorporation of the biceps tendon into the tendon of insertion of the brachialis is followed by a very satisfactory functional result. The technic for this procedure is illustrated in figure 468. The flexor function of the biceps is restored via the ulna rather than the radius. Supination power of the muscle is lost but this produces little or no functional defect. Early and progressive motion within pain limits, but with the elimination of sudden flexion motions of the elbow may be permitted when the wound is healed.

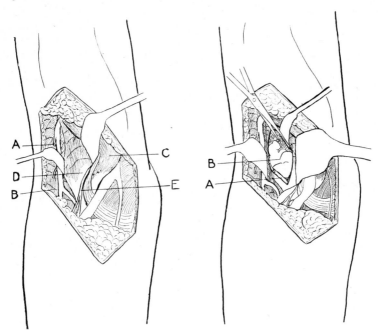

Fig. 467. Exposure and removal of myositis ossificans from brachialis. *Left:* A. The radial nerve, and B. the brachioradialis are retracted laterally, en bloc. C. The biceps is retracted medially. D. The brachialis muscle is exposed in the base of the wound. E. The lateral antebrachial cutaneous nerve is retracted from the field. *Right:* A. The brachialis fibers are spread apart over B., the bony tumor. The latter is removed by sharp dissection. Complete hemostasis is essential.

Incision of the Forearm Fascia for Threatened Volkmann's Ischemia. This procedure is rarely necessary, and by itself seldom results in any real benefit to the local condition. The threat of Volkmann's ischemia usually results from neurovascular spasm due to internal pressure upon the vessels by displaced bone fragments, external compression by improperly applied splints or by vessel compression due to position, *e.g.,* acute flexion of the elbow in the presence of subfascial tension. Exposure of the vessels in threatened Volkmann's ischemia discloses vascular spasm which does not subside immediately following deflation of whatever subfascial tension exists until the mechanical focus of irritation has been removed. Application of warm saline to the spastic vessels usually will hasten their relaxation. Volk-

mann's paralysis has been observed to develop in hemophiliacs due to subfascial tension alone, but under such circumstances fasciotomy is always
strongly contraindicated.

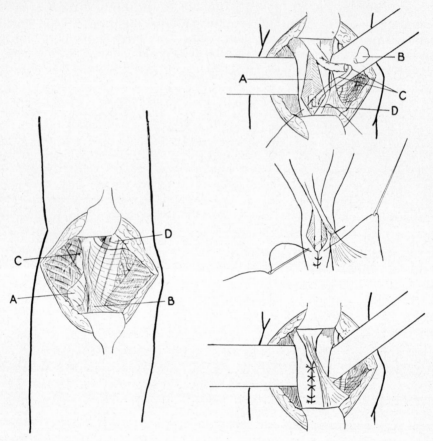

Fig. 468. Repair of biceps avulsion from the radius. A transverse incision produces
adequate exposure and the optimum cosmetic result. *Left:* A. The avulsed tendon end is
located, lying free under the antebrachial fascia. B. Gross retraction is prevented by intact
attachments to the fascia and lacertus fibrosus. C. Brachialis muscle. D. Brachial vessels
and median nerve. *Right:* A. A longitudinal incision is made into the tendon of the
brachialis. B. The devitalized end of the avulsed tendon is excised. C. Placement of a
continuous suture designed to fix the tendon end into the opening in the brachialis
tendon. D. Ulnar (coronoid) cortex removed in the depths of the opening into the
brachialis tendon. *Middle:* The continuous suture is tied and the repair reinforced by
another continuous suture woven through both tendons. *Below:* Completed repair.

The rational management of a threatened Volkmann's lesion consists
primarily of the elimination of all important contributing causes, support of
the local circulation by moderate elevation, and the application of gentle
heat and, at times, reduction of existing vascular spasm by cervical sympathetic block. Incision of the deep fascia of the forearm unaccompanied by
these measures is of little benefit. When subfascial tension continues to pro-

gress in spite of conservative measures and is severe enough to warrant fasciotomy, an incision is made along either side of the forearm and the deep fascia enclosing the flexor muscles incised for a distance of 10 to 15 cm. When possible the skin, but not the fascial incisions, are closed loosely. When the seat of pathology is in the antecubital region the fascia is exposed through a step cut skin incision (Fig. 466). The fascia is opened along the medial border of the biceps as widely as is necessary for the deflation of all subfascial tension. The skin alone is closed but may be left open if closure is accompanied by significant tension.

THE WRIST REGION

Aspiration of Ganglion. This procedure is simple and when it is successful the patient is saved the inconvenience and expense of hospitalization. However, the available evidence indicates it to be successful in only about 33 per cent of cases. The lesion usually is subcutaneous and may be entered easily with a needle introduced through the skin overlying the most prominent portion of the tumor. Tuberculous tenosynovitis may simulate the clinical picture of a ganglion and should be ruled out before aspiration is attempted. Rather thick, amber colored, viscid fluid is recovered from the typical ganglion. This may be replaced by a small amount of some mild sclerosing fluid in an attempt to obliterate the lesion. A compression dressing should be applied for several days following aspiration and the prognosis always should be guarded.

Excision of Ganglion. This procedure offers the best chance for cure. Recurrences following excision are reported in between 15 and 35 per cent of cases. Many such recurrences undoubtedly result from incomplete ablation of the tumor and its connective tissue base. Unless complete removal of both the ganglion and its base is accomplished recurrence is likely. Adequate hemostasis is necessary to the identification and removal of all pathological tissue and for this reason the use of a tourniquet warrants consideration.

A transverse skin incision is made over the presenting tumor. On the dorsum of the wrist care must be taken to avoid damage to the superficial branch of the radial nerve and on the volar surface the radial artery, which is commonly in close proximity to the ganglion, must be protected from injury. The lesion is found to be bounded on either side by tendons which also must be retracted gently away from the field of operation and protected from damage. The tumor is dissected free by a combination of blunt and sharp technic. The connective tissue base from which it originates should be cleared of areolar tissues and excised. If a tourniquet is used it should be released following removal of the tumor and complete hemostasis obtained prior to wound closure.

Operative Management of Spontaneous Rupture of the Extensor Pollicis Longus Tendon. This lesion, characterized by inability to extend the interphalangeal joint of the thumb, usually occurs several weeks to months following a Colles' fracture. The rupture takes place at the level of the previous fracture and retraction of the proximal tendon fragment usually makes end-to-end repair impossible. Continuity between the tendon ends may be restored by the implantation of a free tendon graft (Fig. 451). The usual procedure indicated is one of tendon transfer.

The simplest technical procedure consists of implanting the distal fragment of the ruptured tendon into the tendon of the abductor pollicis longus. A 3 cm. incision is made along the dorsum of the thumb metacarpal and the long abductor tendon exposed. The distal fragment of the ruptured tendon is then identified (traction upon this tendon fragment produces terminal phalanx extension), dissected free from its neighboring tissues and brought over to the exposed abductor tendon. With the terminal phalanx held in hyperextension by an assistant, a side-to-side suture of the two tendons is carried out (Fig. 448). The proximal end of the tendon juncture should remain far enough distal so that it does not encroach upon the abductor tunnel at the radial styloid on motion of the thumb. The wound is closed with fine silk and the thumb immobilized in an extended position for three weeks. Progressive active motion and exercises then are commenced. Following union between the two tendons, contraction of the abductor muscle performs interphalangeal joint extension coincidently with abduction. The results are satisfactory but some defect in terminal phalanx extension is to be expected.

Excision of Palmar Fascia for Dupuytren's Contracture. The object of this operation is to remove every vestige of fascia from the palm as well as every digital extension of the palmar fascia into the fingers. Whenever possible the procedure should be done before gross flexion contractures of the fingers become established. In cases having a marked flexion contracture a preliminary subcutaneous tenotomy of the main fascial bands, followed by mild continuous traction is advisable. This facilitates the excision which should follow within two weeks.

Complete hemostasis and visibility throughout the operative field is a *sine qua non* of adequate fascial excision and this makes the use of a tourniquet almost compulsory. A longitudinal skin incision never should be used in the palm. Oblique or curved incisions following the flexion creases as much as possible provide adequate exposure and optimum prospects for uneventful healing (See Chapter 22 for types of incision in the hand). The first step in the operation is a complete separation of the palmar skin from its deep attachments, leaving no fascial fibers attached to its deep surface. In certain areas this may necessitate shaving the cutaneous layer very thin and buttonholing this layer is to be avoided at all cost. The fascia is then divided transversely at the insertion of the palmaris longus. The severed end is grasped with a strong clamp and pulled distalward in order to place tension upon the fascial septae penetrating into the deep palmar space. In regular progression, proceeding distally, all fascial attachments, including every penetrating septum, are dissected free and the fascia removed, en bloc (Fig. 469). Each penetrating septum should be severed as close to its deep attachment as possible and removed along with the main block of fascia. Additional small incisions along the sides of each proximal phalanx facilitate removal of the fascial extensions into the fingers. Complete removal of all digital extensions of the fascia is of considerable importance to the success of the procedure.

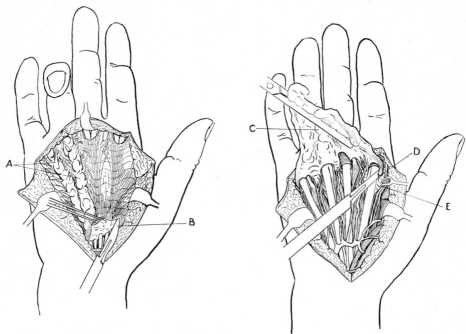

Fig. 469. Removal of palmar fascia for Dupuytren's contracture. *Left:* A. Main contracted fascial bands. B. The skin of the palm is reflected from the fascia which is divided transversely at the insertion of the palmaris longus. *Right:* C. The fascia is grasped with a clamp and pulled distalward while the deep penetrating septa are divided in regular progression. D. Each penetrating septum is exposed and divided as close to its deep attachment as possible. E. The digital vessels and nerves must be protected against damage.

Complete removal of the fascia seldom produces immediate and complete eradication of the existing contractures. All structures are contracted and an overenthusiastic attempt to obtain complete extension at the time of operation, by forcible manipulation of the fingers, is apt to result in fracture or dislocation. A dorsal splint should be applied in the position of maximum extension permitted by the residual contracture. The latter may be relieved progressively by a program of gradually increasing exercises, traction and gentle repeated manipulations.

Healing of the palmar area often is difficult to obtain. The skin flaps are devitalized by loss of subcutaneous fat and operative dissection. Frequently the avascularity of the flaps reduces them almost to the status of free grafts. Such areas of skin, if they are in poor condition to begin with, are much better replaced by healthy full thickness skin grafts taken from the abdominal wall. Drainage of the wound for 24 hours is usually advisable lest a hematoma under skin flap or graft vitiate the benefits of the operation. Gentle and diffuse pressure should be maintained on the palmar surface for 1 to 2 weeks. Immobilization of the hand and metacarpophalangeal joints to promote healing of the palmar wound, coincident with free interphalan-

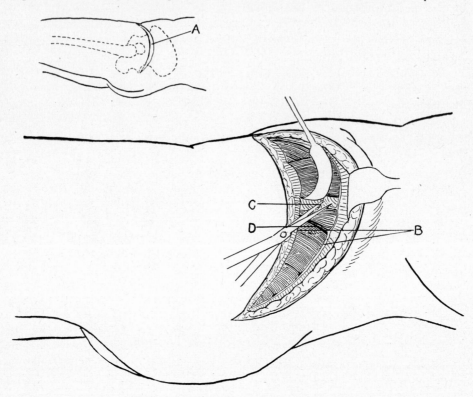

FIG. 470. Gluteal fasciotomy. A. Skin incision. B. Divided fascia, exposing from top to bottom the sartorius, tensor fascia femoris, gluteus medius and gluteus maximus. C. Division of the deep layer of the fascial envelop enclosing the tensor, which, along with all intermuscular septa, must be transected. D. Penetrating intermuscular septum. Some of these structures are visible and others require identification by palpation.

geal motion to prevent adherence of the tendons should be maintained until healing takes place.

THE LOW BACK REGION

Gluteal Fasciotomy. Unilateral fasciotomy is carried out with the patient postured on the unaffected side. Bilateral procedures are done with the patient supine and a small flat sand bag under the buttocks. Local anesthesia presents definite advantages in making possible a subjective localization of the painful areas by the patient. The skin incision extends obliquely backward from a point just distal to the anterior-superior spine to pass midway between the tip of the greater trochanter and the iliac crest and terminate close to the midpoint of the sacro-iliac joint of the same side. This incision is developed down to fascia lata and hemostasis secured. The presenting surface of the fascia is then divided. Excess tension may be evident at this point. Often the cut edges of the fascia snap apart and separate for a distance of an inch or more, and, at times, instantaneous relief from pain is appreciated by the patient. However, one should not be satisfied to stop at this point. Release of tension in the presenting surface of the fascia augments the existing strain upon the remaining intact intermuscular septae and unless they also are divided symptoms may return. Each penetrating septum as well as the deep fascial encasements of the tensor and sartorius muscles must be divided (Fig. 470). Localization is accomplished with a palpating finger and as each tense band is sectioned the exploring finger precedes the scalpel, pushing muscle tissue away from the structures to be divided and feeling for additional tight bands. No attempt should be made to suture the divided fascia. After complete hemostasis has been obtained the subcutaneous tissues and skin are closed with interrupted fine sutures. A many tailed binder applied to the pelvis for a few days following operation acts as an efficient compression dressing. Ambulation and active exercises designed to further stretch the divided fascial bands should commence following healing of the operative wound.

Iliolumbar Fasciotomy. The patient is postured in the prone position. The reduction of vital capacity caused by this position may be neutralized considerably by sand bags, placed under each shoulder and each side of the pelvis, and intratracheal anesthesia supplemented by copious quantities of oxygen. Slight hip flexion reduces the normal lumbar curve and makes more accessible the posterior iliac crests. The skin incision follows the posterior ⅓ of the iliac crest and extends to a point just distal to the posterior-superior iliac spine. This incision is deepened down to bone and the periosteum incised along the same line. The origins of the erector spinae muscles are elevated subperiosteally from the mesial aspect of the ilium until the sacrum comes into view. In a similar manner the gluteal origins are elevated from the outer surface of the bone for a distance of at least 1 inch. Whenever appreciable tension or contracture of the erector spinae is present these muscle origins should be divided transversely as far as the midline. After securing hemostasis, the superficial fascia and skin are closed with interrupted fine sutures. The use of a pelvic binder as a pressure dressing for a few days following the operation reduces the risk of hematoma formation. Ambulation should commence upon healing of the operative wound.

THE HIP REGION

Aspiration of the Trochanteric Bursa. The trochanteric bursa, located on the posterolateral aspect of the greater trochanter and the tendons of the lesser glutei and short rotators of the hip which form its floor, and the overlying tensor and gluteus maximus muscles and their associated fascial strata is subject to all the affections of other synovial structures. One of the most common affections of this bursa is characterized by pain and tenderness centered around an inflamed calcific deposit situated in the tendons forming the floor of the bursa. The general principles and technic for aspiration conform to those outlined in the discussion of calcific deposits in the shoulder tendons (see page 808). At the exact center of tenderness a large bore needle is inserted through the skin and deeper tissues until the bone is reached. It is then withdrawn a few millimeters and the aspiration carried out. If localization of the center of tenderness has been accurate the point of

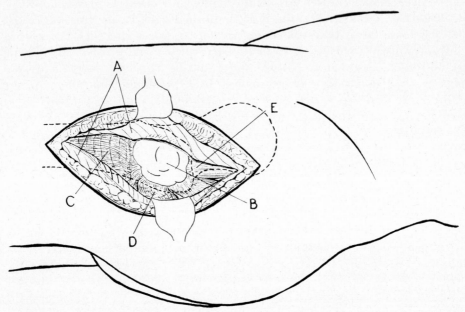

Fig. 471. Exposure of the subtrochanteric bursa. A. Incision through the fascia lata. B. Subtrochanteric bursa. C. Vastus externus. D. External rotator muscles of the hip. E. Gluteus medius.

the needle should be within the tendon cavity containing the calcific material, some of which may be withdrawn into the syringe. If it has not been accurate, or if the patient has moved the leg during the aspiration so that the position of the lesion changed in relation to the point of aspiration it may be necessary to infiltrate the whole area with procaine hydrochloride and probe in various directions with the aspirating needle before the deposit is encountered. Local heat and rest may be required for a short time following the aspiration. If the procedure has been technically adequate, *i.e.,* if some of the irritant material has been recovered, the symptoms may be expected to disappear within 6 to 12 hours.

Incision and Excision of the Trochanteric Bursa. A longitudinal incision is made distalward for a distance of 3 inches from the palpable tip of the greater trochanter. The fascia lata is incised between the posterior border of the tensor fascia femoris and the gluteus maximus. A portion of the uppermost insertion of the latter muscle usually requires incision

before an adequate exposure of the bursal region is obtained. The bursa
is encountered directly under the fascial structures on the lateral aspect of
the most prominent portion of the trochanter (Fig. 471). Localized suppurative lesions warrant a wide incision of the bursa. The wound should be
packed open loosely and allowed to fill in by granulations. Chronic suppurative lesions characterized by fibrosis and thickening of the bursal wall
constitute an indication for complete excision of the bursa. All infected
tissues should be removed including not only the bursa but also any areas
of infected tendon or bone in the bursal floor. The wound should be packed
open loosely and allowed to granulate. After a healthy bed of granulation
tissue has become established rehabilitation may be hastened by the application of skin grafts to the granulating surface.

Snapping Hip. This condition may result from several causes. Exploration of all cases in which the etiology is doubtful therefore should be carried out under local anesthesia. In this way the snapping incidents may be
reproduced by the patient and the true pathologic anatomy identified by
the surgeon at operation, with a certainty that is not always possible under
general anesthesia.

A skin incision similar to that for exposure of the trochanteric bursa
(Fig. 471), but extending for a distance of 2 to 3 inches along the posterior
border of the tensor fascia femoris proximal to the tip of the greater trochanter, is made and deepened to the fascia lata. The skin edges then should
be retracted and the fatty tissues cleared away from the surface of the fascia.
The hip then is moved about prior to incision of the fascia which not uncommonly is the offending agent in the production of the snapping incidents. When a portion of the fascia appears to snap across the trochanter
a simple fasciotomy of the offending area often relieves the condition completely. When the supero-anterior edge of the gluteus maximus is seen to
snap across the trochanter the involved portion of the muscle insertion
should be separated from its fascial attachments as extensively as is necessary to eliminate the snapping, and sutured directly to the bone. When the
posterior border of the tensor fascia femoris is seen to produce the snapping
a releasing incision through its posterior fascial attachments often will produce relief. If the snapping persists after division of these fascial structures
the iliotibial band may be divided just distal to the muscle belly, the distal
portion of the muscle mobilized and transposed to a more anterior point
of insertion where it is sutured firmly to the fascia lata of the anterior thigh
region. Occasionally the tendon of the gluteus medius is seen to snap over
the proximal extremity of the greater trochanter on motion of the hip.
When this condition is encountered the hypermobile portion of gluteus
tendon may be sutured directly to the trochanter over an area sufficient to
obliterate the snapping incidents. Occasionally the mechanical irritation
produced by constantly repeated snapping incidents results in the formation of a thickened and inflamed bursa. Such a structure always should be
excised coincidentally with its cause. The wound is closed in layers with
interrupted sutures. Early motion and a resumption of normal activities

should be encouraged as soon as the wound is healed. Providing the true cause of the snapping has been identified and eradicated the results are uniformly excellent.

THE KNEE REGION

Aspiration of Prepatellar Bursa. This procedure may be carried out easily due to the subcutaneous situation of the bursa. Strict aseptic technic should be followed since the prepatellar is second only to the olecranon bursa in the ease with which organisms introduced by needle or scalpel may produce an established infection. When a diagnostic aspiration is carried out in a case suspected of bursal infection great care should be taken to make sure that the aspirating needle does not slip over the edge of the patella where deeper penetration may introduce organisms into the joint cavity. In most suppurative lesions of this bursa a coincident joint effusion is present. Such an effusion is secondary to the neighboring extra-articular inflammatory process but does not necessarily indicate the presence of a suppurative arthritis. Such a joint never should be aspirated through the inflamed tissues surrounding an infected bursa until the presence of intra-articular infection has been established beyond doubt. Acute trauma to the patellar region may produce a prepatellar bursitis due to hemorrhage into the bursal cavity. In such a case prompt aspiration followed by a compression dressing and a temporary restriction of knee joint motion is indicated.

Incision of the Prepatellar Bursa. This procedure should be carried out promptly as soon as the presence of localized suppuration becomes apparent. Rest, elevation, and local heat to the region should be prescribed until the infection localizes and incision should not be done during the cellulitic or spreading stage of the infection. A transverse incision sufficient to open the bursal cavity from side-to-side gives adequate drainage and the optimum cosmetic result (Fig. 472). The bursal cavity should be packed open loosely and allowed to fill in by granulation tissues. Following drainage for an acute infection the leg should be immobilized in extension and moist local heat applied frequently to the operative area until the infectious process is brought under control. Once a healthy granulating surface becomes established wound healing and rehabilitation of the patient may be greatly hastened by the application of skin grafts.

Excision of the Prepatellar Bursa. A transverse, slightly curved incision (Fig. 472) gives adequate exposure and the optimum cosmetic result. The bursa is encountered directly under the skin and may be excised by a combination of sharp and blunt dissection. If the lesion requiring bursectomy is uninfected, no attempt should be made to remove any of the bursal floor. If the operation is done for a chronic suppurative lesion a complete removal of all infected tissues, including not only the bursa but also the underlying quadriceps fibers or patella, if they are involved in the infectious process, should be carried out. In chronic suppurative lesions the incision should be placed to include and excise existing sinus openings through the skin. Uninfected cases may be closed and allowed early mobilization of the ex-

tremity but infected lesions should have temporary rest and elevation until
the open wound fills in by secondary intent.

Excision of Cystic Lesions from the Popliteal Region. Cystic lesions
of the popliteal region may be enlarged bursae, ganglion like structures
arising from connective tissue origins or herniations of the synovial lining
of the knee joint capsule. The position of such a lesion as evidenced by the

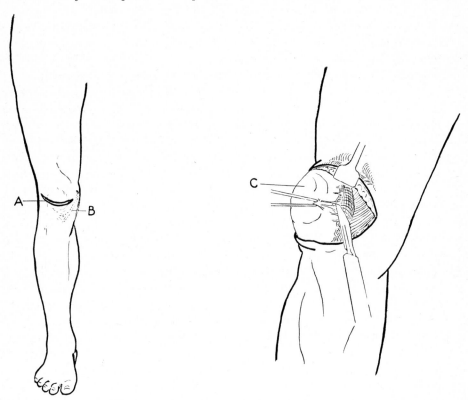

FIG. 472. Excision of the prepatellar bursa. A. Skin incision. B. Infrapatellar branch
of the saphenous nerve which is to be avoided. C. Removal of the bursal walls by sharp
dissection.

location of its presenting portion on clinical examination may be a considerable distance from its point of origin. For this reason an adequate exposure
of the popliteal region always must be available.

A vertical incision across the flexion crease of the knee never should be
made if it can be avoided. For adequate exposure of the popliteal area and
an optimum cosmetic result a step cut incision (Fig. 473) should be made.
The contralateral vertical limbs of this incision may be varied according to
the position of the lesion to be removed. The skin flaps are elevated at the
level of the superficial fascia and the popliteal structures exposed (Fig. 473).
In the presence of a large lesion the anatomical relationships and location
of the normal structures may be considerably distorted. The cyst wall is separated from its surrounding structures by a combination of blunt and sharp

dissection and if rupture of the cyst can be prevented this dissection is facilitated. By severance of all the areolar attachments of the cyst wall and retrac-

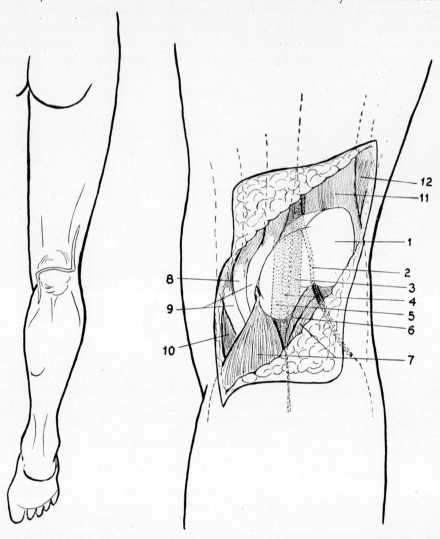

FIG. 473. Exposure of the popliteal structures for the removal of a cyst. *Left:* A step-cut incision gives an excellent exposure and avoids the risk of contractures common to vertical incisions across the flexion crease. *Right:* The skin flaps are reflected at the level of the fascia and the popliteal structures exposed. 1. The cyst. 2. Common peroneal nerve. 3. Tibial nerve. 4. Popliteal vein. 5. Popliteal artery. 6. Plantaris muscle. 7. Gastrocnemius. 8. Semitendinosus. 9. Semimembranosus. 10. Gracilis. 11. Biceps, long head. 12. Biceps, short head.

tion of the normal structures one eventually encounters the point of origin of the lesion. When the cyst arises from a connective tissue base it is likely to be a ganglion and an area of the connective tissue surrounding its point of origin should be removed along with the tumor. Frequently a communication with the joint cavity becomes apparent as the dissection is terminated. All such communications should be divided flush with the knee joint capsule and the residual opening closed tightly enough to prevent joint fluid leakage (Fig. 474). Otherwise a joint fluid sinus rapidly may become established and result in a fluid collection in the operative area equivalent in effect to

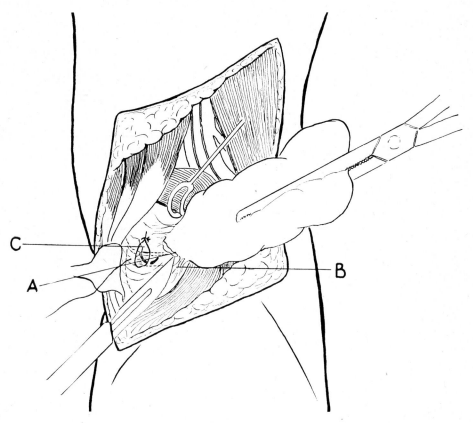

Fig. 474. Removal of a popliteal cyst. The tumor is dissected free from its surrounding structures by sharp dissection. A. Its point of origin is identified and divided, flush with the connective tissue from which it arose. B. All connections with the point of origin should be divided and a portion of the connective tissue surrounding the base of the tumor should be removed. C. Any communication with the knee joint cavity should be obliterated by suture.

the original condition. When such an accumulation of joint fluid does occur following operation, prompt aspiration followed by immobilization of the extended leg with a gentle pressure dressing against the popliteal area is indicated until wound healing occurs. Persistent reaccumulations of fluid may require that the operative area be reopened and the joint aperture adequately closed by suture. Unless the postoperative course is complicated by such a complication mobilization of the knee and gradual resumption of activities may be allowed as soon as the wound is healed.

Repair of Ruptured Quadriceps or Patellar Tendon. An excellent exposure of the whole anterior knee region may be obtained through a median parapatellar incision extending from a point 6 inches proximal to the patella to the tibial tuberosity (Fig. 475). The proximal or distal extent of such an incision is varied according to the level of the pathology to be

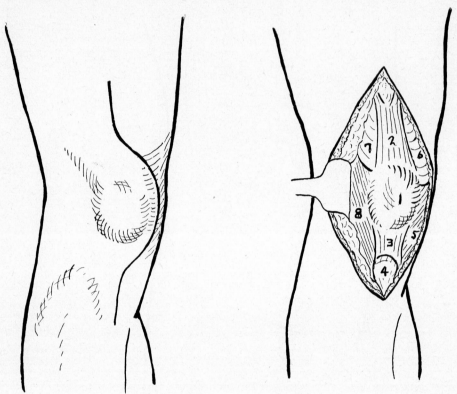

Fig. 475. Exposure of the anterior knee region through a median parapatellar incision. *Left:* The skin incision, extending from the tibial tuberosity to a point 6 inches proximal to the patella. *Right:* The skin flap is reflected at the level of the fascia to expose the anterior structures of the knee. 1. Patella. 2. Quadriceps tendon. 3. Infrapatellar tendon. 4. Tibial tuberosity. 5. Expansion of vastus medialis. 6. Vastus medialis. 7. Vastus lateralis. 8. Expansion of vastus lateralis.

exposed and the working room required. After deepening the incision through superficial fascia the entire flap is undermined and retracted laterally (Fig. 475).

Incised wounds of either tendon may be repaired by end-to-end suture if the operation is carried out before retraction of the proximal fragment and contracture of the quadriceps muscles becomes established. Multiple small mattress sutures produce a more secure repair than a few heavy sutures under tension.

Ruptures through these tendons present a somewhat different problem. A rupture invariably takes place through an area of degenerated tendon tissue so that the ends of each tendon fragment are fibrotic and devitalized from the start. Some of this devitalized tissue must be excised from each fragment before healthy tissues can be made available for repair. Following such an excision it is only with some difficulty that the tendon ends can be approximated or held in apposition against the strong pull of the quadriceps

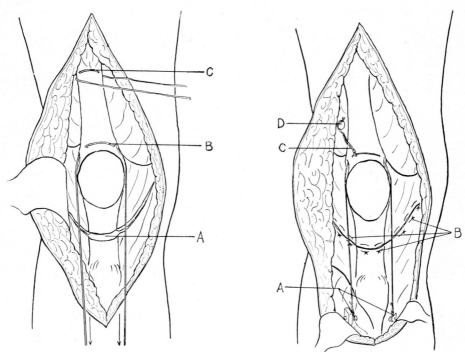

Fig. 476. Repair of ruptured infrapatellar tendon by removable suture. *Left:* Exposure by a median parapatellar incision. A. Rupture through infrapatellar tendon. The devitalized edges of the tear have been excised and the fragments are held in apposition by traction on, B. the main traction suture. C. Placement of main suture in ruptures through the quadriceps tendon and for neutralizing muscle pull following surgical removal of the patella. *Right:* A. A bolt is passed through the tibial crest at the level of the tubercle. An ordinary bone screw, cut off lateral to the nut at the desired length, may be used. The ends of the main suture are wound around either end of the bolt. B. Exact apposition of the tendon ends is insured by a few fine silk sutures. C. A removing wire is attached to the main suture. D. A split lead shot is clamped to the end of the removing wire. This remains palpable through the skin after wound closure.

muscles. Occasionally, especially in long standing cases, the gap between the tendon ends cannot be obliterated by ordinary methods and various forms of grafting procedures or a bridging of the defect by autogenous tendon or fascial materials (Fig. 450) may be required.

Utilization of the removable suture principle has greatly facilitated the surgical management of such tendon lesions. Following exposure of the pathology and excision of the devitalized periphery of the tendon defect a bolt is passed through the crest of the tibia in the region of the tibial tubercle (Fig. 476). If the infrapatellar tendon is ruptured, a heavy wire suture is placed mattress fashion through the quadriceps tendon just proximal to the patella. If the quadriceps tendon is the site of rupture, or if the patella has been removed surgically, the transverse portion of the mattress suture is placed through the quadriceps tendon as far proximal to the site of pathology as possible. The ends of the suture are then pulled distalward until retraction of the proximal fragment has been overcome and the separated tendon ends once again come into apposition with each other. With the knee extended the ends of the suture are pulled tight and then wound around either end of the tibial bolt. All strain is thereby removed from the site of rupture and taken up by the traction suture which extends from healthy tendon proximal to the site of rupture to tibia, bridging the area where repair is to be carried out. Fixation of the tendon ends in apposition is insured by a few fine silk sutures. A removing wire is wound around the transverse portion of the main suture and left projecting about ½ an inch into the subcutaneous fat. For purposes of future localization it is advisable to clamp a small split lead shot to the end of this wire. Such a shot is easily palpable through the skin after the wound has been closed over it and proves of considerable aid in localizing the removing wire when the time for removal arrives. The operative wound is closed in layers, and after it has healed the extended leg is immobilized in a circular plaster encasement from groin to ankle.

The patient is then allowed to walk on the extremity during the period necessary for healing of the repair.

After two months he is readmitted to the hospital, the plaster encasement removed and the skin of the leg cleansed and prepared as for an operative procedure. Using local anesthesia three 1 cm. incisions are made, one over the palpable lead shot attached to the end of the removing wire and one over each palpable subcutaneous end of the bolt. Through the latter incisions the ends of the traction suture are unwound from the bolt or divided with wire cutters. The nut is grasped with a hemostat, a screw driver inserted into the opposite incision and the apparatus dismantled and removed. The lead shot is then located, the end of the removing wire grasped with a clamp through the remaining incision and the main suture removed from the leg. The results are uniformly excellent. The disability period is reduced to a minimum by the maintenance of active function of the leg muscles during almost the whole healing period.

Snapping Knee. This condition usually results from some instability of the biceps tendon. Snapping incidents resulting from a lateral meniscus lesion or from some abnormal instability of the femur on the tibia should be excluded. There may be an exostosis on the fibular head over which the biceps tendon snaps on motion of the knee. Occasionally the tendon may snap over a normal fibular head in a similar manner.

A skin incision is made over the distal 3 inches of the biceps tendon and carried downward to the level of the neck of the fibula. This is deepened with care until the peroneal nerve is identified and protected from unintentional operative trauma. The snapping incidents then may be reproduced under direct vision by motion of the knee. If a slipping biceps tendon is seen to be the offending agent, it is first mobilized and then sutured directly to the fibular head up to a point proximal to that where the slipping incidents occur. If there is an exostosis at the fibular head, it should be removed completely along with a generous portion of its bony base. The wound is closed in layers with interrupted sutures. Ambulation with aid of crutches may be commenced as soon as the wound is healed. Some protection by cane or crutches for a period of several weeks is advisable following attachment of the biceps tendon to the fibula lest a sudden unexpected flexion of the knee disrupt the repair.

THE LEG

Fasciotomy for Threatened Volkmann's of the Calf. This condition may occur in the lower as well as the upper extremity. The basic causes of this condition and the principles of therapy are identical in both locations. When deflation of subfascial tension in the calf is required a postero-medial incision is made over the middle ⅔ of the lower leg. The fascia is incised in such a way as to open completely the space between the gastrocnemius and soleus muscle bellies. If the medial origin of the soleus then is detached from the tibia, the subsoleus space which contains the large vessels and is the most important site of tension, can be opened and deflated. Additional fascial incisions are, at times, necessary in the posterior midline. All blood clot is evacuated from the subfascial spaces. If the posterior tibial nerve has been divided, it is repaired and if the major vessels are ruptured, they must be caught and ligated. When the posterior tibial artery has been divided localization of the bleeding end of the vessel may be extremely difficult due to uncontrollable hemorrhage. Under such circumstances it is advisable to detach the soleus origin from the postero-medial crest of the tibia, and control the intact artery at this level before attending to the more distal pathology.

THE ANKLE AND FOOT

Bunion. The inflamed adventitious bursa situated medial to the exostosis on the head of the first metatarsal in certain hallux valgus lesions may become the seat of a chronic infection with or without sinus formation. When conservative measures fail to control the process, excision of the bursa usually is necessary. The skin incision should include and remove any existing sinus opening. The bursa is encountered directly beneath the skin and is removed completely by sharp dissection. This bursa is most frequently removed in the course of an operation for the correction of the associated hallux valgus.

Retroachillis Bursa. This bursa is seldom encountered except in an inflamed condition resulting from excess pressure on the back of the heel by a tight shoe. It is easily accessible and may be completely removed when conservative measures fail to relieve the symptoms. A midline incision over the back of the heel is to be avoided since it leaves a scar that is exposed to shoe pressure. An incision along either margin of the tendo achillis, curving slightly toward the midline in its proximal portion where it is above the level of shoe pressure (Fig. 477), gives an excellent exposure. Ambulation may commence when the wound is healed.

Achilles Bursa. This bursa rests between the superior surface of the calcaneal tuberosity and the deep surface of the tendo achillis. Chronic inflammation may result from mechanical irritation by an abnormally large

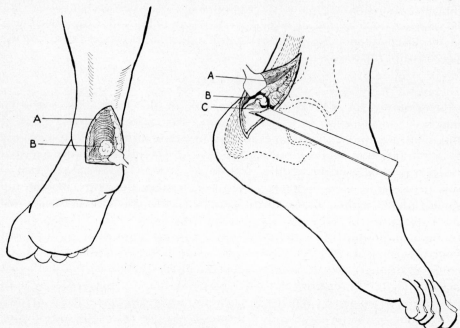

Fig. 477. *Left:* Excision of achilles bursa. A. The skin incision is curved medially to escape midline shoe pressure upon the scar. B. The achilles bursa. *Right:* Excision of the retrocalcaneal bursa. A. A lateral incision is made and the tendo achillis retracted posteriorly. B. The retrocalcaneal bursa is located between the posterosuperior corner of the os calcis and the tendo achillis. C. An enlarged calcaneal tuberosity or arthritic spur should be removed by osteotome along with the bursa.

calcaneal tuberosity or a hypertrophic spur on the tuberosity. Exposure is obtained through a 3 inch incision along the lateral margin of the achilles tendon (Fig. 477). The bursa is removed completely along with any spur or undue prominence of the tuberosity. Ambulation may commence when the wound is healed.

Tailor's Bunion. This lesion is an adventitious bursa which forms between the skin and the external malleolus as the result of chronic mechanical irritation of the region. The condition usually is encountered in its chronic stage and when removal of the cause cannot be accomplished or fails to arrest the condition excision should be done. An incision over the prominence formed by the swollen bursa provides adequate exposure for complete removal of the lesion.

Calcaneal Bursa. Inflammation in this bursa commonly has been associated with some remote infectious process and the formation of hypertrophic spurs projecting downward from the anterior plantar ridge of the calcaneus. An incision 2 to 3 inches long is made along the medial aspect of the heel parallel to the plantar surface. This incision is deepened to bone and the calcaneal ridge from which the plantar muscles and fascia take origin is identified and cleared of soft tissue. The fascial origin is divided and the inflamed bursa located and removed. All spurs or irregularities of the bone are removed by osteotome or rongeur. The wound is closed loosely with fine interrupted sutures and a gentle pressure dressing applied to the plantar surface of the heel. Following wound healing the patient may resume weight bearing and normal activities as rapidly as symptoms permit.

Plantar Fasciotomy. The origins of the plantar muscles and fascia are exposed by the same operative approach as described above under calcaneal bursae. The fascial origin is identified and severed across the full width of the calcaneal ridge. Fascia and muscles are then elevated subperiosteally from the plantar surface of the calcaneus for at least an inch anterior to the ridge. The wound is closed loosely with interrupted sutures and a plantar pressure dressing applied to the area. Following wound healing ambulation is allowed and further stretching of the divided fascial structures is aided by the institution of a program of active exercises.

Slipping Peroneal Tendons. Chronic habitual luxation of the peroneal tendons from their fibular grooves is best treated by operation. Exposure is obtained through a 3 inch incision a little posterior and parallel to the lateral malleolus. The fibrous sheath overlying the tendons is separated along its anterior margin and the tendons retracted forward from their bony grooves. The latter are then deepened with a gouge or curet. The tendons are then replaced in the deepened grooves and their fibrous sheath reattached to the fibula. When stabilization by this technic does not appear to be adequate it may be reinforced by a fascial sling. The fascia is obtained from the thigh (Fig. 446), fashioned as a sling around the peroneal tendons and sutured to the posterior tissues in such a way that anterior excursion of the tendons on dorsiflexion or eversion of the foot is prevented. Gentle, progressive active motion of the foot may be commenced when the wound is healed but unprotected weight bearing should not be allowed for several weeks following repair.

Repair of Ruptured Tendo Achillis. Incised wounds of this tendon are amenable to early repair by multiple fine sutures, with or without reinforcement by autogenous sutures of fascia or tendon (Fig. 450). Ruptures invariably take place through degenerated tendon tissue, some of which must be excised from the end of each tendon fragment before healthy tissues can be made available for approximation. Utilization of the removable suture principle for the repair of these lesions provides the most rapid and best results.

A 10 inch posterior midline incision is made over the tendo achillis. The distal 2 inches of this incision are curved toward the lateral aspect of the os calcis to avoid subsequent shoe pressure upon a midline scar (Fig. 478). The ruptured tendon is exposed over its whole length and the lateral surface of os calcis bared with a periosteal elevator. The devitalized tendon ends are excised. A heavy mattress suture of wire is placed through normal tissues at the musculo tendinous junction (Fig. 478), far proximal to the usual site

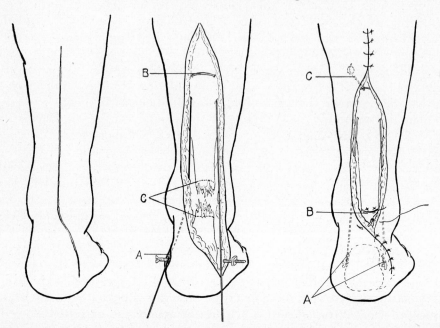

Fig. 478. Repair of ruptured tendo achillis by removable suture. *Left:* A midline incision is made which curves laterally in its distal portion to avoid shoe pressure upon the scar. *Middle:* The ruptured tendon and the lateral aspect of the os calcis are exposed. A. A small incision is made over the medial aspect of the heel. Entering this incision a bolt is passed through the os calcis to emerge in the lateral wound. B. A heavy wire suture is passed through the musculo tendinous junction and its medial end brought through subcutaneous tissues to emerge at A. C. Line of excision of devitalized tendon ends. *Right:* Traction, sufficient to produce apposition of the tendon ends, is applied to the main suture. A. The ends of the suture are wound around either end of the bolt which has been cut off short enough to allow of skin closure over both ends. B. Continued apposition of the tendon ends is insured by a few fine sutures. C. A removing wire, with a split lead shot clamped to its end is attached to the proximal end of the main suture. The skin is closed over this wire but the lead shot remains palpable so that subsequent localization is simplified.

or rupture. A 1 centimeter incision is then made over the medial surface of the os calcis. Through this a drill, and then a bolt is passed through the bone to emerge in the depths of the lateral wound. The medial limb of the main wire suture is then passed through the subcutaneous tissues and brought out through the small medial stab wound. Manual traction is made on both ends of the main suture until the retraction of the proximal fragment has been overcome and the tendon ends lie loosely apposed to each other. The ends of the suture then are wound around the bolt, fixing the proximal

fragment in the corrected position and the tendon ends held in exact apposition by a few fine silk sutures. A removing wire with a small lead shot
clamped to its end is fastened to the proximal transverse portion of the main
suture and the lead shot buried in subcutaneous tissues. The operative
wounds are closed. Both the lead shot on the removing wire and the subcutaneous ends of the bolt are easily palpable.

When the wound is healed a snug fitting plaster boot is applied to the
knee and a walking iron incorporated into it. Unrestricted knee motion is
allowed and the patient is discharged walking. Ambulation is not only allowed but insisted upon during the healing period in order to minimize the
penalties of disuse.

The patient is readmitted after 6 weeks, the plaster removed and the
leg cleansed and prepared as for operation. A 1 centimeter incision is made
over each end of the bolt and over the lead shot, using local anesthesia. Bolt
and suture are removed from the leg in a manner similar to that described
under ruptures of the quadriceps and patellar tendons. The results are
uniformly excellent.

21

THE BLOOD VESSELS

Daniel Elkin, M.D. and Michael E. DeBakey, M.D.

ACUTE VASCULAR INJURIES

Michael E. DeBakey, M.D.

Acute or fresh injuries of major arteries, because they literally threaten both life and limb, have always constituted a serious problem in the surgical management of traumatic conditions. Despite the constant and tireless efforts of numerous investigators and the extensive experience provided by both World Wars, a completely satisfactory solution to this problem has yet to be evolved. Obviously, and this has long been recognized, ideal therapy has as its objective preservation or restitution of vascular function. Unfortunately, as pointed out in a previous consideration of this subject,[5] this desideratum can be attained in only a limited number of cases, for certain definite reasons. Essentially, these reasons may be divided into two categories: (1) those in which the factors are of such vital significance that they seal the fate of the part regardless of any form of therapy; and (2) those which jeopardize the effects of ideal therapy or preclude its institution. These factors are; time-lag, practical technical considerations, the presence of associated injuries, the site of injury, the type of arterial lesion, and the possible occurrence of infection.

The significance of the time-lag, *i.e.,* the time elapsing between wounding and institution of therapy, is obvious. Once this period exceeds the generally accepted limit of 6 to 8 hours, it is doubtful that reparative surgical therapy can influence the end result. The factor of associated injuries, whether they are local or remote, is also of considerable importance. Local wounds, depending upon their extent, may further impair or even completely destroy the regional circulation. More remote wounds may require attention far more urgently, as a lifesaving matter, than does the vascular wound.

Perhaps the most important factors determining end results are the site and type of the arterial lesion. Wounds of certain vessels, such as the popliteal artery, are far more serious than wounds of other vessels, such as the brachial artery. Wounds above the profunda branch in both the femoral and brachial arteries are more likely to be followed by ischemic gangrene than wounds of these vessels below this branch. Accordingly, certain vessels have come to be regarded as critical and others as noncritical, and restorative surgical procedures obviously assume greater importance in the former category of vessels than in the latter. The type of injury (laceration of the vessel, partial or complete severance, contusion and thrombosis, acute spasm, or false aneurysm) also influences the outcome. A small, cleanly incised longitudinal wound, or even an incised transverse wound, may be repaired with greater chances of success than a lacerated wound in which there is much loss of substance.

In vascular injuries, therefore, the circumstances and character of the injury often determine the therapeutic procedure and consequently predetermine the end result. Under certain conditions the only procedure applicable is ligation; it must be done for the basic purpose of controlling hemorrhage. Under other conditions some type of reparative procedure may be employed; since this constitutes ideal therapy, every effort should be made to apply it.

Supplemental Therapeutic Measures. All the established principles of good wound surgery, such as proper resuscitation of the patient and thorough débridement, are essential to the successful management of acute vascular injuries. These principles are discussed elsewhere and require no further elaboration here. There are, however, certain supplemental therapeutic measures that deserve consideration, including blood transfusion, sympathetic block or sympathectomy, anticoagulant therapy, and posture.

The extent of blood loss in acute vascular injuries is often considerable. As a consequence of the reduction in the volume of the circulating blood, the amount of blood flow through the peripheral arteries is also reduced, and the circulation of the part distal to the vascular injury is even further impaired. For these reasons, prompt restoration of the circulating blood volume and of the hemoglobin concentration assumes particular importance.

Vasospasm is a natural response to those forms of trauma which directly or indirectly affect vascular structures.[4] Its extent and degree vary considerably. It may range from localized constriction, with consequent minimal ischemia, to a more extensive and generalized involvement, especially of the collateral circulation, with consequent ischemia of a degree sufficient to produce actual gangrene. Rational therapy in such cases is based upon an attempt to counteract vasospasm and to produce maximum vasodilatation in the involved extremity. Since the disturbance is apparently due to a vasomotor reflex initiated in the traumatized tissues, and since vasoconstrictor impulses are transmitted by way of the sympathetic nerve fibers, interruption of these impulses prevents vasospasm and permits vasodilatation. Vasodilatation may be achieved by débridement of surrounding traumatized tissue, by periarterial stripping of the involved area, by procaine hydrochloride block of the regional sympathetic ganglia, or by sympathectomy. Sympathetic block or sympathectomy, which is probably the most effective method of producing maximum vasodilatation in these cases, should be employed in all types of peripheral vascular injuries accompanied by manifestations of vasospasm. It may be necessary to repeat the block at least once or twice daily for several days. Body warmth is carefully maintained but heat should not be applied to the involved part. As elevation of the part may accentuate ischemia, the extremity should be maintained at heart level, or preferably in a slightly dependent position.

On a theoretical basis, as well as on the basis of experimental and clinical investigations, the use of anticoagulants (heparin and dicoumarol) would appear to be a valuable adjunct in vascular surgery.[20,21] By this means the extension of thrombosis in the peripheral collateral tributaries or the occurrence of thrombosis after operation at the site of repair, which so often spells failure, can be better controlled. It should be realized, however, that anticoagulant therapy is not without danger, especially in the presence of extensive injury. The method requires careful observation and adequate laboratory checks. Clinically, the exact field of usefulness of anticoagulant therapy in acute vascular injuries has not been defined and must await further experience. That it is not essential to successful repair in certain forms of vascular injury is well known. Perhaps it will be found most useful in cases which require bridging of the arterial gap.

Surgical Therapy. LIGATION. In cases in which ligation is promptly indicated, as in wounds of the smaller noncritical vessels or because of the type and character of the injury, it should be done not by ligation in continuity but by placing nonabsorbable ligatures well above and below the site of injury, with excision of the intervening damaged segment in order to eliminate the dangers of secondary hemorrhage, thrombosis, and vasoconstrictor influences. Although it may be theoretically desirable to ligate at such a level as to avoid the creation of a blind pouch,[10,14] the deliberate effort to do so frequently involves extensive dissection and may still further jeopardize the circulation of the injured limb. If the concomitant vein is also injured, it should be similarly ligated; however, if undamaged it should not be disturbed.

SUTURE REPAIR. As has been indicated, the ideal objective in the therapy of vascular injuries is the restoration of the flow of blood through the original channel. This may be achieved, depending upon the character and extent of the injury, by suture repair, end-to-end anastomosis, or vein grafts and prosthetic tubes. The fundamental principles underlying all of these methods of vascular repair have long been well known. They have remained essentially unchanged, except possibly for certain refinements in suture material or in prosthetic devices, since the time of their establishment through the research efforts of numerous investigators, including, particularly, the work of Glück,[7] Jassinowsky,[12] Murphy,[19] Jaboulay and Briau,[11] Dörfler,[6] Payr,[23] Höpfner,[9] Matas,[15,17] Carrel and Guthrie,[2,3,8] and Moure.[18] The reader will find an excellent historical résumé of this phase of the subject in Matas' publications.[15,17]

Suture repair of arterial injuries is particularly indicated in relatively small longitudinal or oblique wounds or in incomplete transections, especially of the larger arteries, such as the carotid, popliteal, common femoral, subclavian and axillary arteries. In complete or incomplete transections in which there is much loss of substance, end-to-end anastomosis should be done unless the defect is so great as to preclude approximation and some means of bridging the defect must be employed.

The essential principles of the suture method of vascular repair are: (1) provisional hemostasis; (2) the use of fine needles and silk; (3) accurate approximation of the intima; and (4) gentle handling of tissues. After the injured vessel is exposed and isolated, provisional hemostasis is obtained by applying small rubber-shod spring artery clamps or by clamping soft rubber tubes snugly against the vessel above and below the site of the wound. All traumatized tissue and blood clots are removed, and ragged tissue and overhanging adventitia are excised, to provide clean smooth wound edges. This should be done with considerable care and gentleness to minimize contusion or other injury to the endothelial edges of the wound. The cleansing of the wound and of the lumen of the vessel is facilitated by use of a stream of normal saline solution or of a 1:1,000 solution of heparin in normal saline solution. Periodic irrigation of the structures throughout the operation is also desirable, to prevent drying of the tissues. Traction or guy sutures are placed at each end of the wound, penetrating all layers of the vessels, to facilitate apposition of the endothelial surfaces and the performance of the suture repair (Fig. 479a). The suture material should be of fine silk (00000 or 000000) directly attached to a fine curved needle. This type of atraumatic arterial suture is available commercially in sealed tubes containing liquid petrolatum.

Various methods of applying the suture to approximate the wound edges have been employed, including single interrupted sutures, interrupted mattress sutures, a continuous over-and-over suture (Fig. 479b), or a continuous mattress suture (Fig. 479c). The continuous over-and-over stitch is the simplest and, in general, gives as good results as any of the others. The sutures should be applied fairly close together (about 1 to 1.5 mm. apart), to prevent leakage between them. After the passage of each stitch gentle traction is applied to the thread, so as to approximate the wound edges snugly, care being taken to provide intima-to-intima contact. Following completion of the repair and removal of the hemostatic clamps above and below the artery, slight leakage at the suture line may be observed. Usually it will stop after the application of gentle pressure with moist gauze over the anastomosis. If this is not effective, it can be controlled with a reinforcing suture.

END-TO-END ANASTOMOSIS. End-to-end anastomosis is indicated in wounds that incompletely or completely transect the vessel unless the loss of substance is so great (more than 2 cm.) that the resultant defect will not permit the ends of the vessel to be brought together without too much tension on the suture line. Under these circumstances, some means of bridging the gap, such as the use of vein grafts or prosthetic tubes, will be necessary. Several methods of end-to-end anastomosis have been employed, including the suture method or the nonsuture method with extra-vasal aids or supporting appliances. The many other methods which have been devised are now only of historical interest.[15,17]

The principles of the suture method of end-to-end anastomosis, which is generally used today, are essentially those developed by Dörfler [6] and perfected by Carrel.[2,3] Following exposure and isolation of the injured vessel, provisional hemostasis is obtained by the application of artery clamps to the artery above and below the site of injury. All traumatized tissue and blood clots are removed and the overhanging adventitia is excised and stripped

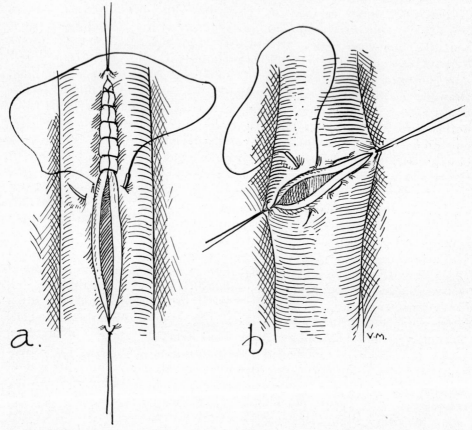

FIG. 479. Technic of suture repair of arterial wounds showing: a. continuous over-and-over type of suture, and b. continuous mattress suture.

away from the edges and the severed ends of the vessel. Irrigation with saline solution or heparin and saline solution is employed, as previously described. The cut ends of the vessel are brought in apposition and three stay sutures are introduced through all layers of the vessel at equidistant points of the circumferences and are tied, care being taken to evert the edges to provide intimal apposition (Fig. 480a). By the application of gentle traction upon these stay sutures the oval outlines of the arterial ends are converted into straight triangular surfaces (Fig. 480b). The new contour facilitates apposition of the surfaces as well as eversion of the edges of the vessel, thus greatly simplifying the performance of suture anastomosis.

Each side of the triangle is sutured consecutively, either by a continuous over-and-over stitch (Fig. 480b and c) or by a continuous mattress suture (Fig. 480d) as described above for lateral arteriorrhaphy, care being taken to provide apposition of the intima. As each segment of the angle is completed, it may be desirable to tie the running suture to the guy stitch.

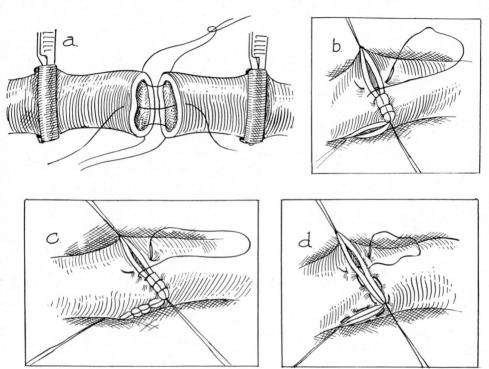

FIG. 480. Technic of end-to-end anastomosis of arteries by suture method showing: a. placement of three stay or guy sutures at equidistant points of the circumference, b. traction upon guy sutures after they have been tied converts oval outline edges of vessels into straight triangular surfaces facilitating suture, c. each side of triangle is sutured consecutively by continuous over-and-over stitch, or d. by continuous mattress suture.

End-to-end anastomosis may also be performed by the nonsuture method, by means of a supporting appliance used to provide intima-to-intima apposition. Of the various types of appliances and technics devised for this purpose the only one that has survived is the method originally developed by Payr in 1900. This method is exactly the same in principle as that recently advocated by Blakemore, Lord, and Stefko,[1] the only difference being that they used vitallium tubes instead of the magnesium alloy tubes employed by Payr. More recently, fibrin tubes have been suggested for this purpose by Swenson and Gross,[2,4] the advantage claimed by these observers being that the tube is gradually absorbed, in a matter of six or seven weeks, and the lumen at the site of the anastomosis is thus able to increase in size with the subsequent growth of the patient. Obviously, this advantage applies particularly to children.

In this method of anastomosis one end of the vessel is threaded through the tube, cuffed back, and fastened with a silk ligature over a groove or a projecting ridge in the tube. The other end of the vessel is then drawn or invaginated over the cuff and secured in position with another ligature. The anastomosis is thus completed and a continuous intimal lining is established (Fig. 481).

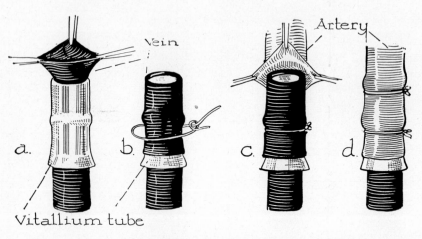

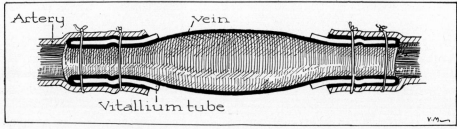

FIG. 481. Technic of end-to-end anastomosis by nonsuture method using vitallium tubes of Blakemore, Lord and Stefko.[1] This drawing shows application of this method of anastomosis for performing vein graft using two tubes but same method may be used for end-to-end anastomosis of arteries using one tube. a. Vein is threaded through tube, b. cuffed back and secured in place with a ligature, c. artery is drawn or invaginated over the cuff, and d. secured in position with two ligatures. The anastomosis thus provides a continuous intimal lining (inset).

The obvious advantages of this method of anastomosis lie in its apparent simplicity and ease of performance. On the other hand, it has certain disadvantages. 1. It utilizes an excess of vessel wall in the performance of the anastomosis and consequently would be impractical in cases in which some loss of substance has already occurred from the original injury. 2. It reduces the caliber of the lumen by the two thicknesses of the vein wall within the tube. In a recent experimental study designed to determine the relative merits of this method of anastomosis and the suture method, the conclusion was reached that in cases in which there is no tension on the suture line and no defect to be bridged, the latter method is superior to the former.[13] Perhaps the nonsuture method of anastomosis will find its greatest field of usefulness in cases in which it is necessary to bridge the defect in the artery by a vein graft.

In cases in which the injury is associated with such extensive loss of substance as to preclude end-to-end anastomosis and in which arterial ligation does not seem promptly indicated, some method of bridging the gap is desirable in order to restore continuity of the artery. This is particularly true of injuries of critical arteries such as the popliteal, common or internal carotid, common femoral, axillary, and brachial arteries. The various methods suggested and practiced for this purpose include the use of vein grafts and prosthetic tubes.[5] In the vein graft method a suitable segment of vein obtained from an accessible site is anastomosed to the proximal and distal ends of the artery by means of either the suture method or the nonsuture method (Fig. 481). In using vein grafts it is desirable to employ a segment without valves, or, if valves are present, to place the vein between the ends of the artery with the valves facing distally. Another technical consideration is that the vein segment be of the exact length required to bridge the gap, to avoid either tension or kinking.

Bridging of the arterial gap by intubation is another method which has been used to provide for temporary maintenance of the blood flow. Its objective is the maintenance of the circulation of the injured limb until more suitable conditions or facilities permit a permanent type of repair or until the collateral circulation has become established. If this objective can be achieved, an emergency procedure, which may be difficult under the happiest circumstances, is converted into an elective one, or the subsequent gradual obliterative thrombosis in the tube, with occlusion of the main vascular channel, will have a much less deleterious effect than if the process had occurred abruptly. In World War I silver tubes were used for this purpose. In World War II glass tubes as well as plastic tubes were employed.[5,22] Unless circumstances or conditions contraindicate the use of heparin, its administration is particularly desirable with this method of provisional restoration of the vascular continuity, since thrombosis, which will invariably occur, should be delayed as long as possible.

REFERENCES

1. BLAKEMORE, H. H., LORD, J. W., JR. and STEFKO, P. L.   The Severed Primary Artery in the War Wounded: A Non-suture Method of Bridging Arterial Defects, *Surgery*. 12:488-508, [Sept.], 1942; also *J.A.M.A.*, 127:685-691, 748-753, 1945.

2. CARREL, ALEXIS.   La technique opératoire des anastomoses vasculaires et de la transplantation des viscéres, *Lyon Méd.*, 93:859, 1902.

3. CARREL, ALEXIS and GUTHRIE, C. C.   Uniterminal and Biterminal Venous Transplantations, *Surg., Gynec. & Obst.*, 2:266-286, [Mar.], 1906.

4. DEBAKEY, MICHAEL.   Traumatic Vasospasm, *Bull. U. S. Army Med. Dept.*, No. 73, 23-28, [Feb.], 1944.

5. DEBAKEY, MICHAEL E. and SIMEONE, FIORINDO A.   Battle Injuries of the Arteries in World War II. An Analysis of 2,471 Cases, *Ann. Surg.*, 123:534-579, [Apr.], 1946.

6. DÖRFLER, JULIUS.   Ueber arteriennaht, *Beitr. zur. klin. Chir.*, 25:781-824, 1899.

7. Glück, Th. Ueber Zwei Fälle von Aortenaneurysmen nebst Bemerkungen über die Naht der Blutgefässe, *Arch. f. klin. Chir.*, 28:548-561, 1883.

8. Guthrie, C. C. *Blood-vessel Surgery and its Applications* (International Monographs), Arnold, London, 1912.

9. Höpfner, Edmund. Ueber Gefässnaht. Gefässtransplantationen und Replantation von amputirten Extremitäten, *Arch. f. klin Chir.*, 70:417-471, 1903.

10. Holman, Emile. Further Observations on Surgery of the Large Arteries, *Surg., Gynec. & Obst.*, 78:275-287, [Mar.], 1944.

11. Jaboulay and Briau, E. Recherches expérimentales sur la suture et la greffe artérielle, *Lyon Méd.*, 81:97, 1896.

12. Jassinowsky, Alexander. Em Beitrag zur Lehre von der Gefässnaht, *Arch. f. klin. Chir.* 42:816-841, 1891.

13. Johns, Thomas N. A Comparison of Suture and Nonsuture Methods for the Anastomosis of Veins, *Surg., Gynec. & Obst.*, 84:939-942, [May], 1947.

14. Leriche, R. and Policard, A. Ligation of Brachial Artery, *Lyon Chir.*, 17:250, 1920; *J.A.M.A.*, 75:639, 1920.

15. Matas, Rudolph. *The Suture in the Surgery of the Vascular System*, The Brown Printing Company, Montgomery, Ala., 1906.

16. Matas, Rudolph. Surgery of the Vascular System, in Keen, W. W. *Surgery: Its Principles and Practice, by Various Authors*, 5:17-350, W. B. Saunders Company, Philadelphia and London, 1921.

17. Matas, Rudolph. Military Surgery of the Vascular System, in Keen, W. W. *Surgery: Its Principles and Practice, by Various Authors*, 7:713-819, W. B. Saunders Company, Philadelphia and London, 1921.

18. Moure, Paul. *Les Greffes Vasculaires et particuliérement leurs applications chirurgicales au rétablissement de la continuité des vaisseaux et des conduits musculomembraneaux*, Octave Doin et Fils, Paris, 1914.

19. Murphy, J. B. Resection of Arteries and Veins Injured in Continuity—End-to-end Suture—Experimental and Clinical Research, *Med. Rec.*, 51:73-88, [Jan. 16], 1897.

20. Murray, Gordon and Janes, J. M. Prevention of Acute Failure of Circulation Following Injuries to Large Arteries. Experiments with Glass Cannulae Kept Patent by Administration of Heparin, *Brit. M. J.*, 2:6-7, 1940.

21. Murray, Gordon. Heparin in Surgical Treatment of Blood Vessels, *Arch. Surg.*, 40:307-325, 1940.

22. Mustard, W. T. The Technic of Immediate Restoration of Vascular Continuity after Arterial Wounds. Indications and Results, *Ann. Surg.*, 134:46-59, [July], 1946.

23. Payr, Erwin. Beiträge zur Technik der Blutgefäss und Nervennaht nebst Mittheilungen über die Verwendung eines resorbirharen Metalles in der Chirurgie, *Arch. f. klin. Chir.*, 62:67-93, 1900.

24. Swenson, Orvar and Gross, Robert E. Absorbable Fibrin Tubes for Vein Anastomoses, *Surgery*, 22:137-143, [July], 1947.

TRAUMATIC ANEURYSM AND ARTERIO-VENOUS FISTULA

Daniel Elkin, M.D.

The wounding of blood vessels results in a progression of changes and varied clinical phenomena which are largely dependent upon the extent of injury to the vessel wall. Traumatization of the arterial wall by passage of a missile near it or from forceful displacement of the vessel may result in no external evidence of damage; rupture of the intima may occur, with thrombosis and sympathetic disturbances, as manifest by a cold pulseless extremity. Extensive injury to the vessels produces a similar deprivation of arterial supply to the extremity with the additional obstruction of the remaining collateral channels by the tension resulting from a hematoma. Bleeding, both external and into the surrounding tissues, with the anemia which results, is also a factor in determining the viability of an extremity. Partial injuries to vessel walls are frequently manifest by similar changes or after a period of several weeks or months, by the development of an arterial aneurysm or an arteriovenous fistula.

Partial division of the arterial wall will result in the formation of a hematoma. The size of the hematoma will depend upon the elasticity of the surrounding structures, the ease with which the blood may escape through an external wound and the extent and type of arterial damage. This hematoma will at first pulsate; as clotting occurs a progressively diminishing area in which unclotted blood is in free exchange with the artery results. Organization of the clot by fibrous tissue progresses with the formation of an ovoid mass. This aneurysmal wall is composed of fibrous tissue and is supported by surrounding structures. The innermost layer of fibroblasts becomes flattened and resembles endothelial cells. The characteristic layers of a true arterial wall are absent. A clot, laminated in nature, forms within the aneurysmal sac, and it also constantly undergoes organization with a tendency toward spontaneous cure of the aneurysm. Unfortunately, this is rarely attained and rupture of the sac is frequent with expansion of the aneurysm. The deposition of calcium in the wall of the sac is occasionally found on roentgenologic examination.

If concomitant wounds of the artery and vein occur an arteriovenous fistula may result. Lateral wounding of the artery and vein, either by a missile which passes between the two vessels or which passes through both vessels with the lateral wounds becoming sealed, may result in a direct shunt of blood from the artery to the vein. An excellent anastomosis of artery and vein may be produced by trauma with little external bleeding particularly if the injured vessels are held in close apposition by a common sheath. In such an instance there is little scar tissue formation. As the vessels enlarge as a result of the fistula, the opening of communication may similarly enlarge. Frequently a false aneurysm is found in association with the arteriovenous connection; the aneurysm may lie between the vein and artery, or may project from a site of injury to either vessel. These false aneurysms do not tend to be as large as in the instances of arterial aneurysms since the decompression afforded by the vein relieves some of the tendency for expansion. Pathologically, the findings are those of two vessels encased in fibrous tissue. The false sac is similar to that previously described except that the tendency for a laminated clot to be present in the sac is less frequent. The wall of the sac is composed of fibrous tissue and contiguous structures. Its lining is that of flattened fibrous tissue. The artery and vein proximal to the fistula are enlarged. The vein distal to the fistula is enlarged but not so markedly as the proximal vein. The distal artery is diminished in size. Section studies of the vessel walls reveal no significant changes.

The Operative Treatment of Arteriovenous Fistula. An arteriovenous fistula is usually the result of trauma but in rare instances may be congenital. The most common cause is a concomitant lateral wounding of an artery and vein which are closely positioned in a common sheath. The femoral and carotid vessels are ideally situated in this respect and are the ones most frequently involved. However, any vessels may be the site of the lesion and involvement of practically all the vessels of the body has been reported. In the presence of a fistula between an artery and vein, blood is short-circuited from the artery directly to the vein. Depending upon the size of the fistula, its location and duration, certain effects upon the heart, the blood pressure and peripheral circulation take place. Following the establishment of a fistula, the heart dilates and the extent of the dilatation depends upon the duration of the fistula and the size of the opening. In large fistulas this dilatation takes place rapidly and eventually results in cardiac failure. The effects upon the heart, the general circulation and the part affected demand that the fistula be eliminated. Prior to operation, a period of bed rest should be carried out, particularly if there is any heart involvement. If actual heart failure is present, preliminary digitalization should be accomplished. The patient's general condition, including his nutrition, should be brought to the highest point. All infection, particularly in the region of the operative site, should be cleared for a period of at least a month.

The time interval between injury and operation is important. In general, the operation should be performed as early as possible after collateral circulation has been established. This, as a rule, will require two or three months and by that time the wound causing the lesion usually will be healed and the danger of infection will have passed. Moreover, in rare instances, small fistulas may heal spontaneously within that time.

Blood donors should be available for every operation and in some instances blood should be ready for transfusion before the operation is begun. The operation should be carried out with greatest care because of the large number of collateral vessels which are usually encountered and because their thinness and friability make them particularly liable to injury which may lead to serious hemorrhage. Bleeding from the smaller collateral vessels may be readily controlled by coagulation. Others should be ligated with fine, nonabsorbable ligatures, and in vessels of any size, ligatures should be reinforced by transfixion sutures.

If the position of the lesion permits, a tourniquet, preferably of the inflatable type, is placed above the operative site but is not inflated unless severe hemorrhage is encountered. Where possible, the skin incision should be made along anatomic lines and care should be taken not to cross skin folds transversely. No matter what type of operation is carried out, the artery proximal to the lesion should first be isolated and a ligature passed around it for control of possible hemorrhage. Ligation of the artery proximal to the fistula alone may temporarily eliminate the bruit and thrill so

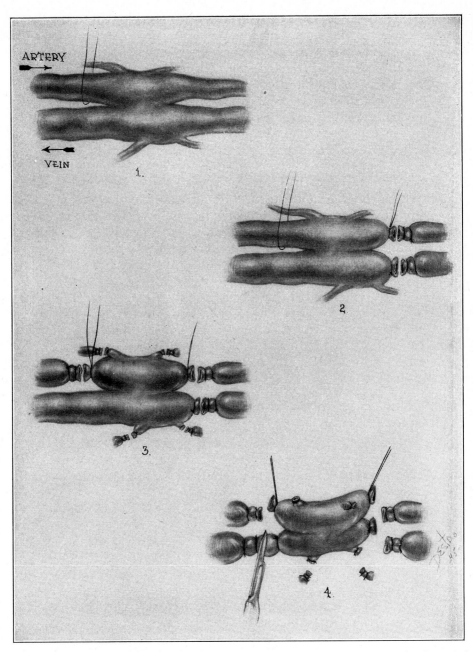

Fig. 482. The four steps in ligation and excision of an arteriovenous fistula: (1) A suture is passed around the proximal artery; (2) The distal vessels are ligated and divided; (3) The proximal artery and the communicating vessels are ligated and divided; (4) The proximal vein is ligated and divided as the last step in the procedure. (From Elkin, *South. M. J.*, 39(No. 4):311-316, 1946.)

characteristic of the lesion, but will not cure the fistula and may lead to gangrene. Likewise, ligation of the four major branches, that is, the proximal and distal arteries and veins may temporarily eliminate the bruit and thrill but will not cure the fistula, since it will readily be reestablished through its collaterals and communicating branches.

In the treatment of arteriovenous fistulas, one of two procedures is most generally employed: first, some type of operation whereby the communication between the artery and vein is obliterated by sutures; or, second, ligation of the vessels leading to and from the fistula and its complete extirpation. It is preferable where possible to preserve the continuity of the artery. This is frequently impossible because the vessels at the site of the lesion are so embedded in scar tissue as to prevent accurate dissection of the communication. Moreover, the opening may be so large that its closure necessitates occlusion of the vessel. Likewise, the presence of a false sac directly communicating with the artery or vein, or transposed between the two vessels, may prevent proper closure with the maintenance of the arterial lumen.

It must be borne in mind that while operative repair is ideal in preserving the continuity of the artery, it is not without danger. Secondary hemorrhage, thrombosis, and recurrence are more apt to follow this procedure than complete excision of the fistula.

Arterial repairs in which scar tissue is utilized may be followed by a false arterial aneurysm.

The operations most frequently performed for this condition are:

    I. Quadruple ligation and division of the main vessels, and excision.

   II. Repair of the arterial opening after removal of a portion of the vein.

  III. Transvenous closure of the opening.

  IV. Repair of the opening in both artery and vein.

   V. Mass ligature of the fistula where I, II, III or IV cannot be carried out.

I. QUADRUPLE LIGATION OF THE MAIN VESSELS, AND EXCISION. *Step 1*. The artery proximal to the fistula is isolated and a ligature passed around it. This ligature is placed for safety should severe hemorrhage be encountered, but is not tied at this time since occlusion of the vessel would interfere with pulsation of the vessels distal to the fistula and make their isolation more difficult as well as obscuring the exact site of the fistula (Fig. 482(1)).

Step 2. The main artery and vein distal to the fistula are isolated, doubly ligated, transfixed and divided (Fig. 482(2)).

Step 3. The artery proximal to the fistula about which a ligature was previously placed is doubly ligated, transfixed and divided. All vessels communicating with the fistula, except for the proximal vein, are then ligated and divided and the fistula is lifted from its bed (Fig. 482(3)).

Step 4. The vein proximal to the fistula is ligated and divided and the fistula is removed. Ligation of the proximal vein is reserved as the last step of the operation in order to provide a passageway for emptying the blood from the fistula. The numerous tributaries demand a careful and painstaking dissection of all vessels in order that the field be kept as free from blood as possible throughout the procedure (Fig. 482(4)).

II. Repair of the Arterial Opening after Removal of a Portion of the Vein. The artery, proximal and distal to the fistula, is exposed and isolated and arterial clamps are applied on either side of the lesion. The vein proximal and distal to the fistula is exposed and ligated and divided on either side (Fig. 483a). All communicating vessels are isolated and

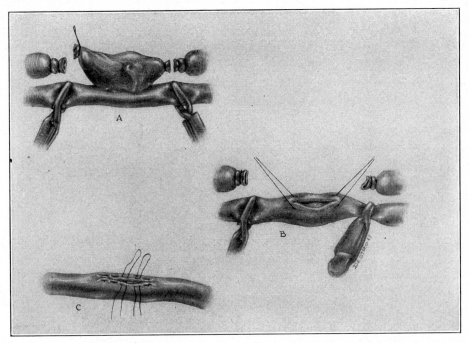

Fig. 483. Repair of an arteriovenous fistula. The arterial opening is closed with sutures after removing a portion of the vein. (From Elkin, *South M. J.* 39(No. 4): 311-316, 1946.)

divided. A portion of the vein is then carefully dissected away from the artery and discarded, thus exposing the arterial opening. The edges of this opening are usually freshened and then closed by interrupted mattress sutures of fine silk, being careful in the first row to approximate intima-to-intima (Fig. 483b, c). Further reinforcing sutures are placed in the adventitia. The clamps are removed and any leaking point is further reinforced. The placing of surrounding muscles directly over the opening will act as a further hemostatic agent. If the carrying out of this procedure results in occlusion of the vessel, that portion should be excised.

III. Transvenous Closure. Exposure of the proximal and distal arteries and veins, followed by ligation and division of the vein, is carried out as in II. Clamps are then applied to the artery above and below the fistula. The vein is ligated and divided proximal and distal to the fistula and opened to expose the communication which is then closed transvenously by inter-

rupted sutures of fine silk. Here too, if the closure results in obliteration
of the artery, it should be excised. The adherent vein may be used to reinforce the suture line (Fig. 484).

IV. REPAIR OF THE OPENING IN BOTH ARTERY AND VEIN. This procedure
is the most difficult to carry out. The proximal and distal artery and vein

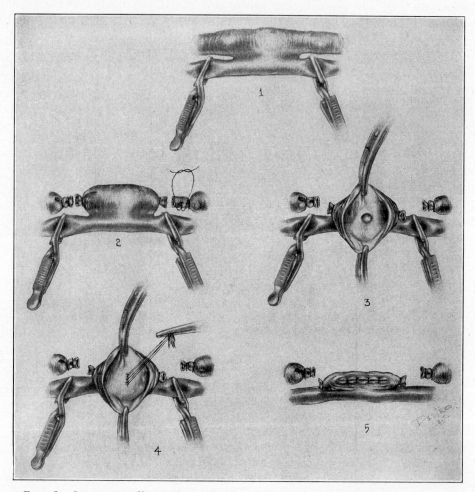

FIG. 484. Steps generally employed in the transvenous or transsaccular repair of an
arteriovenous fistula with preservation of the artery. (From Elkin, *Surg., Gynec. & Obst.,*
82(No. 1):5, 1946. By permission of Surgery, Gynecology and Obstetrics.)

are exposed and occluded by vessel clamps as in III. Communicating vessels
are ligated and divided. If there is a minimum of scar tissue and if the
communication is small, the vessels may be separated, thus exposing the
arterial and venous openings which are closed as in II and the clamps
removed.

V. MASS LIGATURE OF THE FISTULA. On rare occasions it may be impossible, particularly in the presence of severe hemorrhage, properly to isolate

the vessels as described above. Here it may be necessary to obliterate the fistula by a series of mass ligatures. Such a method is undesirable, since adjacent structures, particularly nerves, may be injured and recurrence and secondary hemorrhage are likely to follow.

In any operation upon blood vessels, the most scrupulous attention should be paid to asepsis. Infection of any severity may be followed by secondary hemorrhage. Since this lesion is usually the result of an external wound, the presence of a latent infection should not be overlooked and the postoperative use of penicillin as a prophylactic measure is advised until such time as any evidence of infection has passed.

After operation, if there is a considerable degree of cardiac dilatation, or if there is actual clinical evidence of cardiac failure, bed rest, proper medication and a slow return to work are indicated.

Sympathetic interruption as a means of increasing the circulation is usually not indicated nor necessary in an arteriovenous fistula because of the collateral circulation which develops as a result of the lesion. However, should claudication and evidence of ischemia develop after operation, this procedure should be given serious consideration.

The Operative Treatment of Arterial Aneurysms. An aneurysm is the result of trauma or of disease. In the latter, the usual predisposing causes are syphilis and arteriosclerosis which cause the vessel to give way with a resulting fusiform swelling (a true aneurysm), or to rupture into surrounding tissues with the formation of a pulsating sac, the walls of which are formed by fibrous tissue and surrounding structures. A third type, usually the result of arteriosclerosis, is a dissecting aneurysm in which blood escapes from the lumen of the vessel and dissects between the layers of the artery (usually the aorta) for a variable distance.

Regardless of the cause, those aneurysms amenable to operative treatment may be considered together as the principles underlying this treatment are the same. In general, it consists of (1) measures designed to produce a clot in the aneurysmal sac or to induce the formation of fibrous tissue about it and thus prevent further expansion and rupture, (2) obliteration of the sac by closure of the offending vessel, or (3) extirpation of the aneurysm-bearing portion of the artery.

A variety of methods, many of them unsuccessful, are to be found in the recorded annals of surgical treatment. Compression by various methods (digital, bandaging, instrumental) and the introduction of sclerosing and coagulating agents have been employed. Older operative methods included that of Antyllus (Second Century A.D.) which consisted of ligation of the vessel above and below the sac, the evacuation of its contents and the application of an astringent or of packing. Anel's operation (1710) consisted of ligation of the proximal artery close to the sac. This may still be used, but ischemia, recurrence and even gangrene are likely to follow. Later, John Hunter tied the femoral artery in the canal which bears his name, for aneurysm of the popliteal artery. It was Hunter's idea to bring about clotting and eventual cure and at the same time preserve collateral circulation, a definite improvement on Anel's procedure. In this he was highly successful, except for the frequent recurrence which took place through the circulation he was so anxious to preserve. On occasion, these methods still have a place (Fig. 485). In 1888, Matas described his method of intra-saccular suture of the vessels feeding the aneurysm, which he named endo-

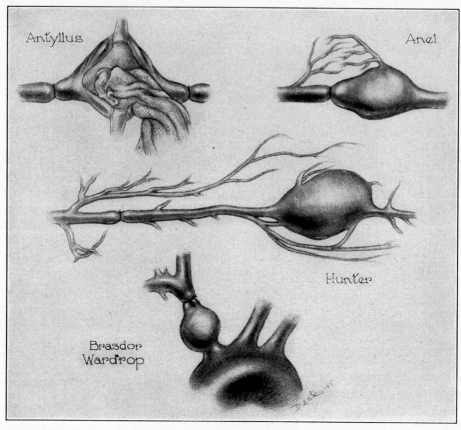

FIG. 485. Diagrammatic illustration of the types of operation employed for the treatment of aneurysms prior to the introduction of endoaneurysmorrhaphy. (From Elkin, *Surg., Gynec. & Obst.,* 82(No. 1):4, 1946. By permission of Surgery, Gynecology and Obstetrics.)

aneurysmorrhaphy. Later Brasdor and Wardrop independently ligated the artery or one of its principal branches on the distal side of the sac in an attempt to slow the circulation through it and thus encourage its clotting. All these methods with the exception of the Matas procedure were frequently followed by infection, hemorrhage, gangrene, or failure to cure the condition. Of them, only the Matas operation has stood the test of time and it is now performed in essentially the same way as that described by its originator.

MATAS ENDO-ANEURYSMORRHAPHY. If the position of the aneurysm permits, blood is emptied from the extremity by elevation, the application of a pressure bandage and finally by application of a tourniquet, preferably of the inflatable variety. The operation may then be performed in a bloodless field. If the application of a tourniquet is precluded by the position of the aneurysm, temporary occlusion of the proximal vessel by the application of an arterial clamp is of aid in performing the operation in a less bloody field.

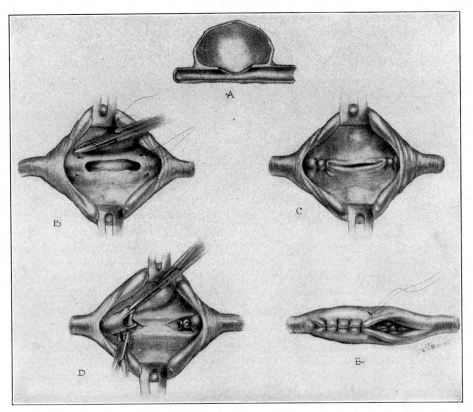

FIG. 486. Diagrammatic illustration of endoaneurysmorrhaphy. (A) Cross section of artery with false sac. (B) Sutures are placed to close the arterial openings within the sac. (C) Sutures tied. (D) Occasionally the vessel is isolated and ligated. (E) Occasionally the sac is obliterated by further sutures. (From Elkin, *Surg., Gynec. & Obst.,* 82(No. 1):6, 1946. By permission of Surgery, Gynecology and Obstetrics.)

The aneurysmal sac is then opened, taking care to avoid any nerves which may be stretched over it. The clot is evacuated and search is made for the openings in the artery. If not readily found, temporary loosening of the tourniquet will disclose their position. Usually one or two figure-of-eight sutures of silk are sufficient to close the opening (Fig. 486). If bleeding occurs after removal of the tourniquet, these can be reinforced by the placing of other sutures. Matas advocated obliteration of the sac by further suturing, but this is difficult because of its friable nature. In some instances the proximal and distal vessels can be dissected from surrounding structures *within the sac* and individually ligated. Closure of the skin and subcutaneous tissues with the application of a snug elastic bandage will bring about obliteration of the sac.

EXCISION OF ANEURYSM. Associated injuries to structures other than the blood vessel frequently make it desirable to remove the sac. This is particularly true if nerve injuries are to be repaired or if a bone graft is contemplated. Following suitable preoperative measures to enhance the circulation, such as proximal intermittent compression of the artery, and suitable tests to insure the adequacy of the collateral circulation, the aneurysm may in many instances be excised with safety.

An incision is made over the course of the vessels involved regardless of the most prominent point of presentation of the aneurysm. The artery is isolated proximal to the false sac with preservation of all branches possible. The artery distal to the aneurysm is similarly ligated and divided. As the sac is approached the artery is doubly ligated, transfixed and divided. Dissection may then be continued distally with ligation of all entering vessels as they are encountered and with final complete removal of the aneurysm. Care must be taken to prevent injury to any nerves which may lie upon or be in close relation with the sac as it is dissected free.

PROXIMAL ARTERIAL LIGATION. Aneurysms in certain locations, namely those in which there are few arterial branches, occasionally respond favorably to proximal ligation alone. This procedure is frequently performed for intracranial aneurysms, aneurysms of the carotid arteries, iliac arteries and the aorta. Ligation with division is the procedure of choice if the competency of the collateral circulation will permit but frequently a partial occlusion must be done as an initial stage to complete occlusion in elderly patients.

MEASURES TO PRODUCE CLOTTING OR INCREASE FIBROUS TISSUE FORMATION. Aneurysms of the aorta are usually not amenable to treatment by any of the methods described. Success has been reported in their treatment by the insertion of a coil of wire into the enlarged vessel and the stimulation of clotting by heating the wire with an electric current.

Large aortic aneurysms which are producing pain or in which rupture is imminent are benefited by extensive mobilization of the vessel with the application of cellophane about the lesion. In this procedure a double purpose is served. Fibrous tissue formation is stimulated with reinforcement of the aneurysmal wall; the sympathetic nerves to the vessel are interrupted with subsequent decrease in pain.

Anesthesia. Fractional spinal anesthesia is preferred for operation upon the lower extremities, since the procedures are usually long and tedious. For operations elsewhere in the body intravenous pentothal sodium, nitrous oxide and oxygen is the anesthetic of choice. In operations on the neck, the introduction of an intratracheal tube insures an open airway and a smoother anesthetic.

VARICOSE VEINS

Michael E. DeBakey, M.D.

General Considerations. The surgical management of varicose veins has as its objective the correction or the elimination of the disturbance in the venous circulation which is a consequence of the varicose state. This disturbance, which occurs principally in the superficial veins of the lower extremity and their tributaries, consists essentially in a slowing down of the return flow of blood from the involved area. It is due primarily to two factors, the dilatation of the veins and the incompetency of their valves. When the individual is in the upright position, these factors contribute to, rather than counteract, the effect of gravity which mitigates against the return flow of blood. The normal return blood flow is further affected by the intermittent, excessive back pressure upon the column of blood in the superficial varicosed veins which is produced by coughing or straining and which is normally counteracted by competent valves. Accordingly, there is a slowing down or even a reversal of the circulation and a tendency toward "pooling" in the varicosed system of veins, with consequent stasis and congestion, which over a long period of time produces undesirable local metabolic disturbances.[1,13,16,34,46,73,76,105]

Obviously reestablishment of original normal function of the involved veins is not possible; rational therapy is therefore directed rather toward the correction or elimination of the disturbance in the venous circulation of the varicose veins. This can be done by obliteration or extirpation of the involved veins, and for this purpose various methods have been devised, ranging from conservative measures to radical surgical procedures. These various methods of treatment, as well as the shifting viewpoints toward their application which have taken place during the past quarter of a century or more, have been adequately reviewed by Ochsner and Mahorner[97] in their comprehensive monograph on varicose veins.

Aside from purely conservative measures, the two basic methods generally employed today, either alone or in combination, are (1) ligation of the varicose vein combined with varying degrees of resection, and (2) obliteration by the injection of a sclerosing solution. At the present time there is a general tendency toward extension of the surgical method. Conservative therapy, consisting essentially in compression by an elastic support, is indicated in those patients in whom active therapy should not be employed, such as persons in advanced age and those with debilitating diseases or with severe arterial disease of the extremity. It is probably better to use conservative therapy, or rather to delay active treatment, in pregnancy until after the puerperium. Active therapy is also better postponed in the presence of cellulitis or other inflammatory states in the involved part until the condition has subsided. The single exception to this practice is the presence of acute phlebitis in varicosities in which high saphenous ligation should be done.

Appropriate treatment is further based upon proper evaluation of the individual case, with particular assessment of such factors as patency of the deep veins, adequacy of the arterial circulation, and competency of the valves in the superficial and communicating veins. Of the various special diagnostic tests devised for this purpose, the Brodie-Trendelenburg test, Perthes' test, and the comparative tourniquet test of Mahorner and Ochsner [70,71] are most widely used. The latter is perhaps the most useful because it combines the advantages of all other tests and provides accurate localization of the sites of incompetent valves as well.

Treatment. As has already been stated, the two principal methods of active treatment are injection of the vein with sclerosing solution and ligation with or without extirpation. As a rule, injection treatment is combined with ligation, for when it is used alone it has been found to be followed by a high incidence of recurrence. It may, however, be employed without ligation for relatively small localized varicosities, particularly in the calf, and in the absence of incompetent valves in the saphenous above or in the communicating veins. It may also be justified as palliative therapy in cases in which operative treatment is contraindicated or, preferably, is delayed.

INJECTION TREATMENT. The following equipment is necessary for injection: (1) several syringes (2 cc. and 5 cc. sizes, preferably with finger and thumb rings and Luer-Lok arrangement); (2) needles (22 to 26 inch gauge); (3) sterile sponges and small felt squares; and (4) compression bandages. A number of sclerosing agents have been advocated, but on the basis of the extensive investigation of Ochsner and his co-workers [93-95] the most efficacious are, in the order given: sodium morrhuate (5 per cent); sodium gynocardate (5 per cent); and quinine urethane. More recently monoethanolamine oleate (monolate) [42,79] and synasol [20] have been recommended as being as efficacious as sodium morrhuate, but without the disadvantage of producing allergic manifestations that occasionally follow the latter agent.

It should be realized, however, that untoward reactions may follow any form of injection therapy. They vary from local inflammatory process or minor allergic manifestations to severe anaphylaxis or fatal embolism.[5,35,43,102,106,113,120] Some reactions are due to imperfections in technic and in postinjection management and others to sensitivity of the patient to the agent employed. Their occurrence is relatively rare and with proper precautions the injection method may be used with reasonable safety.[75,77,84,100]

Some variations exist in the proper procedure for injections, but adherence to the following principles seems desirable: (1) assurance that the needle is in the lumen of the veins; (2) isolation of the particular segment of the vein to be injected; (3) removal of as much blood as possible from the affected segment of vein before injection; and (4) maintenance of compression of the segment of vein following the injection.

With the patient in a sitting position and the leg hanging down or resting on a stool, the engorged segment of vein to be injected is readily

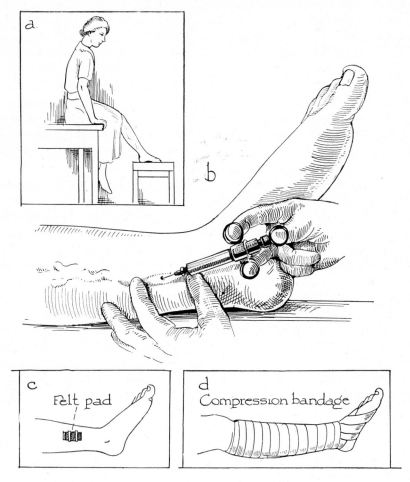

FIG. 487. Technic of injection therapy in varicose veins. a. With the patient in the sitting position and the leg hanging down or resting on a stool, the engorged segment of vein to be injected is readily identified and isolated between the thumb and index finger of the left hand. b. With the fingers maintained in this manner the extremity is brought to a horizontal position on the table and the needle attached to the syringe containing the sclerosing solution is introduced into the lumen of the vein. The left thumb and index finger are then temporarily removed to allow the segment of vein to be emptied of blood. Digital pressure is then reapplied and the sclerosing agent is injected into the isolated segment. c. After the needle is withdrawn, gentle pressure with a small felt or gauze pad is applied over the injected segment and, d. a compression bandage is applied over the leg.

identified and may be isolated between the thumb and index finger of the left hand (Fig. 487a). With the distended segment of vein still between the thumb and index finger, the extremity is brought to a horizontal position on the table and the needle attached to the syringe containing the sclerosing solution is introduced into the lumen of the vein (Fig. 487b). After it has been ascertained, by aspiration of a small amount of blood, that the needle is in the lumen, the left thumb and index finger are temporarily removed, to allow the segment of vein to be emptied of blood. Digital pressure is then reapplied and the sclerosing agent is injected into the isolated segment. This maneuver confines the sclerosing agent to the desired area and provides for its more intimate contact with the endothelial surface. Following the injection, the needle is allowed to remain in situ for about a minute before it is withdrawn, after which gentle pressure with a felt or gauze pad is applied over the injected segment (Fig. 487c). Finally, a compression bandage is applied over the leg and is maintained for a period of four to six weeks (Fig. 487d). It is desirable to inject only one vein at the first sitting, in order to determine the individual's reaction to the agent employed. Thereafter, depending upon the character and extent of the reaction, several injections may be made at one sitting, the distance between each injection varying from 2 to 4 cm. It is also desirable to begin the injections at the lowermost area and work upward with successive injections at intervals of three to five days. Depending upon the size of the affected segment of vein, from 0.5 to 2 cc. of sodium morrhuate solution is used at each site, but the total amount used should not exceed 5 to 10 cc.

OPERATIVE TREATMENT. *High Ligation of the Saphenous Vein.* The procedure of high ligation of the saphenous vein and all of its tributaries at the fossa ovalis is now fairly well standardized and is generally recognized as probably the most important measure in the management of varicose veins.[30,40,48,97,109,115] Unless there are specific contraindications to operation, it should be employed in all cases with involvement of the internal or long saphenous in the thigh. Various combinations of this procedure with other measures have been advocated, depending upon the extent of involvement below this site and the personal preference and experience of the authors. Among those most commonly advocated are retrograde injection of a sclerosing solution into the distal segment, with or without ligation at lower levels (below the point of incompetent communicating veins), and extirpation of the distal segment by "stripping" methods or multiple excision. Although some differences of opinion exist concerning the best method of dealing with the distal segment, there is general agreement upon the importance and the proper performance of the high ligation of the saphenous.

Though the operation may be considered an outpatient, ambulatory procedure, it is desirable to keep the patient under observation in the hospital for twenty-four hours and to perform the procedure in the operating room. Unless ligation is combined with more extensive distal dissections, local infiltration analgesia with 1 per cent procaine hydrochloride solution is adequate. A longitudinal or slightly oblique (descending medialward) skin incision is preferable, beginning at the level of the inguinal ligament about 2 to 2.5 cm. medial to the femoral pulsation and extending downward for a distance of about 10 cm. (Fig. 488a). The saphenous vein is then exposed as it lies in the deeper layers of the superficial fascia and is freed of its surrounding tissues from the saphenofemoral junction to a point 3 to 5 cm. distally. This distance is usually sufficient to expose all of the tributaries (Fig. 488b).[22] Dissection may be facilitated by working proximally toward the saphenofemoral junction. All of the tributaries of the saphenous are

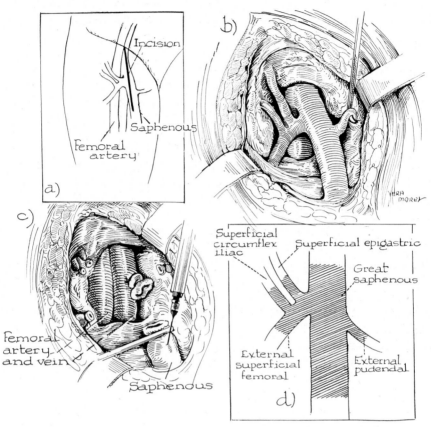

FIG. 488. Technic of high ligation of saphenous vein and its tributaries. a. The incision is made in a longitudinal or slightly oblique direction beginning at the level of the inguinal ligament about 2 to 2.5 cm. medial to the femoral artery pulsation and extending downward for a distance of about 10 cm. b. The incision is carried down through the deeper layers of the superficial fascia exposing the saphenous vein from its junction with the femoral vein to a point 3 to 5 cm. distally, which is usually sufficient to expose all its tributaries. c. The saphenous vein and all its tributaries are ligated and divided, following which the distal end may be injected with a sclerosing solution. d. Diagrammatic illustration of segment of saphenous vein, represented by shaded area, that should be resected in order to provide greater assurance of interrupting all tributaries of the saphenous vein.

identified and individually divided between ligatures (Fig. 488c). The saphenous vein is then ligated as close as possible to the femoral, care being taken not to encroach upon the lumen of the femoral vein. A transfixation tie is applied just distal to this ligature. Considerable variations in the vascular patterns of the saphenous vein and its tributaries in the thigh have been observed,[22,98,107] but the significant fact surgically is that all the tributaries near its terminal end enter the main vein within a distance of 2 to 3.5 cm. from the saphenofemoral junction.[22] The resection (Fig. 488d), therefore, of a segment of the saphenous vein for a distance of about 4 or 5 cm. from its termination in the femoral provides both a reliable means of interrupting all the tributaries and better assurance against subsequent re-establishment of vascular connections with resultant recurrence of varicosities.

Attention is now directed to the distal end of the saphenous, which, as previously indicated, may be handled in various ways. Some observers consider simultaneous ligation and injection preferable. Others do not believe it is necessary. Our experience has inclined us toward the former procedure except in cases in which the varicosed saphenous vein is quite large and tortuous, when, as will be pointed out later, it is handled differently. Simultaneous injection is done by inserting the needle attached to a syringe containing a 5 per cent solution of sodium morrhuate into the lumen of the distal segment of the vein as it is steadied with the clamp that has been allowed to remain in situ during the preceding part of the operation (Fig. 488c). After the injection of 2 to 3 cc. of the sclerosing solution, care being taken to prevent leakage into the wound by placing a gauze pad beneath the vein, a clamp is applied to the vein immediately below the site of puncture and the needle is removed. The vein is then ligated further distally and a transfixation ligature is applied just proximal to the level of ligation. The excess segment of vein proximal to these ligatures, including the portion to which the clamps have been applied, is resected. The wound is then closed in layers with interrupted sutures of fine cotton or silk. A snug compression bandage of sterile cotton waste is applied over the wound and an elastic bandage is applied to the extremity from the toes to the groin.

In the presence of incompetent communicating veins at a lower level of the saphenous in the thigh it is desirable to combine the high ligation with one or more low ligations.[48,52,97,112,119] The additional low ligation is also particularly useful when a communication exists between the greater and lesser saphenous systems. Low ligation is done through a transverse or longitudinal incision, preferably the latter because it more readily permits resection of a few centimeters of the vein, which is considered a more desirable procedure than simple division between ligatures.

Still another variation of these methods of management is the combination of high ligation with complete extirpation of the saphenous in the thigh by means of "stripping" or other means. This more radical procedure, originally advocated by Keller, Mayo, and Babcock, had been largely abandoned because of its high morbidity. Its recent revival [31,33,45,47,54,55,107] is based on the belief that this more direct approach to the problem, *i.e.,* the elimination of the varicosities, provides greater assurance against recurrence and that morbidity may be kept reasonably low by supplementing the procedure with elastic compression bandages and early activity to combat thrombosis and embolism. On the basis of our experience, the method is useful only in selected cases, and particularly in dealing with the markedly dilated and enlarged forms of varicosities involving the long saphenous vein associated with incompetent communicating veins. The procedure is performed under spinal analgesia or general anesthesia. High ligation and resection of the saphenous are first done, as described. The distal end of the saphenous vein is then threaded through the eye of a Mayo vein stripper and the vein is stripped distally to the knee or as far down the thigh as

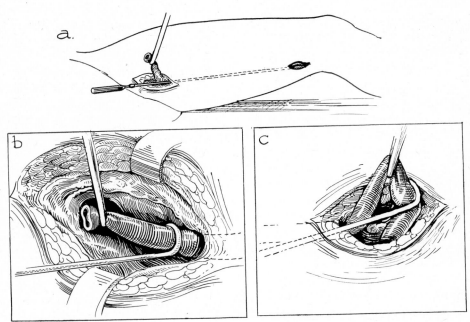

Fig. 489. Technic of stripping of saphenous vein in the thigh using the Mayo stripper. a. High ligation of the saphenous is first done as described in figure 488. b. The distal end of the saphenous vein is then threaded through the eye of the stripper and the vein is stripped distally to free it from its surroundings down as far as possible, which is usually above the knee. c. A small incision is made over the distal end of the stripper and the freed vein is drawn out through it and the distal end is ligated.

possible, after which a small incision is made over the distal end of the stripper and the freed vein is drawn out through it (Fig. 489). It is sometimes necessary to use multiple small incisions down the length of the vein, successively rethreading and stripping the vein through each incision. Some have advocated extending the stripping procedure below the knee to remove the entire length of the saphenous down to the ankle.

The patient is encouraged to walk and to be ambulatory after any of the operations described above, although as already emphasized it is desirable for him to remain in the hospital for the first twenty-four hour period. Early ambulation is considered a desirable and effective measure against the development of propagating thrombi.

Subfascial Ligation of Communicating Veins. In a small proportion of cases (about 2 per cent)[84] with incompetent communicating veins of the legs, still more extensive procedures than those described will be required to secure a satisfactory result. Such cases are characterized by long-standing varicosities which have resisted ordinary measures and which are commonly associated with ulceration. More often than not there is a history of antecedent thrombophlebitis. Under these circumstances it may be found desirable to perform a complete dissection and ligation of the communicating veins of the legs as advocated by Linton,[65-67] though in view of the extensive nature of this procedure considerable care and judgment should be exercised in the selection of patients for its application. On the basis of Linton's anatomic studies, these communicating veins may be classified into three groups, medial, lateral and anterior. The medial group is by far the most commonly involved (80 to 90 per cent) and the anterior group the least (5 per cent). In cases of ulceration, the location of the ulcer generally corresponds with the group of veins involved.

It is well, in applying this particular method of treatment, to follow the steps outlined by Linton and Keeley.[67] It is necessary first to obtain healing of the ulceration which is usually present. In simple cases this may be achieved by conservative management, with elevation of the extremity and application of warm compresses of saline solution. In others, after the large ulcerated surface has been properly cleaned by similar measures, it may be more practicable to cover the granulating area with skin grafts. The second step consists of high ligation and resection of the long saphenous and its tributaries in the fossa ovalis, as already described. This procedure may be combined with low ligation or with retrograde injection, depending upon the indications previously described. The third step consists of a period of observation lasting six weeks or more during which the patient is ambulatory and wears an elastic supporting bandage. By the end of this period the condition of the skin of the lower leg should be in sufficiently good condition to permit the operative procedure of ligation of the communicating veins, which is the next (fourth) step.

The operation is performed under general anesthesia or spinal analgesia. The position of the patient, as well as the site of the incision, depends upon the group of veins involved (Fig. 490). For the medial group, which is most commonly involved, a longitudinal incision is made on the medial aspect of the leg, extending downward from just behind and below the medial edge of the tibia to just behind the internal malleolus. The incision is carried down through the deep fascia to expose the underlying muscles and the flaps are mobilized on each side for several centimeters in order to obtain proper exposure (Fig. 490).

All the communicating veins encountered between these structures are ligated and divided. The most enlarged and most numerous veins are usually found beneath, and in the immediate region of the old ulcer. The wound is closed in layers with interrupted sutures. Immobilization of the leg during the first ten days postoperatively is advised to aid healing and is best obtained by a posterior plaster splint. At the end of this period, graduated activity is begun with vascular exercises such as the Buerger type.

An elastic bandage applied from the toes to the knee should be worn by the patient for several months or even longer.

A much less extensive procedure, but one which will often give satisfactory results, as emphasized by Ochsner,[84] may also be used in some of

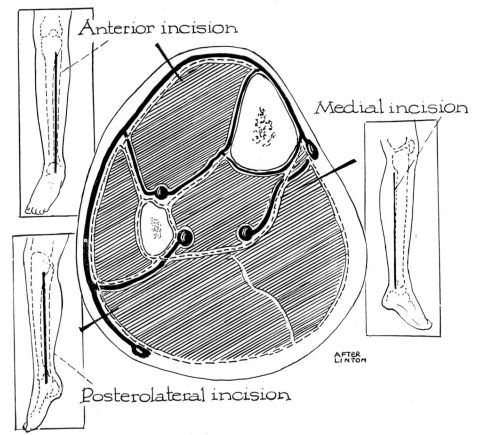

Anterior incision

Medial incision

Posterolateral incision

AFTER LINTON

FIG. 490. Diagrammatic drawing of cross section of leg, illustrating approaches suggested by Linton for ligation of incompetent communicating veins in leg. One of three approaches may be used, depending upon the group of veins involved. The medial incision is used for exposure and ligation of the communicating branches extending from the posterior tibial as well as the medial branches from the interior tibial; the anterior incision is used for exposure and ligation of the central and lateral divisions of the communicating veins of the anterior tibial veins; and the posterolateral incision is used for exposure and ligation of the communicating branches from the peroneal vein.

these cases in which feeder or incompetent communicating veins exist immediately beneath and around the ulcer bed. It consists essentially in exposing the bed through an elliptical incision, with mobilization of the flaps and resection of the superficial veins, and ligating the feeder or communicating veins. In other cases the old ulcer area with underlying indurated fibrotic tissue and surrounding pigmented skin is completely excised and is covered by a skin graft.

Lumbar Sympathectomy. In addition to the indicated methods of treatment described, lumbar sympathectomy may be used in certain types of varicose veins and especially in those associated with chronic postphlebitic syndrome.[2,32,53,61-63,91,108] In our experience it has proved particularly valuable in bettering results of these modes of treatment. It should usually be done as a preliminary procedure to the more extensive operations on the leg. It is particularly useful in cases with excessive sweating in which chronic fungous infection is difficult to control or in cases associated with cyanosis, induration, and much discomfort and pain. Most of these cases are of the postphlebitic type. It has been demonstrated clinically and experimentally [26,86-88] that there is a strong factor of vasospasm in the acute form of thrombophlebitis and that interruption of these vasoconstrictor impulses has a desirable effect. There is reason to believe that in the chronic form of the disease some element of vasospasm persists, and on this basis blocking of the sympathetic pathways would produce beneficial effects.

Sympathectomy provides a warm dry skin, permitting effective control of the fungous infection, and, as a consequence of permanent vasodilatation, improves the circulation. It thus encourages healing, helps to relieve discomfort and edema, and in general improves the local condition for subsequent surgical intervention if this becomes necessary. The procedure recommended for lumbar sympathectomy, which has been described elsewhere,[89] is removal of the lumbar ganglia and chain through an anterolateral extraperitoneal approach under spinal analgesia.

VENOUS THROMBOSIS

General Considerations. Venous thrombosis may arise under a variety of circumstances in any individual, at any time, and in any part of the venous system. It may develop spontaneously in an otherwise apparently perfectly normal active person, but more frequently it develops as a complication of certain conditions and states, such as trauma, operation, parturition, and other serious bed-confining circumstances. Although it may develop in any part of the venous system, it most commonly occurs in the veins of the lower extremities. There is, however, a special and rather uncommon form of the disease in the upper extremities known as axillary thrombosis or effort thrombosis.[28,72,114] Clinically there are also variations in both the manifestations and the course of thrombosis. Depending upon the particular form it assumes, the process may (1) heal completely without any residual, (2) leave the patient with permanent and often crippling disability, or (3) terminate fatally as a result of massive or repeated pulmonary embolization.

Venous thrombosis thus appears to be a disease of protean nature, although to a great extent this impression may be a reflection of incomplete understanding of its etiology and pathogenesis. This same fact also probably accounts for much of the diversity of opinion concerning therapy. A more detailed consideration of these phases of the subject may be found in previous publications [86-88,90-92] and the chief emphasis here will be placed upon those pertaining to its surgical management. For the same reason this discussion will be concerned primarily with thrombosis involving the veins of the lower extremities and pelvis.

Although, as has been indicated above, venous thrombosis may assume a variety of forms, in general it is possible and, for prognostic and therapeutic purposes, it is desirable to distinguish between two main types of the disease, namely, phlebothrombosis and thrombophlebitis.[86-88,90-92] It is believed that in the former the clotting process is due primarily to venous stasis and to alterations in the cellular and fluid constituents of blood which increase the clotting tendency, whereas in the latter it is due to injury to the vascular endothelium from mechanical trauma, chemical injury, or bacterial invasion. Because of the associated inflammatory reaction in thrombophlebitis the clot tends to be firmly adherent to the vein wall and to obstruct its lumen completely. Fragmentation or detachment of the clot, with the consequent occurrence of pulmonary embolism, is therefore less likely to take place, unless suppuration, which is very unusual, intervenes.

On the other hand, in phlebothrombosis, which Homans [50-53] has termed bland or deep quiet venous thrombosis, because of the minimal inflammatory reaction, the clot tends to be lightly adherent to the vein wall and much of its proximal portion forms a loosely floating and incompletely obstructive propagating thrombus. The likelihood of fragmentation or detachment of the thrombus, with consequent pulmonary embolism, is obviously much greater in this form of the disease.

As might be expected, the clinical picture differs considerably in the two forms, there being outspoken manifestations of an inflammatory process in thrombophlebitis and minimal local and systemic reactions in phlebothrombosis. Thus, in thrombophlebitis, the local manifestations of pain, tenderness and swelling and the systemic reactions of fever, leukocytosis and increased pulse rate are quite prominent and the diagnosis, as a result, is relatively simple. Thrombophlebitis is typified by the nonseptic postpartal femoroiliac thrombophlebitis or the classical form of phlegmasia alba dolens. In phlebothrombosis, on the other hand, symptoms and signs are either very mild or are entirely absent, which accounts for Homans' [50-53] application to it of the term deep quiet venous thrombosis. In fact, it may be stated that in general the fixation of the clot is directly proportional to the severity of the clinical manifestation.[50] The more prominent and severe are the manifestations, the more adherent and secure is the clot; the quieter and milder is the process, the less secure is the clot and the greater is the danger of its detachment with resultant pulmonary embolism.

Between these two clinically characteristic forms of the disease there are, as would be expected, intermediate types.[50] It has been clearly demonstrated [9,10,41,56,57,104] that in phlebothrombosis the clotting process begins in the deep veins of the foot and leg. Once the process has begun, it may pursue several courses, depending upon a number of factors, many as yet undetermined, influencing the clotting mechanism. It may remain confined to a relatively small area and heal completely without producing any manifestations of its presence. Conceivably, this occurs quite frequently. It may continue to progress upward into the deep venous radicals of the thigh and the femoroiliac vessels, exciting an inflammatory reaction along its attachment to the vein, fully obstructing these large channels, and resulting in the development of a full-fledged thrombophlebitis. In its progression upward along these deep venous channels, the propagating thrombus may grow as a soft fragile mass lightly adherent at some points but to a great extent floating freely, without causing much obstruction. This type is, of course, the most dangerous, for it constantly threatens to produce pulmonary infarction or embolism. Once the process has begun, it may pursue variable courses, and there is no way at present of determining beforehand either the direction or the extent of its course. This, of course, adds greatly to the difficulty of clarifying the problem and standardizing therapy.

Venous thrombosis may involve the superficial as well as the deep veins of the extremities, whether they are varicosed or not. In them it usually assumes an inflammatory form, with the clot firmly adherent and completely obstructive, though occasionally it may become suppurative.

In addition to these forms of venous thrombosis, which involve the veins of the lower extremities, there is still another important category, in which the veins of the pelvis are primarily involved. This type of thrombophlebitis, which is usually associated with suppuration or with serious infection of the pelvic viscera, is well exemplified by septic postabortal or puerperal thrombophlebitis. This is a particularly serious form because liquefaction of the clot by the infection is likely to occur, and separation of infected emboli produces repeated pulmonary infarction, pneumonitis, and sepsis. The diagnosis is readily apparent, for clinically the manifestations of sepsis are evident; the patient appears acutely ill, with chills, high fever, and a spiking temperature curve.

Treatment. PROPHYLAXIS. Treatment may be divided into prophylactic and active therapy. Prophylaxis consists essentially in the correction or avoidance of those factors which are considered to predispose or favor the development of the thrombotic process, including, particularly, circulatory retardation or venous stasis, cardiovascular disorders, dehydration, physical and chemical disturbances in the blood, trauma, and infection. These factors and their control, which should be self-evident, are considered in detail in previous publications.[27,86,88,90-92] The factor of local circulatory retardation or venous stasis, however, deserves further consideration because of its special importance. The institution of measures directed toward its correction or prevention is particularly important in those conditions or under those circumstances in which venous thrombosis of the lower extremities seems to occur with relatively greater frequency. Such measures include chiefly restoration of normal cardiovascular function, avoidance of increased abdominal tension, avoidance of postures that favor venous stasis in the lower extremities, the use of deep breathing exercises and leg exercises, early activity and ambulation, and the application of elastic compression bandages to the extremities.

Still another prophylactic measure that may be instituted under certain conditions is the administration of anticoagulants such as heparin and dicoumarol. They would seem to be particularly useful in patients with an antecedent or familial history of thrombosis or with other indications of a thrombotic tendency. The use of anticoagulants is not, however, without danger, and close observation of the patient, with repeated laboratory checks, is required when they are employed. For these details of their use, as well as other considerations of their indications, limitations, and contraindications, the reader should consult other publications.[7,8,11,12,21,24,58,81]

ACTIVE TREATMENT. At present, considerable diversity of opinion exists concerning the most satisfactory treatment of venous thrombosis and several schools of thought on the subject have developed. These range from the most conservative to the most radical, with some advocating, to the exclusion of all other specific measures, the use of anticoagulants, such as heparin or dicoumarol, or the use of proximal vein ligation, and with others preferring to utilize these as well as other specific measures, such as sympathetic block to produce vasodilatation, depending upon certain conditions and indications in the individual case. Though the advocates of these different methods have marshalled much evidence to support their opinions, the conclusive demonstration of the superiority of any of these particular forms of therapy must await further evaluation. Moreover, it would serve no useful purpose to present here a discussion of the pros and cons of these various modes of treatment. The reader interested in this phase of the subject should consult other publications.[3,4,7-12,21,27,39,50-53,58,68, 81,88,90-92] Emphasis here will be placed on the method of treatment which, according to our experience, has provided the most satisfactory results.

Uncomplicated Thrombophlebitis. As has been indicated, it is important to distinguish between thrombophlebitis and phlebothrombosis because the therapeutic approach to each condition is different. In thrombophlebitis, with certain exceptions to be indicated, conservative measures combined with induction of vasodilatation in the involved extremity are considered satisfactory. In phlebothrombosis, on the other hand, because of the constant threat of detachment of the clot with consequent pulmonary embolism, it is preferable to employ more radical measures, chiefly the surgical interruption of the vein above the site of involvement.[49]

Conservative measures in thrombophlebitis consist essentially in elevation of the involved extremity and the use of an elastic compression bandage, combined with procaine hydrochloride block of the regional sympathetic ganglia. Elevation of the extremity, by the use of pillows or an inclined plane or, preferably, by elevation of the foot of the bed, and the use of a compression bandage aid the return flow of venous blood and provide for drainage of excess tissue fluid. In addition to these measures, and perhaps the most effective therapeutic procedure in thrombophlebitis, is the production of vasodilatation by means of procaine hydrochloride block of the regional sympathetic ganglia, as originally suggested by Leriche. The rationale of this procedure lies in the clinical and experimental demonstration of the presence of vasospasm resulting from impulses originating in the involved venous segment, probably set up by the inflammatory reaction, and transmitted over the sympathetic pathway.[26,27,85-88,90-92] Such vasospastic influences, which probably affect both arterial and venous systems, may be so marked that the condition appears to be arterial embolism and in occasional

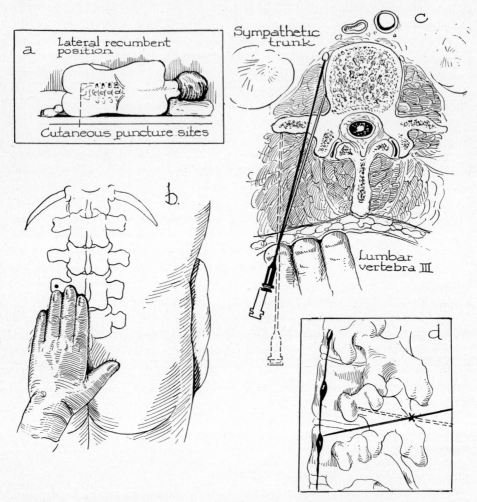

instances actual gangrene has occurred.[14,44,60,69] The mechanism by which it is believed vasospasm contributes to the untoward manifestations has been considered in previous publications.[26,27,85-88,90-92] It suffices to say here that these manifestations can be greatly ameliorated by interrupting the vasoconstrictor impulses with procaine hydrochloride infiltration of the regional sympathetic ganglions. Following this form of therapy there occur dramatic relief of pain, rapid subsidence of fever, and early disappearance of edema, and the patients are usually out of bed in five to six days or less. The blocks are performed daily for several days or until the fever subsides. The technic of sympathetic block is relatively simple (Fig. 491).[25,85,87,92]

Septic Thrombophlebitis. In thrombophlebitis associated with sepsis or with localized infection or suppuration, more radical therapy is indicated. Occasionally too, radical therapy is indicated in thrombophlebitis in which there is an acute and rapid progression of the infection proximally along the vein wall, probably through the perivenous lymphatics, with rapid propagation of the clot. In such cases ligation and division of the main venous channel above the involved segments should be done, to prevent extension of the process and the possible occurrence of septic emboli due to liquefaction and fragmentation of the infected clot. The classical and perhaps the most frequent example of this type of thrombophlebitis is the variety commonly observed as a postabortal complication or observed in the puerperium. Despite the effectiveness of chemotherapy, and the even greater effectiveness of penicillin in the management of puerperal sepsis, septic thrombophlebitis still remains the leading cause of death in postabortal and postpartal sepsis.[17-19]

Whereas the measures described should be employed in every case, in many cases venous ligation is additionally necessary for the effective control of the condition. The value of this procedure, as well as the optimum time and the technical methods of its application, are matters that have received much consideration in the older literature.[23,90] The recent revival of interest in it is probably based to a great extent on the unsatisfactory results obtained by the more conservative forms of management and stems particularly from the work of Collins and his associates.[17-19] Their observations, which have been amply confirmed by others,[78] demonstrate the value of venous ligation in septic or suppurative pelvic thrombophlebitis.

Since there is generally an extensive involvement of the pelvic venous system, including particularly the uterine, hypogastric, common iliac, and ovarian veins, successful management depends upon complete interruption of the venous return from this area. Accordingly, it is necessary in the majority of cases to ligate the ovarian veins as well as the vena cava. This

---

FIG. 491. Technic of lumbar sympathetic block. The patient may be placed in the prone position with a pillow under the lower abdomen or, preferably, in the lateral recumbent position, as shown in a. The cutaneous sites of puncture lie on a horizontal level with, and two and one-half to three fingerbreadths lateral to, the upper part of the spinous processes of the first four lumbar vertebrae. This places the cutaneous puncture sites directly over the transverse processes of the respective vertebrae. c. The needle is inserted vertically until the transverse process is reached (dotted needle). A point on the needle two and one-half to three fingerbreadths above the skin surface is taken and represents the distance the needle will be introduced further. The needle is then directed anteromedially and introduced above or below the transverse process (as shown in d) so that its point impinges against the lateral surface of the body of the vertebra (white needle). The needle is then withdrawn slightly to slip away from the body of the vertebra and inserted until the point on the needle previously made has been reached (black needle). Thus, the distance the needle is finally inserted beyond the transverse process is two and one-half to three fingerbreadths and represents the approximate distances between the transverse process and the site of the sympathetic chain. Because the sympathetic chain lies snugly against the anterolateral surface of the body of the vertebra, it is desirable to keep the point of the needle during insertion close to the lateral aspect of the body of the vertebra until the needle has been introduced the required distance.

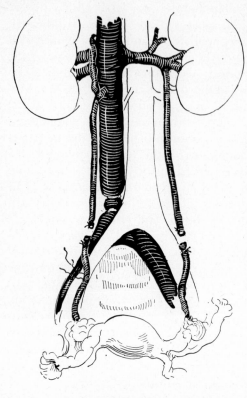

FIG. 492. Diagrammatic drawing showing site of ligation of vena cava and ovarian veins in septic pelvic thrombophlebitis. A transperitoneal approach through a low paramedian incision is used. The right ovarian vein and vena cava are exposed retroperitoneally by mobilizing the cecum and ascending colon medially after incising the peritoneal reflection in the paracolic groove. The right ovarian vessels are ligated and divided just above the pelvic brim, or above the clot if they are found thrombosed, care being taken to avoid injury to the ureter, which is usually nearby. Two heavy ligatures about 1.5 to 2 cm. apart are placed around the vena cava just above its formation by the junction of the iliac veins. The left ovarian vein is exposed by mobilizing medially the sigmoid and descending colon after incising their peritoneal reflection laterally. The left ovarian vessels are ligated and divided, and reperitonealization is accomplished on both sides. The abdominal wound is then closed in layers.

can best be accomplished by a transabdominal approach, which provides ready access to the pelvis, permitting exploration and simultaneous ligation of the vena cava and both ovarian veins above the thrombotic process (Fig. 492).

Section of the lumbar sympathetic chains is advised by Collins, or, if this is considered unwise at the time of operation, daily bilateral lumbar sympathetic blocks with procaine hydrochloride solution should be carried out postoperatively for several days, to counteract the vasospasm which sometimes follows ligation of the vena cava. Other postoperative measures include elevation of the foot of the bed, application of an elastic compression bandage, and early ambulation. Elastic compression bandages, applied from the toes to the groin, should be worn after the patient becomes ambulatory until they are no longer needed to counteract dependent edema. This period varies from several weeks to several months.

Phlebothrombosis. The diagnosis of phlebothrombosis is an immediate indication for radical therapy, *i.e.,* proximal venous ligation, because, as previously emphasized, in this form of venous thrombosis there is a constant threat of detachment of the clot and of consequent pulmonary infarction or embolism. Although this form of therapy is effective in controlling extension of the disease and preventing pulmonary embolism, there may be some difficulty in its practical application in a particular case. This is due primarily to the frequent absence of precise criteria in determining the presence of the disease or in predicting the possible occurrence of embolism. The clinical manifestations of phlebothrombosis are often so mild as to pass unnoticed, and not infrequently the first manifestation of its presence is the sudden occurrence of pulmonary infarction. Because of its insidious development and treacherous nature, the diagnosis, if it is to be made early when therapy is most effective, often must be assumed on the basis of rather minimal findings. These may consist of minor discomfort or slight pain in the foot or calf on movement or palpation, mild swelling in the ankle region, slight dilatation of the superficial veins of the foot, a faint tinge of cyanosis of the toes or nail bed, especially on dependency, and slight elevation of the temperature and especially the pulse. The presence of pain or tenderness in the calf and popliteal area on palpation or on forced dorsiflexion (Homans) is a particularly important sign. Phlebography is a useful diagnostic procedure and when properly performed provides fairly reliable information on the presence or absence of venous thrombosis.[9,10,29,36,37] Unfortunately, it is a procedure that requires considerable experience and skill in both its performance and interpretation and for this reason has not been widely adopted. Furthermore, as clinical experience with the problem of venous thrombosis increases its practical diagnostic value diminishes.

Whether the diagnosis is merely suspected on the basis of these minimal findings or is established on the basis of the occurrence of a nonfatal pulmonary infarct, treatment consists in surgical exploration and division of the main venous channel above the clot. In the majority of instances, the operative site is just below the level of the junction of the superficial femoral vein and the profunda. In other cases, however, the process may have extended to such a level that ligation of the inferior vena cava becomes necessary. It is probably wiser in most cases, and especially in elderly patients, to perform the operation on both sides, since bilateral involvement is not uncommon and since experience has shown that pulmonary infarction or embolism not infrequently arises from the opposite, apparently normal side.

Although the surgical procedure of exposure of the femoral vein and its tributaries in the upper part of the thigh is not difficult, it requires knowledge of the local anatomy and careful operative technic. The patient lies on the table in the supine position, with the upper part of the body elevated to increase venous pressure and thus discourage infarction (Fig. 493a). Local infiltration analgesia (1 per cent procaine hydrochloride solution) is adequate. A longitudinal or slightly oblique incision is made, beginning at the inguinal crease, just medial to the femoral pulsation, and extending downward over the course of the femoral vessels for a distance of 8 to 10 cm. (Fig. 493b). After division of the superficial and deep fascia, the femoral vein and its tributaries are exposed by careful dissection. Because the femoral artery lies somewhat lateral to, but more or less over, the femoral vein, it is necessary to free the artery sufficiently to allow its gentle retraction laterally (Fig. 493c). After the common femoral (*superficial*), femoral, deep femoral (*profunda*), and saphenous veins have been identified and freed, coarse ligatures or, preferably, soft rubber tubes are loosely placed around them to provide a ready means of hemostasis later (Fig. 493c). The superficial vein is then opened between two stay sutures, by a transverse incision in its anterior wall (Fig. 493c).

If no thrombosis is found and if free bleeding occurs from all of the branches, which may be readily determined by successively compressing with

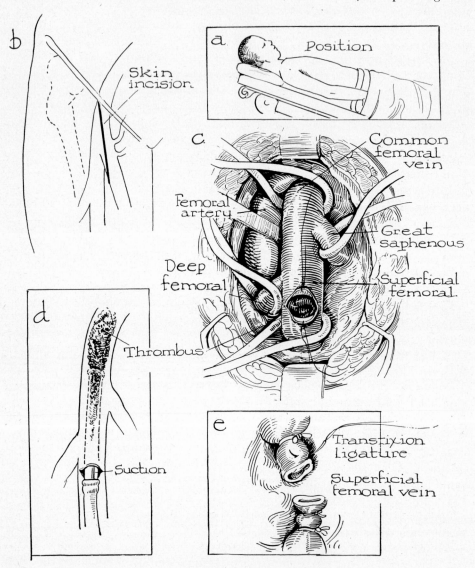

the encircling ligatures or soft rubber tubes all the branches except the one being tested, the vein is merely divided between double ligatures, those nearest the severed end being transfixion ties (Fig. 493e). If a thrombus, usually in the form of a soft, friable, nonadherent mass, is found, it is removed by gentle aspiration with a glass tube introduced into the upper segment (Fig. 493d). The lower segment may be treated in a similar manner. Complete removal of the clot is evidenced by free bleeding when all the branches are compressed but the one under consideration. If it is determined by this means that the profunda contains no clot, the superficial vein is divided between double ligatures as already described. If the deep femoral vein is also occluded, it is preferable to ligate it in continuity. The wound is closed in layers with interrupted sutures.

The postoperative management of these patients is similar to that already described, particularly as regards elevation of the foot of the bed, the use of elastic compression bandages, and early ambulation.

In the more advanced stages of this form of venous thrombosis, consideration must be given to surgical interruption of the vein at a higher level than that of the superficial femoral vein. Although some have advocated ligation of the common femoral following extraction of the clot above, there are certain disadvantages to interruption at this level. For one thing, it does not provide adequate assurance against recurrence of the process above this point, with subsequent pulmonary infarction. For another, as emphasized by Homans,[50] it does not allow an adequate collateral circulation and may therefore be followed by an acute, dangerous venous engorgement of the leg, especially in the presence of fairly extensive thrombosis of the lower venous channels.

For these reasons, and because the method provides a vastly superior collateral circulation, Homans[50] advocated ligation of the common iliac vein in cases of this sort. In a subsequent report,[53] however, he seemed to regard ligation of the vena cava as a more logical procedure under these circumstances, since it offers certain advantages over the former procedure, such as alleviation of the need for bilateral operation, and since it is associated with no greater hazard either in its performance or its sequelae than ligation of the common iliac vein. In fact, it may actually be a simpler procedure than iliac ligation, especially on the left side. This opinion has become increasingly widespread among surgeons interested in this problem.[80,83,99,110,116] Accordingly, it is now recommended that in cases in which deep vein interruption is indicated above the level of the superficial femo-

---

FIG. 493. Technic of exposure and ligation of femoral vein in phlebothrombosis. a. The patient is placed on the table in the supine position, with the upper part of the body elevated to increase venous pressure. b. Under local analgesia a longitudinal incision is made, beginning at the inguinal crease, just medial to the femoral pulsation, and extending downward over the course of the femoral vessels for a distance of about 8 to 10 cm. c. After division of the superficial and deep fascia, the femoral vein and its tributaries are exposed by careful dissection and coarse ligatures or, preferably, soft rubber tubes are loosely placed around them. The superficial vein is then opened between two stay sutures by a transverse incision in its anterior wall. If no thrombus is found and if free bleeding occurs from all of the branches, the vein is divided between double ligatures, those nearest the severed end being transfixion ties. d. If a thrombus, usually in the form of a soft, friable, nonadherent mass, is found, it is removed by gentle aspiration with a glass tube introduced into the upper and then the lower segments, e, following which the two ends of the veins are ligated and divided. If the deep femoral vein is also occluded, it is ligated near its junction with the superficial femoral vein.

ral vein that ligation of the vena cava be the procedure of choice. The available collateral channels which may function following vena caval ligation have been studied by a number of observers,[83,99,117,118] who emphasize their adequacy. It is further evidenced by clinical follow-up observations on these patients, who show remarkably few sequelae. The most extensive

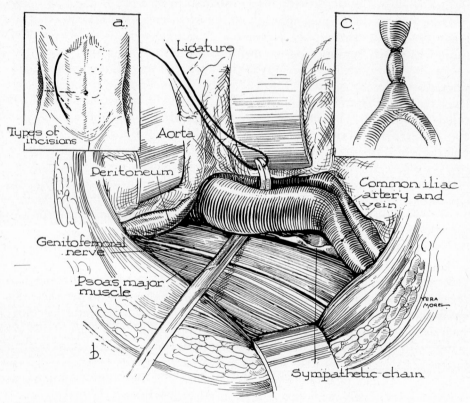

FIG. 494. Technic of extraperitoneal approach for ligation of vena cava. a. The incision which may be of several types, *i.e.*, transverse, oblique, or semilunar, is made in the right anterolateral region of the abdomen. b. The fibers of the external oblique, internal oblique, and transversus abdominis are successively separated in the direction in which they run, following which the parietal peritoneum is mobilized medially to expose the iliopsoas muscle and vena cava. After the vena cava has been gently freed of its surrounding structures, care being taken not to injure its small lumbar branches, coarse ligatures of silk or cotton are passed around the vessel. c. The two ligatures are secured around the vena cava about 1.5 cm. apart with the lower one tied just above the junction of the right and left veins.

clinical and physiologic observations of this kind were made by Ray and Burch, who studied 12 patients for periods up to four and one-half years following vena caval ligation. Their careful observations failed to reveal any detrimental effect from the ligation and showed complete circulatory adjustments.

The approach to the vena cava may be transperitoneal or extraperitoneal. The indications and technic for the former approaches have already been presented. The latter approach, which is preferred for the type of venous thrombosis under discussion here, is quite similar to that used for right lumbar sympathectomy.[89] Spinal or general anesthesia may be used, though the former is preferred. The patient lies in the supine position, with the right side slightly elevated by small pillows beneath the hip and shoulder. The incision, which may be of several types, *i.e.*, transverse, oblique, or semilunar, is made in the right anterolateral region of the abdomen (Fig. 494a). The fibers of the external oblique muscle and its aponeurosis are separated in the direction in which they run, thus exposing the internal oblique muscle. The fibers of this muscle and of the transversus abdominis, which lies immediately beneath it, are then split parallel to their course, thus exposing the peritoneum. The posterolateral and posterior parietal peritoneum, with the right ureter, is mobilized medially by blunt dissection to expose the iliopsoas muscle and the vena cava (Fig. 494b). Usually the vena cava is fairly mobile and easily compressed. It is gently freed of its surrounding structures at the level of the bifurcation of the aorta, care being taken not to injure its small lumbar branches, which can produce troublesome bleeding. A coarse ligature, such as heavy braided silk or No. 8 cotton, is passed around the vessel by means of a curved ligature carrier and is tied securely (Fig. 494b). A second ligature is similarly secured around the vessel about 1.5 cm. higher (Fig. 494c). It is preferable not to open and explore the vessel. The wound is then closed in layers with interrupted sutures.

The postoperative care of these patients is much the same as that already described above, particularly as regards elevation of the foot of the bed, the use of elastic compression bandages, and early ambulation.

REFERENCES

1. ADAMS, JOHN C. Etiologic Factors in Varicose Veins of the Lower Extremities, *Surg., Gynec. & Obst.*, 69:717-725, [Dec.], 1939.
2. ADAMS, RALPH. The Treatment of Varicose Veins and Varicose Ulcers, *Surg. Clin. North America*, 22:933-944, [June], 1942.
3. ALLEN, ARTHUR W. Interruption of the Deep Veins of the Lower Extremities in the Prevention and Treatment of Thrombosis and Embolism, *Surg., Gynec. & Obst.*, 84:519-527, [April 15], 1947.
4. ALLEN, A. W., LINTON, R. R. and DONALDSON, G. A. Venous Thrombosis and Pulmonary Embolism: Further Experience with Thrombectomy and Femoral Vein Interruption, *J.A.M.A.*, 128:397-403, 1945.
5. ATLAS, LAWRENCE N. Hazards Connected with the Treatment of Varicose Veins, *Surg., Gynec. & Obst.*, 77:136-140, [Aug.], 1943.
6. BABCOCK, W. W. A New Operation for the Extirpation of Varicose Veins of the Leg, *New York Med. J.*, 86:153, 1907.
7. BARKER, NELSON W. Anticoagulant Therapy. Modern Concepts of Cardiovascular Disease, *Am. Heart Assoc.*, 15 [No. 11]: [Nov.], 1946, New York.
8. BARKER, NELSON W., CROMER, HORACE E., HURN, MARGARET and WAUGH, JOHN M. The Use of Dicumarol in the Prevention of Postoperative Thrombosis and Embolism with Special Reference to Dosage and Safe Administration, *Surgery*, 17:207-217, [Feb.], 1945.

9. BAUER, G. A Venographic Study of Thromboembolic Problems, *Acta chir. Scandinav.*, 84:1, 1940.

10. BAUER, G. Roentgenological and Clinical Study of Sequels of Thrombosis, *Acta chir. Scandinav.*, (Supp. 74), 86:1-116, 1942.

11. BAUER, G. Heparin Therapy in Acute Deep Venous Thrombosis, *J.A.M.A.*, 131: 196-203, 1946.

12. BAUER, G. Thrombosis. Early Diagnosis and Abortive Treatment with Heparin, *Lancet*, 1:447, 1946.

13. BEECHER, H. K. Adjustment of the Flow of Tissue Fluid in the Presence of Localized Sustained High Venous Pressure as Found with Varices of the Great Saphenous System During Walking, *J. Clin. Investigation*, 16:733, 1937.

14. BERGERET, A., GUILLAUME, A. C. and DeLARUE, J. Gangrène ischemique de membre inférieur par thrombose oblitérante de la totalité des veines. *Ann. d'anat. path.*, 9:536, [May], 1932.

15. BRODIE, SIR B. *Lectures Illustrative of Various Subjects in Pathology and Surgery*, 7:411, Longmans, Green and Co., London, 1846.

16. CHAPMAN, E. M. and ASMUSSEN, E. On the Occurrence of Dyspnea, Dizziness and Precordial Distress Occasioned by the Pooling of Blood in Varicose Veins, *J. Clin. Investigation*, 21:393, 1942.

17. COLLINS, CONRAD G., JONES, JACK R. and NELSON, EDWARD W. Surgical Treatment of Pelvic Thrombophlebitis. Ligation of Inferior Vena Cava and Ovarian Veins. A Preliminary Report, *New Orleans Med. & Surg. J.*, 95:324-329, [Jan.], 1943.

18. COLLINS, CONRAD G. and NELSON, EDWARD W. Phlebothrombosis and Thrombophlebitis in Gynecology and Obstetrics, *Am. J. Obst. & Gynec.*, 52:946-959, [Dec.], 1946.

19. COLLINS, CONRAD G., NELSON, EDWARD W., JONES, J. R., WEINSTEIN, B. B. and THOMAS, P. Ligation of the Vena Cava. A Critical Evaluation Based on a Study of 22 Cases, *New Orleans Med. & Surg. J.*, 99:488-493, [April], 1947.

20. COOPER, WILLIAM M. Modern Treatment of Varicose Veins, with Special Reference to the Use of Synasol as a Sclerosing Agent, *New York State J. Med.*, 44:2483-2487, [Nov. 15], 1944.

21. CRAFOORD, G. Heparin as Prophylactic Against Postoperative Thrombosis, *Acta med. Scandinav.*, 107:116-122, 1941.

22. DASELER, EDWARD H., ANSON, BARRY J., REIMANN, ARTHUR F. and BEATON, LINDSAY E. The Saphenous Venous Tributaries and Related Structures in Relation to the Technique of High Ligation Based Chiefly Upon a Study of 550 Anatomical Dissections, *Surg., Gynec. & Obst.*, 82:53-63, [Jan.], 1946.

23. DEBAKEY, M. E. Discussion of Collins, Jones, and Nelson, *New Orleans Med. & Surg. J.*, 95:328-329, [Jan.], 1943.

24. DEBAKEY, M. E. Dicoumarin and Prophylactic Anticoagulants in Intravascular Thrombosis, *Surgery*, 13:456-459, [March], 1943.

25. DEBAKEY, MICHAEL. Traumatic Vasospasm, *Bull. U. S. Army Med. Dept.*, No. 73, [Feb.], 1944.

26. DE BAKEY, MICHAEL, BURCH, G. E. and OCHSNER, ALTON. Effect of Chemical Irritation of Venous Segment on Peripheral Pulse Volumes, *Proc. Soc. Exper. Biol. and Med.*, 41:585, [June], 1939.

27. DEBAKEY, MICHAEL and OCHSNER, ALTON. Novocain Sympathetic Block Method of Therapy in Thrombophlebitis, *J. M. A. Alabama*, 11:87, 1941.

28. DEBAKEY, MICHAEL, OCHSNER, ALTON and SMITH, MARVIN C. Primary Thrombosis of the Axillary Vein, *New Orleans Med. & Surg. J.*, 95:62-70, [Aug.], 1942.

29. DEBAKEY, MICHAEL E., SCHROEDER, GEORGE F. and OCHSNER, ALTON. Significance of Phlebography in Phlebothrombosis, *J.A.M.A.*, 123:738-744, [Nov. 20], 1943.

30. DE TAKATS, G. E. Ambulatory Ligation of the Saphenous Veins, *J.A.M.A.*, 94:1194, 1930.

31. DE TAKATS, GÉZA. Ligation of the Saphenous Vein. A Report on Two Hundred Ambulatory Operations, *Arch. Surg.*, 26:72-88, [Jan.], 1933.

32. DE TAKATS, GÉZA and FOWLER, EDSON FAIRBROTHER. The Problem of Thrombo-embolism, *Surgery*, 17:153-175, [Feb.], 1945.

33. DE TAKATS, GÉZA and QUINT, HAROLD. The Injection Treatment of Varicose Veins, *Surg., Gynec. & Obst.*, 50:545, [March], 1930.

34. DE TAKATS, G., QUINT, H. and TILLOTSON, B. I. The Impairment of Circulation in the Varicose Extremity, *Arch. Surg.*, 18:671, 1929.

35. DOBSON, LEONARD. Sodium Morrhuate Reactions. Report of Two Severe Reactions During the Injection Treatment of Varicose Veins, *Ann. Surg.*, 111:645-649, 1940.

36. DOS SANTOS, J. La Phlébographie Directe Conception, Technique, Premier Résultats, *J. internat. de chir.*, 3:625, 1938; 8:206, 1947.

37. DOUGHERTY, JOHN and HOMANS, JOHN. Venography: A Clinical Study, *Surg., Gynec. & Obst.*, 71:697, [Dec.], 1940.

38. EGER, S. A. and CASPER, S. L. Etiology of Varicose Veins from an Anatomical Aspect, Based on Dissection of 38 Adult Cadavers, *J.A.M.A.*, 57:196-198, 1942.

39. EVANS, J. A. and BOLLER, R. J. Subcutaneous Use of Heparin in Anticoagulation Therapy, *J.A.M.A.*, 131:879, 1946.

40. FAXON, H. H. Treatment of Varicosities: Preliminary High Ligation of the Internal Saphenous Vein with Injection of Sclerosing Solutions, *Arch. Surg.*, 29:794, 1934.

41. FRYKHOLM, R. The Pathogenesis and Mechanical Prophylaxis of Venous Thrombosis, *Surg., Gynec. & Obst.*, 71:307-312, 1940.

42. GLASSER, S. THOMAS. A New Sclerosing Drug for Varicose Veins—Monolate, *Am. J. Surg.*, 39:120, 1938.

43. GOLDEN, R. F. and HEYERDALE, W. W. Sensitivity to Sodium Morrhuate and Monoethanolamine Oleate (Monolate); Report of a Case, *Proc. Staff Meet. Mayo Clinic*, 15:436, 1940.

44. GRÉGOIRE, R. La Répercussion de l'inflammation des veines sur le système artériel collatéral, *Mém. Acad. de chir.*, 64:363, [April 27], 1938.

45. HARKINS, HENRY N. and SCHUG, RICHARD. The Surgical Management of Varicose Veins: Importance of Individualization in the Choice of Procedure, *Surgery*, 11:402-421, [March], 1942.

46. HELLER, R. E. The Pathologic Physiology of Varicose Veins, *Surg. Gynec. & Obst.*, 71:566, 1940.

47. HODGE, G. B., GRIMSON, K. S. and SCHRIBEL, H. M. Treatment of Varicose Veins by Stripping, Excision and Evulsion, *Ann. Surg.*, 121:737-749, [May], 1945.

48. HOMANS, J. The Operative Treatment of Varicose Veins and Ulcers, Based upon a Classification of These Lesions, *Surg., Gynec. & Obst.*, 22:143, 1916.

49. HOMANS, JOHN. Thrombosis of the Deep Veins of the Lower Leg Causing Pulmonary Embolism, *New England J. Med.*, 211:993, 1934.

50. HOMANS, JOHN. Deep Quiet Venous Thrombosis in the Lower Limb. Preferred Levels for Interruption of Veins; Iliac Sector or Ligation, *Surg., Gynec. & Obst.*, 79:70-82, [July], 1944.

51. HOMANS, JOHN. Diseases of the Veins, *New England J. Med.*, 231:51, [July 13], 1944.

52. HOMANS, JOHN. The Surgery of the Veins of the Legs: Varicosity and Some Problems in Thrombosis, *Rhode Island M. J.*, 28:565-569, 1945.

53. HOMANS, JOHN. Diseases of the Veins, *New England J. Med.*, 235:163-167, 193-198 and 249-253, [Aug. 1, 8 and 22], 1946.

54. HORGAN, EDMUND. Varicose Veins, with Special Reference to Treatment by Ligation, Stripping, and Injection, *Surgery*, 3:528, 1938.

55. HOWARD, N. J., JACKSON, C. R. and MAHON, E. J. Recurrence of Varicose Veins Following Injection: A Study of the Pathologic Nature of the Recurrence and a Critical Survey of the Injection Method, *Arch. Surg.*, 22:353, 1931.

56. HUNTER, W. C., SNEEDEN, V. D., ROBERTSON, T. D. and SNYDER, G. A. C. Thrombosis of Deep Veins of Leg. Its Clinical Significance as Exemplified in 351 Autopsies, *Arch. Int. Med.*, 68:1-17, 1941.

57. HUNTER, W. C., KRYGIER, J. J., KENNEDY, J. C. and SNEEDEN, V. D. Etiology and Prevention of Thrombosis of the Deep Leg Veins, *Surgery,* 17:178-189, [Feb.], 1945.

58. JORPES, J. ERIK. Anticoagulant Therapy in Thrombosis, *Edinburgh M. J.,* 53:222, 1946; also *Surg., Gynec. & Obst.,* 84:677, [April 15], 1947.

59. KELLER, W. L. A New Method of Extirpating the Internal Saphenous and Similar Veins in Varicose Conditions: A Preliminary Report, *New York Med. J.,* 82:385, 1905.

60. LÄWEN, A. Arteriospasmus bei akuter massiver Thrombose der v. Femoralis, *Zentralbl. f. chir.,* 61:1681-1685, 1934.

61. LERICHE, R. Traitement chirurgical des suites éloignées, des phlébites et des grands oedémes non médicaux des membres inférieurs, *Bull. et mém. Soc. nat. de chir.,* 53:187, [Feb. 19], 1927.

62. LERICHE, R. Sur l'importance de la périphlébite dans la genése des accidents tardifs consécutifs aux oblitérations veineuses, *Bull. et mém. Soc. nat. de chir.,* 53:561-565, 1927.

63. LERICHE, RENÉ. *Les embolies de l'artére pulmonaire et des artéres des membres; physiologie pathologique et traitement,* Masson & Cie, Paris, 1947.

64. LERICHE, R. and KUNLIN, J. Traitement immédiat des phlébites post-opératoires par l'infiltration novocainique du sympathique lombaire, *Presse méd.,* 42:1481, 1934.

65. LINTON, ROBERT R. The Communicating Veins of the Lower Leg and the Operative Technic for Their Ligation, *Ann. Surg.,* 107:582-593, 1938.

66. LINTON, R. R. A New Surgical Technic for the Treatment of Postphlebitic Varicose Ulcers of the Lower Leg, *New England J. Med.,* 219:367-373, 1938.

67. LINTON, ROBERT R. and KEELEY, J. KENNETH. The Postphlebitic Varicose Ulcer. Surgical Treatment with Special Reference to the Communicating Veins of the Lower Leg, *Am. Heart J.,* 17:27-39, 1939.

68. LINTON, R. R. Diagnosis and Treatment of Thromboembolic Disease, *M. Clin. North America,* 1068, [Sept.], 1946.

69. MAGENDIE, J. and TINGAUD, R. Phlébite a forme pseudoembolique—Phlébite bleue de Grégoire, *Bordeaux chir.,* 3 and 4:112, 1945.

70. MAHORNER, H. R. and OCHSNER, ALTON. A New Test for Evaluating Circulation in the Venous System of the Lower Extremity Affected by Varicosities, *Arch. Surg.,* 33:479, 1936.

71. MAHORNER, H. R. and OCHSNER, ALTON. The Modern Treatment of Varicose Veins as Indicated by the Comparative Tourniquet Test, *Ann. Surg.,* 107:927, 1938.

72. MATAS, R. On So-called Primary Thrombosis of Axillary Vein Caused by Strain: Report of Case with Comments on Diagnosis, Pathogeny, and Treatment of this Lesion in its Medico-legal Relations, *Am. J. Surg.,* 24:642, 1934.

73. MAYERSON, H. S., LONG, CARROL H. and GILES, E. J. Venous Pressures in Patients with Varicose Veins, *Surgery,* 14:519-525, [Oct.], 1943.

74. MAYO, C. H. Treatment of Varicose Veins, *Surg., Gynec. & Obst.,* 2:385, 1906.

75. MCPHEETERS, H. O. Saphenofemoral Ligation with the Immediate Retrograde Injection, *Surg., Gynec. & Obst.,* 81:355-364, [Oct.], 1945.

76. MCPHEETERS, H. O., MERKERT, C. E. and LUNDBLAD, R. A. The Mechanics of the Reverse Flow of Blood in Varicose Veins as Proved by Blood Pressure Readings, *Surg., Gynec. & Obst.,* 55:298, 1932.

77. MCPHEETERS, H. O. and RICE, C. O. Varicose Veins; Complications Direct and Indirect, *J.A.M.A.,* 91:1090, 1928.

78. MEIGS, JOE V. and INGERSOLL, FRANCIS M. Thrombophlebitis and Phlebothrombosis in Gynecologic Patients; the Prophylaxis, Recognition and Treatment, *Am. J. Obst. & Gynec.,* 52:938-945, [Dec.], 1946.

79. MEYER, NATHANIEL E. Monoethanolamine Oleate—a New Chemical for the Obliteration of Varicose Veins, *Am. J. Surg.,* 40:628-629, 1938.

80. MOSES, WILLIAM R.   Ligation of the Inferior Vena Cava or Iliac Veins. A Report of Thirty-six Operations, *New England J. Med.*, 235:1, 1946.

81. MURRAY, GORDON.   Anticoagulants in Venous Thrombosis and the Prevention of Pulmonary Embolism, *Surg., Gynec. & Obst.*, 84:665-668, [April 15], 1947.

82. NEUMANN, R.   Ursprungszentren und Entwicklungs formen der Bein-Thrombose, *Virchows Arch. f. path. Anat.*, 301:708-735, 1938.

83. NORTHWAY, ROBERT O. and BUXTON, ROBERT W.   Ligation of the Inferior Vena Cava, *Surgery*, 18:85-94, 1945.

84. OCHSNER, ALTON.   *Varicosities of the Lower Extremity. Lewis' Practice of Surgery*, W. F. Prior Co. Inc., Hagerstown, Md., Vol. XII, Chap. 5a, 1944.

85. OCHSNER, ALTON and DeBAKEY, MICHAEL.   Treatment of Thrombophlebitis by Novocaine Block of Sympathetics; Technique of Injection, *Surgery*, 5:491-497, [April], 1939.

86. OCHSNER, ALTON and DeBAKEY, MICHAEL.   Thrombophlebitis and Phlebothrombosis, *The Southern Surgeon*, 8:269-290, [Aug.], 1939.

87. OCHSNER, ALTON and DeBAKEY, MICHAEL.   Thrombophlebitis. The Role of Vasospasm in the Production of the Clinical Manifestations, *J.A.M.A.*, 114:117-123, [Jan. 13], 1940.

88. OCHSNER, ALTON and DeBAKEY, MICHAEL.   Therapy of Phlebothrombosis and Thrombophlebitis, *Arch. Surg.*, 40:208-231, [Feb.], 1940.

89. OCHSNER, ALTON and DeBAKEY, MICHAEL.   Peripheral Vascular Disease. A Critical Survey of its Conservative and Radical Treatment, *Surg., Gynec. & Obst.*, 70: 1058-1072, [June], 1940.

90. OCHSNER, ALTON and DeBAKEY, MICHAEL.   Therapeutic Considerations of Thrombophlebitis and Phlebothrombosis, *New England J. Med.*, 225:207-227, 1941.

91. OCHSNER, ALTON and DeBAKEY, MICHAEL.   Intravenous Clotting and Its Sequelae, *Surgery*, 14:679-690 [Nov.], 1943.

92. OCHSNER, ALTON and DeBAKEY, MICHAEL.   *Thrombophlebitis and Phlebothrombosis in Lewis' System of Surgery*, Vol. 12, Chapter 5b, W. F. Prior Co., Hagerstown, Md., 1945.

93. OCHSNER, A. and GARSIDE, E.   The Intravenous Injection of Sclerosing Substances, *Ann. Surg.*, 96:69, 1932.

94. OCHSNER, A. and MAHORNER, H.   Comparative Value of Intravenous Sclerosing Solution, *Arch. Surg.*, 29:397, 1934.

95. OCHSNER, A. and MAHORNER, H.   Histologic Effects of Intravenous Sclerosing Solutions and Subcutaneous Tissues, *Arch. Surg.*, 30:573, 1935.

96. OCHSNER, A. and MAHORNER, H.   The Modern Treatment of Varicose Veins, *Surgery*, 2:889, 1937.

97. OCHSNER, ALTON and MAHORNER, H.   *Varicose Veins*, C. V. Mosby Co., St. Louis, 1939.

98. OGDEN, ERIC and SHERMAN, R. STANTON.   Physiologic Considerations in the Care of Patients with Varicose Veins, *Arch. Surg.*, 52:402, 1946.

99. O'NEIL, E. EVERETT.   Ligation of the Inferior Vena Cava in the Prevention and Treatment of Pulmonary Embolism, *New England J. Med.*, 232:641-646, [May 31], 1945.

100. PENNOYER, G. P.   Injection Treatment of Varicose Veins, *Ann. Surg.*, 91:416, 1930.

101. PERTHES, G.   Über die Operation der Unterschenkelvaricen nach Trendelenburg, *Deutsche med. Wchnschr.*, 21:253, 1895.

102. PRIOLEAU, W. H.   Complications Connected with the Treatment of Varicose Veins in the Legs, *J. South Carolina M. A.*, 37:204-206, 1941.

103. RAY, C. THORPE and BURCH, GEORGE.   Vascular Responses to Ligation of the Inferior Vena Cava in Man, *Arch. Int. Med.*, (In press).

104. ROSSLE, R.   Über die Bedentung und die Entstehung der Wadenvenenthrombosen, *Virchows Arch. f. path. Anat.*, 300:180-189, 1937.

105. SEIRO, V.   Blood Pressure and Circulation in Veins of Lower Extremities, *Acta chir. Scandinav.*, 80:41, 1937.

106. SHELLEY, HAROLD J. Allergic Manifestations with Injection Treatment of Varicose Veins. Death Following an Injection of Monoethanolamine Oleate, *J.A.M.A.*, 112:1792-1794, [May 6], 1939.

107. SHERMAN, R. STANTON. Varicose Veins. Anatomic Findings and an Operative Procedure Based upon Them, *Arch. Surg.*, 120:772-784, [Nov.], 1944.

108. SMITHY, H. G. Complicating Factors in the Surgical Management of Varicose Veins with Special Reference to Interruption of Sympathetic Nerve Impulses as an Adjunct in Treatment, *Surgery*, 17:590-605, [April], 1945.

109. TAVEL, E. Behandlung der Varicen durch die Ligatur und die kunstliche Thrombose, *Cor.-Bl. f. Schweiz, Aerzte*, 34:617, 1904.

110. THEBAUT, BEN R. and WARD, CHARLES S. Ligation of the Inferior Vena Cava in Thromboembolism. Report of 36 Cases, *Surg., Gynec. & Obst.*, 84:385-400, [April], 1947.

111. TRENDELENBURG, J. Über die Unterbindung der Vena saphena magna bei Unterschenkelvaricen, *Beitr. z. klin. Chir.*, 7:195, 1890-1891.

112. VAUGHN, ARKELL M. Multiple Retrograde Saphenous Vein Ligation and Phlebectomy with Aid of Malleable Intraluminal Guide, *Surgery*, 21:851-860, [June], 1947.

113. VAUGHN, ARKELL M. and LEES, WILLIAM M. Fatal Pulmonary Embolism Following Varicose Vein Injection. Report of a Case and Review of the Literature, *J.A.M.A.*, 118:1293-1296, [April 11], 1942.

114. VEAL, J. R. and McFETRIDGE, E. M. Primary Thrombosis of the Axillary Vein, *Arch. Surg.*, 31:271, 1935.

115. VEAL, J. R. and VAN WERDEN, B. D. The Physiologic Basis for Ligation of Great Saphenous Vein in the Treatment of Varicose Veins, *Am. J. Surg.*, 40:426, 1938.

116. VEAL, J. ROSS, HUSSEY, HUGH HUDSON and BARNES, EARL. Ligation of the Inferior Vena Cava in Thrombosis of the Deep Veins of the Lower Extremity, *Surg., Gynec. & Obst.*, 84:605, [April 15], 1947.

117. WARREN, J. V. and WEENS, H. S. Venographic Studies Following Ligation of the Inferior Vena Cava (To be published). (Quoted by Thebaut and Ward.)

118. WEINSTEIN, B. B. Discussion of COLLINS, C. G., JONES, J. R. and NELSON, E. W., *New Orleans Med. & Surg. J.*, 95:324, 1942-43.

119. WRIGHT, A. DICKSON. Treatment of Varicose Veins, *Brit. M. J.*, 1:665-668, 1940.

120. ZIMMERMAN, LEO M. Allergic-like Reactions from Sodium Morrhuate: in Obliteration of Varicose Veins, *J.A.M.A.*, 102:1216-1217, [April 14], 1934.

22

SURGERY OF THE HAND AND ITS TENDONS

Harvey S. Allen, M.D. and Sumner L. Koch, M.D.

A few principles of good surgical technic are applicable to every phase of hand surgery and should be stressed at the outset. They concern particularly the preparation of the field of operation, the anesthetic, the use of a bloodless field, the equipment in the operating room, the use of compression bandages and splints and postoperative care.

THE PREPARATION OF THE FIELD OF OPERATION

To attain the surgical cleanliness that reduces the risk of infection to a minimum and favors rapid wound healing, we have found nothing so effective as soap and water cleansing, whether for operations of election or immediately after extensive injuries. For the first group of cases washing with soap and water for at least twenty minutes, careful cleansing of the nails and protection of the cleansed hand and forearm with a sterile dressing are the essential steps carried out the day before operation. In the operating room the hand is uncovered and washed again for ten minutes with large squares of soft sterile cotton, plain white soap and sterile water. Finally the soap suds are rinsed off with sterile water. We have used no chemical antiseptics in preparation of the operative field for a number of years and have come to believe that the method described, combined with good technic in the operating room, provides the most favorable conditions to insure wound healing without infection.

THE ANESTHETIC

A general anesthetic is usually preferred. Sodium pentothal, because of ease of induction, has definite advantages. It can often be used alone, particularly for incision of the infected hand; or it can be combined with ethylene or nitrous oxide. Occasionally a local anesthetic, such as procaine hydrochloride in 0.50 per cent solution and without adrenalin, can be used to advantage for removal of simple tumors, ganglia and similar conditions. We purposely avoid the use of a local anesthetic in the presence of infection and have seen so many serious local complications following the use of freezing anesthetics that we believe they have no place in the surgery of the hand. For the more serious and extensive surgical operations on the hand we use a general anesthetic, preferably ethylene or nitrous oxide.

THE BLOODLESS FIELD

No single aid is of more importance to the surgeon operating upon the extremities than a bloodless field. It permits accurate visualization of structures essential for function. It avoids the necessity for and the trauma of constant sponging. It can make the work of the surgeon precise and exact instead of difficult and uncertain. It can be secured effectively with the ordinary blood pressure apparatus.

A few layers of gauze are first laid about the arm to protect the underlying skin. The blood pressure cuff is applied smoothly, not tightly. A bandage is then applied over the cuff so as to cover it completely and prevent the rubber bag from "herniating" from beneath the cloth band when the cuff is inflated to 260 mm. of mercury.

We have not found it necessary to bandage the extremity with a taut rubber bandage from finger tips to upper arm to empty it of blood. Just before the operation is begun the extremity is elevated for a moment to allow it to empty itself of blood. The cuff is then inflated to 260 mm. This pressure is maintained until the dissection is completed. The pressure is then released and any bleeding vessels caught and ligated. The extremity is then elevated again, the cuff reinflated and repair carried out. The pressure is finally released only after the operation is completed and the final compression bandage has been applied. Though we have seen cases in which nerve palsy has followed the use of rubber bandages and a pneumatic tourniquet inflated to a pressure of 15 pounds, we have never seen this complication following the use of a blood pressure cuff in the manner described.

THE OPERATING EQUIPMENT

An arm board which can be attached to the operating table and whose outer end is supported firmly on a separate pedestal gives firm support to the extremity during the operation. Fine instruments, particularly small "mosquito" hemostats, small tissue forceps—"Adson forceps"—and small retractors—"Senn retractors"—are essential for accurate and painstaking work. The finest suture material that gives the required tensile strength is advantageous in that it leaves a minimum of foreign material in the tissues.

For suturing tendons, No. 6 or No. 8 silk (Champion scale) on small straight needles is most frequently used. For securing apposition of tendon ends and for nerve sutures, 6-0 or 8-0 silk swaged on fine curved needles, such as the ophthalmologists use for cataract operations, has proved very satisfactory. For ligating blood vessels very fine white silk, and for fascial closure the same silk on small curved needles is preferred.

It is hardly necessary to add that incisions must be parallel to flexion creases and not across them, that gentle handling of tissues, avoiding trauma of important structures, such as tendons and nerves, careful hemostasis, the use of warm salt solution as an irrigating solution, combined with suction to remove excess fluid, and finally accurate suture of the deep fascia to provide a protecting and retaining layer of fibrous tissue over sutured tendons and nerves are all of help in achieving a good result.

COMPRESSION BANDAGES AND SPLINTS

Over the sutured wound a large mass of gauze fluff is bandaged with compression before the blood pressure cuff is deflated. As the last step of the dressing, a splint is added to hold the extremity in the desired position— the position which provides maximum relaxation of sutured nerves or tendons. Light aluminum splints, cut from sheet aluminum No. S ½ H and 0.064 inch in thickness have proved very satisfactory from the standpoint of weight and tensile strength. If desired, such splints can be sterilized for incorporation in a sterile dressing. At a later stage they can be fitted with felt and straps to give freedom from rigid pressure and permit easy application and removal. Ordinarily the postoperative dressing is left unchanged for from four to six days, unless some definite indications arise for inspecting the wound. At the first dressing any tight skin sutures can be divided and a part of the bulky dressing removed. Constant cleanly care to avoid the possibility of adding infection is as important in the postoperative care as in the operating room.

POSTOPERATIVE CARE

After wound healing has taken place there often remain swelling, inflammatory reaction and induration which cause discomfort and pain and delay the return of function. No form of physical therapy is more helpful at this stage than soaking the hand in warm soapy water for ten or fifteen minutes three times daily, massaging it gently with a soft wash cloth and carrying out active and passive movements through as wide a range as possible without causing undue swelling and pain. Warmth, moisture and gentle massage are the most effective measures for stimulating the circulation and the flow of blood through the tissues—the most important factor in restoring injured tissues to normal. Forceful movements, vigorous massage and, particularly, mobilization of joints with the aid of an anesthetic have in our experience more often proved harmful than helpful, and have too often delayed recovery instead of hastening it.

COMPOUND INJURIES OF THE HAND

First Aid. The successful outcome of a hand injury is often jeopardized by improper first aid. Great harm can be done by pouring strong antiseptics into the wound; they not only injure tissues but discolor them and can make difficult identification of important structures.

First aid should be limited to the simple application of sterile dressings. Bleeding can be controlled by applying pressure over the sterile dressings. A splint should be added to the dressing and the patient immediately transferred to a well equipped emergency room.

Diagnosis. Diagnosis of the extent of the injury to the hand can often be made without removal of the first aid dressings or manipulation of the wound. Probing a wound to determine the extent of damage to nerves or tendons is a dangerous practice. Tendon damage can be correctly estimated by testing the motion at the joints of each finger. Nerve injury can be recognized by testing the sensation of the fingers with a cotton applicator. Loss of sensation indicates damage to the median, ulnar or digital nerves. If the hand has been crushed an x-ray examination should be made to ascertain the extent of bone injury.

General Considerations. The important objectives of treatment are conversion of the wound into a clean wound, its repair and closure, and early restoration of function of the part.

Before determining a definite plan of treatment several factors should be considered. The type of injury is an important consideration. A clean cut wound sustained in a factory or home is very different from one resulting from a human bite. In the latter case primary repair of the deeper structures and skin should not be undertaken. The interval of time between the injury and definitive care is very important. The "golden period" of time in which it is safe to repair divided nerves and tendons without danger of subsequent infection is considered to be from two to four hours. After this time it is better simply to cleanse and débride the wound, approximate skin edges without tension and provide rest for the part. Other factors than the time interval, however, may contraindicate definitive operation during the "golden period." The most important of these is the type of first aid administered to the wound. If there has been manipulation, probing or undue exposure of the wound, or if there has been a previous and ineffectual attempt at surgery of this wound, it is not wise to attempt repair of the deeper divided structures. If the wound has been properly cared for during the first few hours, it is entirely logical to undertake the repair of deeper structures, to unite divided nerves and tendons and to close the wound without drainage. Only in unusual circumstances a few strips of rubber tissue are inserted for drainage.

Treatment of Compound Injuries of the Hand. Simple lacerations with exposure of deeper structures only require closure. A superficial loss of skin and subcutaneous tissue should be replaced immediately with a graft of part thickness skin. With the aid of anesthesia such a graft can be secured from the volar surface of the forearm with a razor blade or scalpel.

CRUSHED FINGER TIPS. There may be severe crushing of the distal phalanx resulting in a "bursting" type of wound along the lateral aspect of the pulp, or there may be actual loss of part of the finger. It is important to accomplish closure of these wounds without sacrificing more of the digit; it is equally important not to suture the wound under tension.

Where the skin is pale and bloodless, it is wise to excise the crushed skin and replace it with a skin graft. An x-ray examination should be made to determine the possibility of a fracture of the distal phalanx. Since union of such fractures is slow the prognosis after a crushing injury should be guarded.

In case of actual amputation of the finger tip, closure may be accomplished under a local anesthetic. After preparation of the wound the jagged subcutaneous tissue and skin are excised. If the bone is bare and extends beyond the soft tissue, it may be removed just proximal to this level. The adjacent soft tissue is brought over the end of the bone and the remaining defect is closed by a skin graft.

In the case of amputation at a higher level the digital nerves are identified, drawn into the wound and 3 to 4 mm. removed, so that nerve ends do not become adherent to the scar at the tip of the finger.

Closure of amputated finger tips by undermining the skin edges and suturing them under tension results in slow healing of the wound and a sensitive stump. Suture of the flexor and extensor tendons over the end of the bone always produces disability because the sutured tendons are fixed and restrict free movement of adjacent tendons.

If the thumb is injured it is imperative that all possible length be preserved. Simple amputation should never be considered in order to obtain closure. If it is impossible to close the end of the stump by approximation of soft tissues and application of a graft, other methods such as the application of a flap of skin and subcutaneous tissue from the abdominal wall should be considered. The hand and arm are supported by a plaster cast to relieve tension on the wound edges. The pedicle of the flap may be divided after three weeks.

CRUSHING INJURIES. Typical of crushing injuries to the hand is the "wringer injury." It may be of any degree from contusion with hematoma formation beneath the subcutaneous tissues to actual avulsion of the tissues from the hand and forearm. The most severe wound is most commonly found on the dorsum of the hand.

Whether the injury is caused by a wringer or by some other mechanism, it is always difficult immediately after injury to judge correctly as to the vitality of the crushed tissues. If one has erred in judgment and attempted to save flaps of tissue which show definite evidence of necrosis after an interval of 48 or 72 hours it is wise not to delay unduly excision of the necrotic tissue. To wait for spontaneous separation and development of the low-grade infection which invariably accompanies tissue necrosis only prolongs convalescence and delays healing.

It is after crushing injuries, too, that gas gangrene is most likely to develop. The possibility of such a complication should always be kept in mind, particularly if the injury has occurred out of doors and the wound has been contaminated with soil or street dirt.

If the skin is not broken there may be only swelling as a result of hemorrhage, or the skin may be lifeless and parchment-like. Even in the former case the overlying skin may eventually become gangrenous and slough. When first seen, the hand should be cleansed, covered with a sterile compression pressure dressing and supported by a splint to maintain the hand in the position of function. This prevents an accumulation of fluid and aids the return of circulation in the part. If the skin is lifeless or has been avulsed from the hand, repair of the wound should be carried out immediately. Under a general anesthetic the wound is cleansed and the flaps of tissue evaluated as to their viability. All avascular and colorless tissue is removed to the level of actual bleeding and the resulting defect closed with an intermediate

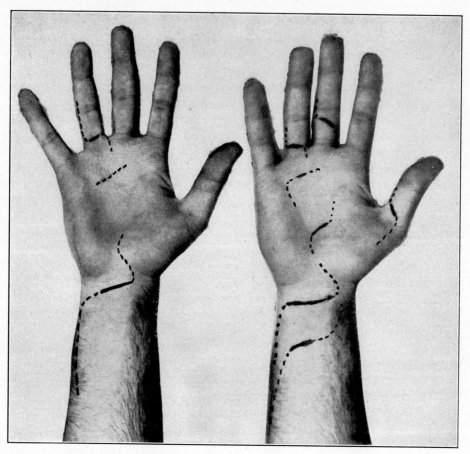

FIG. 495. Methods of enlarging accidental wounds to provide adequate exposure. The dotted lines represent the enlarging incisions. (From Mason, *Surg., Gynec. & Obst.,* 70(2A):392-402, 1940. By permission of Surgery, Gynecology and Obstetrics.)

thickness skin graft. Occasionally a pedicled flap may be required to obtain a satisfactory closure.

Repair of Divided Nerves and Tendons. The repair of divided nerves and tendons is a major procedure and should be performed under general anesthesia. The operation is invariably time consuming and difficult; adequate assistance and suitable equipment are essential for a successful result. Divided tendons separate and the proximal or distal segments may retract a considerable distance from the site of the wound. Adequate exposure by extension of the wound must be obtained in order to identify and suture the injured structures. Divided nerves do not separate as widely as do tendons, but in most instances the wound must be enlarged to obtain adequate exposure.

Correctly placed incisions are important in any operation on the hand (Fig. 495) if one is to avoid scar contractures. If enlargement of the wound is necessary a midline incision should be avoided whenever possible and lateral extensions made at each end of the wound. The extended incision should either follow the lines of skin cleavage or be made along the lateral surface of the hand, the wrist or the fingers. The angles created by enlarging the wound should be made as wide as possible to avoid necrosis at the corners.

In some cases it may be possible to expose the ends of the retracted tendons through a new incision along the lines of skin cleavage or along the lateral aspect of the wrist or digits and at a calculated distance proximal to the site of injury. The retracted tendons are then drawn into the original wound and united to the distal segments.

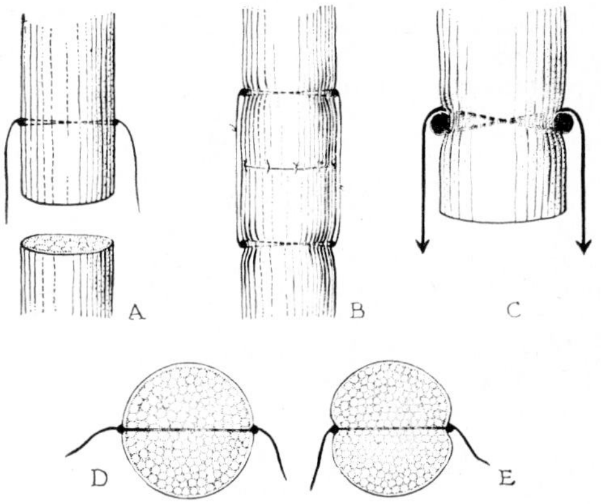

The original wound should be enlarged whenever necessary. A well planned incision will result in less trauma than ineffectual "blind fishing" deep within the hand or wrist for the retracted ends of the nerves or tendons.

Divided nerve and tendon ends are usually covered by a clot and surrounded by hemorrhagic areolar

FIG. 496. Method of tendon suture in which the longitudinal pull of the suture is converted into a transverse pull across the center of the tendon. (From Mason, *Surg., Gynec. & Obst.*, 70(2A):392-402, 1940. By permission of Surgery, Gynecology and Obstetrics.)

and sheath tissue. Certain identification of the injured structures may require exposure beyond the level of hemorrhagic discoloration. If a number of tendons and nerves have been divided, identifying sutures may help to avoid confusion at the time of closure.

After the injured structures have been identified the wound is checked for hemorrhage and repair of the nerves and tendons undertaken. Relaxation of the structures to be sutured is accomplished by manipulation of the hand and digits. Tension at the line of suture or early motion jeopardizes firm healing; unless satisfactory relaxation can be obtained and maintained, tendon suture should not be undertaken.

The tendon suture is carried out as shown in figure 496. Silk is used as the suture material. After the retention sutures have been inserted and tied, fine sutures on an atraumatic needle are used to appose the ends accurately. Only the very edge of the tendon is included in this suture.

If the fibrous tendon sheath within the digit has been divided, either by the injury or by enlarging the wound, it must be repaired so as to hold the tendon in place when tension is put upon it. For the same reason, careful repair of the deep fascia and the carpal ligaments must be made before the wound is closed.

To prevent the formation of adhesions about the site of tendon repair it is wise to surround the sutured tendon with areolar tissue or a thin layer of subcutaneous fat from the forearm. Foreign materials such as amniotic membrane, foil and fibrin film have proved ineffective in preventing the formation of adhesions.

Tendons divided within the digits can be successfully repaired. If both the sublimis and profundus tendons have been divided within the fibrous tendon sheaths, it is wise to remove the sublimis tendon and suture only the deep tendon. If one attempts to suture both tendons dense adhesions invariably form between the two tendons and prevent the free gliding movement essential for function. An intact profundus tendon alone is adequate for carrying out flexion of a digit. Mason has shown that after suture of the tendon within the tendon sheath, it is helpful to excise a segment of the fibrous sheath directly over the site of suture (Fig. 497) so as to secure a covering of vascular subcutaneous tissue for the sutured tendons and prevent constriction of the tendon callus—the spindle shaped thickening which develops at the line of suture.

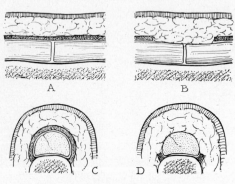

FIG. 497. Excision of window of fibrous digital sheath to provide subcutaneous fatty roof for healing tendon. A is longitudinal and C is cross section of finger before excision. B and D are corresponding sections following excision of fibrous sheath. The healing tendon is in contact with fatty areolar tissue. (From Mason, *Surg., Gynec. & Obst.*, 70(2A):392-402, 1940. By permission of Surgery, Gynecology and Obstetrics.)

The divided nerves, whether in the hand or in the fingers, should be united after tendons have been sutured. If the ends of the nerves are difficult to identify because of hemorrhagic discoloration of all the tissues, the wound must be enlarged in order to follow them into normal tissue. Ragged and torn nerve ends are cut across cleanly without unnecessary sacrifice of length. Nerves are sutured with small atraumatic needles and fine silk. Only the nerve sheath is caught by the suture, and unnecessary tension is avoided by flexion of the wrist or fingers. The nerves are aligned as nearly as possible in their original position and relationship. To insure correct approximation and avoid rotation, it may be possible to identify a divided blood vessel on each of the ends.

After repair of the deeper structures the fascia should be accurately reunited, the skin closed and the hand splinted in a position to provide relaxation for the divided structures. The tensile strength of a sutured tendon is very slight during the first few days following repair. By the third or fourth week it becomes sufficient to permit motion without danger of partial sepa-

ration. During this period the inflammatory reaction about the site of operation, with its tendency to form restricting adhesions of sutured tendons to
surrounding tissues, has time to subside. Splinting of repaired flexor tendons
should be maintained for a minimum of three weeks and of the extensor
tendons for four weeks.

LATE REPAIR OF NERVES AND TENDONS

If one can confidently anticipate healing of the wound by primary union,
nerves and tendons should be repaired immediately following injury, but in
many cases complicating factors make the outcome uncertain. If immediate
repair of the deep structures is not considered advisable it is wise to obtain
healing of the skin and subcutaneous tissues as quickly as possible and
undertake the repair of the divided structures later. The indications for
repair and the prognosis of healing following secondary repair of divided
nerves and tendons depend on several factors.

Condition of the Soft Tissue Wound at the Time of Repair. In a
wound which has healed primarily and with a minimum of inflammatory
reaction the repair of the deeper structures can be safely performed as early
as three weeks after injury. If healing of the wound has been delayed by the
presence of infection there is thickening and hardening of the soft tissues and
repair must be delayed until the danger of recrudescence of the infection has
passed and until the soft tissues are free from inflammatory reaction and
induration. This may require weeks and even months, and during this
period of waiting simple physical therapy, such as soap and water washing
with a soft washcloth for ten to fifteen minutes three times daily, combined
with passive and active movement at all the joints, can aid materially in
hastening subsidence of inflammatory reaction. If nerve injury is present a
splint should be provided to prevent constant overstretching of paralyzed
muscles.

Repair of deeper structures cannot be successfully carried out if the
covering tissues are defective. If the site of injury is covered by paper-like
epithelium it must be replaced by normal skin and subcutaneous tissue
before repair of the deeper tissues can be undertaken.

Condition of the Small Joints of the Hands. After injury to the
nerves and tendons, and loss of active movement at the small joints of the
hand, fixation may develop rapidly unless constant effort is directed toward
maintaining mobility. Tendon repair cannot be successfully performed if
joints are fixed in flexion or extension. Throughout the period following
injury passive movement at the joints should be maintained. If fixation has
taken place the joints can often be mobilized by a combination of elastic
traction with easily removable splints and physical therapy; and, in some
cases of fixation in extension, by surgical division of the collateral ligaments
of the metacarpophalangeal joints.

The Site of Injury. The tendons on the dorsum of the hand which are
surrounded by paratenon respond well to repair. When divided they do

not retract as far as tendons confined within tendon sheaths, such as the tendons over the dorsum of the wrist and the flexor surface of the fingers. In case of sheath enclosed tendons, the divided ends may be widely separated and often the proximal end is curled upon itself.

The Time Element. The longer the interval between injury and repair, the firmer is the myostatic contracture of the affected muscle and the more

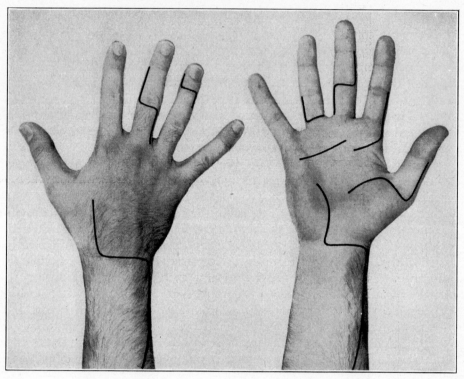

FIG. 498. Skin incisions in the hand should avoid the midline and should follow as closely as possible the lines of skin creases. They should be planned so as to produce flaps which overlie the site of nerve and tendon suture. (From Mason, *Surg., Gynec. & Obst.,* 70(2A):392-402, 1940. By permission of Surgery, Gynecology and Obstetrics.)

difficult it becomes to approximate tendon ends. Unless the separated ends of the tendon can be brought together and sutured without tension, a tendon graft to bridge the defect should be used. After from four to six weeks the tendon ends are invariably fixed to the surrounding structures and can only be freed by sharp dissection. Collapsed tendon sheaths can sometimes be opened, in other cases it is necessary to dissect free the "roof" so as to leave a smooth floor on which the repaired tendon can lie.

In any operation for the repair of nerves and tendons the incision is planned so as to permit adequate exposure of separated ends of the divided structures (Fig. 498). It is usually not difficult to approximate divided tendons if operation is carried out three or four weeks after injury. The tendon ends are not fixed and the muscles have not undergone a firm myostatic contracture in this period of time. A neuroma is invariably present at the proximal end of the divided nerves; it must be excised in thin sections until normal appearing nerve bundles are present over the entire cut surface, and any

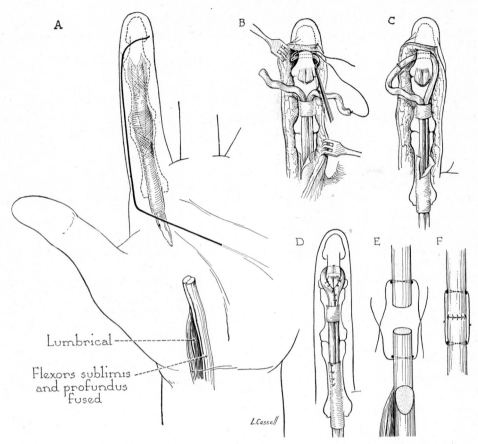

Lumbrical

Flexors sublimis and profundus fused

L.Cassell

FIG. 499. Technic of substituting a free tendon graft for hopelessly injured flexor tendons. (A) Incision. (B) After fibrosed flexor tendons have been excised free grafts are drawn through the carefully preserved tendon sheath and a guide suture is carried around the distal phalanx through a shallow tunnel made with a sharpened aneurism needle. (C) The free ends of the two tendons are smoothly united; by tension on the tendon first drawn through the tunnel, the two grafts are drawn taut, and the line of suture comes to lie in the midline on the dorsum of the distal phalanx. (D) Fine silk sutures between tendon graft and stump of profundus help to make attachment of graft to distal phalanx secure. (E), (F) Suture of proximal segment of flexor profundus. Incision in finger is closed before suture of graft to profundus is carried out. (From Koch, *Quarterly Bull.,* Northwestern Univ. Medical School, 19:265, 1945.)

scar tissue present over the end of the distal segment must also be excised before the ends are approximated.

Delayed tendon repair can be performed in all parts of the hand except within the fibrous tendon sheaths of the fingers; there suture of the ends is seldom successful. In this location a tendon graft is preferable.

Tendon Grafts. Because of the wide separation of the divided tendon ends, which invariably takes place after division of the flexor tendons within the digital sheath, a graft may be needed to bridge the defect if flexion contracture of the affected digit is to be avoided.

The remains of the divided tendon are freed in the finger and palm and the greater part of the distal segment of the flexor profundus is removed. Any sheath tissue which can serve as a retaining ligament to hold the tendon graft in place is preserved. Tendon grafts of required length are taken from the extensor digitorum longus on the dorsum of the foot. An adequate incision is needed for exposure of the tendons so as to avoid traumatizing them and stripping away their thin covering of areolar tissue. At times it is possible to use as a graft, the uninjured portion of the flexor sublimis or the palmaris longus tendon.

The tendon graft is inserted and attached to the distal phalanx, as illustrated (Fig. 499). That part of the digital fibrous sheath which has been saved is used to hold the tendon in place over the middle and proximal phalanges. If no sheath tissue remains, a free slip of tendon is drawn around each phalanx and its ends united so as to form a new annular ligament.

The tension at which the graft should be sutured is difficult to determine with exactness. If the hand is well flexed at the wrist and the fingers flexed at the metacarpophalangeal joints the graft and the proximal segment of the tendon should come together at normal and without forceful tension.

INFECTIONS OF THE HAND

A thorough knowledge of the anatomy of the hand is necessary to diagnose correctly and to foresee the possible extensions of an infectious process. The relationship of a localized infection to the various nerves, tendons and joints is of greatest importance. The pitfalls in treating surgical infections of the hand may be summed up as follows: (1) incorrect diagnosis as to the site of the infection; (2) incorrect incision; and (3) inadequate incision.

A general anesthetic is advisable for incision and drainage of infections of the hand. Drainage is maintained by the use of a soft nonadherent type of material such as fine meshed gauze impregnated with petrolatum. The drains are left in place for 48 to 72 hours. Following the operation the hand is supported on a splint in the position of function and a large sterile dressing is applied. Gauze is placed between the digits to prevent maceration. The dressings are moistened with sterile solution at six hour intervals throughout the day and night. The hand and forearm are elevated and placed under an electric baker or a heated cradle to maintain constant external heat. Antibiotics and chemotherapeutic agents are used when indicated.

Superficial infections, such as furuncles or carbuncles, are most often found on the dorsum of the hand, and after localization has occurred should be drained in the usual manner.

Infections confined to specific sites in the hand require incision and drainage and it is in such cases that familiarity of the anatomy of the hand is essential to proper care.

Felon. This infection follows a minor penetrating wound into the distal closed space of the digit. The pulp becomes tense, hard and exquisitely tender. If these findings are present, the diagnosis of a felon should be made and the affected area incised. Any delay or ineffectual attempt at drainage may allow an osteomyelitis of the distal phalanx to develop. A felon is drained by making an incision along the lateral border of the distal closed space of the finger. The scalpel is carried across the fibrous septa which extend from the skin to the periosteum of the bone. This method provides adequate drainage, but is not a "through-and-through" wound. The bone is never curetted. "Fishmouth" incisions are avoided because they invariably leave a deep painful scar.

If osteomyelitis has developed, adequate drainage as described must be provided. Healing is delayed until any necrotic bone separates. Curetting of the bone is likely to add injury and cause extension of the infectious process. A diagnosis of osteomyelitis from an x-ray film is often incorrectly made because of the decalcification associated with infection of the soft tissues and disuse. Amputation is rarely indicated because of osteomyelitis.

Paronychia. To drain a paronychia an incision is made at each side of the proximal end of the nail and the flap of eponychium between them is raised from the nail. The proximal third of the nail itself is also removed to permit the drainage of pus from under the nail. Gauze saturated with petrolatum is used to hold the flap of skin back and allow drainage. In early, well treated cases there is no residual damage to the nail or to its bed.

Collar-button Abscess or "Frog-felon." This may develop under a callus on the palm of the hand or after a penetrating injury. The process is characterized by pain, tenderness and swelling of the hand out of proportion to the superficial local wound. The purulent material is found to lie in two compartments, above and below the deep fascia of the palm. If only the more superficial pocket is drained the infection will continue to progress. An incision is made over the site of the infection in the direction of lines of skin cleavage of the palm. After the more superficial pocket is evacuated it is often possible to see a sinus leading to the deeper collection of pus. The incision is then continued through the deep fascia where a large amount of pus is often encountered. In making this deeper incision care is needed to avoid injury of the nerves and tendons.

Tendon Sheath Infections. Such infections are always serious and can result in crippled functionless fingers. They usually result from a penetrating injury over or near the anatomical position of the tendon sheaths. The finger is held in slight flexion, there is uniform swelling of the entire finger, tenderness over the entire sheath, and wincing and pain on an attempt at extending the finger. These are the four cardinal points of diagnosis so often stressed by Kanavel.

The correct treatment of these infections is early incision and drainage (Fig. 500). Infections of the tendon sheaths of the index, middle and ring fingers are drained through an incision over the lateral surface of the digit and through a second palmar incision, parallel to the distal flexion crease, to expose the proximal end or the cul-de-sac of the tendon sheath. Because of the marked swelling of the digit in the presence of a tendon sheath infection a deep incision is needed to expose the tendon sheath. Unless one has a bloodless field one may fail to open the sheath. In incising the finger the

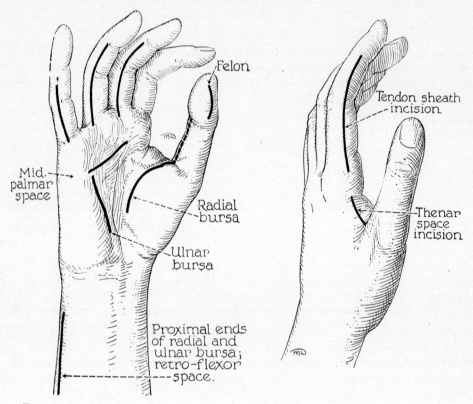

Fig. 500. Incisions for drainage of tendon sheaths and fascial spaces of the hand. (From Kanavel and Mason, *Cyclopedia of Medicine, Surg., and Specialties,* 7:27, 1945, F. A. Davis Co., Philadelphia.)

lateral extensions of the flexion creases of the digit can be used as landmarks. After the skin and deep fascia have been divided, the digital nerves and vessels are identified and retracted dorsally. The fibrous tendon sheath is opened along the side from the distal phalanx to the level of the web. In the second incision over the proximal end of the tendon sheath in the palm one must identify the digital nerves and vessels which lie on each side close beside the tendon sheath.

TENDON SHEATH INFECTIONS OF THE THUMB AND LITTLE FINGER. In infections of the tendon sheath of either the thumb or little finger, one must anticipate an extension of the infection throughout the length of the synovial lined radial and ulnar bursae. The greatest amount of pus will be found in the retroflexor space within the forearm. The incisions are placed as illustrated in the diagram, and in making them the digital nerves and vessels must be identified and protected. The incision for draining the forearm is made just volar to the subcutaneous margin of the ulna; the ulnar nerve and vessels are retracted volarward and the retroflexor space is entered dorsal to the nerve and blood vessels.

Middle Palmar Space Infections. These infections result from a penetrating wound of the middle palmar space or from an extension of infection from the tendon sheath of the middle or ring fingers. They are characterized by local tenderness, by loss of the concavity of the palm, by swelling of the entire hand, more marked on its dorsal surface. The incision for drainage is made over the anatomical location of the space and parallel to the distal flexion crease. The digital nerves and flexor tendons are identified. The pus lies between and beneath the tendons of the middle and ring fingers.

Thenar Space Infections. Such infections result from a penetrating wound of the thenar space or from extension of a tendon sheath infection of the index finger. The infection is characterized by a ballooning of the web space between the thumb and index finger and by forced abduction of the thumb from the hand. The incision is made over the dorsal aspect of this web space and parallel to the web. The pus lies volar to the adductor muscles of the thumb.

Human Bite Infections. These are virulent, rapidly spreading infections and are usually not seen early in their course. It is important to be aware of each step in the advance of these infections and treat them as they develop. If the infection involves the joints a poor prognosis for function is indicated, for there will result a suppurative arthritis and osteomyelitis of the adjacent ends of the bones. Infection at the level of the metacarpophalangeal joint may dissect along the expansions of the extensor tendon and it may then extend into the lumbrical canal and along this pathway into the palm. Such an extension results in an abscess within the mid-palmar or thenar space. If the interphalangeal joints are involved the pus may rupture through the joints to the volar surface and into the tendon sheath.

Osteomyelitis of the Bones of the Hand. Following severe infections, crushing injuries or burns to the dorsum of the hand, the extensor tendons may become necrotic and the dorsum of the phalanges exposed. When this occurs the surgeon may follow two courses: the first is to provide careful aseptic dressings and immobilization and to wait for sequestration to occur spontaneously; the other method is surgical excision of the dry necrotic bone. The resulting defect is then carefully dressed to encourage the formation of granulation tissue over which split thickness skin grafts may be applied. Amputations should not be undertaken in the presence of an open infected wound or osteomyelitis.

CHRONIC INFECTIONS

Tuberculous Tenosynovitis. Tuberculosis of the tendon sheath may occur within any sheath-lined space on the volar or dorsal surface of the hand or wrist. In the early stages of this disease it may be confused with a simple ganglion. At first the tuberculous infection involves the parietal layer of the tendon sheath. Gradually it becomes distended with fluid, rice bodies may be formed in large numbers and the visceral sheath of the tendon is involved, and still later the process may extend to adjacent bones and joints, particularly to the wrist and carpal joints. The thickened sheaths are purple-red in color, the thickened visceral layer of the sheath is markedly adherent to the tendon. With increasing involvement the tumor mass produces swelling both proximal and distal to the carpal ligaments. The presence of the thickened tendon sheaths and rice bodies produces the characteristic physical finding of crepitation on movement of the fingers.

The correct treatment is surgical excision of the involved tendon sheaths. Incisions are planned so as to expose the affected area as widely as possible. If the infection is on the volar surface of the wrist the sheaths of the thumb and little finger may be involved because of the continuity of the radial and ulnar bursae. In such a case a complete operation would involve removal of the diseased tendon sheaths from the thumb, the little finger, the palm, the wrist and the forearm. The incision is made along the flexion crease of the thumb as far as the wrist, transversely to the ulnar side of the forearm, and proximally to the level of the musculo-tendinous junctions within the forearm. The deep fascia is opened and carefully freed so that it can be accurately sutured at the close of the operation. The median and ulnar nerves are identified and retracted to prevent damage to them during the dissection. The thickened tendon sheath is opened along the midline. Each involved tendon is taken in turn, the sheath opened and the thickened inflamed synovial tissue removed by sharp dissection. If the involvement is so extensive that necrosis of the tendon has occurred, the necrotic portions are removed and replaced by grafts.

When the diseased tissue in the wrist and palm has been dissected away, any extension into the thumb and little finger is removed. The incisions are placed along the sides of the affected digits, the digital nerves are identified and retracted dorsally. The fibrous tendon sheath is opened along the lateral side of the digit and the infected sheath tissue is then removed.

Within the digits the fibrous tendon sheath is reunited. In the palm and forearm the deep fascia is united and the carpal ligament at the wrist is carefully repaired. The skin is closed in the usual manner.

Tuberculous infection may involve the tendon sheaths of the middle, ring and index fingers. Removal of the sheaths of these digits requires two incisions, one for the finger and one to expose the proximal end of the tendon sheath within the palm. The latter incision on the palm is made transversely and the nerves and vessels lying close to the side of the tendon sheaths are identified and protected during the dissection.

BURNS AND FREEZING INJURIES TO THE HANDS

Early Care. The immediate treatment of these injuries is the careful cleansing and simple removal of obviously devitalized tissues. An anesthetic is seldom required. The hand is covered completely with fine meshed petrolatum gauze, and over this a dressing is placed so as to separate the fingers and cover the entire hand. A compression dressing is then applied and the hand placed on a splint in the position of function.

Unless there are definite signs of infection this large dressing is left intact for ten days without changing. At the time the dressings are removed, the areas of part thickness loss will be healed; the areas of whole thickness loss will be covered with moist necrotic tissue. This necrotic tissue may be removed by one of four methods: The least desirable is the liquefaction resulting from a superimposed infection which not only causes separation of necrotic tissues but further destruction of living tissue as well; a second method is the daily application of sterile dressings saturated with Dakin's solution; a third is surgical excision under general anesthesia; and the fourth, débridement by a chemical agent such as by pyruvic acid. The earlier the devitalized tissue can be removed and the resulting open wound covered with skin grafts, the better will be the final functional result.

Later Care. As soon as the devitalized tissue of a deep burn is separated the wound should be dressed daily with dressings saturated with Dakin's solution and covered with a compression dressing. When the raw surface is surgically clean and covered with red granulation tissue a graft of intermediate thickness should be applied over the entire wound. It should be possible to cover the affected area by the tenth to fourteenth day following the injury; in some cases it may be possible to do so even earlier. Exposed tendons and joints provide a complication most difficult to overcome. If the tendons appear of normal color and have a thin layer of areolar tissue over them, healing will take place following grafting. Grafting should not be delayed because of the presence of necrotic tendon or bone, for where the remainder of the wound appears clean, it should be grafted to the level of the necrotic tissue. After sequestration of these structures has occurred, the remaining area can be grafted.

Contractures Following Burns of the Hand. Burn contractures of the hand can be corrected by complete excision of the scar tissue and the application of normal covering tissue. Whether a graft of skin alone will suffice, or whether a flap of skin and subcutaneous tissue is required depends on the depth of the original injury and whether bare tendons, nerves and blood vessels are left exposed in the floor of the wound when scar excision is complete. A scar which is recent and red or tender should not be excised, but the operation should be delayed until inflammatory reaction and induration have been reduced to a minimum.

At operation, scar tissue is carefully excised until healthy tissue can be seen over the entire field. The nerves and tendons must be identified and protected throughout the operation; often these structures are completely surrounded by the scar tissue. After all scar tissue is entirely removed, it should be possible to extend or to flex the contracted digits. An exact pattern of the defect is made and a whole thickness skin graft, cut from the pattern, taken from the inner aspect of the thigh or lower abdomen. This graft is accurately sutured over the defect on the hand. A dressing is applied to insure uniform pressure over the graft and complete rest, with the finger in complete extension if the graft is on palm, and with the fingers in semiflexion if the graft is on the dorsum; it is maintained until healing is complete.

Pedicled flaps may be necessary to replace the scar tissue produced by a burn and are essential if secondary tendon grafting is contemplated. A pedicled flap is usually raised in two stages from the abdominal wall. When the flap is ready for transfer the scar is excised from the hand, the flap raised from the abdominal wall and sutured over the defect on the hand. The hand and arm are immobilized by a plaster of paris cast to prevent motion which might cause tension at the suture line. After three weeks the pedicle is divided and suture of the wound on abdomen and hand completed.

RADIATION INJURIES TO THE HAND

Radiation burns or ulcers are often seen on the hand. The patient seeks medical help because of keratoses, persistent deep pain or the presence of an indolent wound. Additional x-ray therapy or radium applications have frequently aggravated the original injury.

In the early stages irregular areas of atrophic skin are found on the dorsum of the fingers and hand. Later keratoses and areas of telangiectasia gradually develop and frequently the finger nails become deformed. Small indolent ulcers may appear over these areas and these ulcers are often the site of malignant change.

In the early stages, satisfactory treatment can be accomplished by removal of the keratoses and simple closure. In the advanced stages, the skin is thin and frequently breaks down following mild trauma. The entire area of atrophic skin should be excised and replaced by a skin graft. Usually grafts of intermediate thickness are satisfactory, but if ulceration and the inevitable concomitant infection have not yet developed one would prefer to apply a graft of whole thickness skin. If ulceration has developed the ulcers and surrounding skin are prepared for operation by a few days of cleanly care. The entire area is completely excised and the defect covered with a graft. If malignant changes have occurred, wider excision or even amputation must be considered.

DUPUYTREN'S CONTRACTURE

The essential pathological change is a thickening and contraction of the palmar fascia occurring most often in males in the fifth and sixth decades. The cause is not known. There is both thickening and hardening of the palmar fascia, dimpling of the skin and, late in the disease, contracture of the fingers into the palm. The ring finger is the most commonly affected. The characteristic position of the involved fingers is that of flexion at the metacarpophalangeal and proximal interphalangeal joints with hyperextension at the distal interphalangeal joint.

Surgical excision, to be successful, requires careful and complete removal of the entire affected fascia and its prolongations into the involved fingers. The initial incision is made transversely across the palm, usually at the level of the distal flexion crease (Fig. 501). The palmar skin is carefully dissected away from the underlying fascia, both proximally and distally. A second incision is made along the flexion crease of the thumb, and after the skin is freed from the underlying fascia, the fascia is completely exposed within the palm. The fascia is divided transversely at the base of the palm and is dissected distalward. As it is raised care is taken to identify the digital nerves and vessels. As the dissection is continued toward the metacarpophalangeal joints it is advisable to divide the thickened fascia directly over the line of each tendon and dissecting lateralward to each side of the tendon to watch and protect the digital nerves and blood vessels. In the same manner, the extensions of the palmar fascia dorsalward to the volar interosseus membrane, the fascial septa on each side of the flexor tendons are excised. After the affected fascia in the palm has been removed the continuation of the

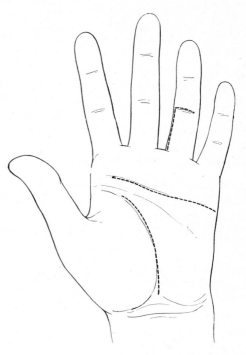

FIG. 501. Skin incisions in the hand and fingers for excision of the palmar fascia for Dupuytren's contracture.

fascia into the involved fingers is excised. A fibrous mass is often found to lie under the palmar skin of the proximal phalanx. An inverted L-shaped incision is made along the flexion crease of the proximal interphalangeal joint or farther distalward, and extended proximally to the web. The digital nerves are identified and the thickened extension of the fascia is dissected away from the overlying skin and underlying tendon sheath.

Frequently the excision of hopelessly involved callused skin and the extension of fingers long held in flexion leaves a considerable defect in the covering skin at the completion of the operative excision. In such a case the attempt to bring wound edges together only results in reformation of the contracture. The use of a whole thickness graft to fill the defect in these hands has given excellent results, in our experience.

THE GANGLION

This is the most common tumor seen on the hand or wrist and its usual site is over the dorsum of the wrist. These tumors are cystic masses which invariably arise from the joint capsule of the wrist or carpus. Operative removal can usually be carried out under local anesthesia. A transverse incision is made over the site of the tumor and the cystic mass is carefully freed down to its base; great care is used to protect the extensor tendons. If the ganglion involves the joint capsule complete excision may require removal of a small portion of the capsule. The entire ganglion, including its base, must be excised if recurrence is to be avoided. The wound is closed in layers, with care to provide a covering of soft tissue over the exposed extensor tendons.

Similar cystic enlargements are found in other locations. The volar surface of the wrist on the radial aspect is a common site. In removing such a ganglion, the radial artery and veins must be protected. Small tense cystic tumors are also found within the flexor tendon sheath over the base of the proximal phalanx and over the dorsum of the hand overlying the distal interphalangeal joint.

23

THE SKIN AND SUBCUTANEOUS TISSUE

Frank Glenn, M.D.

INFECTIONS

Furuncle. The most common abscess associated with the skin and sub-cutaneous tissue is the furuncle, or boil. The infection enters the skin, in-volves the hair follicle or sebaceous gland, and is caused by the *Staphylo-coccus aureus*. As the bacteria grow, they elaborate a toxin that causes necrosis of the surrounding tissue before the protective mechanisms become established. As time elapses and the infection extends, there is a greater response on the part of the tissue and the necrosis of tissue subsides. There remains in the center where the infection entered, a complete slough of necrotic material. Surrounding this is a zone of further injury with a re-sponse on the part of the tissues to provide a wall of leukocytes. Peripheral to this there is an area commonly known as the pyogenic membrane—here the protective mechanisms of the body are most active.

The surgical treatment of a furuncle consists of incision of the area within the circumference of the pyogenic membrane to permit the free drainage of pus and necrotic material. When this is accomplished extension of the infection because of "pus under pressure" is overcome.

A furuncle may be treated by: (1) chemotherapy; (2) carbolization of its central and necrotic portion; (3) incision; (4) excision; (5) x-ray therapy. A combination of these methods is frequently indicated.

(1) CHEMOTHERAPY. The systemic administration of penicillin in doses of 30,000 units every three hours for early furuncle has been followed by rapid resolution of the process. When pus has already developed, surgical drainage is required in addition. Multiple furuncles, which are so trouble-some, are reduced in severity and in many instances aborted.

(2) CARBOLIZATION. Carbolization of the central or necrotic portion of a furuncle by using a metal stick dipped in carbolic acid can be accomplished with little discomfort. If this is done meticulously and thoroughly, drainage of adequate degree that decompresses the deep abscess cavity of the furuncle will be established.

(3) INCISION. Incision under anesthesia affords by and large the more satisfactory means of decompression. For small furuncles a simple incision, and for large ones a cruciate incision that extends to but not beyond the zone of the pyogenic membrane, is adequate. The surgeon, furthermore, can explore the furuncle and determine that small adjacent abscesses are drained.

(4) EXCISION. Block excision is seldom justified and leaves an unsightly scar.

(5) X-RAY THERAPY. Furuncles may be aborted by x-ray therapy in their incipient stages in some instances. It has been advocated for multiple furuncles in an area such as the back of the neck or buttocks. Any patient with furunculosis requires a complete medical investigation.

Carbuncle. The carbuncle, like the furuncle, is most frequently caused by *Staphylococcus aureus;* however, the infection is much more virulent and extensive. The route of the infection is through the skin; necrosis of the subcutaneous tissue may be extensive over a fairly large area with little response on the part of the protective mechanisms of the body. Individuals with lowered resistance, such as those who have diabetes or nephritis, are quite susceptible. As necrosis takes place in the subcutaneous tissue the fibrous trabeculae that extend throughout form compartments which become tense and distended with purulent material and rupture one into another and sometimes to the surface where the superficial are only partly drained by what appear as multiple openings in the skin. Thus the process can extend over large areas in the subcutaneous tissues before the infection is overcome sufficiently by the tissue response. Like the furuncle, once a zone of reaction such as the pyogenic membrane is established the process may be limited. Carbuncles in the debilitated are associated with extensive lymphangitis, cellulitis, septicemia, bacteremia, and metastatic abscesses, and may be the cause of death. In individuals with reasonable health adequate treatment is followed by recovery.

The presence of a carbuncle implies that the individual is lacking in the ordinary mechanisms for protection against bacterial invasion. Although such patients frequently are not favorable subjects for radical surgical procedures, nevertheless cure remains dependent upon the thorough and complete extirpation of the carbuncle. The surgical treatment of the local process should be preceded by careful evaluation of the patient and such preoperative preparation as may be indicated, such as the control of diabetes with insulin. Chemotherapy should be instituted to aid the suppression of the infection and the prevention of a bacteremia following surgery. Penicillin, 30,000 units intramuscularly, is given every three hours. Initial dosage by intravenous administration may well be used to establish immediately a satisfactory blood level.

General anesthesia is required for those with large carbuncles. The operative site requires the same careful preparation as any surgical procedure because the danger of introducing a virulent secondary invader is a very real one. Incisions that extend beyond the involved tissue and give free drainage are required. These may be curvate, stellate, or made in parallel. Necrotic tissue should be excised. In order to accomplish this it is sometimes better to excise the entire carbuncle using the scalpel or the electro-cutting apparatus. In the treatment of carbuncles the primary objective is to overcome the infection, and repair of the defect is secondary. Incomplete excision often results in the extension of the infection. The electro-cutting and coagulating machines enable one to excise involved tissue rapidly and to control hemorrhage with the coagulation current. In using the scalpel catgut ligatures and packing will suffice. Wounds following the removal

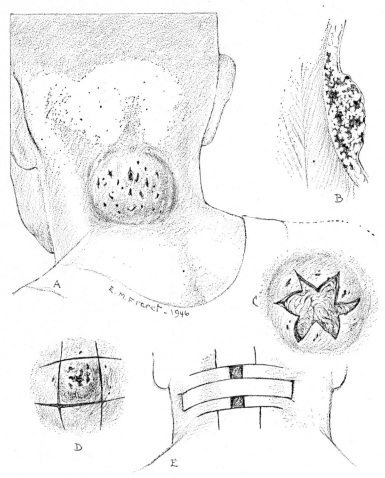

FIG. 502. Carbuncle. (A) Frequent location of a carbuncle. (B) In the subcutaneous tissue fibrous trabeculae form compartments that become tense and distended with purulent material as infection progresses. These rupture one into another and sometimes to the surface; thus multiple sinuses of the long standing carbuncle that afford inadequate drainage. (C) Cruciate incision with undercutting of periphery and minimal excision of the central necrotic portion, followed by loose packing with gauze containing a chemotherapeutic agent such as penicillin. (D) A type of incision that permits excision of central portion and reflection of peripheral flaps. (E) Following subsidence of infection, such flaps (D), can be partially approximated. Large defects may require skin grafting.

of as much necrotic tissue as possible should be loosely packed with gauze and kept moistened with penicillin solution (250 units per cc.). X-ray therapy has been used in the early phases of a carbuncle with good results, there following a definite subsidence of the extension of the infection.

Tuberculosis of the Skin (*Lupus Vulgaris*). Tuberculosis of the skin is a slowly progressive and extremely chronic disease. It is not limited to individuals with pulmonary disease and frequently is not properly diagnosed. Any persistent chronic ulcerative lesion of the skin that exhibits hypertrophy, as the process of repair takes place, should be considered as possible tuberculosis, and a biopsy taken. However, the classical and very troublesome lesions of the face, *lupus vulgaris*, usually do not require biopsy for diagnosis. These are seen most frequently in young people with other easily recognizable lesions of tuberculosis.

The surgical treatment of tuberculosis of the skin should be undertaken only after prolonged general health measures, and for lesions of the face only after very careful deliberation and by the most skilled. Complete excision of all infected skin and subcutaneous tissue can be accomplished by including 2 to 3 cm. of skin beyond the margin of the lesion and using meticulous sharp dissection to remove the underlying subcutaneous tissue or base of the ulcerated area. The immediate skin grafting of these defects is becoming more popular and the results are good if all tuberculous tissue has been removed. However, the most satisfactory results have followed skin grafting of the granulating surface two weeks after the primary operation. X-ray therapy is of no value. The use of streptomycin locally, employing dressings kept moist with a solution of 5000 units per cc. has recently been reported, but its value is not yet established.

Actinomycosis. Actinomycosis in cattle is known as lumpy jaw. It occurs in man where it gives rise to a granuloma that forms a sinus or fistula and discharges a thin pus which contains yellow sulphur-like granules. These are large enough to be recognized on dressings from actinomycotic lesions. The Actinomyces are commonly found in the mouth, and special studies in normal people have revealed a high incidence of the organisms about carious teeth and in tonsillar crypts. This probably accounts for the frequency with which cervico-facial actinomycosis occurs.

The organisms cause a granulomatous type of reaction wherever they become lodged. Following an acute granuloma the central portion liquefies and burrows into surrounding uninvolved tissue. The chronic sinus tracts become indurated and brawny as the result of connective tissue response to the actinomycosis and secondary infection. Multiple sinuses or fistulae form along the burrowing tracts; from these is discharged a thin, purulent material containing characteristic small white flake-like material and sulphur granules.

Three types of actinomycosis are commonly considered according to the region involved: (1) cervico-facial; (2) abdominal; and (3) thoracic. Between 60 and 70 per cent of all patients with actinomycosis have these primary demonstrable lesions about the face and neck. The correct diagnosis of the disease is dependent upon the examiner keeping in mind the tendency of actinomycosis to produce discharging sinuses in the neck and lower face. Abdominal lesions are most frequently associated with the appendix and cecum. Following operation for appendicitis, and especially ruptured acute appendicitis, actinomycosis may develop. Whether it causes the appendicitis or develops as a result of the escape of fecal contents into the peritoneal cavity is not known. Lesions of this disease may appear anywhere in the abdomen, leading to multiple sinus tract formation and subphrenic and other intra-abdominal abscesses. Thoracic involvement usually follows the other two forms and may represent a general systemic extension. Intracranial lesions may develop by direct extension of the infection from the face or from Actinomyces carried from some more distant area by the blood.

Early actinomycosis responds favorably to a combination of chemotherapy and surgery. A period of treatment of from two to eight weeks, during which both sulfadiazine and penicillin are used continuously and concomitantly, should precede the attempted surgical eradication of all granulomata and sinus tracts. In the blood a sulfadiazine level of 4 to 5 mgm. per 100 cc. should be maintained. Penicillin may be administered by various routes but intramuscular injection of 30,000 units at intervals of four hours has many advantages. The nature of the presenting lesions and the material discharged from the sinus openings then subside. The complete and meticulous removal of all sinus tracts and granulomatous tissue should next be undertaken. Although curetting of such sinus tracts is sometimes followed by cure, the direct attack with sharp dissection and excision of involved tissue should be employed when possible. Gauze wet with physiologic saline solution makes a satisfactory primary dressing. Twenty-four to forty-eight hours later penicillin in saline (500 units per cc.) may be used. As soon as fresh granulation tissue appears these wounds may be closed by delayed suture of skin graft. The chemotherapy, consisting of penicillin and sulfadiazine, is continued for a minimum of four weeks after operation.

Granuloma Pyogenica. Following a small circumscribed infection in the skin or subcutaneous tissue, or the implantation of a foreign body in these tissues, a draining sinus with an exuberant granulation tissue may form. The granulomatous tissue is a response to (a) infection, or (b) reaction to a foreign body. It is self limiting, chronic, and persistent. It may result from parasites, especially in the tropics. Occasionally a draining sinus from a deeper level may lead to a similar process. This localized granulation tissue with a varied and rich bacterial flora has been labelled granuloma pyogenica.

Excision of the granuloma and irritating focus under local anesthesia is readily accomplished and gives good results in small lesions where primary closure of the wound may be done. For larger lesions and those with a high degree of infection, local and systemic therapy may be used in preparation for excision. Sometimes primary closure may not be feasible because of infection, and for these cases delayed closure or skin graft after further local chemotherapy gives the most satisfactory results.

Decubitus Ulcer. The experience accumulated during World War II in the Medical Corps of the United States Army has rendered the conservative treatment of decubiti untenable. The large bed sore in civilian practice is relatively rare but it continues to occur, especially in patients maintained in body casts for a prolonged period of time, or have lesions of the spinal cord. It has been demonstrated that the large decubitus ulcer provides an exit for the serum proteins and at the same time possesses a suitable culture medium for bacterial growth. The toxin produced by the bacteria when absorbed into the system is detrimental to well being. It is therefore of great

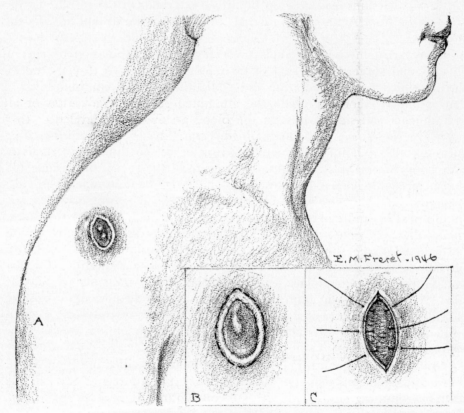

FIG. 503. (A) Granuloma pyogenica. (B) Outline of incision for complete removal. (C) Secondary or delayed closure is sometimes preferable if infected tissue is incompletely removed or if a virulent organism has been isolated from the wound.

importance that the decubitus ulcer be treated surgically as early as possible. This holds equally true for the debilitated patient as well as the more vigorous.

Patients with decubiti who are debilitated should be provided with an adequate caloric fluid and vitamin intake, and attempts should be made to restore the individual to nitrogen balance. Concomitantly, suitable chemotherapy, such as penicillin or one of the sulfa drugs used systemically and locally, should reduce the degree of infection. As soon as the patient's condition will permit the undertaking of a surgical procedure such *as is required* to correct the decubitus operation should be embarked upon. In those instances in which the lesion is small, the operation is not a demanding one, but when they are large the procedure may require hours; such patients should receive infusions and transfusions during the surgical procedure for these in particular are the most debilitated.

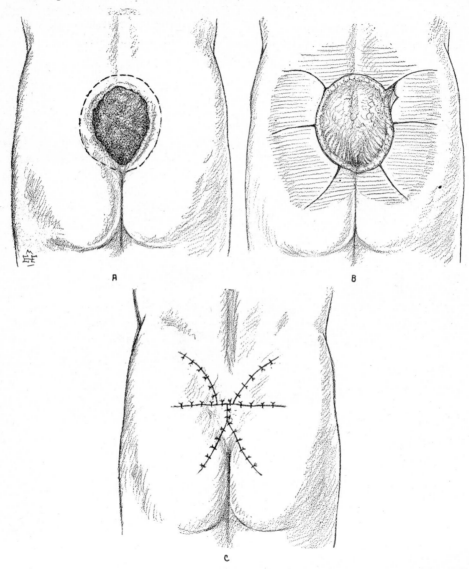

FIG. 504. Decubitus. (A) A typical decubitus ulcer over the sacrum with considerable scar tissue at the periphery of the ulcer. The dotted line indicates incision down to normal tissue. In this step some normal skin may be removed. (B) Flaps are made and undermined 10 to 15 cm. beyond the limit of the ulcer. (C) The flaps have been approximated. The wound is drained by a rubber tissue drain placed through a stab wound apart from the suture line.

Croce, Schullinger, and Shearer have advocated the raising of *full* thickness skin flaps about the ulcer, employing curvilinear incisions along the iliac crest above and the buttocks below, and rotating the flaps centripetally to cover large defects after completely excising the ulcer and its peripheral scar tissue. All bleeding points are secured with fine ligatures of plain catgut, and the flaps are united in their new position with interrupted sutures of double zero chromic catgut. The skin margins are approximated with interrupted sutures of fine silk. A stab wound is made some distance from a

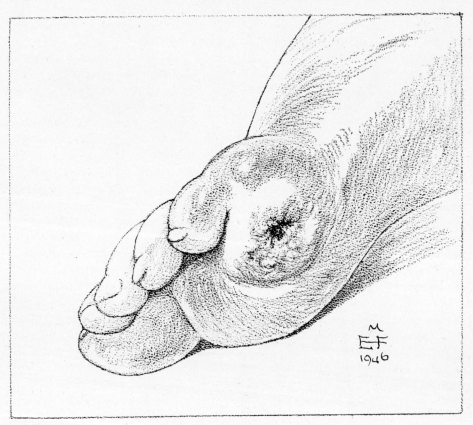

FIG. 505. A perforating ulcer at the metatarsophalangeal joint in a patient with arteriosclerosis and diabetes.

suture line and rubber tissue placed for a drain. Pressure dressings of mechanic's waste or sea sponge are placed over the flaps in order to prevent separation of the opposing surfaces. The drain is removed on the third or the fifth day and the patient is mobilized within ten to fourteen days.

The use of pinch grafts may be sufficient for those small decubital ulcers that are seen following the use of casts on extremities or the trunk. However, excision of the base of the ulcer and undermining of the surrounding tissue in a cleavage plane enables one to close the defect with ease and to secure a minimum amount of scarring and disfigurement.

Epidermophytosis. Epidermophytosis (athlete's foot), and infection of the skin caused by fungi, involves the feet of a fair percentage of our population.

It is also seen on the hands and other regions of the body. Its chief significance to the surgeon is that it provides a portal for the entry of "secondary
invaders" of a virulent nature, such as certain strains of streptococci. These
in turn lead to a disabling lymphangitis, adenitis, and sometimes a serious
septicemia and even bacteremia. The persistence of epidermophytosis predisposes to recurrent attacks of lymphangitis and phlebitis caused by secondary invaders. The eradication of this prevalent skin infection is dependent
upon cleanliness and good skin hygiene and the generous use of suitable
fungicides, including foot powders containing formaldehyde. Fungi are
frequently secreted about nails and calluses and these serve as a source of
reinfection. Epidermophytosis with cellulitis and suppuration is treated by
general systemic measures, chemotherapy, and incision and drainage of encapsulated pus.

Perforating Ulcer. Over the plantar aspect of the foot at the metatarsophalangeal joint in patients suffering from chronic disease, ulceration
frequently occurs. The majority of these patients suffer from one of the
chronic diseases, such as arteriosclerosis, diabetes, syphilis, and the degenerative diseases of the nervous system. These ulcers may occur any place on the
plantar aspect of the foot or toes. Because surgical treatment is seldom completely successful, considerable judgment is required in undertaking even
the simplest operative procedure. Bed rest and careful toilet of the ulcer,
keeping it clean with soap and water, will be followed by improvement in
many instances. Saline dressings may stimulate granulation tissue on some
of the more indolent lesions. Thereafter mildly irritative ointments, such as
1 per cent scarlet red, weak boric acid, or balsam of Peru, are effective in
encouraging epithelization. Simple excision of the ulcer and skin grafting
have been used with some success. When pedicle grafts are used the result
is much better than when simple split thickness grafts or pinch grafts are
applied. Following the excision of the lesion extensive procedures such as
lumbar sympathectomy have been used with limited success. Because many
of these patients are suffering from degenerative disease of one kind or
another, extensive surgical procedures should not be hastily undertaken.
They should be guarded against such a procedure which, if unsuccessful, may
further cripple them. These geriatrical problems are best treated by conservative measures.

BENIGN TUMORS

The benign tumors of the skin and subcutaneous tissue include fibroma
and neurofibroma (Von Recklenhausen's disease), lipoma, angioma, lymphangioma, and endothelioma. Fibromata are usually single, whereas neurofibromata occur both as isolated tumors or as multiple ones (Von
Recklenhausen's disease). Pigmentation is frequently an accompanying
stigma. Both disfigurement and pain are the cause for patients seeking their
removal. Angiomata may be divided into hemangiomata and lymphangi-
omata. These may be simple lesions or extensive complex tumors. Hemangiomata if superficial may be easily dealt with, whereas the deep and

cavernous tumors may not be removable. Regardless of their appearance, their removal should not be approached as a minor surgical problem. Hemangiomata about the face are most likely to penetrate deeply. Small "port wine" tumors are removed by a number of methods, including carbon dioxide snow, radiotherapy, and injection of sclerosing solutions. However, simple excision and closure of the defect with care gives the most satisfactory result. Benign tumors depend upon complete removal for cure and it is all important that excision be complete. Most of these superficial lesions can be operated upon under local anesthesia. Sufficient surrounding skin should be excised and well undermined in order that the wound may be readily approximated without tension.

Neurofibroma. Neurofibromata arise from the peripheral nerves. They may be single or multiple. They are firm, usually freely movable, and may or may not be associated with pain. The diffuse occurrence of these tumors, as in Von Recklenhausen's disease, precludes their complete removal. However, those that cause pain, paresthesia, paresis, or pressure should be removed surgically as individual lesions. Generally speaking, they are extremely slow growing and may produce no symptoms over a period of years, and then for some reason or reasons not evident they rapidly begin to increase in size. It is then that symptoms appear too late for the patient to seek relief.

The majority of these tumors is benign, although there is a definite tendency for those of long standing to show sarcomatous changes. All such tumors, therefore, should be carefully examined microscopically following their removal. Those tumors that involve the nerves must be removed with great care, exercising every precaution to preserve all nerve trunk tissue. In order to accomplish this, where possible a tourniquet should be used in order to maintain a bloodless operative field. Meticulous surgery is to be employed, using fine silk or cotton ligatures and sutures. When considerable injury has resulted to a nerve trunk with marked disappearance of function, resection with end-to-end anastomosis may be done.

Lipoma. Simple lipomata, the most benign of tumors, arise most frequently in the subcutaneous tissue, although they may be found in any part of the body. They vary in size from very small to extremely large tumors, sometimes sufficient to fill most of the chest cavity. Common sites for lipomata are the neck, back, buttocks, and axilla. They may be multiple and seemingly sometimes involve most of the subcutaneous fat of the body, a condition known as adiposis dolorosa, or Dercum's disease. The single lipoma is usually without a true capsule. It grows slowly and may produce symptoms by direct pressure or deformity.

The removal of these tumors, when superficial, is a simple surgical procedure. The lines of elasticity should be followed when incisions are made to expose them. The larger tumors frequently have a main blood supply that enters some place about their base. This should be identified and secured as the tumor is excised. Care should be exercised to remove all of the tumor because recurrences do grow where part of the tumor is left. Meticulous

a more formidable procedure may be required. Any amputation stump that is painful should be considered for revision and simple nerve section will seldom give complete relief.

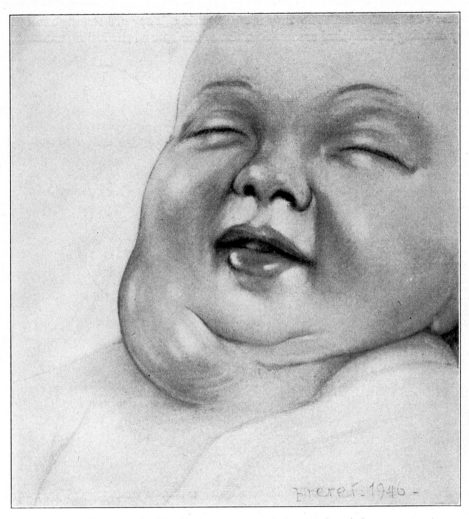

FIG. 507. Cystic lymphangioma in the neck of an infant.

The second lesion is neuroma of the skin which is associated with superficial scars and often with keloid formation, and may occur in the intact derma as well. Excision of the scar or the skin where pain and tenderness are greatest with primary repair of the defect is required.

The third is a rare albeit a fascinating lesion—the neuromyoarterial glomus of the skin. It is an arteriovenous anastomosis richly supplied with nerve fibers which render it very sensitive to painful stimuli. They are encountered beneath the nail and in the skin. Treatment consists of simple excision.

Epithelial Tumors. Among the benign epithelial tumors, *papillomata* may for the sake of convenience be grouped as hard or soft. The first group is seen in elderly people and represents proliferation of keratinized cells, and may be small flat lesions or grow to resemble a horn. On the exposed areas of the skin and scalp they are disfiguring. They are readily removed by excising an elliptical area of skin about the base of the lesion, extending

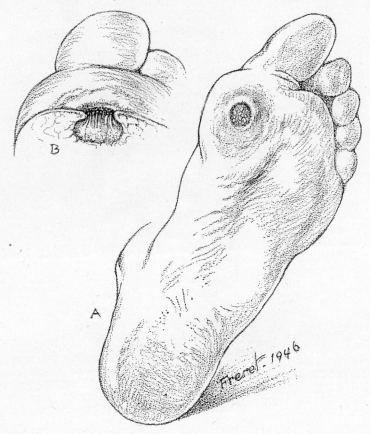

Fɪɢ. 508. Plantar wart. This lesion is actually larger than its presenting surface appears. Its excision must be complete to effect a cure.

the incision so that the subcutaneous fat may be removed. The soft papillomata make up the common warts. These occur on irritated surfaces of the skin of the fingers and hands most frequently but are to be found anywhere on the skin. They are best treated by prevention with hygienic measures. Removal by electrocoagulation is more readily accomplished for multiple small verrucae than excision.

The *plantar wart* that develops on the sole of the foot is at times difficult to distinguish from a simple callus. The presenting surface is smaller than the base from which it arises in the granular layers of the skin. They appear as single and multiple lesions and if untreated they may prove disabling.

It has been suggested that they represent a viral infection. Treatment by irradiation has been successfully employed; however, patients are seen from time to time with ulceration of the area after such therapy. Complete surgical excision of the lesion followed by electrodesiccation of the wound surface has proved most satisfactory. Care must be exercised to remove the lesion completely or it will rapidly grow much larger than it was primarily (Fig. 508).

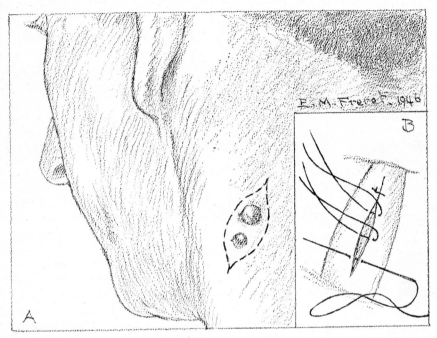

FIG. 509. Mole of the neck. After moles are excised with an adequate elliptical area of skin, the defect can be closed with interrupted arterial silk sutures. Such wounds should leave a hair-line scar.

The *venereal wart, condyloma acuminatum,* is a very exuberant one and may involve the entire perineal region. It is not limited to surfaces irritated by urethral and vaginal discharges but is seen with any irritating discharge from the rectum or perineal sinuses. Multiple rectal fistulae associated with ulcerative colitis may cause very large condylomata. These cauliflower-like verrucae are best treated by electro-surgical removal. This can be done under local anesthesia and as a step procedure. When removal of these lesions is attempted by simple surgical excision there is likely to be an extension of the process. Any direct treatment will be of temporary value if the source of the irritating discharge is not controlled.

There are a variety of superficial lesions of the skin referred to as moles and dermoid patches. Those on the face are removed for cosmetic reasons. The simple excision of these with a scalpel under local anesthesia is the method of choice. The careful reapproximation of the skin with very fine suture material should leave a minimal scar. Indeed, such a scar is preferable to those that remain after the use of the electro-surgical apparatus.

Xanthomata are depositions of yellow material, the result of faulty lipoid metabolism. They are seen as small yellow tumors on the eyelids and not infrequently are found along the course of tendons, especially in the hand. When they are of sufficient size to be troublesome, they should be excised. They tend to be multiple and may recur. Individuals with a tendency to form these depositions should be carefully studied from the standpoint of fat metabolism. Multiple lesions should lead one to consider Christian's syndrome of bony defects of the cranium, diabetes, and exophthalmos, a disease of children.

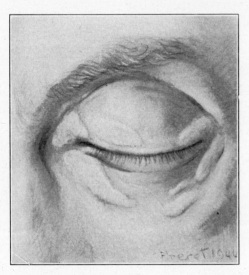

FIG. 510. Xanthomata of the eyelids. Surgical excision requires meticulous dissection for removal and careful approximation of the skin to avoid unsightly scars.

In the excision of these lesions about the face, the skin should be incised along the periphery and a flap dissected to expose the deposited material. Following its complete removal the flap is replaced and the skin margins approximated with interrupted sutures of arterial silk.

Callus, or thickening of the skin, is to be seen wherever there is continuous pressure or friction on skin directly over a bony prominence. These lesions are not true neoplasms. They are seen on the palm of anyone doing manual work; they lead to no disability in themselves, although they are a factor in the formation of "collar button" abscesses of the hand. On the feet where pressure and irritation are more constant and prolonged, they are much larger and lead to pain and discomfort. Occasionally the area may become infected. Surgical removal, although relieving discomfort for the time, accomplishes little unless the cause is corrected. Rather than resorting to repeated trimming of the calluses, ill-fitting shoes or loss of arch support leading to pressure directly over the heads of the metatarsals should be dealt with. Pads so placed as to reduce pressure over the involved areas and removal of that part of the callus that causes discomfort will give the greatest relief.

A *subungual corn or callus (onychoma)* may appear on the toes or fingers and may be associated with an exostosis of the terminal phalanx. In some cases it is due to occupation. Considerable pain and disability result from these. They are to be distinguished from melanomata of the same location or distribution. Surgical treatment consists of excision of the callus and closure of the wound with suture. X-ray examination is sometimes indicated to demonstrate the presence or absence of an exostosis. Any bony prominence should be excised if it is present; otherwise there will be a recurrence.

Glomus Tumor. The subungual tumor so well described by Masson often persists undiagnosed. It is one of the most painful lesions of the finger and

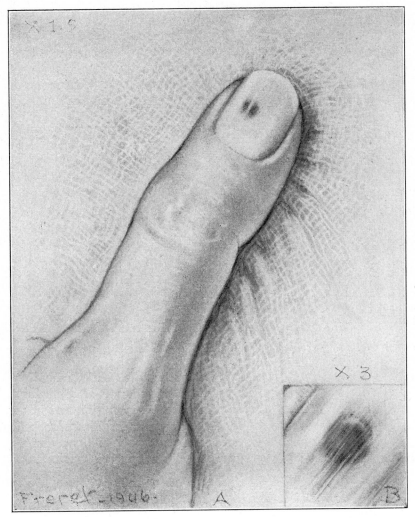

FIG. 511. Glomus tumor. Subungual glomus tumor in a young man. Pressure on the nail caused partial blanching of the tumor.

is fortunately infrequently encountered. A neuromyoarterial tumor, it consists of an arteriovenous anastomosis richly supplied with nerve fibers which probably accounts for its extreme sensitivity. The diagnosis is made upon observation of a bluish nodule beneath the nail associated with pain that radiates up the arm and may be extremely severe. The pain may be initiated by slight trauma or appear spontaneously. Such a lesion may be so painful as to prevent the use of the extremity.

Removal of the tumor gives complete relief. This usually requires removal of the nail or a sufficient part of it to give adequate exposure of the tumor in the soft tissue. It is then excised en bloc.

MALIGNANT EPITHELIAL TUMORS

Squamous Cell Epithelioma. This tumor is to be kept in mind wherever an exposed or irritated skin surface exhibits scaling and crusting that recurs. As this process continues, as the tumor grows, it produces a flat excavated ulcer, the base of which is indurated. Here microscopic examination demonstrates masses of carcinomatous cells extending down into the subcutaneous

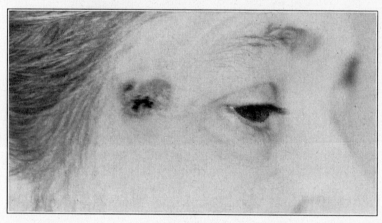

FIG. 512. Squamous cell epithelioma of the face—an early lesion.

tissue. These destroy whatever they traverse in their path, including bone and cartilage, and therefore about the face produce disabling and very disfiguring lesions. Fortunately the tumor is slow in growth and in metastasizing. Usually it extends to the regional lymph nodes. However, before extending to the lymph node it extends well beyond the evident border of the lesion in the skin, a fact to remember in the surgical treatment of this epidermoid carcinoma.

Complete surgical removal requires excision of the skin 2 to 3 cm. beyond the apparent margins of the lesion and an equal distance beyond the evident tumor tissue beneath its base. General anesthesia is frequently indicated and will enable the surgeon to do a more complete operation. Meticulous sharp dissection removing the tumor en bloc without regard to the resulting defect should be employed. Closure of the wound is of secondary importance and may be effected by sliding skin flaps, or skin grafting. Incomplete surgical excision is to be deplored and always guarded against. Irradiation, favored by some, is very popular and in early lesions without metastases has many cures to its credit. However, while appearing to have produced a cure it may obscure a deep extension of the tumor that involves vital structures. The same may be said for incomplete surgical excision followed by skin grafting.

Basal Cell Epithelioma (Rodent Ulcer). As the name implies, this tumor grows from the basal cells of the skin and extends by expansion with a well defined border. When first recognizable it appears as a pea-like nodule in the skin of the face or exposed areas of the body. As it grows the central portion ulcerates and the borders become elevated. It destroys tissue it invades, although it is an extremely slowly growing tumor, especially in its early

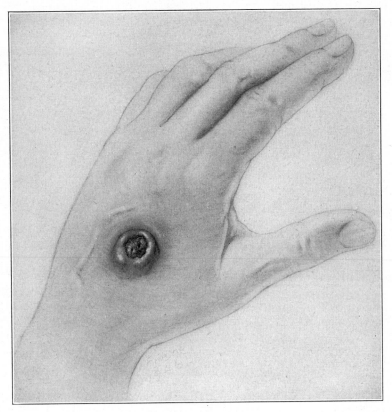

FIG. 513. Squamous cell carcinoma of the hand of an aged man. The lesion is unmistakable at this stage.

stages. It is a malignant tumor and erodes all structures as it extends. In its early phase its complete removal is easily achieved, and before it invades deep or important structures it is well controlled or cured by x-ray therapy. As in all tumors its surgical excision with a wide margin provides the most satisfactory treatment. Metastasis and recurrence are the result of neglect and inadequate therapy.

Columnar Epithelioma and Gland Cell Carcinoma. There are many lesions of the skin that have been classified both as precancerous and low-grade malignant tumors. One of these is often seen as a small rounded growth in the skin known as the cylindroma or columnar epithelioma. Another is the gland cell carcinoma or hair matrix carcinoma, a distinctly more malignant growth that may develop into a rodent ulcer. All of them should be excised in their early stages when simple excision is readily accomplished and should afford a cure.

Scar Carcinoma. In the scar that follows injury, burns, or surgery, there may grow exuberant connective tissue that microscopically appears to range from inflammatory reaction to neoplasia. Keloid is an example, and excision and meticulous closure of the wound will usually give a minimal scar. Irradiation during wound healing will also reduce the tendency to keloid formation. Scars of long standing that are exposed to frequent or constant

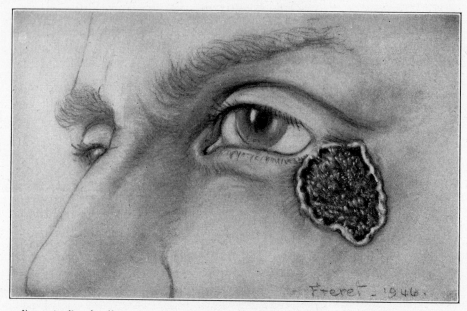

FIG. 514. Basal cell carcinoma (rodent ulcer) of the face. This is a neglected lesion and one that requires radical excision followed by skin graft.

irritation may become the site of malignant epitheliomata and require the excision of both tumor and scar followed by skin grafting.

Melanoma (Malignant Pigmented Nevus). Melanoma, or melanosarcoma, the most malignant of all tumors, commonly arises from the skin but may be found wherever there are tactile corpuscles. They are closely associated with the benign nevus or mole and resemble the latter both grossly and microscopically. There is a high incidence of pigmented nevi in our population; most of these are congenital in origin and innocent. Irritation of these by clothing or any other cause may be followed by growth and change from the harmless pigmented spot to a rapidly growing malignant tumor. Pack and Livingston found that over 50 per cent of melanomata develop in nevi that have been present since infancy. A pigmented nevus that increases in size, becomes darker in color, ulcerates, or becomes sensitive should be considered as having undergone malignant activation. Foot has called attention to the wide variation of the histology of these tumors and to the fact that some may have very little or no pigment and are therefore amelanotic melanomata. Rapid growth of metastasized tumors are frequent examples of this.

Melanomata extend by the lymphatics to the adjacent skin, regional lymph nodes, and by the blood stream to all parts and all structures of the

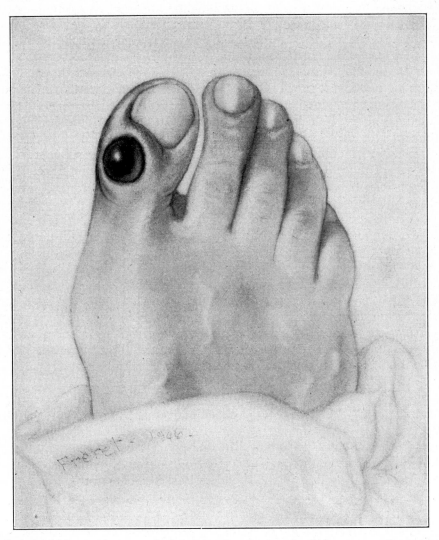

FIG. 515. Melanosarcoma on the large toe that developed without a preceding nevus.

body. The local extension about the primary tumor is usually of little significance. Considerable time may elapse between the onset of the local growth of the tumor and its spread by the blood stream, and there are reports in the literature that this interval may vary from three months to six years. Distant metastases are most commonly to the liver, lungs, and bones, but any organ or tissue may be involved. Extensive spread of the tumor to the gastrointestinal tract is not infrequent.

No other malignant lesion of the skin has presented so difficult a problem in treatment because extension of the tumor *may* take place before its activity is suspected. Because over 50 per cent of these malignant tumors have their origin in the simple nevus of long standing, it is evident that removal of pigmented moles which are being irritated and therefore stimulated to activity should be insisted upon. Complete removal of the nevus is important because cutting across such tissue and subjecting it to the trauma of operation may stimulate it to activity. A margin of 1 cm. beyond the periphery is usually adequate; however, nests of cells similar to those of the nevus may be located in the block excised. In the excision of benign nevi the defect that remains is closed after undercutting the adjacent skin and approximating it with interrupted sutures. If, however, the lesion is a malignant one, then the surgeon should use a more radical approach and remove a wider margin of skin and subcutaneous tissue without concern for correction of the defect. If necessary, skin grafting should be done. If the melanoma occurs on the finger or toe, or has developed in or about the nail bed as a "melanotic whitlow," amputation of the digit or even the extremity in certain instances should be done. Whenever a melanoma has been excised locally or amputation of a digit or extremity done, then a radical and meticulous resection of the lymphatics which drain that area should be performed within a period of one or two weeks. The advisability of this procedure has been demonstrated by the finding of tumors in resected lymph glands and the apparent prolongation of life in those who have been subjected to such a procedure.

Melanosarcomata do not respond favorably to irradiation and are much more resistant than squamous cell tumors in general. This treatment should not be used for those which can be removed surgically because in addition to being of little value it renders later surgery more difficult.

The radical resection of lymph nodes has recently been given greater consideration in the treatment of melanosarcoma. Ten to fourteen days are allowed for the malignant cells to travel from the site of the primary tumor in the foot after its removal to the inguinal lymph nodes, and then the inguinal resection is done. The technic of removal of lymph nodes of the groin (*i.e.* radical groin dissection) is described in Chapter 16.

Melanotic whitlow and *subungual melanoma* are of great importance and require early diagnosis because they are often the most malignant of the melanosarcomata. They appear adjacent to or under the nail. Usually they are painful but not always, and they tend to ulcerate early and extend into the nail bed. Unfortunately, they are often subjected to treatment which stimulates them to further activity. The melanosarcoma is one of the most malignant tumors and when located about the nail of a digit requires at least amputation of the finger or toe followed by radical lymph gland resection of the axilla or groin (see melanosarcoma).

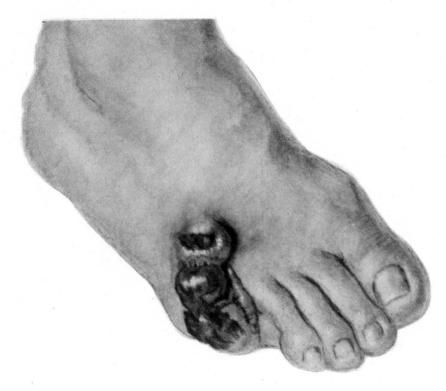

FIG. 516. Local recurrence of melanosarcoma following amputation of the fifth toe.

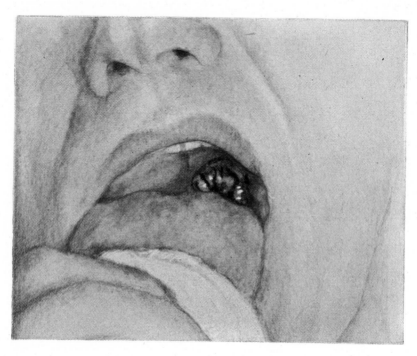

FIG. 517. Melanosarcoma metastasis at the base of the tongue one year after removal of primary lesion on the toe.

CYSTS AND FISTULAE

Sebaceous Cyst. This cyst arises from the detritus of an obstructed sebaceous gland. It is to be found any place in the subcutaneous tissue, most commonly on the back of the neck, the face, and back. The cyst consists

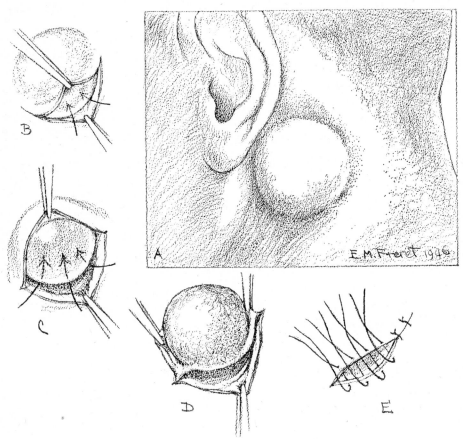

FIG. 518. (A) Sebaceous cyst of the neck. (B) Incision following the elastic lines of the skin. (C) Skin dissected from the cyst. (D) Dissection completed. (E) Approximation of the skin with arterial silk after mobilizing skin flaps.

of an outer fibrous wall and an inner layer of squamous epithelium, and contains partially dehydrated sebaceous material. Although some may reach a large size, many of them rupture and become secondarily infected. Once ruptured, they present a painless nodule in the subcutaneous tissue. Infected, they usually exhibit the manifestations of inflammation.

Treatment consists of simple excision, employing a linear or curved incision following the elastic lines of the skin to one side of the cyst and then reflecting a flap and dissecting the cyst from it (see Fig. 518). If the cyst is large and if the skin overlying the central portion of it is extremely thin, it is sometimes advantageous to excise an elliptical portion of skin over the most prominent part of the cyst. In any event care should be exercised to prevent rupture of the cyst, but if it does occur the wound should be irrigated with saline solution and a small rubber drain inserted as the wound is closed. When an elliptical area of skin has been excised, it is well to undermine the skin at the margin of the wound so that it can be approximated without tension. Local anesthesia is used and only a minimal amount of buried suture material is necessary; skin margins should be approximated with meticulous care with interrupted sutures of arterial silk.

Cysts and fistulae arising from developmental defects occur frequently in the skin and subcutaneous tissue. These include dermoid, urachal, and pilonidal cysts and are readily recognized and dealt with. In addition there is another group located in the cervical region which is more complex and presents problems in both diagnosis and treatment.

Dermoid Cyst. This is a congenital type of cyst arising from displaced epithelium and is found where there has been an infolding of the skin rudiment. It is commonly unilocular. Its wall is made up of skin with a layer in reverse order and therefore contains the products of sebaceous and sweat glands. It may also contain disintegrated epidermal cells and even teeth, hair, or bone, resembling, therefore, teratomata that are derived from epiblast or mesoblast. The common site of occurrence is the floor of the mouth, over the orbit, and in various places in the neck, as well as the mediastinum and occasionally the ovary.

Treatment consists of complete surgical excision, which can be done in the majority of cases occurring in the surface structures under local anesthesia. Failure to remove these cysts frequently is followed by their rupture and secondary infection which produces a draining sinus that tends to persist until it is extirpated completely.

Urachal Cyst. The urachus, the remnant of the umbilical cord that extends from the bladder to the umbilicus, may persist as a patent duct or have patent segments which are known as urachal cysts. If the duct is patent it discharges urine and serves as a portal of entry for infection. It should be excised, the defect in the bladder carefully closed, and the remainder of the wound closed in such a manner as to provide an anatomical reconstruction of the abdominal wall. The urachal cyst, which represents a patent segment of the urachus, may exist unrecognized. These require removal only when they produce symptoms.

Pilonidal Cyst and Sinus. Overlying the sacrococcygeal hiatus in the midline, a dimpling, one or more openings, or a cystic tumor mass represent most likely a pilonidal sinus or cyst. A high percentage of our population has the manifestations of this developmental defect. Only a few, however, produce symptoms, and although these may appear at any age they are commonly seen in the young shortly after puberty or in early adult life along with the development of secondary sexual characteristics.

Subcutaneous Fistulae of Congenital Origin. There are a number of cysts and fistulae that are the result of faulty embryological development. The majority of these occur in the cervical region and are associated with the branchial arches of early intra-uterine life. They appear in the midline or the lateral aspect of the neck anywhere between the mandible and the sternum. One of the most common is the sublingual inclusion cyst in the

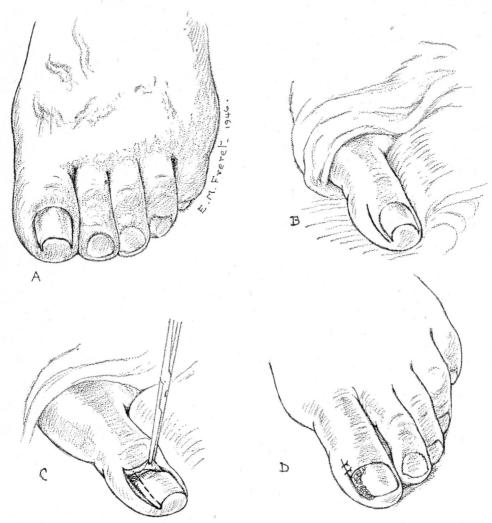

FIG. 519. Ingrown toe nail. (A) The nail margin cuts into the soft tissue; infection follows. (B) Incision is lateral to expose the nail margin. (C) With the nail margin exposed, the dotted line indicates block excision of the nail with underlying bed and matrix to be excised. (D) Partial suture of the defect is sometimes feasible and reduces convalescence. Gauze lightly packed in the wound permits healing by secondary intention and is preferable where considerable infection has been present.

midline; another the thyroglossal cyst which extends from the foramen cecum to the level of the thyroid where it may be palpated beneath the skin. Other cysts, usually branchial cleft remnants, are located in the lateral portions of the neck. These may have openings into the pharynx or to the skin. Some of them have no openings and become quite large, producing symptoms. Once incised, ruptured, or incompletely removed, they become secondarily infected. Their removal should be considered as a major surgical procedure and is to be undertaken only by those with a good understanding of the anatomy and embryological development of the cervical structures. The technic of removal of these fistulae or cysts is discussed in Chapter 6.

MISCELLANEOUS LESIONS

Ingrown Toe Nail. The ingrown toe nail may cause considerable pain and disability. The edges of the nail grow obliquely and curve down into the soft tissue. The nail margin injures the soft tissue; irritation and trauma are followed by infection. Shoes which are too narrow or too tight contribute

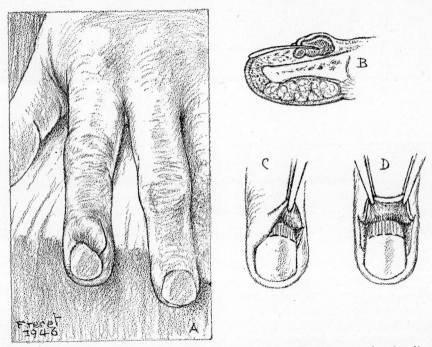

Fig. 520. (A) Paronychia, with swelling, redness, pain, and tenderness, showing line of incision if infection is superficial. (B) Untreated, the infection extends about the base of the nail. (C) and (D) Exposure of the base of the nail. Dotted line indicates part of nail to be excised when infection has extended beneath it, as seen in (B).

to this condition, as well as repeated cutting of the nail so short that the soft tissue is pressed against it, both across its cut portion and along its margin. In some people there is a congenital tendency for the nail to grow out obliquely. Foot wear is an important etiological factor and probably accounts for the higher incidence of this condition in girls and young women.

Early cases are best treated by adoption of proper shoes with adequate toe room and the placing of cotton under the nail in an effort to raise the nail margins and reduce the pressure on the soft tissue. If suppuration is present, rest, hot wet dressings, and soaks will aid in clearing the infection.

Where there is marked deformity of the nail or there has been a failure to respond to conservative treatment, the radical operative treatment alone will give relief. This operation is done under local anesthesia by blocking the digital nerves with 1 per cent procaine solution, using a small rubber tube tourniquet. The nail margins with the underlying bed and matrix are excised en bloc. If the process is an old and neglected one with infected granulation and scar tissue in the soft part, then this too should be excised. Complete excision of the nail bed should be done with great care. Partial suture of the defect is sometimes feasible, and aids in early recovery. Gauze lightly packed in the wound permits healing by secondary intention and is preferable where considerable infection has been present.

Paronychia. This infection takes place usually through a torn hang-nail or some injury to the cuticle. There is swelling, pain, and tenderness with redness of the

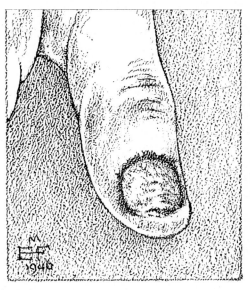

FIG. 521. Onychia, with irregular, furrowed, deformed nail.

skin about the nail. These become more marked but fluctuation is seldom evident. An adequate incision is made parallel to the line of the nail which will liberate encapsulated pus and afford drainage. If not treated, infection extends proximally and beneath the base of the nail, leading to the formation of a subungual abscess. Spontaneous rupture of such an abscess usually leads to loss of the nail. If only the base of the nail is involved, the undermined portion may be cut away, leaving the remainder of the nail to protect the fingertip. In the treatment of these infections digital nerve block is adequate, although general anesthesia is preferred by some surgeons. (See also Chapter 22.)

Onychia. A persistent inflammation of the matrix of the nail, onychia or onychitis, often occurs in the aged and those with chronic disease. The soft tissue about the nail is red, swollen, and tender. Suppuration rarely takes place; ulceration may be followed by deformity or loss of the nail. Conservative measures and treatment of the systemic disease, such as diabetes and syphilis, commonly relieves this troublesome condition. Chronic granulation tissue may require excision. Deformity of the nail may also require partial or complete removal of the nail. (See also Chapter 22.)

INDEX